Paramedic Care: Principles & Practice

Fifth Edition

Volume 4
Trauma Emergencies

BRYAN E. BLEDSOE, DO, FACEP, FAAEM, EMT-P
Professor of Emergency Medicine
University of Nevada, Las Vegas School of Medicine
University of Nevada, Reno School of Medicine
Attending Emergency Physician
University Medical Center of Southern Nevada
Medical Director, MedicWest Ambulance
Las Vegas, Nevada

RICHARD A. CHERRY, MS, EMT-P
Director of Training
Northern Onondaga Volunteer Ambulance
Liverpool, New York

LEGACY AUTHOR

ROBERT S. PORTER

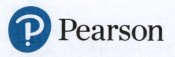 Pearson

330 Hudson Street, NY, NY 10013

Publisher: Julie Levin Alexander
Publisher's Assistant: Sarah Henrich
Editor: Sladjana Repic Bruno
Editorial Assistant: Lisa Narine
Development Editor: Sandra Breuer
Copyeditor: Deborah Wenger
Director, Publishing Operations: Paul DeLuca
Team Lead, Program Management: Melissa Bashe
Team Lead, Project Management: Cynthia Zonneveld
Manufacturing Buyer: Maura Zaldivar-Garcia
Art Director: Mary Siener
Cover and Interior Designer: Mary Siener
Managing Photography Editor: Michal Heron

Vice President of Sales & Marketing: David Gesell
Vice President, Director of Marketing: Margaret Waples
Senior Field Marketing Manager: Brian Hoehl
Marketing Assistant: Amy Pfund
Senior Producer: Amy Peltier
Media Producer and Project Manager: Lisa Rinaldi
Full-Service Project Manager: iEnergizer Aptara®, Ltd.
Composition: iEnergizer Aptara®, Ltd.
Printer/Binder: LSC Communications
Cover Printer: Phoenix Color
Cover Image: ollo/Getty Images, Rudi Von Briel/ Getty Images

Notice

The author and the publisher of this book have taken care to make certain that the information given is correct and compatible with the standards generally accepted at the time of publication. Nevertheless, as new information becomes available, changes in treatment and in the use of equipment and procedures become necessary. The reader is advised to carefully consult the instruction and information material included in each piece of equipment or device before administration. Students are warned that the use of any techniques must be authorized by their medical advisor, where appropriate, in accordance with local laws and regulations. The publisher disclaims any liability, loss, injury, or damage incurred as a consequence, directly or indirectly, of the use and application of any of the contents of this book.

Library of Congress Cataloging-in-Publication Data

Names: Bledsoe, Bryan E., author. | Cherry, Richard A., author. | Porter, Robert S., author.
Title: Paramedic care : principles & practice | Bryan E. Bledsoe, Richard A. Cherry, Robert S. Porter.
Description: Fifth edition. | Boston : Pearson Education, Inc., 2016- | Includes bibliographical references and index.
Identifiers: LCCN 2016009904 | ISBN 9780134449746 (pbk. : alk. paper) | ISBN 0134449746 (pbk. : alk. paper)
Subjects: | MESH: Emergencies | Emergency Medical Services | Emergency Medical Technicians
Classification: LCC RC86.7 | NLM WB 105 | DDC 616.02/5—dc23 LC record available at http://lccn.loc.gov/2016009904

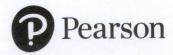 **Pearson**

ISBN 10: 0-13-444974-6
ISBN 13: 978-0-13-444974-6

22 2022

This text is respectfully dedicated to all EMS personnel
who have made the ultimate sacrifice. Their memory
and good deeds will forever be in our thoughts and prayers.

BEB, RAC

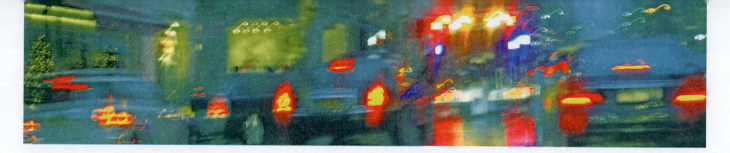

Contents

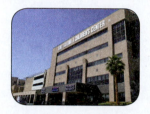

1 Trauma and Trauma Systems   1

2 Mechanism of Injury   17

3 Hemorrhage and Shock   57

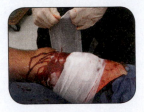

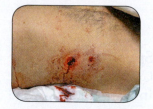

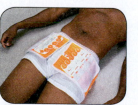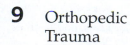

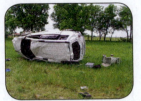

11 Special Considerations in Trauma 328

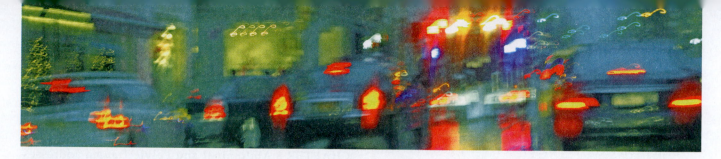

Preface to Volume 4

Until the late 1960s, the highest level of medical care available outside the hospital was Red Cross First Aid. In 1966, the National Academy of Sciences commissioned a research study to examine the inadequacies of emergency medical care in this country. The findings of this study were published in a document called *Accidental Death and Disability: The Neglected Disease of Modern Society.* This document, commonly referred to as "The White Paper," was the impetus for development of EMS and emergency medicine as we know it today.

The initial emphasis of prehospital training was trauma care. Prehospital personnel received considerable training in bandaging, splinting, and rescue techniques. In the 1980s, prehospital trauma care was again improved through the development of Basic Trauma Life Support (BTLS) and Prehospital Trauma Life Support (PHTLS) training. These courses provided EMTs and paramedics with the additional information needed to care adequately for the trauma patient in the field.

Under the current *National EMS Education Standards* and the accompanying *Paramedic Instructional Guidelines*, paramedics are responsible for a much more detailed understanding of trauma emergencies. The publication of *Paramedic Care: Principles & Practice, Volume 4, Trauma* takes prehospital trauma care to the highest level yet. This volume details the anatomy, physiology, and pathophysiology of trauma. Although trauma is a surgical disease, and in many instances definitive care must be provided in the operating room, there is a significant amount of care that can be provided by prehospital personnel to help reduce both morbidity and mortality.

This volume addresses the various types of trauma based on the body systems involved. It is important to remember that many trauma patients have multiple injuries involving multiple body systems. Because of this, it is essential to consider the "whole patient" and not become distracted by a single injury.

Overview of the Chapters . . . and what's new in the 5th edition?

CHAPTER 1 Trauma and Trauma Systems introduces the paramedic student to trauma, the concept of trauma systems, and trauma triage protocols. It has been shown that trauma victims have the best chances of survival if they are cared for in a facility that routinely provides trauma care. In addition, certain patients will require very specialized trauma care, and it is often the responsibility of the paramedic to ensure that the patient gets to the correct facility.

New in the 5th Edition: Emphasis on the evolving role of **prevention of trauma** in EMS, preventing trauma being easier and less costly than treating trauma. There is emphasis on evaluating for possible spine injury and deciding, based on spinal protocols, which patients require spinal precautions.

CHAPTER 2 Mechanism of Injury presents the kinetics and biomechanics of blunt and penetrating trauma and details the effects of trauma on the various body tissues. This chapter encourages the paramedic to evaluate the physics and mechanism of injury to help determine likely injuries.

New in the 5th Edition: This chapter **discusses both blunt trauma and penetrating trauma**, which were separate chapters in the prior edition. There is a new section on **hybrid vehicles** and dangers they present during collision analysis: electrocution and unexpected movement. A new section on **quaternary blast injuries** has been added to the discussion of blast injuries.

CHAPTER 3 Hemorrhage and Shock makes clear that regardless of the mechanism of injury, the final common denominator in most trauma patients is the fact that they are losing blood. Severe blood loss can result in the development of shock. The body's physiologic responses to hemorrhage and shock are complex. This chapter details the physiologic and pathophysiologic response to hemorrhage and shock so that the paramedic can recognize the process early and intervene appropriately.

New in the 5th Edition: A discussion of the recently increased use of **tourniquets** with emphasis on their dangers and their use only as a last resort. A new section introduces the drug **tranexamic acid (TXA)** as an antifibrinolytic that can mitigate deterioration of the blood clotting system that occurs with some trauma, reducing trauma mortality especially during long transport times. There is expanded information on **fluid resuscitation** for patients in hypovolemic shock and the varied responses that can be expected. Text regarding **the pneumatic anti-shock garment (PASG) has been deleted; its use is no longer recommended.**

CHAPTER 4 Soft-Tissue Trauma explains that this is by far the most common form of trauma. Although most soft-tissue injuries are not life threatening, many can be. This chapter provides a detailed review of the anatomy and physiology of the integumentary system, a discussion of the pathophysiology of soft-tissue trauma, and a detailed discussion of soft-tissue treatment, including bandaging.

CHAPTER 5 Burns discusses the unique pathophysiology of burn injuries. The incidence of burn injuries is declining, but burn patients require specialized care. This chapter discusses the anatomy, physiology, and pathophysiology of burn injuries, including thermal, electrical, chemical, and radiation burns and inhalation injuries, with emphasis on management of the burn patient.

CHAPTER 6 Head, Neck, and Spinal Trauma reviews the anatomy of the head, face, neck, and spine and of the nervous system, including a review of the pathophysiology of brain and spinal cord injury. Emphasis is placed on recognizing head, neck, and spinal injuries early and on protecting the airway. The chapter also reviews prehospital spinal precautions and spinal clearance protocols.

New in the 5th Edition: This chapter **combines two formerly separate chapters** on head, face, neck, and spine injury and on nervous system trauma.

CHAPTER 7 Chest Trauma details the impact of chest trauma on the body. Thoracic anatomy and physiology are unique and can require specialized treatment procedures. Special emphasis is placed on recognition and treatment of chest injuries, especially tension pneumothorax.

CHAPTER 8 Abdominal and Pelvic Trauma addresses the anatomy and physiology of the abdomen and pelvis and discusses trauma pathology by organ and organ system. The chapter emphasizes the importance of maintaining a high index of suspicion when treating a trauma patient with possible internal injury.

New in the 5th Edition: Information about gunshot wounds has been expanded to address, especially, **high-velocity military-type gunshot wounds** that are now occurring more often in civilian settings. Text regarding **the pneumatic anti-shock garment (PASG) has been deleted; its use is no longer recommended.**

CHAPTER 9 Orthopedic Trauma notes that this type of trauma is second only to soft-tissue trauma in frequency. In this chapter, the student learns about various types of musculoskeletal trauma with special emphasis on treatment and pain control.

New in the 5th Edition: **References to nontraumatic injuries have been deleted** as they are covered in the medical chapter "Nontraumatic Musculoskeletal Disorders" (Volume 3, Chapter 13)

CHAPTER 10 Environmental Trauma details the impact of the environment on the body. A review of relevant physics, chemistry, and biology is followed by a discussion of specific environmental emergencies heat and cold disorders, drowning and diving emergencies, and high-altitude illness.

CHAPTER 11 Special Considerations in Trauma ties together the underlying concepts regarding specific types of trauma addressed in the prior chapters. An early emphasis in the chapter is injury prevention. The chief emphasis of the chapter is on recognizing all potential injuries, including multisystem injuries, and reviews the effects of hemorrhage and shock. There is further emphasis on aggressive treatment, as well as transport to a hospital capable of providing the required care.

New in the 5th Edition: The spinal precautions section was revised to deemphasize automatic full spinal immobilization and to emphasize the **range of spinal precautions based on the NEXUS criteria, the Canadian C-Spine rule, or similar protocols.**

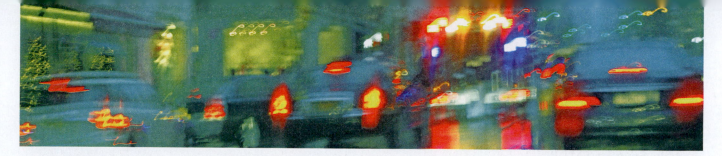

Acknowledgments

Chapter Contributors

We wish to acknowledge the remarkable talents of the following people who contributed to this five volume series. Individually, they worked with extraordinary commitment. Together, they form a team of highly dedicated professionals who have upheld the highest standards of EMS instruction.

Paul Ganss, MS, NRP (Volume 1, Chapter 2)

Michael F. O'Keefe (Volume 1, Chapter 5)

Wes Ogilvie, MPA, JD, LP (Volume 1, Chapter 7)

Kevin McGinnis, MPS, EMT-P (Volume 1, Chapter 9)

Jeff Brosious, EMT-P (Volume 1, Chapter 10)

W.E. Gandy, JD, NREMT-P (Volume 1, Chapter 15)

Darren Braude, MD, MPH, FACEP (Volume 1, Chapter 15)

Joseph R. Lauro, MD, EMT-P (Volume 2, Chapter 6)

Brad Buck, NRP, CCEMT-P (Volume 3, Chapter 10)

Bryan Bledsoe, DO, FACEP, FAAEM, EMT-P (Volume 4, Chapter 10)

Andrew Schmidt, DO, MPH (Volume 4, Chapter 10)

Justin Sempsrott, MD (Volume 4, Chapter 10)

David Nelson, MD, FAAP, FAAEM (Volume 5, Chapter 4)

Mike Abernethy, MD, FAAEM (Volume 5, Chapter 10)

Ryan J. Wubben, MD, FAAEM (Volume 5, Chapter 10)

Louis Molino, NREMT-I (Volume 5, Chapter 11)

Dale M. Carrison, DO, FACEP, FACOEP (Volume 5, Chapter 14)

Dan Limmer, AS, NRP (Volume 5, Chapter 14)

Deborah J. McCoy-Freeman, BS, RN, NREMTP (Volume 5, Chapter 15)

BEB, RAC

Instructor Reviewers

The reviewers of *Paramedic Care: Principles & Practice, Fourth Edition, Volume 2* have provided many excellent suggestions and ideas for improving the text. The quality of the reviews has been outstanding, and the reviews have been a major aid in the preparation and revision of the manuscript. The assistance provided by these EMS experts is deeply appreciated.

Fifth Edition

Michael Smith, MS, Educator, Kilgore College, Longview, TX

Edward Lee, A.A.S., BS, Ed.S., NRP, CCEMT-P, EMT Paramedic Program Coordinator, Trident Technical College, Summerville, SC

Ryan Batenhorst, BA, NRP, EMS-I, Program Director, Paramedic Program, Southeast Community College, Milford, NE

Brett Peine, BS, NRP, Director, Southern State University, Joplin, MO

Fourth Edition

John L. Beckman, AA, BS
FF/EMT-P I/C
Addison Fire Protection District
Technology Center of DuPage
Addison, IL

Bryon Bellinger, NREMT-P, BA, RN
Lead Instructor Paramedic Specialist Program
Indian Hills Community College
Ottumwa, IA

Brian Bird, AS, EMS
Firefighter/Paramedic
Santa Fe Fire Department
Santa Fe, NM

L. Kelly Kirk, III, AAS, BS, EMT-P
Director of Distance Education, Paramedic
Randolph Co. Community College/Davidson County EMS
Asheboro, NC/Lexington, NC

Gregory M. Reardon, BS, NREMT-P
Paramedic, Adjunct Faculty Cecil College/Maryland Fire and Rescue Institute
Baltimore Washington International Airport Fire and Rescue Department
Baltimore, MD

Billy Respass, NCEMT-P
EMS Programs Instructor
Beaufort County Community College
Washington, NC

Mike Smertka, EMT-P
Assistant EMS Instructor
Graduate Student of Medicine/Medical University of
Silesia
Katowice, Poland

Kelly Weller, MA, RN, LP, EMS-C
EMS Program Director
Lone Star College-Montgomery
Conroe, TX

We also wish to express appreciation to the following EMS professionals who reviewed the third edition of Paramedic Care: Principles & Practice. Their suggestions and perspectives helped to make this program a successful teaching tool.

Mike Dymes, NREMT-P
EMS Program Director
Durham Technical Community College
Durham, NC

Ginger K. Floyd, BA, NREMT-P
Assistant Professor
Austin Community College EMS Professions
Austin, TX

Darren P. Lacroix, AAS, EMT-P
Del Mar College
Emergency Medical Service Professions
Corpus Christi, TX

Greg Mullen, MS, NREMT-P
National EMS Academy
Lafayette, LA

Deborah L. Petty, BS, EMT-P I/C
Training Officer
St. Charles County Ambulance District
St. Peters, MO

B. Jeanine Riner, MHSA, BS, RRT, NREMT-P
GA Office of EMS and Trauma
Atlanta, GA

Aaron Weitzman, BS, NREMT-P
Lieutenant (ret.)
Faculty, Emergency Medical Services
Baltimore City Community College
Baltimore, MD

Brian J. Wilson, BA, NREMT-P
Education Director
Texas Tech School of Medicine
El Paso, TX

Photo Acknowledgments

All photographs not credited adjacent to the photograph or in the photo credit section below were photographed on assignment for Brady/Prentice Hall/Pearson Education.

Organizations

We wish to thank the following organizations for their assistance in creating the photo program for this project:

Michael J. Grant, President & CEO
Ambitrans Medical Transport, Inc., Punta Gorda, FL

Debbie Harrington, BS, NREMT, Director
Community Relations, Ambitrans Medical Transport, Inc.

Companies

The following companies assisted in our photo program by donating EMS products to use in our photo shoots:

Persys Medical. NIO and BIG interosseous

Pyng Medical. FAST interosseous

Teleflex Corp. LMAs

Photo Coordinators/ Technical Advisors

Thanks to the following for valuable assistance directing the medical accuracy of the shoots and coordinating models, props, and locations for our photos:

Skippi Farley, EMT-P

Rodney VanOrsdol, FF/EMT-P

Photographers who have contributed to this project

Michael Gallitelli, Michal Heron, Kevin Link and Richard Logan

Photographer for the Fifth edition

Maria Lyle/Maria Lyle Photography
Sarasota, Florida

Models

Thanks to the following people from the Flower Mound Fire Department, Flower Mound, Texas, and from Winter Park Fire-Rescue, Winter Park, Florida, who provided locations and/or portrayed patients and EMS providers in our photographs.

FAO/Paramedic Wade Woody

FF/Paramedic Tim Mackling

FF/Paramedic Matthew Daniel

FF/Paramedic Jon Rea

FF/Paramedic Waylon Palmer

FF/EMT Jesse Palmer

Captain/EMT Billy McWhorter

Linda Kirk, Director, Winter Park Towers, Winter Park, FL

Andrew Isaacs

Richard Rodriguez

Tod Meadors

Jeff Spinelli

Mark Vaughn

Victoria Devereaux

Teresa George

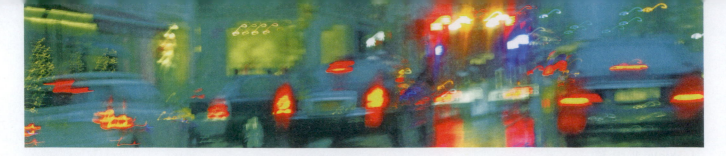

About the Authors

BRYAN E. BLEDSOE, DO, FACEP, FAAEM, EMT-P

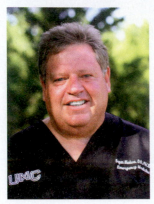

Dr. Bryan Bledsoe is an emergency physician, researcher, and EMS author. Presently he is Professor of Emergency Medicine at the University of Nevada School of Medicine and an Attending Emergency Physician at the University Medical Center of Southern Nevada in Las Vegas. He is board-certified in emergency medicine and emergency medical services. Prior to attending medical school, Dr. Bledsoe worked as an EMT, a paramedic, and a paramedic instructor. He completed EMT training in 1974 and paramedic training in 1976 and worked for six years as a field paramedic in Fort Worth, Texas. In 1979, he joined the faculty of the University of North Texas Health Sciences Center and served as coordinator of EMT and paramedic education programs at the university.

Dr. Bledsoe is active in emergency medicine and EMS research. He is a popular speaker at state, national, and international seminars and writes regularly for numerous EMS journals. He is active in educational endeavors with the United States Special Operations Command (USSOCOM) and the University of Nevada at Las Vegas. Dr. Bledsoe is the author of numerous EMS textbooks and has in excess of 1 million books in print. Dr. Bledsoe was named a "Hero of Emergency Medicine" in 2008 by the American College of Emergency Physicians as a part of their 40th anniversary celebration and was named a "Hero of Health and Fitness" by *Men's Health* magazine as part of their 20th anniversary edition in November of 2008. He is frequently interviewed in the national media. Dr. Bledsoe is married and divides his time between his residences in Midlothian, TX, and Las Vegas, NV.

RICHARD A. CHERRY, MS, EMT-P

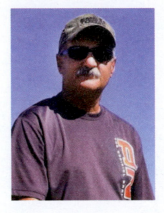

Richard Cherry is the Director of Training for Northern Onondaga Volunteer Ambulance (NOVA) in Liverpool, New York, a suburb of Syracuse. He recently retired from the Department of Emergency Medicine at Upstate Medical University where he held the positions of Director of Paramedic Training, Assistant Emergency Medicine Residency Director, Clinical Assistant Professor of Emergency Medicine, and Technical Director for Medical Simulation. His experience includes years of classroom teaching and emergency fieldwork. A native of Buffalo, Mr. Cherry earned his bachelor's degree at nearby St. Bonaventure University in 1972. He taught high school for the next ten years while he earned his master's degree in education from Oswego State University in 1977. He holds a permanent teaching license in New York State.

Mr. Cherry entered the emergency medical services field in 1974 with the DeWitt Volunteer Fire Department, where he served his community as a firefighter and EMS provider for more than 15 years. He took his first EMT course in 1977 and became an ALS provider two years later. He earned his paramedic certificate in 1985 as a member of the area's first paramedic class.

Mr. Cherry has authored several books for Brady. Most notable are *Paramedic Care: Principles & Practice, Essentials of Paramedic Care, Intermediate Emergency Care: Principles & Practice,* and *EMT Teaching: A Common Sense Approach.* He has made presentations at many state, national, and international EMS conferences on a variety of teaching topics. He and his wife, Sue, run a summer horse-riding camp for children with special needs on their property in West Monroe, New York. He also plays guitar in a Christian band.

A GUIDE TO KEY FEATURES

Emphasizing Principles

LEARNING OBJECTIVES

Terminal Performance Objectives and a separate set of Enabling Objectives are provided for each chapter.

KEY TERMS

Page numbers identify where each key term first appears, boldfaced, in the chapter.

Chapter 1

Introduction to Paramedicine

Bryan Bledsoe, DO, FACEP, FAAEM

STANDARD
Preparatory (EMS Systems)

COMPETENCY
Integrates comprehensive knowledge of EMS systems, the safety and well-being of the paramedic, and medical–legal and ethical issues, which is intended to improve the health of EMS personnel, patients, and the community.

⌄ Learning Objectives

Terminal Performance Objective: After reading this chapter your should be able to discuss the characteristics of the profession of paramedicine.

Enabling Objectives: To accomplish the terminal performance objective, you should be able to:

1. Define key terms introduced in this chapter.
2. Compare and contrast the four nationally recognized levels of EMS providers in the United States.
3. Describe the requirements that must be met for EMS professionals to function at the paramedic level.
4. Discuss the traditional and emerging roles of the paramedic in health care, public health, and public safety.
5. List and describe the various health care settings paramedics may practice in with an expanded scope of practice.

KEY TERMS

Advanced Emergency Medical Technician (AEMT), p. 3
community paramedicine, p. 4
critical care transport, p. 7
Emergency Medical Responder (EMR), p. 3

Emergency Medical Services (EMS) system, p. 2
Emergency Medical Technician (EMT), p. 3
mobile integrated health care, p. 4

National Emergency Medical Services Education Standards: Paramedic Instructional Guidelines, p. 5
Paramedic, p. 3
paramedicine, p. 4

1

---

more rapid are the pulse and respiratory rates.

3.0 and 3.5 kg. Because of the excretion of extracellular

As newborns make the transition from fetal to pulmonary circulation in the first few days of life, several important

Table 11-1 Normal Vital Signs

	Pulse (Beats per Minute)	Respiration (Breaths per Minute)	Blood Pressure (Average mmHg)	Temperature	
Infancy:					
At birth:	100–180	30–60	60–90 systolic	98–100°F	36.7–37.8°C
At 1 year:	100–160	30–60	87–105 systolic	98–100°F	36.7–37.8°C
Toddler (12 to 36 months)	80–110	24–40	95–105 systolic	96.8–99.6°F	36.0–37.5°C
Preschool age (3 to 5 years)	70–110	22–34	95–110 systolic	96.8–99.6°F	36.0–37.5°C
School-age (6 to 12 years)	65–110	18–30	97–112 systolic	98.6°F	37°C
Adolescence (13 to 18 years)	60–90	12–26	112–128 systolic	98.6°F	37°C
Early adulthood (19 to 40 years)	60–100	12–20	120/80	98.6°F	37°C
Middle adulthood (41 to 60 years)	60–100	12–20	120/80	98.6°F	37°C
Late adulthood (61 years and older)	*	*	*	98.6°F	37°C

*Depends on the individual's physical health status.

TABLES

A wealth of tables offers the opportunity to highlight, summarize, and compare information.

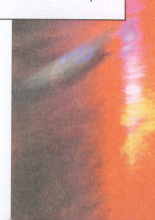

components of the rule of threes. Whenever BVM ventilation is difficult, however, the rule of threes should be employed.

- *Three providers.* One provider on the mask, one on the bag, and one for cricoid pressure.

- *Three inches.* A reminder to place the patient in the sniffing position (elevate the head three inches) if not contraindicated.

- *Three fingers.* Three fingers on the cricoid cartilage to perform cricoid pressure.

- *Three airways.* In a worst-case scenario, the airway can be maintained, if necessary, with an oropharyngeal airway and two nasopharyngeal airways (one in each nostril).

CONTENT REVIEW

Content review boxes set off from the text are interspersed throughout the chapter. They summarize key points and serve as a helpful study guide—in an easy format for quick review.

PHOTOS AND ILLUSTRATIONS

Carefully selected photos and a unique art program reinforce content coverage and add to text explanations.

index, and middle finger of one hand. If a lesser-trained provider is performing the maneuver, you should confirm that they are in the correct position (Figure 15-47).

Use caution not to apply so much pressure as to deform and possibly obstruct the trachea; this is a particular danger in infants. The necessary pressure has been estimated as the amount of force that will compress a capped 50-mL syringe from 50 mL to the 30 mL marking. In the event that the patient actively vomits, it is imperative to release the pressure to avoid esophageal rupture. Similarly, if cricoid pressure is being performed during intubation, reduce or release the pressure if the intubator is having difficulty visualizing the vocal cords.

Optimal BVM Ventilation Using the Rule of Threes

The *rule of threes* was developed to help providers recall the components of optimal BVM ventilation. Many patients can be easily oxygenated and ventilated without using all

- *Three PSI.* A gentle reminder to use the lowest pressure necessary to see the chest rise.

- *Three seconds.* A reminder to ventilate slowly and allow time for adequate exhalation.

- *Three PEEP.* Or up to 15 cm/H_2O positive-end expiratory pressure (PEEP) as needed to improve oxygen saturations.

Bag-Valve Ventilation of the Pediatric Patient

The differences in the pediatric patient's anatomy require some variation in ventilation technique. First, the child's relatively flat nasal bridge makes achieving a mask seal more difficult. Pressing the mask against the child's face to improve the seal can actually obstruct the airway, which is more compressible than an adult's. You can best achieve the mask seal with the two-person BVM technique, using a jaw-thrust to maintain an open airway.

For BVM ventilation, the bag size depends on the child's age. Full-term neonates and infants will require a pediatric BVM with a capacity of at least 450 mL. For children up to 8 years of age, the pediatric BVM is preferred, although for patients in the upper portion of that age range you can use an adult BVM with a capacity of 1,500 mL if you do not maximally inflate it. Children older than 8 years require an adult BVM to achieve adequate tidal volumes. Additionally, be

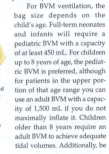

Thyroid cartilage (Adam's apple)

Cricothyroid membrane

Trachea

Esophagus

Cricoid cartilage occluding esophagus

FIGURE 15-47 Cricoid pressure.

Summary

The scene size-up is the initial step in the patient care process. Sizing up the scene and situation begins at your initial dispatch and does not end until you are clear of the call. As the call unfolds, you should be making constant observations and adjustments to your plan of action. Remember that your safety and the safety of your partner are paramount—it is hard to effectively treat both yourself and others.

Scene size-up should be practiced so much that it becomes second nature to you. It is like noticing veins on people in public after you begin starting IVs. (You have all done it—looked across the room at the back of someone's hand and noticed what nice veins they had.) Sizing up a scene is no different. After a while, you begin to notice mechanisms of injury and other important details almost subconsciously. But be careful and do not get complacent! Always make it a point to pause for just a few seconds and consciously look around the scene before proceeding into any situation.

Scene size-up is not a step-by-step process, but a series of decisions you make when confronted with a variety of circumstances that are often beyond your control. It is a way to make order out of chaos, keep yourself and your crew safe, and ensure that all necessary resources are focused on patient care and outcomes. With time and experience, you will learn to perform a scene size-up quickly and focus on important issues. Your careful size-up lays the foundation for an organized and timely approach toward patient care and scene management. And always remember that scene size-up is not a one-time occurrence. It is an ongoing process.

SUMMARY

This end-of-chapter feature provides a concise review of chapter information.

airway management in every patient, you should learn and use advanced skills such as intubation, RSI, and cricothyrotomy. You must maintain proficiency in all airway skills, especially the more advanced techniques, through ongoing continuing education, physician medical direction, and testing with each EMS service. If you cannot do this, it is in the patient's best interest to focus on less sophisticated airway skills. If you anticipate that every airway will be complicated, apply basic airway skills before using advanced procedures, and perform frequent reassessments, you will give the patient his best chance for meaningful survival.

You Make the Call

You and your paramedic partner, Preston Connelly, are assigned to District 4, a quiet suburban neighborhood, on a warm Saturday in June. At 2:00 P.M., you are dispatched to care for a choking child at the Happy Hotdog Restaurant on Main Street. On your way to the location, the dispatcher advises you that they are currently giving prearrival choking instructions to the bystanders at the scene. On arrival, you find a frantic mother who tells you that her 6-year-old son was eating a hot dog and drinking a soda when he started coughing and gasping for air. She keeps yelling for you to do something. Bystanders surround the child and are attempting to perform the Heimlich maneuver without success. On your primary assessment, you find a 6-year-old boy lying on the floor, unconscious and apneic, with a pulse rate of 130. There is cyanosis surrounding his lips and fingernail beds, with a moderate amount of secretions coming from his mouth. There are no signs of trauma. You and Preston immediately start management of this child.

1. What is your primary assessment and management of this child?

2. What are your first actions?

3. What are your options for managing the airway after the obstruction is relieved?

4. What are the major anatomic differences between pediatric and adult patients in terms of airway management?

See Suggested Responses at the back of this book.

YOU MAKE THE CALL

A scenario at the end of each chapter promotes critical thinking by requiring students to apply principles to actual practice.

REVIEW QUESTIONS

These questions ask students to review and recall key information they have just learned.

Review Questions

1. When you couple the physical assessment findings with the patient's medical history, you are able to derive a list of _____
   a. clinical diagnostics.
   b. field prognoses.
   c. chief complaints
   d. differential field diagnoses.

2. The pain, discomfort, or dysfunction that caused your patient to request help is known as the
   _____
   a. primary problem.
   b. nature of the illness.
   c. differential diagnosis.
   d. chief complaint.

3. You are assessing a patient who complains of cardiac-type chest pain that is felt in the jaw and down the left arm. This pattern of pain is known as
   _____
   a. sympathetic pain.
   b. tenderness.
   c. referred pain.
   d. associated pain.

4. Your patient has smoked 2 packs of cigarettes each day for the past 35 years. He is a _____ pack/year smoker.
   a. 35
   b. 70
   c. 730
   d. 25,550

5. The CAGE questionnaire is used as an evaluation tool to assess a patient with what type of history?
   a. Alcoholism
   b. Lung disease
   c. Allergies
   d. Pregnancy

6. What interviewing mnemonic should be used for each presenting problem a patient has?
   a. SAMPLE
   b. DCAP–BTLS
   c. OPQRST–ASPN
   d. AEIOU–TIPS

7. The mnemonic GPAL is used to evaluate a patient's
   a. alcoholism.
   b. allergies.
   c. pregnancy history.
   d. endocrine dysfunction.

Match the following elements of the present illness of the patient with a chief complaint of chest pain with their respective examples:

1. O   a. Pain is 6 on a scale of 1–10
2. P   b. Patient also complains of shortness of breath and nausea
3. Q   c. Pain had a sudden onset
4. R   d. Pain began 2 hours ago
5. S   e. Pain worsens while lying down
6. T   f. Patient denies dizziness
7. AS   g. Pain goes through to the back
8. PN   h. Pain is heavy and vise-like

See Answers to Review Questions at the back of this book.

6. Which radio frequencies may be used by cities and municipalities for their ability to better transmit through concrete and steel?
   a. UHF
   b. VHF
   c. 800-mHz
   d. none of the above

7. Which frequency band is typically used by county and suburban agencies due to its ability to transmit over various terrains and longer distances?
   a. UHF
   b. VHF
   c. 800-mHz
   d. none of the above

8. What is the name of the basic communications system that uses the same frequency to both transmit and receive?
   a. Multiplex
   b. Duplex
   c. Simplex
   d. Complex

9. A communications system that uses a different transmit and receive frequency allowing for simultaneous communications between two parties is called
   _____
   a. multiplex.
   b. duplex.
   c. simplex.
   d. complex.

10. _____ communications systems are capable of transmitting both voice and electronic patient data simultaneously.
    a. Multiplex
    b. Duplex
    c. Simplex
    d. Complex

See answers to Review Questions at the back of this book.

References

1. Department of Homeland Security. SAFECOM. (Available at http://www.dhs.gov/safecom/)
2. National EMS Information System (NEMSIS). The NEMSIS Technical Assistance Center (TAC). (Available at http://www.nemsis.org/./.)
3. American College of Emergency Physicians (ACEP). "Automatic Crash Notification and Intelligent Transportation Systems." *Ann Emerg Med* 55 (2010): 397.
4. National Emergency Number Association (NENA). National Emergency Number Association. (Available at: http://www.nena.org)
5. Association of Public-Safety Communications Officials (APCO). [Available at: http://www.apco911.org/]
6. Department of Transportation, Research and Innovative Technology Administration. Next Generation 911. (Available at: http://www.its.dot.gov/ng911/.)
7. Centers for Disease Control and Prevention. Recommendations from the Expert Panel: Advanced Automatic Collision Notification and Triage of the Injured Patient. (See NHTSA summary at http://www.nhtsa.gov/Research/Biomechanics+&+Trauma/Advanced+Automatic+Collision+Notification+-+AACN)
8. Wilson, S., M. Cooke, R. Morrell et al. "A Systematic Review of the Evidence Supporting the Use of Priority Dispatch of Emergency Ambulances." *Prehosp Emerg Care* 6 (2002): 42–29.
9. Billittier, A. J., 4th, E. B. Lerner, W. Tucker, and J. Lee. "The Lay Public's Expectations of Prearrival Instructions When Dialing 911." *Prehosp Emerg Care* 4 (2000): 234–237.
10. Munk, M. D., S. D. White, M. L. Perry, et al. "Physician Medical Direction and Clinical Performance at an Established Emergency Medical Services System." *Prehosp Emerg Care* 13 (2009): 185–192.
11. Cheung, D. S., J. J. Kelly, C. Beach, et al. "Improving Handoffs in the Emergency Department." *Ann Emerg Med* 55 (2010): 171–180.
12. Chan, T. C., J. Killeen, W. Griswold, and L. Lenert. "Information Technology and Emergency Medical Care during Disasters." *Acad Emerg Med* 11 (2004): 1229–1236.
13. DREAMS Ambulance Project. (See article at: https://www.ems1.com/ems-products/technology/articles/1183110-DREAMS-revolutionizes-communication-between-ER-and-ambulance/.)
14. Haskins, P. A., D. G. Ellis, and J. Mayrose. "Predicted Utilization of Emergency Medical Services Telemedicine in Decreasing Ambulance Transports." *Prehosp Emerg Care* 6 (2002): 445–448.

Further Reading

Bass, R., J. Potter, K. McGinnis, and T. Miyahara. "Surveying Emerging Trends in Emergency-related Information Delivery for the EMS Profession." *Topics in Emergency Medicine* 26 (April–June 2004): 2, 93–102.

Fitch, J. "Benchmarking Your Comm Center." *JEMS* 2006: 98–112.

McGinnis, K. K. "The Future of Emergency Medical Services Communications Systems: Time for a Change." *N C Med J* 68 (2007): 283–285.

McGinnis, K. K. *Future EMS Technologies: Predicting Communications Implications.* National Public Safety Telecommunications Council, National Association of State EMS Officials, National Association of EMS Physicians, June, 2010.

McGinnis, K. K. "The Future Is Now: Emergency Medical Services (EMS) Communications Advances Can Be as Important as Medical Treatment Advances When It Comes to Saving Lives." *Interoperability Today* (SafeCom, U.S. Department of Homeland Security), Volume 3, 2005.

McGinnis, K. K. *Rural and Frontier Emergency Medical Services Agenda for the Future.* National Rural Health Association Press: October 2004.

REFERENCES

This listing is a compilation of source material providing the basis of updated data and research used in the preparation of each chapter.

FURTHER READING

This list features recommendations for books and journal articles that go beyond chapter coverage.

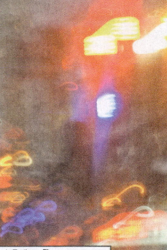

cleaning, p. 70
Code Green Campaign, p. 78
disinfection, p. 70
exposure, p. 70
isotonic exercise, p. 61
pathogens, p. 65
personal protective equipment (PPE), p. 66
sterilization, p. 70
stress, p. 74
stressor, p. 74
Tema Conter Memorial Trust, p. 78

CASE STUDY

This feature at the start of each chapter draws students into the reading and creates a link between text content and real-life situations.

Case Study

Howard is a 15-year veteran of a high-volume, inner-city EMS service. When he first started his career, Howard thought he knew what he was getting into, but the years have taught him differently.

Right now, Howard is in the spotlight for saving the life of a police officer who was shot in a hostage situation. "That call forced me to reflect on a few important things," he says. "Two years ago, I had a minor heart problem, and it was a good wake-up call. Since then I've been lifting weights and running, so I was able to get to the officer with enough strength to carry him to safety.

"Another thing is that I always use personal protective equipment. I never go to work without steel-toed boots and I never leave the ambulance without a pair of disposable gloves. Can you believe there are still paramedics who knock the concept of infection control? If any one of my partners sticks a needle into the squad bench in my ambulance, they know I'll speak up."

Howard, a mild-mannered, nondescript man, doesn't realize that his young colleagues regard him as a role model. They've seen him handle himself at chaotic scenes as well as when a situation demands sensitivity, patience, and gentleness. "Howard is the man I'd want to tell bad news to my mother," one of his partners says. "He can handle people involved in just about any circumstance—death situations, panicked parents, lonely elderly people, and even hostile drunks. I've never seen anyone treat others with such dignity and respect. He's the best partner anyone could want, especially when we have to manage patients who are thrashing around. But that was not always so, was it, Howard?"

"No, it wasn't," Howard replies. "There was a time when no one wanted to work with me. I was a rebel, and I figured there was only one way to do things: my way. But an incident that occurred a few years ago changed all that. It's a long story. But the upshot is that when I recovered from the stress, my outlook had been altered. I realized that though I couldn't save the world, I could save myself. That's when I learned how to deal with the effects of a stressful job. I started eating right, lost a lot of weight, and adopted a new attitude. Anyway, if I can maintain my own well-being, I can do a lot more to help others. Right? Isn't that what we're about?"

Introduction

The safety and well-being of the workforce is a fundamental aspect of top-notch performance in EMS.[1] As a paramedic, it includes your physical well-being as well as your mental and emotional well-being. If your body is fed well and kept fit, if you use the principles of safe lifting, observe safe driving practices, and avoid potentially addictive and and insidious infections. If you let your spirit appreciate the fear and sadness on other faces, you will find ways to combat your prejudices and treat people with dignity and respect. By doing all these things, you will also be able to promote the benefits of well-being to your EMS colleagues.

Death, dying, stress, injury, infection, fear—all these threaten your wellness and conspire to interfere with your good intentions. However, you can do something about

PROCEDURE SCANS

Visual skill summaries provide step-by-step support in skill instruction.

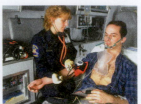

Procedure 7-4 Reassessment

7-4a Reevaluate the ABCs.

7-4b Take all vital signs again.

7-4c Perform your focused assessment again.

7-4d Evaluate your interventions' effects.

laryngospasm may be occurring. Airway and breathing management requires constant reevaluation.

oxygenation. Lip cyanosis indicates central hypoxia (overall oxygen status), whereas peripheral cyanosis indicates decreased oxygen to the tissues. Pallor and coolness sug-

---

Special Features

the present illness. Common sense and clinical experience will determine how much of the following history to use.

Preliminary Data

For documentation, always record the date and time of the physical exam. Determine your patient's age, sex, race, birthplace, and occupation. This provides a starting point for the interview and establishes you as the interviewer. Who is the source of the information you receive about your patient? Is it the competent patient himself, his spouse, a friend, or a bystander? Are you receiving a report from a first responder, the police, or another health care worker? Do you have the medical record from a transferring facility?

After you have gathered the information, you should establish its reliability, which will vary according to the source's knowledge, memory, trust, and motivation. Again, reconfirm the information with the patient, if possible. This is a judgment call based on your experience. For example, if the patient information you received from a particular EMT first responder has been accurate in the past, you probably will trust it again. On the other hand, if the nurse at a physician's office has repeatedly provided you with erroneous information, you probably will doubt its accuracy.

scious patient, the chief complaint becomes what someone else identifies or what you observe as the primary problem. In some trauma situations, for instance, the chief complaint might be the mechanism of injury, such as "a penetrating wound to the chest" or "a fall from 25 feet."

Patho Pearls

The renowned Canadian physician Sir William Osler said, "Listen to the patient, and he will tell you what is wrong." This advice is as true today as it was 100 years ago. A great deal of information can be determined from a skillful history taking. As you listen to a patient's medical history, try to understand the underlying pathophysiologic processes that might cause the symptoms the patient describes. This will help you to fully comprehend the disease process or processes affecting the patient.

For example, consider the following case. Mrs. J. Franklin is a 72-year-old pensioner, twice widowed, who lives in an older section of town. She summons EMS with what initially seem like vague complaints. She reports to the dispatcher, when queried, that she is "just sick." You arrive and begin an assessment, starting with a pertinent history. The patient reports that her symptoms began about two weeks ago after several family members came to her house with dinner, which included a baked ham. Since that time, she has developed some fatigue, progressive dyspnea, and occasional chest pain. She now reports that she often wakes up at 3:00 A.M. with breathing trouble that resolves when she walks around the room or

PATHO PEARLS

Offer a snapshot of pathological considerations students will encounter in the field.

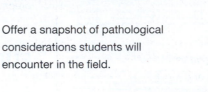

FIGURE 2-11 Patients may be transported by ground or air. Medical helicopter transport was introduced in the 1950s during the Korean War. (© Ed Effron)

Legal Considerations

Emergency Department Closures. Numerous factors have resulted in emergency department closures and ambulance diversions. This can have a significant impact on the EMS system. All systems must address this situation so that patient care does not suffer.

In 1974, in response to a request from the DOT, the General Services Administration (GSA) developed the "KKK-A-1822 Federal Specifications for Ambulances." This was the first attempt at standardizing ambulance design to permit intensive life support for patients en route to a definitive care facility. The act defined the following basic types of ambulance:

- **Type I (Figure 2-13).** This is a conventional cab and chassis on which a module ambulance body is mounted, with no passageway between the driver's and patient's compartments.
- **Type II (Figure 2-14).** A standard van, body, and cab form an integral unit. Most have a raised roof.

Vietnam, and success of military evacuation procedures led to their use in civilian ambulance systems. In 1970, the Military Assistance to Safety and Traffic (MAST) program was established. This demonstration project set up 35 helicopter transportation programs nationwide to test the feasibility of using military helicopters and paramedics in

LEGAL CONSIDERATIONS

Offer a snapshot of pathological considerations students will encounter in the field.

An important part of patient assessment is gathering information that is accurate, complete, and relevant to the present emergency. To begin, you must identify the patient's chief complaint. Although dispatch probably will have given you an idea of what the emergency is about, it is

Cultural Considerations

Eye contact is a major form of nonverbal communication. Short eye contact is often seen as friendly, whereas prolonged eye contact may be interpreted as threatening. Thus, timing is an important factor in how a person interprets eye contact.

One's culture also influences how eye contact is interpreted. Eye contact can mean respect in one culture and disrespect in another. Often, Asians will avoid eye contact even when they have nothing to hide. Eye contact between people of different sexes is problematic in Muslim cultures, in which a prolonged look in the face of a member of the opposite sex might be misinterpreted. Because of this, people in Middle Eastern countries might look a person of the same sex in the eye and not look into the eyes of a person of the opposite sex.

If you work in a culturally diverse community, you should learn the customs of eye contact and other forms of nonverbal communication of those you might encounter during the course of your work.

unexpected but important facts. For example, instead of asking your patient with abdominal pain, "Did you have breakfast today?" which can be answered with either a "yes" or a "no," ask: "What have you eaten today?"

- *Use direct questions when necessary.* Direct questions, or **closed questions,** ask for specific information. ("Did you take your pills today?" or "Does the abdominal pain come and go like a cramp, or is it constant?") These questions are good for three reasons: They fill in information generated by open-ended questions. They help to answer crucial questions when time is limited. And they can help to control overly talkative patients, who might want to tell you about their gallbladder surgery in 1969 when their chief complaint is a sprained ankle.
- *Ask only one question at a time, and allow the patient to complete his answers.* If you ask more than one question, the patient may not know which one to answer and may leave out portions of information or become confused. Equally important is having one person do the interview. Don't force your patient to discern questions from multiple interviewers.
- *Listen to the patient's complete response before asking the next question.* By doing so, you might find that

CULTURAL CONSIDERATIONS

Provide an awareness of beliefs that might affect patient care.

ASSESSMENT PEARLS

Offer tips, guidance, and information to aid in patient assessment.

Provocation/Palliation
What provokes the symptom (makes it worse)? Does anything palliate the symptom (make it better)? In many

Assessment Pearls
Chest pain is a common reason that people summon EMS. However, the causes of chest pain are numerous. In emergency medicine or EMS, we often look to exclude the most serious causes before determining whether chest pain is of a benign origin. Internal organs do not have as many pain fibers as do such structures as the skin and other areas. Pain arising from an internal organ tends to be dull and vague. This is because nerves from various spinal levels innervate the organ in question. The heart, for example, is innervated by several thoracic spinal nerve segments. Thus, cardiac pain tends to be dull and is sometimes described as pressure. It also tends to cause referred pain (i.e., pain in an area somewhat distant to the organ), such as pain in the left arm and jaw. Dull pain that is hard to localize (or to reproduce with palpation) may be due to cardiac disease. One sign often seen with patients suffering cardiac disease is Levine's sign. With Levine's sign, the patient will subconsciously clench his fist when describing the chest pain. Levine's sign is associated with pain of a cardiac origin (e.g., angina or acute coronary syndrome).

Ask about any activity, medication, or other circumstance that either alleviates or aggravates the chief complaint.

Quality
How does your patient perceive the pain or discomfort? Ask him to explain how the symptom feels, and listen carefully to his answer. Does your patient call his pain crushing, tearing, oppressive, gnawing, crampy, sharp, dull, or otherwise? Quote his exact descriptors in your report.

Region/Radiation
Where is the symptom? Does it move anywhere else? Identify the exact location and area of pain, discomfort, or dysfunction. Does your patient complain of pain "here," while holding a clenched fist over the sternum, or does he grasp the entire abdomen with both hands and moan? If your patient has not done so, ask him to point to the painful area. Identify the specific location, or the boundary of the pain if it is regional.

Determine whether the pain is truly pain (occurring independently) or **tenderness** (pain on palpation). Also determine whether the pain moves or radiates. Localized pain occurs in one specific area, whereas radiating pain

---

the result of a head injury; hypothermia, severe hypoxia, or drug overdose. Bradycardia is a common finding in the well-conditioned athlete, but it may be found in almost anyone. Treat bradycardia only if it compromises your patient's cardiac output and general circulatory status.

Tachycardia usually indicates an increase in sympathetic nervous system stimulation as the body compensates for another problem, such as blood loss, fear, pain, fever, drug overdose, or hypoxia. It is an early indicator of shock and may indicate ventricular tachycardia, a life-threatening cardiac dysrhythmia.

The pulse's quality can be weak, strong, or bounding. Weak, thready pulses indicate a decreased circulatory status, such as shock. Strong, bounding pulses may indicate high blood pressure, heat stroke, or increasing intracranial pressure. The pulse location may be another indicator of your patient's clinical status. The presence of a carotid pulse generally means that his systolic blood pressure is at least 60 mmHg. The presence of peripheral pulses indicates a higher blood pressure; their absence suggests circulatory collapse. Practice locating each of the pulse locations (Figure 5-12). As with other vital signs, take your patient's pulse frequently in the emergency setting and note any trends.

To take the pulse of a conscious adult or large child, the most accessible and commonly used location is the radial artery. With the pads of your first two or three

Pediatric Pearls
In infants and small children, use the brachial artery or auscultate for an apical pulse. Remember that auscultating an apical pulse does not provide information about your patient's hemodynamic status. To locate the brachial artery, feel just medial to the biceps tendon. Auscultate the apical pulse just below the left nipple.

fingers, compress the radial artery onto the radius, just below the wrist on the thumb side (Procedure 5-1b). In the unconscious patient, begin by checking his carotid pulse. To locate the carotid pulse, palpate medial to and just below the angle of the jaw. Locate the thyroid cartilage (Adam's apple) and slide your fingers laterally until they are between the thyroid cartilage and the large muscle in the neck (sternocleidomastoid).

First, note your patient's pulse rate by counting the number of beats in 1 minute. If his pulse is regular, you can count the beats in 15 seconds and multiply that number by 4. If his pulse is irregular, you must count it for a full minute to obtain an accurate total. Also note the pulse's rhythm and quality.

Blood Pressure
Blood pressure is the force of blood against the arteries' walls as the heart contracts and relaxes. It is equal to cardiac output times the systemic vascular resistance. Any

---

PEDIATRIC PEARLS

Offer tips, guidance, and information on how to deal with pediatric patients encountered in the field.

CUSTOMER SERVICE MINUTE

Shows how extending extra kindness and compassion can make an important difference to patients and families coping with an emergency.

Customer Service Minute
Following Up. Last week, a man took his dog to the vet for an upper respiratory infection. The dog was pretty sick, but the vet assured the owner that she was not critical, and with antibiotics she would be better in a few days, so he brought her home. The next day, the veterinarian called to find out how the dog was doing. She called every day until the dog was back to normal. Needless to say, the man was delighted in the service he received from that vet.

Physicians' offices, dentists' offices, and veterinary offices often call their patients a few days following a visit to see how things are going. Why don't we? Before you leave your patient and the family, why not ask them for permission to call the next day or in a few days to see how they're doing? If they say no or are hesitant to give permission, drop it. If they give permission, call them and see if there is anything you can do for them.

The follow-up has many benefits. You get to reconnect with the people in your community. It is great for public relations. It is educational because you can see whether your diagnosis was accurate. It's a winner from every angle. When they hang up, they'll be thinking, "Wow!"

Introduction
Patient assessment means conducting a problem-oriented evaluation of your patient and establishing priorities of

your patient en route to the hospital to detect changes in patient condition.

Your proficiency in performing a systematic patient assessment will determine your ability to deliver the highest quality of prehospital **advanced life support** (ALS) to sick and injured people. Paramedic patient assessment is a straightforward skill, similar to the assessment you might have performed as an EMT. It differs, however, in depth and in the kind of care you will provide as a result.

Your assessment must be thorough, because many ALS procedures are potentially dangerous. Safely and appropriately performing advanced procedures such as administration of drugs, defibrillation, synchronized cardioversion, needle decompression of the chest, or endotracheal intubation will depend on your assessment and correct field diagnosis. If your assessment does not reveal your patient's true problem, the consequences can be devastating.

As always, common sense dictates how you proceed in the field. When you assess the responsive medical patient, the history reveals the most important diagnostic information and takes priority over the physical exam. For the trauma patient and the unresponsive medical patient, the reverse is true. However, trauma may cause a medical emergency, and, conversely, a medical emergency may cause trauma. Only by performing a thorough patient assessment can you discover the true cause of your patient's problems. This chapter provides problem-oriented patient assessment examples based on the information and techniques presented in the previous six chapters.

IN THE FIELD

Provides extra tips that can help ensure success in real-life emergency situations.

In the Field
The Tools of Your Trade: The Ophthalmoscope
An **ophthalmoscope** (Figure 5-27) is a medical instrument used to examine the internal eye structures, especially the retina, located at the back of the eye. Although it is most often used to diagnose eye conditions, you can discover information that may be relevant to other medical and traumatic events.

The ophthalmoscope is basically a light source with lenses and mirrors. It has a handle, which houses the batteries, and a head, which includes a window through which you visualize the internal eye; an aperture dial, which changes the width of the light beam; a lens dial to bring the eye into focus; and a lens indicator, which identifies the lens magnification number (i.e., 0 to +40 or 0 to –20). You examine the eye by looking through a monocular eyepiece into the eye of your patient. You can view different depths of the eye at different magnifications by rotating a disk of varying lenses within the instrument itself.

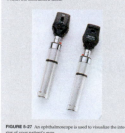

FIGURE 5-27 An ophthalmoscope is used to visualize the interior of your patient's eyes.

eye while the patient continues to fix his gaze on an object in the distance. Adjust the lens disk as needed to focus on the retina. Farsighted patients will require more "plus" diopters (black or green numbers), whereas nearsighted patients will require more "minus" diopters (red numbers) to keep the retina in focus.

Try to keep both your eyes open and relaxed. The optic disk should come into view when you are about 1.5 to 2 inches from the eye while you are still aiming your light 15 to 25 degrees nasally. If you are having difficulty finding the disk, look for a branching (bifurcation) in a retinal blood vessel. Usually the bifurcation will point toward the disk.

Follow the vessel in the direction of the bifurcation and you should arrive at the optic disk. The disk should appear as a yellowish-orange to pink round structure. Within the center of the disk there should be a central physiologic cup, which normally appears as a smaller, paler circle. The cup should be less than half the diameter of the disk. An enlarged cup may indicate chronic open-angle glaucoma. Indistinct borders or elevation of the optic disk may indicate papilledema, which is a marker of increased intracranial pressure.

Next, look at the arteries and veins of the retina. The arteries are usually brighter and smaller than the veins. Spontaneous venous pulsations are normal. Abnormalities of the retina such as hemorrhages, arteriovenous (AV) nicking, and cotton wool spots may indicate local or systemic disease such as retinal vein occlusion, hypertension, or many other conditions.

Finally, look at the fovea and surrounding macula. This area is where vision is most acute. It is located about two disk diameters temporal to the optic disk. You may also find the macula by asking the patient to look directly into the light of your ophthalmoscope. Prepare for a fleeting glimpse as this area is very sensitive to light and may be uncomfortable for your patient to maintain. A "cherry red" macula with surrounding pallor of tissue in the setting of acute painless monocular visual loss indicates a central retinal artery occlusion. Irreversible damage occurs

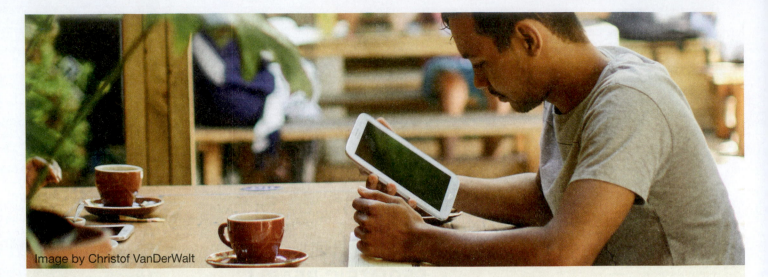

Image by Christof VanDerWalt

MyBRADYLab®

Our goal is to help every student succeed.
We're working with educators and institutions to improve results for students everywhere.

MyLab & Mastering is the world's leading collection of online homework, tutorial, and assessment products designed with a single purpose in mind: to improve the results of higher education students, one student at a time. Used by more than 11 million students each year, Pearson's MyLab & Mastering programs deliver consistent, measurable gains in student learning outcomes, retention, and subsequent course success.

Highlights of this Fully Integrated Learning Program

- **Gradebook:** A robust gradebook allows you to see multiple views of your classes' progress. Completely customizable and exportable, the gradebook can be adapted to meet your specific needs.

- **Multimedia Library:** allows students and instructors to quickly search through resources and find supporting media.

- **Pearson eText:** Rich media options let students watch lecture and example videos as they read or do their homework. Instructors can share their comments or highlights, and students can add their own, creating a tight community of learners in your class.

- **Decision-Making Cases:** take Paramedic students through real-life scenarios that they typically face in the field. These cases give students the opportunity to gather patient data and make decisions that would affect their patient's health.

**For more information,
please contact your BRADY sales representative at 1-800-638-0220,
or visit us at www.bradybooks.com**

ALWAYS LEARNING

PEARSON

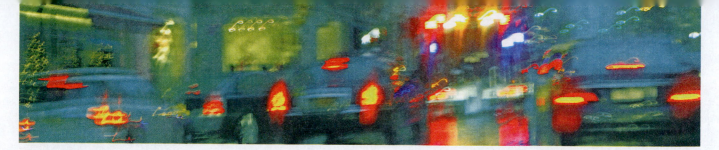

Chapter 1
Trauma and Trauma Systems

Bryan E. Bledsoe, DO, FACEP, FAAEM, EMT-P

Robert S. Porter, MA, Paramedic

STANDARD
Trauma (Trauma Overview)

COMPETENCY
Integrates assessment findings with principles of epidemiology and pathophysiology to formulate a field impression to implement a comprehensive treatment/disposition plan for an acutely injured patient.

⌄ Learning Objectives

Terminal Performance Objective: After reading this chapter you should be able to describe the operation of a functional trauma care system and discuss the roles and responsibilities of paramedics within a trauma care system.

Enabling Objectives: To accomplish the terminal performance objective, you should be able to:

1. Define key terms introduced in this chapter.

2. Describe the epidemiology of trauma in general, and with respect to trauma that results in requests for emergency medical care.

3. Apply the five-step public health model to injury prevention.

4. Describe the capabilities of the various levels of designated trauma centers.

5. Given a variety of scenarios, conduct trauma assessments that result in categorization of patients as critical, unstable, potentially unstable, or stable (CUPS system).

6. Discuss the role of time to definitive care in the outcomes of trauma patients.

7. Apply trauma triage criteria to identify patients who should be transported to a trauma center.

8. Describe the purposes of data collection in injury prevention, the trauma registry, and quality improvement.

KEY TERMS

Case Study

On a sunny and warm midsummer day, the annunciator sounds and requests that the quick response vehicle with paramedic Earl Antak and the Hamilton Area Volunteer Ambulance respond to a bicycle/auto collision 3 miles south of Amble Corners. It is a 10-minute trip for Earl, and about the same for the volunteer ambulance service. While the vehicles are en route, the dispatcher radios that the sheriff's department is on scene and has reported an unresponsive bicyclist.

Arriving at the collision scene, Earl notes that sheriff's deputies have secured the scene and are directing traffic. As he begins his scene size-up, Earl notices that several cars are parked along the highway's shoulder. Earl also sees a bicycle with a mangled front wheel resting against the open door of one of the cars. A deputy is attending to a young adult who is lying on the roadside about 45 feet in front of the car. As Earl studies the scene more closely, he observes that the car's open door has been bent forward and that glass from the car door is strewn along the highway.

The deputy tells Earl that the person he is attending to is named John. He reports that John was unresponsive when the deputy arrived but is now responsive, though somewhat confused. Earl's general impression is that the patient is a thin but well-developed male in his early 20s. He is wearing a bicycle helmet, shorts, and a T-shirt. He has several abrasions to his right shoulder, arm, and forearm, as well as to his right thigh. His helmet is badly scraped and deformed. Earl asks the deputy to continue manual head stabilization while Earl applies a cervical collar.

Earl's primary assessment suggests possible spine injury from the mechanism of injury and reveals that John is responsive and oriented to person but not to place or time. A witness reports that John was riding along at about 20 miles per hour when "this lady opened her door right in front of him." John flew through the door window and onto the pavement. Now John asks, "How's my bike?" His radial pulse is strong, with a rate of about 100, and his respirations are about 22 and full. Both lung fields are clear, and his skin is warm and very wet. At the end of the primary assessment, Earl categorizes John as U (unstable) on the basis of his period of unconsciousness, will expedite further assessment and care, and plans to transport John to the regional trauma center with neurosurgical capability.

The rapid trauma assessment reveals a small deformity just medial to the right upper anterior shoulder and some crepitus and pain with any movement of the right upper extremity. There is a large abrasion to the right thigh. Extremity evaluation reveals limited sensation to touch and limited strength in all limbs, pain on motion with the right upper limb (suspected clavicle fracture), but otherwise equal and strong pulses with good capillary refill and all limbs warm to the touch. There are no signs of soft-tissue injuries to the head and John denies any pain other than to his right shoulder and thigh, a "twinge of pain" in his neck, and a sensation of "pins and needles" in his extremities. When vital signs are taken, John's pulse is still strong at 100, his respirations remain 22 and unlabored, and his blood pressure is 132/84 mmHg.

As the volunteer ambulance arrives, Earl uses his smart phone to contact medical direction for trauma center assignment. He is directed to Mercy Hospital, the regional trauma center, and speaks to the trauma triage nurse. Earl tells the nurse that John meets the system's trauma triage criteria—initial unresponsiveness and a serious mechanism of injury—and relates his assessment findings, Glasgow Coma Score, and patient's vital signs. Because ground transport time is projected to be 45 minutes, and because the mechanism of injury puts this patient within the guidelines for air transport, he requests a helicopter intercept.

After about 8 minutes at the patient's side, Earl and the EMTs from the volunteer ambulance have loaded him into the ambulance. As transport begins, Earl establishes a 16-gauge IV access site, begins to administer normal saline at a to-keep-open rate, and continues to provide frequent reassessments. He notices that John can no longer remember what happened to him or the name of the paramedic. John then begins to mumble incoherently.

Earl and the ambulance intercept with a Central State Medevac helicopter at a predesignated landing zone, a parking lot at the county community college. The flight paramedic greets Earl, takes his report, and quickly begins her assessment. She readies John for flight and Earl helps load him into the helicopter. Within minutes of the ambulance's arrival, the helicopter takes off for Mercy Hospital.

Later that day, Earl gets a follow-up phone call from the flight paramedic thanking him for providing good care for the patient and an informative patient report. She says that the patient had a fracture of the right clavicle, an epidural hemorrhage that required emergency surgery, and a C2 and C3 fracture managed by immobilization. Because of the patient's age and excellent physical condition, he is expected to recover quickly.

Introduction to Trauma and Trauma Care

Trauma, by definition, is a physical injury or wound caused by an external force or forces. It is the third leading cause of death in the United States today behind cardiovascular disease and cancer. For Americans between the ages of 1 and 44 years, trauma is the number-one cause of death, accounting for 47 percent of all lives lost for this age group. Trauma is a major cause of life years lost in the United States because it tends to affect younger people more commonly than other disease processes (Table 1-1). In addition to lives lost, trauma costs more than $400 billion annually in medical costs and lost productivity.

Trauma accounts for more than 170,000 deaths per year, with motor vehicle collisions responsible for about 34,500 and gunshot wounds for another 31,500.[1] Despite reductions in motor vehicle collision and violence-related death rates, the overall trauma and injury mortality rates have been inching steadily upward over the past decade. This is due in part to an aging population that is more vulnerable to the untoward effects of trauma. Other trauma deaths can be attributed to falls, blasts, burns, stabbing, crush injuries, drowning, and sports injuries.

Each year, approximately 42 million Americans will present to hospital emergency departments with trauma. Of these, 2 million patients will require hospital admission. The National EMS Information System (NEMSIS) reports that trauma accounts for around 30 percent of all EMS calls. Of these, 47 percent are for falls, 28 percent are for on-road motor vehicle collisions, 13 percent are for other forms of blunt trauma, 3 percent for off-road motor vehicle collisions, and 2 percent for intentional lacerations/stabbings. Other requests for EMS responses, such as vehicle/pedestrian collisions, accidental lacerations/stabbings, and intentional and unintentional firearm injuries, account for less than 1 percent of EMS calls.[2]

Patho Pearls

Likelihood of Lethal Injury. You will note that on-the-roadway vehicle collisions account for about 28 percent of responses and cause about 34,500 deaths annually. Intentional and unintentional firearm injuries account for fewer than 1 percent of EMS responses, yet cause 31,500 deaths per year. Thus, if you are called to a gunshot wound, it is more likely that the injury will be life threatening than if you were called to an auto crash. Another way of stating this is that a gunshot wound is far more likely to be lethal than an auto crash.[2]

EMS plays an important role in modern trauma care. Thus, it is essential that the paramedic understand the design and purpose of the trauma care system, participate in injury prevention, and provide the trauma patient with proper assessment, aggressive care, and rapid transport to the most appropriate facility. The remainder of this chapter will detail these responsibilities as it further defines trauma, explains components of trauma care systems, identifies differing trauma center capabilities, and more fully defines the role of the paramedic as a prehospital provider in the modern trauma system.

Trauma

Trauma can range from slight abrasions resulting from a slide into first base to fatal, multiple-system injuries resulting from a high-speed automobile-versus-pedestrian collision. Trauma is generally divided into two major categories, blunt and penetrating, based upon the general mechanism of injury. **Penetrating trauma** occurs when an object enters the body and exchanges energy directly with human tissue, thereby causing injury. **Blunt trauma** occurs as a result of a nonpenetrating injury—typically blunt force. Many of the trauma patients encountered in EMS will have some

Table 1-1 Life Years Lost by Disease (2010 Data)

Disease	Life Years Lost (%)
Trauma	30%
Cancer	16%
Heart disease	12%
HIV/AIDS	2%

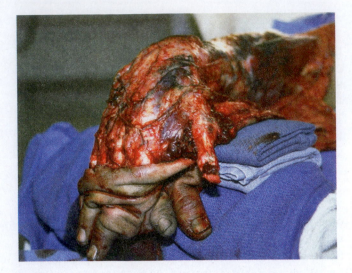

FIGURE 1-1 In prehospital care, it is essential that gruesome, non-life-threatening injuries do not distract you from more subtle, life-threatening problems.

(© Edward T. Dickinson, MD)

component of both mechanisms of injury. These two trauma categories are discussed in greater detail in the chapter "Mechanism of Injury."

On primary assessment, visible injuries can often distract or mask the actual severity of the patient's condition. Extremity injuries, for example, rarely cause death. However, they can be obvious and grotesque (Figure 1-1). Life-threatening problems, such as internal bleeding and shock, can occur with only subtle signs and symptoms. Thus, when assessing a trauma patient, you must look beyond obvious injuries for evidence that indicates a more serious or life-threatening condition. If suspected, it is essential to ensure aggressive care and rapid access to the appropriate hospital or trauma center.

Serious and life-threatening injuries typically occur in less than 10 percent of all trauma patients. Most patients with life-threatening trauma will have sustained internal injury—most commonly to the head or torso (chest, abdomen, or pelvis). Generally speaking, these patients cannot be adequately stabilized in the prehospital setting. Oftentimes, the most prudent care may be establishment of an airway, assurance of adequate ventilation, hemorrhage control and rapid transport to definitive trauma care. Definitive trauma care is best provided at an accredited trauma center with rapid access, if required, to emergent surgical care.

Fortunately, most trauma patients do not have serious or life-threatening injuries. For these patients, prehospital care includes thorough on-scene assessment and care followed by conservative transport to the nearest appropriate hospital. The role of the paramedic is to determine, if possible, the difference between those trauma patients with serious, life-threatening conditions and those who are less seriously injured. This process is guided by prehospital trauma triage criteria (discussed later in this chapter). These criteria include multiple factors, such as mechanism of injury, physical examination findings, age, the presence of other medical conditions, and other findings. Using the trauma triage guidelines will help ensure that the prehospital trauma patient is properly routed to the most appropriate level of trauma care based on his condition.

Trauma as a Disease

The initial impetus to develop a modern EMS system was to improve prehospital trauma care. This began with a white paper titled "Accidental Death and Disability: The Neglected Disease of Modern Society." This was followed by subsequent passage of the Highway Safety Act of 1966. The white paper was one of the first documents to classify trauma as a "disease." Modern medicine has developed and applied a five-step approach to prevent or reduce the impact of disease. Often referred to as the "public health care model," the five steps are surveillance, risk identification, intervention development, implementation, and evaluation. This model emphasizes the importance and efficiency of prevention of a disease. In the case of trauma and other diseases, it is much easier and less expensive to try to prevent the disease rather than treat it.

Surveillance

Surveillance is the process of collecting data in order to identify the existence, significance, and characteristics of disease. The study of disease based on such surveillance is referred to as **epidemiology**). For example, we know, based on surveillance programs, that trauma is the number-one cause of death for Americans between the ages of 1 and 44, accounting for more than 170,000 deaths annually. We also know that for every trauma death (mortality), another two patients will survive with a significant disability (morbidity), and another 20 will require an EMS response and subsequent emergency department care. Further, we know that more than 120,000 persons die yearly because of accidental injury, with 34,500 of those deaths resulting from motor vehicle collisions alone. Falls account for another 24,000 unintentional deaths, drowning 4,000 deaths, and burns 4,000 deaths. Intentional death accounts for 30,000 lives lost from suicide and about 20,000 from homicide. About 60 percent of these intentional deaths are caused by firearms—most commonly, handguns (Figure 1-2). Thirty percent of EMS responses are to trauma calls.[3]

CONTENT REVIEW

➤ Trauma as a Disease: The Public Health Model
- Surveillance
- Risk analysis
- Intervention development
- Implementation
- Evaluation

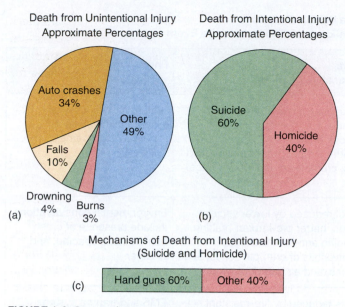

Death from Unintentional Injury
Approximate Percentages

Auto crashes
34%

Other
49%

Falls
10%

Drowning
4%

Burns
3%

(a)

Death from Intentional Injury
Approximate Percentages

Suicide
60%

Homicide
40%

(b)

Mechanisms of Death from Intentional Injury
(Suicide and Homicide)

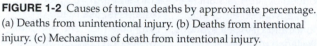

Hand guns 60% | Other 40%

(c)

FIGURE 1-2 Causes of trauma deaths by approximate percentage. (a) Deaths from unintentional injury. (b) Deaths from intentional injury. (c) Mechanisms of death from intentional injury.

Risk Analysis

Risk analysis is a process to examine a disease and determine the various factors that affect its development, course, and consequences. Males, for example, account for more than 65 percent of all trauma deaths and 75 percent of trauma mortality between the ages of 16 and 24. Alcohol is related to around 50 percent of traffic fatalities and is also considered a major contributing factor in off-road vehicle and boating crashes, falls, drownings, and homicide/suicide. Clearly, human behavior plays an important role in trauma. The high number of deaths in young men might be attributed to risk-taking behavior, alcohol consumption, and a general disregard for safety.

A helpful tool to identify risk elements associated with trauma is the **Haddon Matrix** (Figure 1-3). The Haddon Matrix is used to identify risk factors for disease using a three-by-three matrix. When applied to trauma, it separates and defines causes and contributing factors and helps to identify factors that can be modified to reduce the incidence, severity, and outcome of trauma. The Haddon Matrix identifies elements occurring prior to the incident (pre-event), during the incident (event), and after the incident (post-event). It also examines the victim (host), causative elements (agent), and factors surrounding the incident (environment). In a motor vehicle collision, for example, the event is the collision, the host is the driver and other vehicle occupants, the agent is the energy exchange

between the automobile interior and its occupants, and the environment is the roadway and weather and lighting conditions.[4]

Pre-event factors are those things that occur well before the collision and cause, influence, or prevent the outcome (injury). Pre-event host factors may include defensive driver training, traffic law compliance, and behaviors regarding drinking and driving (or texting) and using safety equipment (seat belts or helmets). Pre-event host factors also include the patient's general health (age, preexisting disease, medications, and physical conditioning), mental status, and absence of distractions. The agent, which is actually the exchange of kinetic injury, can be reduced before the collision by factors such as improved auto design, antilock brakes, air bags, proper use of child seats, and crumple zones and air bags. The environment can be improved by better highway design (improved traffic flow patterns, keeping high-speed oncoming traffic separated, lines painted on the roadway, increased intersection visibility, appropriate and clear signage, and better barrier engineering), lowered highway speeds, and traffic law enforcement.

Event factors exist during the crash. Host-related event factors include the occupant's health at crash time, fatigue and alertness, any influence of alcohol or other drugs, and seat belt use. The agent (impact) is reduced by lower vehicle speeds, better pre-impact braking (including the beneficial effects of antilock brakes), the presence and effectiveness of crumple zones in the vehicle, seat belt use, and air bag deployment. Environmental event considerations include such things as crash barriers deflecting an auto away from a bridge abutment, an open space or barrier between lanes preventing the auto from crossing into oncoming traffic, and weather that may reduce visibility, reduce vehicle control, and extend stopping distances.

Post-event factors are those that either worsen or improve the victim's outcome after the energy exchange. For the host, they include his knowledge of what to do after the crash: first aid, not to move if he has spinal symptoms or pain, and how to access the EMS system (911, OnStar). Post-event host elements also include the victim's

Haddon Matrix

	Host	Agent	Environment
Pre-event			
Event			
Post-event			

FIGURE 1-3 A Haddon Matrix for risks and preventive measures regarding disease (including trauma) often assumes a three-by-three construction.

Haddon Matrix for a Vehicle Collision:
Analysis of Factors that May Ameliorate or Exacerbate the Event

	Host: Driver/Occupants	Agent: Causative Elements	Environment: Surrounding Factors
Pre-event: **Before the collision**	Defensive driver training, traffic law compliance, behaviors regarding drinking and driving and using safety equipment (seat belts or helmets), general health, alertness, absence of distractions.	Kinetic energy exchange reduced by better auto design such as anti-lock brakes, lap belts and shoulder straps, proper use of child seats, crumple zones, and air bags.	Better highway design, lowered highway speeds, traffic law enforcement.
Event: **The collision**	Effects on occupant influenced by health at crash time, rest state, alertness, influence of alcohol or other drugs, seat belt use, air bag deployment.	Impact reduced by lower vehicle speeds, better pre-impact braking (including anti-lock brakes), effectiveness of crumple zones, seat belt use, and air bag deployment.	Environmental considerations include presence of crash barriers, lane spacing, and weather.
Post-event: **After the collision**	Outcome after crash worsened or improved by knowledge of what to do: first aid, not moving, accessing EMS, physiological ability to deal with blood loss and shock based on health, condition, and medications.	Effects reduced by fire-resistant fuel systems, advanced automatic collision notification (AACN) systems, video surveillance of crash area, priority dispatch of right resources, and speed of reaching the scene.	EMS and trauma system responses, use made of teachable moment, effect of weather on collision victims after the crash.

FIGURE 1-4 A Haddon Matrix identifying preventive elements for motor vehicle collisions.

ability physiologically to deal with blood loss and shock based on the person's general health and conditioning and the effects of medications such as beta-blockers and anticoagulants. Potential agent effects are reduced by fire-resistant fuel systems and advanced automatic collision notification (AACN) systems such as OnStar. Post-crash environmental factors include video surveillance of high-traffic and frequent crash areas and priority dispatch to ensure that the right resources arrive quickly at the scene. Post-event environmental factors also include the EMS system and trauma system responses and possibly a teachable moment (future incident prevention). Finally, post-event environmental factors include the effects that adverse weather (cold, heat, wind, and precipitation) has on collision victims (Figure 1-4).

Intervention Development

Intervention development is the development or modification of programs to reduce both the incidence and the seriousness of trauma. In an auto crash, we can see preventive opportunities in almost all components of the Haddon Matrix. For example, safer highway design, such as barriers that deflect traffic or absorb impact energy, can improve morbidity and mortality in motor vehicle collisions. Improved auto technology, such as better braking systems, crumple zones, and passive restraint systems, can reduce injuries and deaths. Educational programs that encourage drivers to use their seat belts and drive rested

and distraction-free, avoid substances that impair mental status, and drive defensively all reduce the number and seriousness of collisions and resulting injuries. EMS was, in fact, a post-event intervention that was developed through this health care approach to provide better care for injured patients after trauma has occurred.

As technology progresses, more accurate information regarding auto crash dynamics is available through General Motors's OnStar, Ford's SYNC, BMW's Assist, and other advanced automatic collision notification (AACN) systems. These devices transmit vehicle data regarding the vehicle's initial speed (velocity), strength and direction of gravitational equivalent forces (G-forces), air bag deployment, and vehicle location through GPS (global positioning system). This information helps public-safety dispatch more accurately direct the needed services to the collision scene and can also help responders anticipate the degree of injury and better prepare for patient assessment and care.

Implementation

Implementation is the act of placing an intervention into practice. It can include enforcing traffic laws, reducing speed limits in hazardous areas, modifying highways to be safer, building safer autos, establishing gun safety programs and workplace safety codes, implementing behavior change and safety education, or continuing to improve the EMS system. As health care providers, paramedics have a responsibility to promote, teach, and teach by example—all actions that help reduce trauma. Paramedics are also responsible to identify ways to provide better trauma patient care.

An important and very effective intervention for trauma is the use of a "teachable moment." We often treat individuals who have been injured because of carelessness or a disregard for safety. In a supportive, nonjudgmental manner, we can suggest that a modest and positive behavior change can prevent an event like this from repeating itself. We all learn from our mistakes; using a teachable moment can reduce the likelihood of another similar trauma event occurring.

Evaluation

Evaluation is the process of repeating the surveillance that took place before an intervention to identify benefits of the intervention. For example, we know that the highway death toll has dropped from 56,000 per year when the Highway Safety Act was passed (in 1968) to just under 30,000 per year in recent times. This occurred despite the fact that more people are on the roadways, traveling greater distances, and at faster speeds. This significant reduction in motor vehicle collision (MVC) mortality demonstrates intervention effectiveness over the past four decades. However, people still die as a result of drunk driving, failure to wear seat belts, falling asleep at the wheel, excessive speed, distraction by cell phone use, and other modifiable risk factors and behaviors. Using the public health care model, we must continue to search out risk factors, develop and implement interventions, and evaluate our system's performance. We also need to apply the public heath care model to other types of trauma: falls, gunshot wounds, burns, sports injuries, recreational injuries, and others. Injury prevention is an evolving role of the modern EMS system.

The Trauma Care System

Development of the modern-day trauma care system mirrors the development of the public health care model just discussed. In the mid- to late 1960s, several medical groups investigated the death toll on U.S. highways. Their studies revealed that vehicle collision victims suffered not only from their crash-related injuries, but also from the lack of an organized approach to bringing these victims into the health care system. Studies also demonstrated that most hospitals at that time were inadequately equipped and staffed to care for crash victims.

More than two decades later, the American College of Surgeons recognized that the system caring for severely injured trauma victims was still inadequate and successfully worked to achieve passage of the Trauma Care Systems Planning and Development Act of 1990. This act helped to establish guidelines, funding, and state-level leadership and support for trauma systems.

Recent statistics have shown that with the most common type of trauma system activation, a patient with a blunt trauma, less than 1.5 percent of adults and less than 0.1 percent of children required urgent surgical intervention. (For penetrating trauma, the surgical intervention rates are considerably higher.)

The overall rate of surgical intervention for trauma may be low, but the injuries that do require an operation (e.g., internal hemorrhage sites, organ rupture) are often difficult to identify in the field and, once identified, can be complex and require a skilled and experienced trauma surgical team. This means that proper hospital care for serious trauma should include the immediate availability of skilled surgical intervention. Although patients with life-threatening injuries account for less than 10 percent of all trauma patients, and although even fewer need emergent surgery, immediate surgical care remains important for some patients and can drastically reduce trauma mortality and morbidity in selected circumstances.

Care for seriously injured patients can be expensive and complicated. A well-designed EMS system allocates trauma resources in a way that provides these patients with the most efficient and effective care. Such a system uses hospitals with special resources and a commitment to trauma care. These hospitals are designated as trauma centers.

Trauma Center Designation

The current model for a trauma system includes four **trauma center** levels, with a differing ability and commitment to provide trauma care at each level, with Level I centers offering the highest level of care (Table 1-2).

Table 1-2 Criteria for Trauma Center Designation

Level I—Regional Trauma Center

Commits resources to address all types of specialty trauma 24 hours a day, 7 days a week.

Level II—Area Trauma Center

Commits the resources to address the most common trauma emergencies with surgical capability available 24 hours a day, 7 days a week; will stabilize and transport specialty cases to the regional trauma center.

Level III—Community Trauma Center

Commits to special emergency department training and has some surgical capability, but will usually stabilize and transfer seriously injured trauma patients to a higher-level trauma center as needed.

Level IV—Trauma Facility

In remote areas, a small community hospital or medical care facility may be designated a trauma receiving facility, meaning that it will stabilize and prepare seriously injured trauma patients for transport to a higher-level facility.

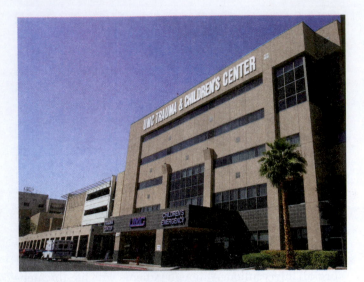

FIGURE 1-5 University Medical Center in Las Vegas, Nevada. As a Level I trauma center, it provides trauma care for a large geographic area. (© Dr. Bryan E. Bledsoe)

A Level I, or regional, trauma center, is a hospital, usually a medical university teaching center, prepared and committed to handle all types of specialty trauma (Figure 1-5). These centers provide neurosurgery, often provide microsurgery (limb replantation), and care for multisystem trauma. They also provide leadership and resource support to other trauma center levels within the regional trauma system through system coordination, data collection, research, and continuing medical and public education programs. When population density or available resources do not permit a commitment to Level I trauma center requirements, a Level II trauma center may act as a regional trauma center.

A Level II, or area, trauma center has a high commitment to trauma care but not as great as a Level I facility. It has surgical care capability available at all times for incoming trauma patients. Level II centers can handle all but the most seriously injured specialty and multisystem trauma patients. (Some of these services may be on call rather than in-house.) Staff at these facilities can stabilize those patients in preparation for transport to a Level I trauma center.

A Level III, or community, trauma center is a general hospital with a commitment to special staff training and resource allocation for trauma patients. These centers are located in smaller communities generally situated in rural areas. They are well prepared to care for most trauma victims and to stabilize and triage more seriously injured ones for transport to higher-level trauma centers.

A Level IV trauma facility, sometimes called a "critical access hospital," is often in a rural area. These facilities are capable of stabilization and care of trauma patients before transport, often by helicopter, to a more distant, higher-level trauma center. In these areas, trauma incidence does not support resource allocation great enough to meet the requirements of a trauma center, so, by default, some other type of health care facility is identified as a trauma transport destination.

Trauma system design should be flexible enough to meet regional needs. In urban and suburban areas, there are often just a few trauma centers to ensure that each receives adequate patient volume to maintain staff proficiency and to ensure that resources are being used effectively. In rural regions, a Level III center may act as a regional trauma center because the incidence of serious trauma does not support any greater commitment. In some areas, a Level IV facility may be all that is available and thus becomes the default destination for seriously injured trauma patients. Consult your EMS system plan and protocols to ensure that you follow the intended patient flow patterns in your region.

Specialty Centers

Beyond classification as trauma centers, certain medical facilities may be designated as specialty centers, such as neurocenters, burn centers, pediatric trauma centers, and centers specializing in hand and limb replantation by

Legal Considerations

The Cost of Trauma Care. Trauma systems and trauma hospital designations are an important element of prehospital care. Trauma triage protocols help direct each trauma patient to a facility that can adequately care for that patient's injuries. However, in the 21st century, several confounding factors are complicating these systems. For example, trauma care is a cost for which hospitals are often not adequately reimbursed. In fact, they might actually lose money while providing such care. In a time of shrinking health care dollars, many hospitals have found that they can no longer afford to provide costly trauma care. This is a contributing factor to the overall reduction in the number of trauma centers in many parts of the country.

Concurrently, skyrocketing malpractice insurance premiums have driven many physicians—especially neurosurgeons—from trauma practice. Trauma patients are often difficult to care for, and patient outcome is often determined more by the injury than by the care provided. Nevertheless, many physicians and surgeons are perceiving that malpractice allegations come more frequently from trauma patients than from other classes of patients and, because of this, have elected not to provide trauma care. This, of course, creates a significant problem for EMS.

With trauma centers closing and physicians closing their practices to trauma, ambulances must often travel greater distances to get their patients to a proper facility. Although these issues are community issues, EMS personnel must stay informed and involved to ensure that their patients receive the best possible care at the closest appropriate facility.

microsurgery. One other specialty service is hyperbaric oxygenation, which is sometimes used in the treatment of carbon monoxide poisoning and problems associated with scuba diving.

Specialty centers have made a commitment of trained personnel, equipment, and other resources to provide services not usually available at a general or trauma hospital. These centers are also more likely to provide specialized intensive care and state-of-the-art injury management that your patient would not find at other facilities. Be aware of specialty services available in your system as well as protocols defining when patients should be directed to them.

Your Role as a Paramedic

As a paramedic, your tasks in the trauma system are likely to begin with an appropriate patient assessment and then triage of trauma patients using standards and guidelines established by your medical direction system (trauma triage criteria), followed by expeditious patient care and then transport to the closest appropriate medical facility (Figure 1-6). For those patients who meet trauma triage criteria, the appropriate facility is the nearest trauma center.

Trauma Assessment

Trauma patient assessment follows the general patient assessment format for all patients but differs from medical patient assessment in some very important ways. These include addressing an increased likelihood of scene hazards, analyzing the mechanism of injury, considering the impact the environment may have on the patient and his subsequent assessment and care, establishing scene oversight, applying trauma triage guidelines, and determining the appropriate patient destination. In trauma assessment, you often treat patients with serious and/or life-threatening

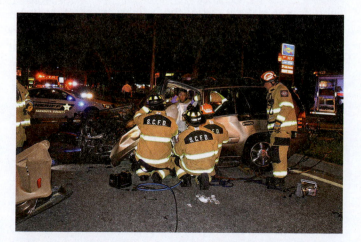

FIGURE 1-6 Your role as a paramedic attending a trauma patient is to ensure the ABCs and prepare the patient for rapid transport.
(© Ed Effron)

injury (necessitating a rapid trauma assessment) or ones with limited injury to a specific body area (such as an isolated forearm fracture and necessitating only a focused trauma assessment). In spite of its special aspects, assessment of trauma patients proceeds much as it does for the medical patient. Its steps include the scene survey, primary assessment, secondary assessment (rapid or focused trauma assessment), and periodic reassessments.

Scene Survey

The scene survey emphasizes scene safety and scene evaluation and identifies factors that may help or hinder scene oversight and efficient delivery of assessment and care. Critical scene survey elements are scene safety, mechanism of injury evaluation, environment impact consideration, and scene oversight.

Scene Safety

Because trauma scenes are often located outdoors, in industrial facilities, and/or involve machinery, the environment is more likely to have associated hazards. These can include traffic hazards from oncoming vehicles, the risk of electrocution from downed power lines, laceration hazards from jagged metal and broken glass, toxic substance exposure from smoke and spilled fluids (e.g., gasoline), a confined space (adverse atmosphere) as in silos and tanks, rough unstable terrain, slippery surfaces, and/or a violent scene. Scene safety is of paramount importance for you, your crew, your patient, and bystanders. Many scene hazards may go unnoticed unless you actively look for them. If the scene is not safe and you cannot make it so, do not enter it and prevent others from doing so. Request additional resources to ensure a safe scene and then await their arrival.[5]

Mechanism of Injury Analysis

The **mechanism of injury (MOI)** is the circumstances and events by which an injury occurs. As you assess the scene, try to mentally re-create the incident from available evidence. Attempt to identify the strength and direction of the forces involved in the incident. Try to determine the area or areas of the patient's body most likely to have been affected by these forces. In an automobile collision, for example, the mechanism of injury includes the energy exchange between the auto and what it struck, between the patient and the interior of the vehicle, and between the various tissues and organs as they are compressed or otherwise injured. Close inspection of the collision site and vehicle can provide evidence regarding the collision and the forces involved. (See the chapter "Mechanism of Injury.")

Information you gather regarding the scene and the mechanism of injury allows you to develop an **index of suspicion** for possible injuries. This index is a mental summation of suspected injuries based on your event analysis.

For example, an adult pedestrian struck by a car can be expected to have lower extremity fractures. Further, if the auto was moving at 20 miles per hour or less, the fracture severity is often less than if it were moving at 55 miles per hour. Also, the probability of internal injury at lower speeds is less than it would be at higher speeds. By evaluating the MOI, you can often predict the body structures and organs injured and the degree of injury.

In addition to examining the MOI, examine trauma patients for current signs of physical injury, during both the primary and the secondary (rapid or focused) trauma assessment. Current research suggests that MOI alone is not as good a trauma severity predictor as was once thought. At best, the MOI is only an indirect indicator of injury severity. For example, modern vehicle design and restraint systems are better able to absorb and disperse energy from significant vehicle collisions. Because of this patients often survive with only limited injuries. Thus, it is important to carefully examine the patient's signs and symptoms including vital signs, Glasgow Coma Scale, and level of consciousness, as well as analyzing the mechanism of injury.

Physical signs and symptoms that suggest serious trauma include the presence of shock or traumatic brain injury. Because shock and traumatic brain injury cause the greatest trauma mortality, carefully look for the earliest evidence of these conditions. It is important to note that the body compensates well for internal blood loss and can often hide the signs of serious injury until late in the shock process. If you have any reason to suspect that a patient has sustained serious internal injury, including traumatic brain injury, carefully monitor the vital signs and level of consciousness and rapidly transport the patient. Otherwise, provide frequent reassessments to ensure detection of progressing signs of shock and traumatic brain injury as soon as possible.

Environmental Impact Consideration

It is important to anticipate the effect of environmental factors on assessment and care. Adverse weather, as with a severe thunderstorm, may expose you and the patient to wind, precipitation, and cold. It may be beneficial to have the fire department provide tarps and/or windscreens to protect you and your patient from adverse conditions. Some conditions, such as a blizzard or extreme heat, may merit moving the patient to the ambulance earlier in the assessment process than you normally would. Always evaluate any extreme of heat or cold, precipitation (snow, sleet, rain), strong winds, and direct sunlight for any possible adverse impact on patient assessment and care. Try to identify the resources needed to address environmental hazards.

Scene Oversight

Scene organization and oversight are critical to effective scene safety and patient access, disentanglement, assessment, care, extrication, and transport. If you are first on the scene, establish scene oversight (command) and report your scene findings to dispatch. When additional resources arrive, transfer command and begin patient care. If the Incident Command System is already in place and operating, report to the incident commander and begin your assignment (usually patient care).

Primary Assessment

The primary assessment of a trauma patient varies slightly from that of a medical patient. The primary assessment of a trauma patient includes forming an initial patient impression; determining the need for spinal precautions; evaluating and securing the airway, breathing, and circulation; and determining patient priority for care and transport. As with a medical patient, quickly determine the patient's level of consciousness and mental status and chief complaint or complaints. This information will allow you to form an initial impression of the patient's condition. This will subsequently expand in depth and specificity as patient assessment continues.

The need to evaluate the patient for possible spinal injury is specific to trauma patient assessment. This requires that the patient not have normal mental status, and have no spinal point tenderness, no neurological deficits, and no distracting injuries. Patients who do not meet these criteria should be considered for spinal precautions.

Assessment and management of the airway, breathing, and circulation mirror medical patient assessments, although looking for significant hemorrhage is more involved than with a medical patient. Note that you should assess circulation first if you suspect the patient is in cardiac arrest (the American Heart Association's CAB formulation).

At the end of the primary assessment, you will assign the patient a preliminary priority for further assessment, care, and transport using the CUPS system or a similar triage scheme. The CUPS system classifies patients as **C**ritical, **U**nstable, **P**otentially unstable, or **S**table. Patients who do not make it out of the primary assessment (e.g., you are unable to secure the airway, breathing, or circulation) are considered critical (C). Those who present with limited injuries and are breathing well and have strong pulses are considered stable (S). Those in between are either unstable (U) or potentially unstable (P).

Secondary Assessment

Stable patients should receive a focused trauma assessment. This is simply an application of the elements of a detailed patient assessment, looking particularly at the area of suspected injury and/or chief complaint. Based on this, you will confirm injury and provide the required care. Reassessment monitors the patient for changes in vital signs and level of consciousness to detect deterioration in the patient's status.

Potentially unstable or unstable patients receive a rapid trauma assessment that includes a quick evaluation of major body regions (a quick head-to-toe exam) and focused assessments when the mechanism of injury, patient complaint, or finding from the rapid trauma assessment suggests injury. Emphasis is placed on the Glasgow Coma Scale (GCS) as a tool for predicting the severity of patient injury. However, the GCS requires adequate training and practice to employ accurately and consistently. The GCS, along with other factors, is used to help make the priority determination for patient care and transport.

Reassessment

Periodic reassessments permit you to trend any patient improvement or deterioration. They include any primary and secondary assessment elements that revealed signs or symptoms and a set of vital signs every 15 minutes for stable patients and every 5 minutes for unstable patients.

The Golden Period

Time is a critical consideration for the survival of many seriously injured trauma patients. Research has demonstrated that, for certain patients, survival rates increase dramatically as time from initial injury to surgery decreases. The current goal for incident-to-surgery time is about 1 hour, often referred to as the **Golden Period**. The Golden Period used to be called the Golden Hour, but the name has evolved to reflect the fact that the science behind the Golden Hour has not been validated. For most trauma patients, minutes or even a few hours do not change survival rates. However, because a few trauma patients will require urgent surgical intervention, it is good EMS practice to minimize scene and transport times in serious trauma cases.

Factors such as response time and the time needed to access a patient, to extricate a patient (in some cases), to assess and care for a patient, and to transport a patient to the trauma center all consume a portion of the Golden Period. Many of these time-consuming factors are beyond your control. Thus, it is vital to keep to a minimum time spent on factors over which you do have control.[6] Ideally, you should provide the primary and secondary assessments, emergency stabilization, patient packaging, and initiation of transport in less than 10 minutes. When distances or traffic conditions present prolonged ground transport times, consider reducing these by calling for an air medical service, if available, and if your patient's condition falls within the guidelines for air transport.[7]

Air medical service, usually provided by helicopter, has added a tool to the race against time for the seriously injured trauma patient (Figure 1-7). Helicopters travel much faster than ground transport and often in a straight line from the crash site to the trauma center. Recognize, however, that helicopters normally serve a greater geographic

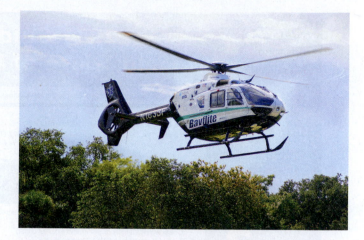

FIGURE 1-7 A helicopter air ambulance (HAA) can sometimes reduce transport time from the accident scene to the trauma center. *(© Ed Effron)*

area than ground-based EMS and are often some distance from the trauma scene. Remember that it takes a finite amount of time for the helicopter crew to receive the call, check weather, board the helicopter, and complete the start and liftoff process. Always consider these factors in your request for air medical service and compare them to normal ground transport times considering that ground ambulance is already on scene. Often, immediate transport from the scene by ground ambulance will actually get the patient to the hospital faster than a helicopter dispatched after scene arrival.[8]

Be aware, also, that air medical transport is not appropriate in many cases. A trauma patient must be in relatively stable condition for air transport to be used. This is because the limited space within the aircraft and its associated engine noise make in-flight care difficult. Further, a combative patient may endanger the flight crew and aircraft safety. Adverse weather conditions can also limit the use of air medical transport. In many cases, ground transport is as fast or faster. Finally, air medical transport services are very expensive and can be used most effectively only as part of a comprehensive EMS trauma system. The use of air medical services is evolving with a trend toward tightening the medical criteria for which flights are authorized. Follow local protocols about when and how to request and use air medical transport.[9]

The Decision to Transport

The Centers for Disease Control and Prevention has introduced revised criteria for prioritizing trauma patients for care and transport: 2011 Guidelines for Field Triage of Injured Patients[10] (Figure 1-8). These criteria, often known as **trauma triage criteria**, identify the GCS, physical findings (vital signs), and the anatomy of the injury as elements of the trauma care and transport decision tree,

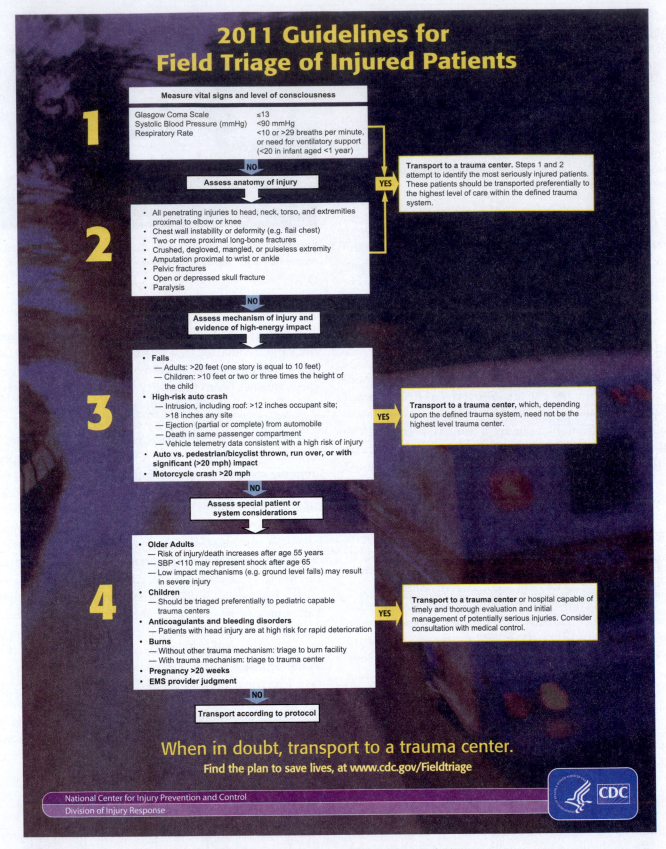

FIGURE 1-8 Guidelines for Field Triage of Injured Patients, Centers for Disease Control, 2011.

followed by mechanism of injury and special considerations such as age.

As mentioned earlier, the mechanism of injury (at least as related to auto collisions) is not as good a predictor as one might think. Modern vehicle design sacrifices vehicle structure to protect the occupants. Consequently, vehicle damage may suggest the degree of energy absorption rather than actual energy transfer to the patient. During the primary assessment (scene survey), however, determination of the mechanism of injury remains the first element of patient assessment to determine patient acuity. Because the Glasgow Coma Scale and vital sign evaluation are performed during the secondary assessment, MOI often provides preliminary information necessary to determine patient priority (CUPS) at the conclusion of the primary assessment.

The decision to either transport a trauma patient immediately or attempt more extensive on-scene care can be difficult. Trauma triage criteria are designed to help guide decision making. As a rule, you should immediately transport patients who display key clinical and anatomic findings or experience certain mechanisms of injury quickly, with intravenous access, endotracheal intubation, and other time-consuming procedures attempted en route. The 2011 Guidelines for Field Triage of Injured Patients (review Figure 1-8) lists the indicators for immediate transport.[11]

When applying trauma triage criteria, it is best to err on the side of caution. Even if a patient does not meet the stated physical findings for rapid transport, consider all factors in decision making. Remember, you see the patient only minutes after the injury. At this point, the patient may not yet have lost enough blood internally to exhibit signs of shock. If in doubt, consider rapid transport to a trauma center, and frequently reassess vital signs and level of consciousness.

The criteria listed in the Guidelines for Field Triage are, by design, sensitive for injury and thus may lead to "over-triaging" trauma patients. The criteria ensure that patients with significant and serious injuries but with very subtle signs and symptoms are not missed during assessment. Application of these criteria may cause you to transport some patients to trauma centers who ultimately will be determined not to require this high level of care. However, transporting a patient to a trauma center who may not need its resources is far better than not transporting a patient who truly does needs those services. (See the chapter "Special Considerations in Trauma" for further discussion of trauma patient assessment.)

Injury Prevention

Prevention is the best and most cost-effective way to reduce trauma morbidity and mortality. It is easier and much less costly to reduce the number of intoxicated drivers on the

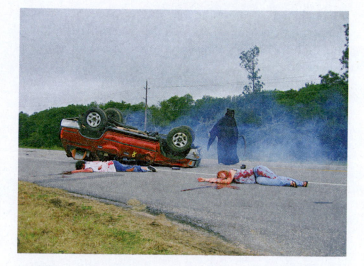

FIGURE 1-9 Public education programs such as the "Shattered Dreams" program can increase people's awareness of the role of the EMS system and of the importance of safe behaviors.

(© Austin County, Texas, EMS)

highway than to care for them and their victims after they have been injured in crashes. This is especially true when you consider the loss of life associated with drunk driving and the cost of rehabilitation for its victims.

Programs promoting defensive driving, seat belt use, undistracted driving, and use of designated drivers encourage people to drive more safely and responsibly. Other programs, such as "Let's Not Meet by Accident" and "Shattered Dreams" (Figure 1-9), increase society's awareness of trauma systems as well as an appreciation for safety-oriented behaviors.[12] Safety programs for off-road vehicles, boating, and firearm use also raise safety awareness and promote injury prevention. The EMS system has a responsibility to support such programs and to promote their development where they do not exist. As an EMS provider, you should participate in these programs and encourage your peers to take part in them as well.[13]

Technical developments such as better highway design, air bag restraint systems, and vehicles constructed to absorb crash energy have also played major roles in reducing the yearly highway death toll. Paramedics have a responsibility to support such development and use of new designs and technologies as a way of further reducing trauma deaths and injuries.[14]

Data and the Trauma Registry

As discussed earlier in this chapter, and as with all emergency medical services, surveillance is the only way to determine which trauma care practices and procedures benefit patients and which that do not. In trauma systems, there is a health care surveillance process called the **trauma registry**. It is a uniform and standardized data collection process by regional trauma centers. These data are analyzed to determine the types of patients and injuries treated, determine how well the system is performing, and identify factors that may either lessen or increase patient survival.

It is important to support the trauma registry and research efforts by ensuring that all prehospital care reports accurately and completely describe assessment findings, patient care, reassessment results, and times associated with calls. Consider taking part in and supporting prehospital research projects. Research can help establish the value of existing and new field techniques and equipment and can ultimately help reduce patient morbidity and mortality.

Quality Improvement

Trauma system quality improvement (QI), or quality management (QM), is another way of examining system performance with the aim of providing better patient care. In the QI process, certain indicators are monitored and examined to determine whether designated system care standards are being met. For trauma system QI, these include trauma triage criteria application, field skill performance, response times, assessment, care, transport, and the appropriateness of trauma patient destinations. QI also examines select calls to determine whether documentation accurately reflects assessment results and care given. If system standards are not being met, strategies may be developed to improve performance through such steps such as continuing education programs, EMS equipment modifications, or protocol revisions. It is important to remember that true QI is not punitive and does not look to identify fault with individual providers. It is, however, an effective method to assess system quality and provide for its improvement. As a prehospital trauma team member, always become actively involved in, and encourage peer participation in, these or similar programs.

Summary

Trauma remains one of modern society's greatest tragedies. It often results in death and disabling injuries. Unlike many medical conditions, it affects those who have their most productive years ahead of them. A well-designed and well-implemented trauma system offers a way of lessening the incidence and impact of trauma. The system consists of varying levels of trauma centers possessing increasing levels of commitment to immediate and intensive trauma care. The well-designed and well-implemented trauma system also has prevention programs that encourage safe practices and behaviors. Finally, such a system has trauma triage protocols that guide paramedics in prioritizing and transporting trauma patients.

As a paramedic, you are a part of the trauma care system. You are charged with evaluating trauma patients by comparing their mental status, physical signs of injury, vital signs, and injury mechanism to pre-established trauma triage criteria. This comparison helps you determine which patients should enter the trauma system and which could be best cared for with less emergent care and transport. In the presence of severe, life-threatening trauma, you must ensure rapid trauma assessment, time-critical on-scene care, and expedited transport to an appropriate facility, a trauma center, to provide your patients the best chances for survival.

You Make the Call

Just as you are about to move a seriously injured 12-year-old patient who has been in a bicycle/auto collision, her mother, Janet, emerges from the crowd. She is quite distraught and becomes even more so when you tell her that you'll be transporting her daughter to the Great Meadows Trauma Center on the far side of town. Janet informs you that she is a "lab tech" at Livingston Community Hospital, just a few minutes from your location, and wants her child transported there.

1. What authority does Janet have regarding the decision to transport her daughter?

2. What will you tell her regarding your choice for a hospital destination?

See Suggested Responses at the back of this book.

Review Questions

1. The leading cause of death for people between the ages of 1 and 44 in the United States is _____
   a. cancer
   b. stroke
   c. trauma
   d. cardiovascular disease

2. Of the following, which intervention will most likely contribute the most to the survival of your trauma patient?
   a. Apply supplemental oxygen.
   b. Control any significant external hemorrhage.
   c. Rapidly transport the patient to the emergency department.
   d. Initiate intravenous therapy.

3. Which trauma center designation is applied to a hospital that commits to special emergency department training and has a degree of surgical capability in house, but usually stabilizes and transfers seriously injured patients to a higher-level trauma center?
   a. Level I
   b. Level II
   c. Level III
   d. Level IV

4. Which specialty service is important for the ongoing treatment of carbon monoxide poisoning or problems related to scuba diving?
   a. Neurocenter
   b. Hyperbaric oxygenation chamber
   c. Burn center
   d. Pediatric trauma center

5. When determining the mechanism of injury, you will assess the _____
   a. dynamic forces involved in the collision.
   b. person who caused the collision.
   c. number of patients.
   d. need for additional resources.

6. When will you begin considering the mechanism of injury for a trauma patient?
   a. During the scene size-up
   b. During the rapid trauma assessment
   c. During the focused trauma assessment
   d. During reassessments

7. The objective time frame, describing the period from the incident to the patient's arrival at surgery, is known in EMS as the _____
   a. Platinum 10 Minutes.
   b. Golden Period.
   c. Trauma Hour.
   d. Trauma Transport Time.

8. After arriving on scene for a multisystem trauma that has no need for extrication, within how many minutes is it recommended for you to assess, stabilize, and initate transport of the patient?
   a. <15
   b. <20
   c. <10
   d. <25

9. Limitations of air medical transport via helicopter include all of the following *except* _____
   a. limited space within the aircraft.
   b. loud engine noise.
   c. mandated landing zone requirements.
   d. inability to handle patients with a complicated airway.

10. In the quality improvement process, a committee will look at selected care modalities to determine whether designated program standards of care are being met. These modalities are also called _____
    a. criteria.
    b. pointers.
    c. indicators.
    d. recommendations.

See Answers to Review Questions at the end of this book.

References

1. Centers for Disease Control and Prevention. Deaths: Final Data for 2009, table 18. (Available at www.cdc.gov/nchs/fastats/injury.htm.)
2. National EMS Information System. "Report: Frequency of Injury Related to EMS Encounter by Cause." 2012. (Available at www.nemsis.org.)
3. Centers for Disease Control and Prevention. "10 Leading Causes of Deaths, United States—2008." Atlanta, GA, 2010. (Available at www.cdc.gov.)
4. Laraque, D., B. Barlow, and M. Durkin. "Prevention of Youth Injuries." *J Nat Med Assoc* 91(10) (1999): 557–571.
5. Reichard, A. A., S. M. Marsh, and P. H. Moore. "Fatal and Nonfatal Injuries among Emergency Medical Technicians and Paramedics." *Prehosp Emerg Care* 15(4) (2011): 511–517.
6. Gonzalez, R. P., et al. "On-Scene Intravenous Line Insertions Adversely Impacts Prehospital Time in Rural Vehicle Trauma." *Am Surg* 74(11) (2008): 1083–1087.
7. Ringburg, A. N., et al. "Helicopter Emergency Medical Services (HEMS): Impact on On-Scene Times." *J Trauma* 63(2) (2007): 258–262.
8. Sullivent, E. E., M. Faul, and M. M. Wald. "Reduced Mortality in Injured Adults Transported by Helicopter Emergency Medical Services." *Prehosp Emerg Care* 15(3) (2011): 295–302.

9. Talving, P., et al. "Helicopter Evacuation of Trauma Victims in Los Angeles: Does It Improve Survival?" *World J Surg* 33(11) (2009): 2469–2476.

10. National Center for Injury Prevention and Control. "Guidelines for Field Triage of Injured Patients." 2011. (Available at www.cdc.gov/fieldtriage.)

11. Smith, R. M. and A. K. Conn. "Prehospital—Scoop and Run or Stay and Play?" *Injury* 40 Suppl 4 (2009): S23–S26.

12. City of Frisco Police Department. "Shattered Dreams." Texas 2012. (Available at www.ci.frisco.tx.us/departments/police.)

13. Sleet, D. A. "Reducing Motor Vehicle Trauma through Health Promotion Programming." *Health Educ Q* 11(2) (1984): 113–125.

14. Rasouli, M. R., et al. "Preventing Motor Vehicle Crashes Related Spine Injuries in Children." *World J Pediatr* 7(4) (2011): 311–317.

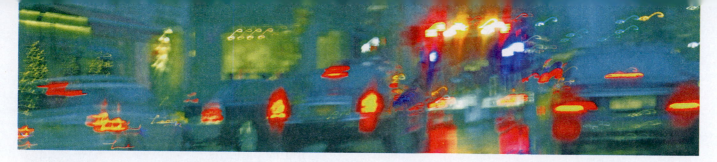

Chapter 2
Mechanism of Injury

Bryan E. Bledsoe, DO, FACEP, FAAEM, EMT-P

Robert S. Porter, MA, EMT-P

STANDARD
Trauma (Trauma Overview)

COMPETENCY
Integrates assessment findings with principles of epidemiology and pathophysiology to formulate a field impression to implement a comprehensive treatment/disposition plan for an acutely injured patient.

⌄ Learning Objectives

Terminal Performance Objective: After reading this chapter, you should be able to relate the kinetics and mechanisms of injury associated with blunt trauma to patients' potential for injury.

Enabling Objectives: To accomplish the terminal performance objective, you should be able to:

1. Define key terms introduced in this chapter.

2. Discuss the laws of inertia, energy conservation, force, and kinetic energy as they relate to kinetics of impact.

3. Associate the application of energy to various body tissues with the biomechanical forces produced to predict injury patterns.

4. Describe the events that occur in motor vehicle impacts.

5. Discuss the various vehicular restraints and safety mechanisms, and identify the potential for injuries in vehicle collisions.

6. Describe injury patterns associated with various types of vehicle impacts, and the

   association between vehicle damage and injury potential.

7. Given a variety of scenarios, conduct a vehicle collision analysis.

8. Modify a collision analysis to account for the characteristics of motorcycle and off-road vehicle collisions.

9. Describe the forces that cause injuries in patients who have fallen and the criteria that constitute a severe fall.

10. Describe the mechanisms of blast injury, blast-injury patterns, and special blast-injury care considerations.

11. Discuss the phases of the blast injury to include common injury patterns in each phase.

12. Describe basic injury patterns and assessment considerations for an injured patient participating in a sporting event.

13. Describe the considerations for the cause and assessment of crush injuries and compartment syndrome.

14. Apply the laws of inertia and energy conservation to the kinetics of penetrating trauma.

15. Discuss how force and kinetic energy exchange relate to the potential for injury.

16. Apply principles of ballistics to the prediction of injury patterns, to include special weapon types.

17. Associate the application of low-, medium-, and high-velocity penetrating mechanisms to various body tissues with the biomechanical forces produced to predict injury patterns.

18. Describe special concerns for EMS provider safety that are associated with penetrating trauma.

19. Given a penetrating trauma scenario, reconstruct events to gain additional information that can help predict injury patterns.

20. Describe the special considerations in assessment and management of penetrating trauma to the face and chest, and of impaled objects.

KEY TERMS

acceleration, p. 21

axial loading, p. 27

ballistics, p. 42

blast wind, p. 36

blunt trauma, p. 22

caliber, p. 43

cavitation, p. 43

crumple zone, p. 28

deceleration, p. 21

drag, p. 43

dyspnea, p. 39

emboli, p. 39

energy, p. 20

epistaxis, p. 38

exsanguination, p. 34

flechettes, p. 36

force, p. 20

hemoptysis, p. 39

incendiary, p. 37

index of suspicion, p. 21

inertia, p. 20

kinematics, p. 20

kinetic energy, p. 21

kinetics, p. 20

mass, p. 20

mechanism of injury, p. 19

motion, p. 20

oblique, p. 28

ordnance, p. 36

overpressure, p. 35

oxidizer, p. 35

penetrating trauma, p. 22

percutaneous cricothyrotomy, p. 53

perforating trauma, p. 41

pericardial tamponade, p. 49

pneumothorax, p. 39

pressure wave, p. 35

profile, p. 43

projectile, p. 42

resiliency, p. 48

trajectory, p. 43

velocity, p. 20

yaw, p. 43

zone of injury, p. 47

Case Study

A call comes in to City Ambulance Unit 2, staffed by paramedic Kris and BLS provider Bob. The dispatcher reports multiple injuries in a two-car collision on the freeway at interchange 20. Because of backed-up traffic, the dispatcher directs the unit to use the freeway exit ramp to access the scene.

Police arrive at the scene and provide Unit 2 with an update while they are en route. A green auto traveling at freeway speed has collided with a red car stalled at the interchange. The wreck involves three injured parties—one in the red car and two in the green one.

When Unit 2 reaches the scene, the police have secured it and are directing traffic around the vehicles involved. Kris and Bob approach the vehicles and begin the scene size-up, noting that about 50 feet now separate the two vehicles. The green car has severe front-end damage. There are two "spider-web" cracks in the windshield, the steering column is deformed, and, as an older-model car, it has no air bags. The police officer in charge reports that neither person in the car was wearing a seat belt. The red car has severe rear-end damage, but the windshield is intact. The driver in this vehicle wore a seat belt and the head rest is in the up position. Before acting, Kris calls for another ambulance to back up Unit 2. Kris and Bob now proceed to the green car, where they expect to find the worst injuries.

Kris and Bob perform primary assessments on the two occupants of that vehicle. The driver has suffered chest trauma from impact with the steering wheel. Although she is experiencing difficult and painful breathing, her airway is clear. She is oriented to time, place, and person and denies any period of unconsciousness. Her pulses are strong, regular, and at a moderate rate, and she appears to be breathing adequately. The physical exam reveals a forehead contusion, a reddened anterior chest with crepitus, and clear breath sounds bilaterally.

The passenger is unconscious and cannot be aroused. She has shallow, rapid breaths and a rapid, barely palpable pulse. Her forehead is badly contused with minor lacerations and moderate bleeding. There are some contusions to her knees, and her thighs appear noticeably shortened. The rapid trauma assessment reveals instability of the pelvis and both femurs.

A police officer who has been trained as an Emergency Medical Responder indicates that the driver of the red car is conscious and alert. Although "shaken up," he has a blood pressure of 126/84 mmHg and a pulse of 86. He is breathing normally at a rate of 20. As the paramedic in charge, Kris asks the officer to stay with the driver until the second ambulance arrives.

Meanwhile, Bob has told the driver of the green car not to move. He then places a cervical collar on the passenger and they safely move her to the soft stretcher. They then load her into the ambulance.

When the second ambulance arrives, Kris briefs that crew and assigns them the remaining patients, the two drivers. Kris and Bob then rush the passenger, who is the most critical patient, to a nearby trauma center. En route, vital signs reveal a blood pressure of 72 by palpation and a weak radial pulse of 130. The legs look ashen, feel cool to the touch, and show no palpable pulses. Capillary refill time is 3 seconds in the upper extremities, longer in the lower ones. The pulse oximeter reading is 82 percent.

Kris gives a brief report to medical direction and receives orders in response. She starts a large-bore IV and quickly administers a 250-mL bolus of normal saline. She will check the patient's response and administer repeat boluses as needed. After administering the first bolus of saline, Kris readies intubation equipment and ventilates the patient using a bag-valve mask. She attempts oral intubation with the patient's head held fixed in the neutral position. When the effort proves unsuccessful, Kris withdraws the tube, ventilates the patient again, and tries to insert an LMA. LMA insertion is successful and Kris infuses another 250-mL bolus of fluid. Lung sounds are clear, chest excursion improves, capnography displays a proper waveform, and oximetry readings begin to rise.

The patient arrives at the trauma center with one more fluid bolus having been administered, for a total of 750 mL of fluid infused; an end-tidal CO_2 reading of 35 mmHg; and an oxygen saturation of 96 percent. An orthopedist is called and uses external fixation to stabilize the pelvis. A major bleeding pelvic artery is embolized to halt its hemorrhage. The patient recovers after a few weeks of hospitalization and months of rehabilitation. She will walk again with only slight reminders of the injuries and the care she received.

Based on the speed of impact and the vehicle damage, the second ambulance crew decides to transport the other two patients to the trauma center. The driver of the green car has two fractured ribs, minor pulmonary contusions, a C-spine cleared by CT scan, and no neurologic deficit. She stays overnight for observation and is released the next afternoon with some medication for rib fracture pain. The other driver has a clear C-spine and returns home shortly after the emergency department evaluation.

Introduction to Mechanism of Injury

Trauma results from the exchange of energy between an object and the human body (Figure 2-1). This energy exchange causes a chain reaction within the affected body tissues. These forces can crush, stretch, tear, and otherwise injure and destroy essential body structures and organs, resulting in injury and death. At its most fundamental level, trauma is a disease. It is typically classified as either blunt or penetrating, based on the **mechanism of injury**, the manner by which the injury occurred. Often, patients have some component of both injury types. For example, a stabbing victim may fall down a flight of stairs, sustaining both penetrating and blunt trauma. As another example, a motorcycle rider who loses control of his bike and impales himself on a fence pipe will have sustained both blunt and penetrating trauma. In this

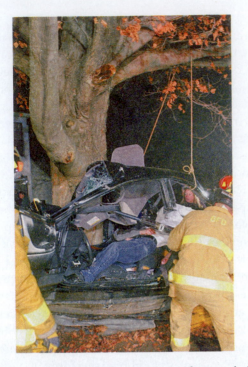

FIGURE 2-1 The mechanism of injury can reveal a great deal of information regarding the patient's condition. Trauma results from the physical exchange of energy from an object or surface transmitted through the skin into the body's interior.

(© Mark C. Ide/Science Source)

chapter we will detail the kinematics of trauma with application to both blunt and penetrating trauma.

Kinematics of Trauma

Kinetics is the branch of physics dealing with objects in motion and energy exchanges that occur as these objects collide. Impacts and collisions are the fundamental causes of trauma. These collisions and impacts deliver energy to the patient, causing injury. **Kinematics**, a similar term, is the branch of physics (mechanics) that studies the motion of a body or a system of bodies without consideration given to its mass or the forces acting on it. An understanding of kinetics and kinematics will help to determine and anticipate the results of auto collisions and other forms of impacts.[1]

The two basic principles of kinetics are the law of inertia and the law of energy conservation. Further, kinetic energy and force formulas help to quantify the energy exchange between a moving object and the human body. These laws and formulas best describe what occurs during impact and helps us understand trauma.

Inertia

The law of **inertia**, as described by Sir Isaac Newton and known as Newton's first law, describes how objects in motion behave. The first part of the law of inertia states: "A body in **motion** will remain in motion unless acted upon by an outside force." For example, consider an auto traveling at 65 miles per hour. To stop the auto, you must apply a force, whether slowing the car gradually with the brakes or slowing it rapidly by colliding with a large tree. The amount of energy exchange needed to stop the car is the same whether the brakes are applied or the car hits the tree. The rate of energy exchange (gradual versus rapid) is a major factor in causing trauma.

The second part of the law of inertia states: "A body at rest will remain at rest unless acted upon by an outside force." For example, an auto stopped at a stop sign can be moved forward using the force of the auto engine—or the auto can move forward from the force of another car hitting it from behind. In both cases, energy from an "outside force" (either the engine or the second vehicle) is transferred to the auto and it moves forward. Again, as with the prior example, the amount of energy exchanged remains basically the same. It is the time interval over which the energy is transferred that determines the severity of trauma.

Energy Conservation

Energy, in the strict physical sense, is defined as the ability to do work. The law of energy conservation states: "Energy can neither be created nor destroyed. It can only be changed from one form to another." In an auto crash, the changing of energy from one form to another is what deforms the auto and may cause injury to the occupants. By examining this energy exchange, one can appreciate the processes and forces that cause injury.

As an auto slows gradually for a stop sign, the brakes develop friction to slow the turning wheels, thus producing heat. Stated another way, the energy of motion is transformed into heat energy. During an auto crash, however, the energy of motion is converted at a much faster rate and is converted into several forms of energy: the sound of impact, deformation of the auto's structural components, heat released from twisting steel, and forces sustained by the occupants as they collide with the vehicle interior. Eventually, as all the energy of motion is finally converted to other energy forms, the auto and its occupants come to rest.

Force

Newton's second law of motion describes the forces at work during a collision. It states that **force** is related to an object's **mass** (weight) and the rate of its change in **velocity** (speed). (Although mass and weight are technically not identical, we will consider them so for this discussion.) The force formula is summarized as:

$$\text{Force} = \frac{\text{Mass (Weight)} \times \text{Acceleration (or Deceleration)}}{2}$$

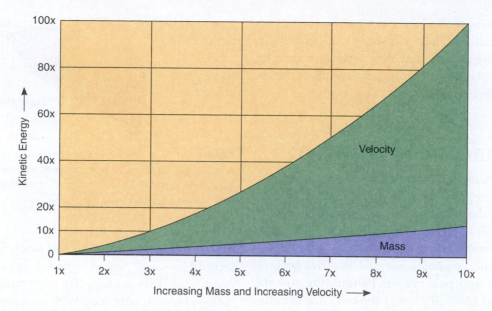

FIGURE 2-2 Increasing mass directly increases kinetic energy, whereas increasing velocity exponentially increases kinetic energy.

The force formula emphasizes the importance of the rate at which an object changes speed, either increasing (**acceleration**) or decreasing (**deceleration**). Gradual changes in speed (low acceleration or deceleration) generate small forces and are usually uneventful. Normal deceleration, such as slowing for a stop sign, covers about 140 feet (from 65 miles per hour to a stop at a braking rate of 22 feet/10 miles per hour of speed). Because the kinetic energy of a moving vehicle is changed over a great distance (and over several seconds), it rarely causes injury. However, colliding with a large tree and slowing from 65 miles per hour to a stop in a matter of inches and a fraction of a second (high deceleration) produces tremendous force and devastating injuries.

Kinetic Energy

Kinetic energy is the energy of an object in motion. It is a function of the object's mass and its velocity (Figure 2-2). The kinetic energy of an object while in motion is measured by the following formula:

$$\text{Kinetic Energy} = \frac{\text{Mass (Weight)} \times \text{Velocity (Speed)}^2}{2}$$

It is important to examine the formula elements carefully. Changes in an object's mass or velocity have different effects on the object's kinetic energy. This formula illustrates that when you double an object's weight, you double its kinetic energy. It is twice as damaging to be hit by a 2-lb ball as to be hit by a 1-lb ball. It is three times as damaging to be hit by a 3-lb ball, and so on (a linear relationship).

As velocity (speed) increases, however, there is a larger increase in kinetic energy. Being hit with a 1-lb ball traveling at 20 miles per hour is four times as injurious as being hit with the same ball moving at 10 miles per hour. Double the speed, and the energy is quadrupled. If the speed increases to 30 miles per hour (tripling), the energy released (and the expected trauma) is nine times greater. This concept plays a key role in understanding the enormous energy released in high-speed motor vehicle crashes as well as the devastating effects of a gunshot wound resulting from a small bullet traveling extremely fast.

Kinetic energy is the measure of how much energy an object in motion has, not necessarily how much injury it will cause. The force formula explains how that energy is delivered to the structure of a vehicle, the occupants, and the organs and tissues affected. Once an object has significant kinetic energy, the rate of deceleration (or acceleration) subsequently determines the force of impact and the severity of the resulting injuries.

When significant kinetic energy is applied to the human body, it results in trauma. *Trauma* is defined as a wound or injury that is violently produced by some external force.

Kinetics of Impact

To properly care for trauma victims, it is important to understand how energy exchange affects the human body. The study of this energy exchange, called the *kinetics of impact*, can provide insight into the events that produce injury (the mechanism of injury). The manner in which this energy exchange damages human tissue is referred to as the *biomechanics of trauma*. Understanding the kinetics of impact and the resulting biomechanics of trauma can help you develop an anticipation of the nature and severity of likely injuries—called the **index of suspicion**. Using the index of suspicion, prehospital personnel can more effectively focus trauma assessment, triage, and care.

In the following section we examine the kinetics of impact, biomechanics of trauma, vehicle collisions, blast injuries, penetrating injuries, and other types of trauma to develop an understanding of these mechanisms of injury and their effects on the human body.

Biomechanics of Trauma

Concepts of the biomechanics of trauma explain the injury process by examining the forces of kinetic energy as they progress through the body. As with the kinetics of impact, the biomechanics of trauma are bound by the laws of physics: inertia, force, and energy conservation.

As noted earlier, trauma is divided into two general categories: blunt and penetrating. **Penetrating trauma** occurs as an object physically enters the body and directly or indirectly injures tissue. **Blunt trauma** occurs when kinetic energy forces, but not the object, enter the body and damage tissue.

During the normal blunt impacts of everyday life, such as sitting in a chair or being jostled in a crowd, little to no damage occurs. However, as an object's kinetic energy and the rate of velocity (acceleration or deceleration) increase, a blunt impact begins to cause injury. Blunt trauma can occur when a person in motion strikes a stationary object (as at the end of a fall) or when a moving object strikes a stationary person (as when someone is struck with a baseball).

Trauma involves a continuous series of collisions as outside forces cause the tissues within the body to rapidly accelerate or decelerate. During the process, compressing, stretching, and shearing forces may cause tissue injury. *Compression* injury occurs when impact abruptly stops a portion of the body while inertia causes the remaining structures to continue in motion. The result is one tissue or organ being pushed into another, compressing it and damaging small blood vessels, connective tissue, and cell structures within.

Stretch is the opposite of compression. Here, the tissues and fibers that hold organs and other structures together are pulled and injured or torn. Stretch occurs as one part of the body is pulled away from another, as between the vertebrae during a hanging. Another example of stretch is the hollow organ filled with fluid or air. During impact, tissue compression brings the anterior and posterior surfaces of the hollow organ closer together, increasing the pressure within. This pressure is opposed by the decelerating anterior organ wall and the inertia of the posterior organ wall. However, there are no such opposing forces from the organ's sides. The increasing air or fluid pressure pushes outward, stretching the lateral organ wall. This is much like compressing a fluid-filled balloon beneath your foot. With increasing force, the side walls of the balloon are stretched and can rupture, stretching and tearing the walls and spilling the contents.

Shear injury occurs along edges of the impacting force or at organ attachments. As the impacting force slows a part of the body, tissue along the impact border continue in motion. The opposing forces—one slowing the structure, the other (inertia) resisting the slowing—tear the tissue in a fashion similar to the blades of scissors, with tissues sliding in opposite directions along parallel planes. With organ attachment, the attaching tissues resist the motion of the dense organ and can tear into the tissue (Figure 2-3).

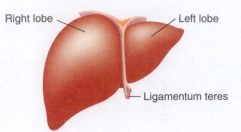

Right lobe   Left lobe

Ligamentum teres

FIGURE 2-3 Shear. With rapid deceleration, as in an auto crash, the liver moves forward at the original speed while the supporting ligamentum teres remains in its fixed position, possibly slicing into the liver (a shearing injury).

Patho Pearls

Compression, Stretch, and Shear. For an example of these biomechanical forces of compression, stretch, and shear at work, let us examine an auto collision. In a frontal impact, the car stops abruptly, setting off the driver-side air bag. While the auto slows, the driver's entire upper body continues to move forward. *Unfortunately, in our example, the occupant's forward speed is not reduced by seat belt use.* As the driver's chest hits the deployed air bag, the skin's surface drastically slows its forward motion. However, the remaining chest contents—the ribs and intercostal muscles, lungs, heart, great vessels, esophagus, spine, and posterior chest wall—continue their forward motion. As the ribs and intercostal muscles, then the lungs and heart, the great vessels and esophagus, and finally the spine and posterior chest wall collide with one another, kinetic energy of the moving chest changes form, injury may occur, and the chest comes to a rest.

If all body tissue and organs were of a consistent density, elasticity, and strength and were uniformly attached, any injury pattern would be consistent and very predictable.[1] However, this is not the case. Skin and muscle tissue are very strong and well able to withstand compression and stretch. Bone is extremely strong but resists bending and may fracture. Lung tissue consists of delicate microscopic air sacs (alveoli)

CONTENT REVIEW

➤ Forces of Blunt Trauma
- Compression
- Stretch
- Shear

that are very susceptible to injury by rapid, strong compression, especially when they are filled with air. Finally, hollow organs, such as the heart, stomach, bowel, and urinary bladder, are very tolerant of trauma forces unless they are distended with fluid or air. Then they are more likely to rupture. Solid organs vary in their ability to withstand the forces of trauma. The spleen and brain are very delicate and damage easily. The kidneys, liver, and pancreas are held together rather strongly by the nature of their tissue and by a firm capsule surrounding them. However, as impact energy and the forces directed to these structures increase, there is a greater likelihood of injury.

Organ attachment also plays an important role in the biomechanics of trauma. The heart is a dense muscle filled with a dense fluid, blood. When deceleration forces occur, the heart has more mass and inertia than the less-dense lung tissue surrounding it. It easily displaces lung tissue and moves violently against the aorta and venae cavae. Because the thoracic aorta is firmly attached to the posterior thoracic wall, the heart twists against this vessel. This action may rupture the aorta or tear its internal lining and create a dissection. The liver is held firmly in the right upper abdominal quadrant by the ligamentum teres. With strong deceleration, this ligament may lacerate the liver like a wire cheese cutter cutting cheese. Other organs, like the kidneys, are attached by structural regions called pedicles, traversed by blood vessels, which anchor the organ. With severe acceleration or deceleration forces, this attachment may stretch and tear, damaging blood vessels, causing internal hemorrhage, and disrupting blood flow to the organ.

Patho Pearls

Trauma and the Laws of Physics. The laws of physics play a significant role in the pathophysiology of both blunt and penetrating injuries. In blunt trauma, the energy tends to be more widely distributed than with penetrating injuries. In addition, as discussed in this chapter, solid organs are at greater risk of injury following blunt trauma than hollow organs are because they tend to absorb more of the energy of impact. Whenever a patient has sustained a blunt force injury to the abdomen, it should increase your index of suspicion of solid-organ injury.

Injuries to the liver, spleen, pancreas, or even the kidneys can result in massive blood loss.

It is important to remember, also, that some hollow organs will begin to react in a way similar to solid organs when they are full or distended. For example, the urinary bladder may be full at the time of injury. Blunt force trauma may result in its rupture, with subsequent spillage of urine into the abdomen. Thus, questions about recent meals, alcohol and fluid intake, and similar factors must be taken into consideration when caring for a victim of blunt trauma.

At the trauma center, surgeons may elect to manage some blunt-force injuries conservatively, and others with immediate surgical repair.

Mechanism of Injury as a Predictor of Trauma Severity

Assessment of the mechanism (or mechanisms) of injury can provide important information regarding the likelihood of patient injuries. However, research has found that some mechanisms are good predictors of injury severity, whereas others are not. The Centers for Disease Control and Prevention has identified several mechanisms of injury as good predictors of the need for trauma center care (Table 2–1). A systematic study of the ability of mechanism of injury to predict trauma center need found that death of another vehicle occupant, fall distance, and extrication time were good predictors of trauma center need. The study also found that passenger compartment intrusion, ejection, and vehicle deformity were moderate predictors of trauma center need (Table 2–2).[1-3] In this table, *sensitivity* is the probability of the test (mechanism of injury) to accurately predict trauma center need, whereas *specificity* is the probability that the test (mechanism of injury) will be negative for a patient who does not experience the given mechanism of injury. Mechanism of injury must be considered along with other physical and anatomic criteria in determining injury severity.

Table 2-1 Centers for Disease Control and Prevention's 2011 Mechanism of Injury Criteria for Trauma Center Transport

Falls	Adults: >20 feet (1 story = 10 feet)
	Children: >10 feet or 2–3 times the height of the child
High-risk auto crashes	Intrusion (including roof): >12 inches occupant side; 18 inches either side
	Ejection (partial or complete) from automobile
	Death of passenger in same passenger compartment
	Vehicle telemetry data consistent with a high risk for injury
Auto versus pedestrian crashes	Thrown, run over, or with significant (>20 mph) impact
Bicycle crashes	Thrown, run over, or with significant (>20 mph) impact
Motorcycle crashes	>20 mph

Table 2-2 Mechanism of Injury as a Predictor for Trauma Center Need

Mechanism of Injury	Triage Criteria	Sensitivity	Specificity
Motor vehicle crash	Death of Occupant	3%	99.5%
	Extrication >20 minutes	11%	98%
	Intrusion >12 inches	19%	95%
	Ejection	3%	99%
	Deformity >20 inches	27%	89%
	Speed >40 mph	47%	76%
	Rollover	13%	87%
Fall	Fall >12 feet	4%	99%
Pedestrian/bicyclist struck by car	Thrown or run over	65%	45%
	Struck at speed >5 mph	93%	24%
Motorcycle crash	Speed >5 mph	87%	29%
	Rider separated from motorcycle	83%	19%

(Modified from: Lerner, E.B. , et al. "Does Mechanism of Injury Predict Need?" *Prehosp Emerg Care* 15 (2011): 518–525.)

Blunt Trauma

Blunt trauma most commonly results from motor vehicle collisions involving automobiles, motorcycles, bicycles, pedestrians, or off-road vehicles (e.g., all-terrain vehicles, watercraft, snowmobiles). It can also result from falls, explosions, crush injuries, and sports injuries. Examination of the biomechanics of injury for each of these mechanisms can help to identify likely injuries (indexes of suspicion).[4]

Vehicular Collisions

Vehicular collisions—sometimes called motor vehicle collisions or motor vehicle crashes (MVCs)—account for a large proportion of EMS responses. Each year, more than 100,000 serious collisions occur on U.S. roadways and some 34,500 people lose their lives in these collisions, and many more are seriously injured or permanently disabled. Paramedics must be prepared to offer rapid assessment and appropriate care to victims of these collisions.[3] To this end, it is important to recognize the various types of vehicular impacts, identify possible mechanisms of injury, and form an index of suspicion for specific injuries. Analysis of the types of impacts and the events associated with them helps in developing an index of suspicion.

Events of Impact

There are various types of vehicle impacts (frontal, lateral, oblique, rear-end, rollover). Each type generally progresses through a series of five events:

1. *Vehicle collision.* Vehicle collision begins when a vehicle strikes an object (or an object strikes the vehicle). The vehicle's kinetic energy causes damage as it is converted to mechanical and heat energy as the vehicle comes to a stop. Mechanical energy is the energy that is possessed by an object because of its motion or its position. Heat energy is the movement of molecules and atoms within an object. Forces developed in the collision depend on the initial velocity (kinetic energy) and stopping distance (rate of deceleration). If an auto slides into a snowbank and slows gradually, damage is usually limited. If an auto strikes a concrete retaining wall and stops abruptly, however, the deceleration rate and vehicle damage are typically much greater. The degree of auto deformity is often an indicator of the strength and direction of forces experienced by its occupants.

2. *Body collision.* An auto collision slows or stops a vehicle, but not necessarily the occupants. Body collision occurs when an occupant remains in motion and subsequently strikes the vehicle's interior. The vehicle and its interior have slowed dramatically during the collision, but an unrestrained occupant remains at or close to the speed at the time the collision occurred. As the occupant impacts the interior, his kinetic energy is transformed into initial tissue deformity (mechanical injury). If the vehicle collision causes intrusion into the passenger compartment, this displacement may further subject occupants to impact forces. Restraints (seat belts and supplemental restraint systems) slow and cushion occupants along with the slowing of the vehicle during the collision, thereby decreasing the occupant's rate of deceleration, impact force strength, and seriousness of expected injuries.

CONTENT REVIEW

➤ Events of Vehicle Collision
- Vehicle collision
- Body collision
- Organ collision
- Secondary collisions
- Additional impacts

3. *Organ collisions.* Organ collision results as an occupant contacts the vehicle's interior and/or restraints and slows or stops. Tissues behind the contacting surface of the occupant's body collide, one into another, as the body comes to a stop. This can cause compression, stretch, and shear injuries as tissues and organs press violently against each other. In this process, organs may also twist or decelerate, tearing at their attachments or at blood vessels. The result is blunt trauma.

4. *Secondary collisions.* Secondary collisions occur when the occupant is struck by loose objects within the vehicle. During the collision, objects within the vehicle, including unrestrained passengers, continue to travel at the vehicle's initial speed. They can then strike the occupant, who has come to rest (or whose speed is slowing) within the auto. It is important to consider the possibility of any secondary collisions and their effects on occupants when developing an index of suspicion for injuries.[5]

5. *Additional impacts.* Additional impacts may occur when a vehicle undergoes a second impact, such as striking another vehicle or a light pole. This second impact may cause additional injuries or increase the seriousness of those already received. For example, consider someone who has sustained a femur fracture. It initially takes a great deal of energy to break the bone. However, once the bone is broken, the energy needed to move those bone ends and cause additional injury to adjoining nerves and blood vessels is much less. It is important to always consider what effect any additional impacts may have on the initial injuries and overall patient condition.

Restraints

Restraints such as seat belts (lap belts and shoulder straps), air bags, and child safety seats have a significant effect in minimizing the injuries associated with auto collisions. They have played a substantial role in reducing collision-related deaths over the past several decades. When approaching a collision scene, try to determine whether the occupants were using restraints (and used them properly) when determining possible injuries.

EMS providers should recognize the value of seat belt use. All personnel must employ seat belts when driving and while in the patient care area of the vehicle. Securing the lap belt firmly provides positive positioning so drivers and other crew members are not as adversely affected by the gravitational-equivalent forces (G forces) sometimes associated with emergency driving.

SEAT BELTS   Lap belt and shoulder strap use prevents the wearer's continuing movement during a vehicle collision. A belted occupant slows with the auto rather than moving rapidly forward and suddenly impacting the stopped or dramatically slowed interior. An occupant's ultimate deceleration rate is thus reduced, lessening the likelihood of serious injury from collisions within the vehicle. Lap belts and shoulder straps also lessen the chances that the wearer will be ejected from the vehicle.

Although lap belts and shoulder straps significantly reduce injury severity, their improper use may cause some, although usually much less serious, injuries. They must be used together. A lap belt worn alone does not restrain the chest, neck, or head from continuing forward. These body regions may impact the dashboard, steering wheel, or air bag, resulting in chest, neck, and head injuries. Sudden body folding at the waist during extreme impacts when only a lap belt is worn may result in intraabdominal or lower spine injuries. If the lap belt is worn too high, abdominal compression and spinal (T12 to L2) fractures may result. If worn too low, it may cause hip dislocations. When used with the lap belt, the shoulder strap restrains the chest and prevents the body from folding at the waist. If the shoulder strap is worn alone, it may cause severe neck contusions, lacerations, possible spinal injury, and even decapitation in more violent collisions.

When both lap and shoulder belts are worn properly, injury may still occur. In very strong impacts, the shoulder strap may cause chest contusions and, in some cases, rib, sternum, and clavicle fractures. Seat belts do not restrict head and neck movement. In rapid deceleration, the head's weight may cause the neck to flex well beyond its normal range of motion, possibly causing connective tissue (ligament) and vertebral injury. The lap belt and shoulder strap do not protect against intrusions into the passenger compartment. In severe collisions, the dashboard may displace into the front seat, crushing and/or trapping an occupant's lower extremities.

SUPPLEMENTAL RESTRAINT SYSTEMS (SRS)   Supplemental restraint systems (SRS) (also called air bags) work much differently than seat belts and are extremely effective for frontal collisions. They inflate explosively on auto impact, filling a fabric container with gas just prior to occupant impact. This produces a cushion to absorb the energy exchange of rapid deceleration. SRS ignition depends on several detectors sensing a very strong frontal deceleration, as can occur only with serious vehicle impact. Only after these detectors all agree does the explosive agent ignite. Ignition instantaneously fills the bag with gas, slightly before or just as the occupant collides with it. Explosive gases escape quickly as the occupant compresses the bag, cushioning impact much like the inflated bags used by pole-vaulters and movie stunt performers. Like seat belts, supplemental restraint systems are credited with dramatically reducing vehicular trauma and death.

Supplemental restraint systems are positioned in the steering wheel. If present in a vehicle, there will be a "SRS" insignia on the windshield and/or on the steering wheel. Air bags are also located in the dashboard for the front seat passenger. Most SRS systems permit deactivation of the passenger SRS units to accommodate children or will deactivate the air bag when passenger weight is not detected. Steering wheel and dash-mounted supplemental restraint systems offer significant protection only in frontal impact collisions. This protection is only for the first impact, and not for subsequent ones.

Supplemental restraint systems may cause injury during ignition and rapid inflation, especially if seat belts are not properly used. As the bag inflates, especially from the steering wheel, it may impact the driver's fingers, hands, and forearms, possibly causing dislocations and fractures. Air bag inflation may also cause nasal fractures, minor facial lacerations, and contusions in persons of small stature seated very close to the steering wheel (less than 12 inches), or dashboard (less than 18 inches). Watch for small-stature occupants wearing glasses, because the air bag inflation may cause orbital or eye injuries as the glasses break and are forced into the face and eyes. The residue from SRS inflation may cause some irritation of the eyes. This can usually be relieved with gentle irrigation. Whenever a supplemental restraint system has deployed, check beneath it for steering wheel or dashboard deformity, which is indicative of extreme impact forces and more likely injury to the driver or passenger.

Children secured in safety seats and placed in the front seat may sustain serious injury with air bag inflation. Passenger air bags have inflated in minor impacts and pushed infant and child safety seats into the seat back with tremendous force. In some cases, infants and children have been severely injured or killed by air bag inflation. For this reason, it is essential that parents secure child safety seats in the backseat when a passenger SRS is in place (and is not disabled).

Auto manufacturers are installing supplemental restraint systems in the headliners and seat sides, adjacent to the doors, for protection in lateral impact collisions. Lateral impacts account for a very high mortality rate that may be mitigated with lateral-impact and head-protection SRS.

Undeployed air bags may present a hazard at the auto crash scene. Their unexpected inflation may cause serious injury to the patient or rescuer. Fire, rescue, and extrication personnel should be trained in SRS deactivation and should deactivate any undeployed devices at the crash scene.

CHILD SAFETY SEATS   Children's anatomy makes their protection in vehicle collisions difficult. Normal restraint systems are designed for adults and not for children because a child's size changes so quickly with increasing age. Small children should be placed in appropriate child safety seats to ensure their relative safety during an auto impact. For infants and very small children (up to two years of age), the child safety seat is positioned in the rear seating area, facing backward and held firmly to the seat with the lap belt or lower anchors and tethers for children (LATCH) child restraint anchoring system. This positioning best distributes frontal impact forces and prevents unrestrained infant movement. As a child grows in size, the child safety seat is turned facing forward and used as a small seat. The lap belt then crosses the child at the waistline with a four-point restraint system holding the child firmly in the seat.

Children held in an adult's lap or arms are *not* protected during a collision. The holder may grasp the child too tightly during impact or, more likely, will not (or cannot) hold on tightly enough. If not held, the child becomes an unrestrained moving object and impacts the vehicle interior, suffering serious, possibly fatal, injury.

HEAD RESTS   Head rests are designed to prevent unopposed rearward motion of the head during a rear-end collision. As a slowing or stopped vehicle is rapidly pushed forward, the torso moves forward with the auto seat. If there is no head rest or the head rest is pushed down, inertia causes the occupant's head to remain still, effectively flinging the head back (extended) in relation to the torso. If the head rest is up, however, it causes the head to move with the seat and the rest of the body. This prevents the violent backward head rotation and neck extension. A properly positioned head rest significantly reduces the incidence of injury to the spinal column, neck ligament, and neck muscles (often called "whiplash" injury). In rear-end collisions, always check the head rest position and its relationship to a patient's height.

When evaluating auto impact results, be sure to look for and inquire about restraint use. Determine whether lap belts and shoulder straps were used and used properly, if any SRS deployed during the collision, if child car seats were properly positioned and secured, and if head rests were in the up position. Properly employed restraints will likely reduce the severity of vehicle occupant injury.

PASSENGER COMPARTMENT INTRUSION   Passenger compartment intrusion occurs when collision forces push through the vehicle's structure into the passenger compartment. Intrusion suggests that increased kinetic forces may have reached the patient, thus increasing the likelihood of serious injury. Passenger compartment intrusion associated with lateral impact is frequent because the associated crumple zone (within the vehicle door) is very limited. Lateral impact is also associated with a very high occupant mortality rate.

Types of Impact

There are five general types of auto impacts:

- Frontal (most common)
- Lateral
- Oblique
- Rear-end
- Rollover[5]

FRONTAL IMPACT Frontal impact is the most common type of impact (Figure 2-4) and produces four pathways of patient travel:

1. *Restrained pathway.* Use of lap belts and shoulder straps restrains movement of the occupants and causes them to decelerate with the vehicle. This limits any interior impact and the energy associated with it. As noted earlier, there may be injury associated with improper lap belt placement (intraabdominal injury, lumbar spine injury, and hip dislocation) and with the shoulder belt (contusions and possible rib fractures). These injuries are far less serious than those expected without restraint use. Supplemental restraint system deployment, likewise, reduces the impact forces and resultant injuries, although they may induce minor hand, arm, and facial injuries.

2. *Up-and-over pathway.* In the up-and-over pathway, the unrestrained occupant tenses his legs in preparation for the collision. With the vehicle slowing, the unrestrained body's upper half pivots forward and upward. The steering wheel impinges the femurs, possibly causing bilateral fractures. In addition, the steering wheel compresses and decelerates the abdominal contents, causing hollow-organ rupture and liver laceration. Traumatic compression may also force abdominal contents against the diaphragm, causing it to rupture and allowing organs to enter the thoracic cavity. As the body continues forward, the lower chest impacts the upper steering wheel and may account for the same thoracic injuries seen with the down-and-under pathway (see the discussion that follows). Deployment of supplemental restraint systems will mitigate deceleration associated with steering wheel impact and significantly reduce the expected injuries.

The same forward motion propels the head into the windshield, leading to head injury. Neck injury may result from hyperextension, hyperflexion, or the compression forces of windshield impact. As the body is thrown upward and forward, the head contacts the windshield. The weight and inertia of the rest of the body tries to push the head through the windshield. The result is a compression force on the cervical spine called **axial loading**. This loading may result in injury to the vertebral column and supporting structures. A large proportion of vehicular deaths in unrestrained occupants are attributed to the up-and-over pathway.

3. *Down-and-under pathway.* In the down-and-under pathway, the unrestrained occupant slides downward as the vehicle comes to a stop. The knees contact the firewall under the dashboard and absorb the initial impact. Knee, femur, and hip dislocations or fractures are common. Once the lower body slows, the upper body rotates forward, pivoting at the hip, and crashing against the steering wheel or dash. This resembles the up-and-over pathway, although the points of contact are higher up on the adult anatomy. Chest injuries such as flail chest, blunt cardiac injury, and aortic tears can result. If the neck contacts the steering wheel, tracheal and vascular injury may occur. An injury process frequently associated with chest-versus-steering-wheel impact is the "paper bag" syndrome. The driver takes a deep breath when anticipating impact. Then, he involuntarily closes his glottis. The resulting impact with the steering wheel compresses the chest and drastically increases pressure within the chest, airway, and alveoli. Lung tissues (alveoli, bronchioles, and larger airways) can rupture, much like an inflated paper bag caught between clapping hands. Pneumothorax and pulmonary contusion may result.

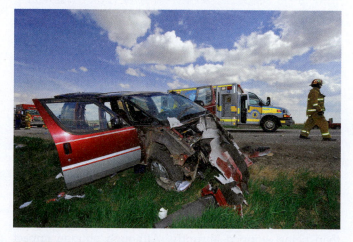

FIGURE 2-4 Frontal impact often results in a significant exchange of energy and serious injuries.

(© Kevin Link/Science Source)

4. *Ejection.* The up-and-over pathway may lead to ejection of an unrestrained occupant. Such a victim experiences two impacts: (1) contact with the vehicle interior and windshield and (2) impact with the ground, tree, or other object. Ejection deprives the occupant of the protections offered by the vehicle design and supplemental restraint systems. This mechanism of injury is responsible for about 27 percent of vehicular fatalities. Although ejection may occur with other types of impact, it is most commonly associated with frontal impact and the unrestrained vehicle occupant.

Recognize that a frontal impact collision interposes more vehicle structure between the point of impact and the passenger compartment. Modern vehicle design uses this region of the vehicle (called the **crumple zone**) to absorb impact forces, making collapse of vehicle structures more gradual, reducing forces transferred to the occupants and thus limiting occupant injury. Supplemental restraint systems also perform best in frontal impact collisions. Air bags have a greater space to fill between the vehicle interior (steering wheel and dash) and the occupants when compared to the space that exists between side doors and the occupants in lateral impacts. Patients in vehicle collisions involving some older vans do not benefit from these energy-absorbing crumple zones. In these circumstances, the apparent vehicle damage may more accurately reflect the forces delivered to the occupants and occupant injuries than in a frontal impact collision.

LATERAL IMPACT   The kinetics of lateral impact are the same as for frontal impact, with two exceptions. First, occupants present a different profile (turned 90 degrees) to the collision forces. Second, as already noted, the physical space and amount of structural steel between the impact site and the vehicle interior (the crumple zone) is greatly reduced (Figure 2-5). The reduced crumple zone results in

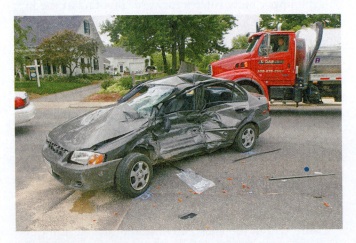

FIGURE 2-5 A lateral impact collision presents the least amount of crumple zone between the vehicle's exterior and its passenger compartment.

(© Mark C. Ide/Science Source)

a greater likelihood of intrusion into the passenger compartment. Lateral impacts account for only one-quarter of all auto collisions, yet they are responsible for a higher percentage of vehicular fatalities. When a lateral impact occurs, the index of suspicion for serious and life-threatening internal injuries must be higher than vehicle damage alone might suggest.

With lateral impacts, there is an increase in upper and lower extremity injuries. The clavicle, humerus, pelvis, and femur may fracture on the impact side. Rib fractures can occur laterally on the impact side instead of anteriorly. Cervical spine injury can occur as the body is pushed laterally (away from impact by the bending vehicle door) while the head remains stationary. Note that the head's center of mass is forward of the cervical spine. As the chest is pushed sideways by the vehicle door, the head turns rapidly toward the impact. Vertebral fractures may occur with the rapid lateral and twisting motion. The head may strike the window. Lateral compression, affecting the torso, may cause diaphragmatic rupture, pulmonary contusions, splenic injury (to the driver), liver injury (to the passenger), and much more. Injury to the aorta may occur with lateral impact as well. The heart, which is not firmly attached in the mediastinum, can move violently toward the impact as the body accelerates away from it. This twists the aorta, tearing its inner layer, the intima. Blood seeps between the connective tissue layers and the vessel begins to delaminate (dissect). The dissecting aorta may rupture immediately or over the next few hours.

Evaluation of lateral impact collisions should take into consideration any unrestrained passenger opposite the impact site. If the driver's side is struck and the passenger is not belted, the passenger becomes an object, causing secondary collision to the driver shortly after initial impact.

As noted earlier, lateral impact collisions often displace vehicle structure inwardly. This intrusion is suggestive of greater forces directed to the passenger compartment and a greater likelihood of serious injury. Lateral impact may also result in ejection through the side windows.

OBLIQUE IMPACT   In **oblique** impact, the auto is struck at an angle rather than directly to the front, side, or rear (Figure 2-6). Oblique impact includes four subcategories: left front, right front, left rear, and right rear. The vehicle profile that contacts the impact forces can create a combination of lateral and either frontal or rear-end injury types. If the impact forces are not directed to a vehicle's center of mass, the impact will cause rotation. With rotation, acceleration (or deceleration) is greatest farther from the auto's center and closest to impact. With these collisions, the vehicle may be deflected from the path of travel rather than being stopped abruptly. Although oblique impact injuries can be serious, they are frequently less so than the vehicle damage might suggest. With impact deflection,

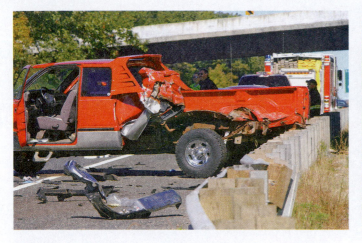

FIGURE 2-6 In oblique impacts, the energy exchange is more gradual and there may be less injury than vehicle damage suggests. There may, however, be multiple impacts.

(© Mark C. Ide/Science Source)

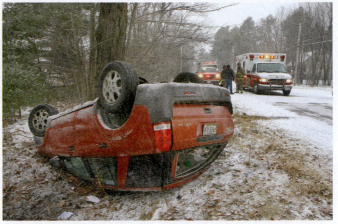

FIGURE 2-8 Rollover crashes result in multiple impacts and, possibly, multiple injury mechanisms.

(© Daniel Limmer)

the occupant's stopping distance is usually much greater, deceleration is more gradual, and injuries are generally less serious.

Note that rotation can occur with any collision type, though it is more commonly associated with oblique impact.

REAR-END IMPACT   In rear-end impact, the collision force pushes the auto forward (Figure 2-7). Within the vehicle, the energy of the collision propels the occupant forward. As discussed earlier, if the head rest is not up, the head is unsupported and remains stationary, possibly causing cervical spine injury. Once acceleration slows, the head snaps forward and the neck flexes. This rapid and extreme hyperextension followed by hyperflexion may result in severe connective tissue and cervical spine injuries. There is also an injury risk when the auto finally stops moving and an unrestrained occupant is thrown forward. However, rear-impact collisions usually result

in limited injuries, especially if the head rest is positioned properly.

ROLLOVER   Auto rollover is normally caused by a change in elevation and/or affects a vehicle with a high center of gravity (such as a sport utility vehicle) (Figure 2-8). As the vehicle rolls, it impacts the ground at various points, and the occupant experiences a collision with each vehicle impact. These collisions can be especially violent because of limited crumple zones (such as the vehicle roof) and the lack of supplemental restraint systems and internal padding at some of the impact points. The types of injuries expected with a rollover relate to the specific vehicle impacts involved. Remember, any injury occurring with the first collision is likely to be compounded with subsequent collisions or impacts. A common rollover result is ejection or partial ejection with a limb, torso, or head trapped between the rolling vehicle and the ground—especially for unrestrained occupants. Mortality increases significantly when occupant ejection occurs. Thus, seat belts are especially effective in reducing ejection and injury during rollover.

Vehicle Collision Analysis

Vehicle collisions often produce hazards not only to the vehicle occupants, but also to bystanders and care providers. Be alert for these hazards during the scene size-up. Such hazards may include hot engine, exhaust, and transmission parts; hot fluids, such as radiator coolant or engine oil; caustic substances, such as battery acid and automatic transmission or power steering fluids; and the sharp, jagged edges of torn metal and broken glass. Spilled fluids, such as motor oil and gasoline, may provide a slippery surface or fire danger as well. Also remain aware of dangers from traffic moving near the crash site or from downed electrical power lines. Finally, survey the scene to evaluate

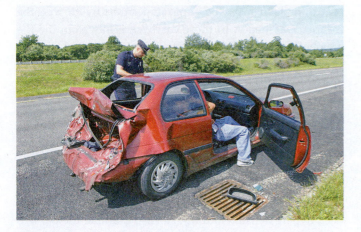

FIGURE 2-7 In rear-end impacts, there is generally good protection for the body, except for the head and neck.

(© Mark C. Ide/Science Source)

the terrain. Consider whether it is uneven or slippery and whether this will have any impact on patient access and movement. Ensure that the scene is safe before attempting rescuer entry. It is not good enough to simply observe for scene hazards at a vehicle crash site. You must rule them out.

Hybrid vehicles are becoming more popular and more common. These special vehicles supplement their normal gasoline or diesel propulsion system with an electric generation, storage, and drive system. These vehicles pose two additional hazards to EMS personnel beyond what would be suspected with a standard automobile. The electrical propulsion system uses direct current at somewhere between 36 and 550 volts and carries a danger of electrocution. This danger is relatively limited, though, because the high-voltage components are well protected, and direct current tends to flow from one battery post to the other, rather than seeking ground.

The second additional hazard posed by hybrid vehicles is unexpected movement. The electrical propulsion system may engage when the vehicle does not appear to be running. The driver's foot may depress the accelerator or may be withdrawn from the brake during assessment or care. If the ignition is on, this may cause the hybrid to accelerate. This danger can be eliminated if the ignition key is removed (or a proximity-ignition fob is moved more than 16 feet from the steering column). Ensure that fire service or other properly trained rescue personnel disable the drive system of a hybrid vehicle.[6]

During the scene size-up, evaluate the vehicle to determine the direction of impact and the amount of vehicle damage. Based on vehicle damage, visualize the direction of forces expressed on vehicle occupants and the strength of those forces. Recognize that the front and rear structures of modern autos are designed to crumple and absorb kinetic forces during impact. Although moderate-speed impacts may severely damage the vehicle, the occupants may escape with little injury. Occupants in lateral and roll-over impacts do not benefit from such crumple zones and frequently suffer injuries more directly related to the vehicle damage and the kinetic forces the damage suggests.

When evaluating a collision, consider the relative sizes (weight) of involved vehicles or objects. A large, heavy vehicle impacting a smaller, lighter one will experience lesser acceleration or deceleration forces than the smaller vehicle. There is likely to be more severe vehicle damage to the smaller vehicle and more serious injuries to its occupants. Similar considerations apply with objects impacted by vehicles. For example, a large, well-rooted tree that does not move will cause much more damage during an impact than will a fence post that shears off.

After examining a vehicle's exterior, look at the passenger compartment (Figure 2-9). Determine whether there is any passenger compartment intrusion, which indicates

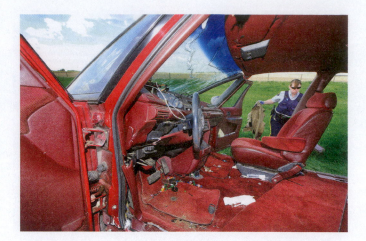

FIGURE 2-9 Study the interior of a crashed vehicle carefully to identify the strength and direction of forces expressed to the patient.
(© Kevin Link/Science Source)

the presence of forces greater than those that could be absorbed by the crumple zones. Quickly look for signs of passenger–interior impacts. A spider-webbed windshield suggests a severe impact between the occupant's head and the glass. Note, however, that spider-webbing sometimes indicates window frame alteration during impact rather than occupant contact. A deformed steering wheel (including deformity under a deflated air bag) suggests injury to the driver's chest or upper abdomen. A dented dash suggests knee injury or forces transmitted to the femur or hip. Deformities of the accelerator, brake, or clutch pedals suggest foot injury. A deployed and deflated SRS may indicate facial, chest, forearm, or hand injury.

In very severe collisions, the resultant forces may push the dashboard and firewall into the passenger compartment, trapping and crushing the lower extremities against the seat. In such cases, parts of the vehicle, such as foot pedals, turn indicator arms, shift levers, and instrument panel knobs or switches may be physically embedded in the victim. This complicates extrication because the seat and dash must be separated carefully to free the trapped passenger. In these cases, carefully examine the area before and while any extrication equipment is used. Frequently reassess the patient during extrication to ensure that the process does not result in unnecessary harm to the patient.

Assess whether restraints were used or supplemental restraint systems were used and deployed. Use of these devices may limit the injury severity in frontal impacts. Conversely, their nonuse or failure to deploy may suggest more severe injuries. Check the positions of head rests in rear-impact collisions. Their proper positioning may limit neck hyperextension and injury. Also examine the passenger compartment interior for intrusion. Any intrusion suggests stronger forces of impact and failure of the crumple zones to protect the occupants.

IMPAIRMENT When evaluating motor vehicle trauma, consider the possibility of alcohol or drug intoxication or impairment. Statistics obtained from states that require mandatory postcollision alcohol and drug testing after fatal auto collisions reveal that more than half of the involved drivers were intoxicated. Substance use also contributes to many off-road-vehicle collisions, all-terrain vehicle collisions, boating collisions, snowmobile collisions, and drownings.

Whenever alcohol or other intoxication or impairment is suspected, assessment and examination must be even more diligent than usual. Remember, alcohol and other substances reduce the patient's reaction time and alertness, and may mask signs and symptoms of injury. Intoxication may be hard to differentiate from signs of head injury. It also anesthetizes the patient somewhat to trauma pain. These factors make the mechanism of injury analysis and the resultant index of suspicion even more important. Otherwise, significant injuries may be overlooked or assumed to be due to alcohol intoxication.

When examining the collision scene, try to mentally visualize the events surrounding the collision. Is there evidence of the driver trying to stop before or to avoid the impact? If not, might the impact have been due to distraction, falling asleep,[7] a medical condition such as heart attack or stroke, or the possibility of suicide? Compare your mental re-creation of the collision to the patient's description of what occurred to try to assess the patient's recall of the incident and thus the reliability of the information he provides.

VEHICULAR MORTALITY Careful analysis of motor vehicle trauma reveals that certain body regions are especially prone to life-threatening injury. A study of the incidence of mortality and the associated location of trauma provides the findings in Table 2–3.

Blunt trauma to the head and body cavity accounts for 85 percent of vehicular-related mortality. For this reason, following the primary assessment and attention to the airway, breathing, and circulation, the rapid trauma assessment should emphasize evaluation of the head, neck, thorax, abdomen, and pelvis. Look carefully at areas where the index of suspicion suggests injury. Examine the head, neck, chest, abdomen, and pelvis first to identify any evidence of life-threatening injuries.

COLLISION EVALUATION Paramedics must be proficient in trauma patient assessment, especially because of the high incidence of serious injury associated with auto collisions. Whenever responding to a motor vehicle collision, analyze the five types of collisions associated with vehicle impact. In each case, consider these questions:

- How did the objects collide?
- From what direction did they come?
- At what speed were they traveling?
- Were the objects similarly sized or grossly different? (For example, did a car and a semi-truck collide?)
- Were any secondary collisions or additional transfers of energy involved?

In analyzing the mechanisms of injury, also consider the cause of the collision.

- Did wet pavement or poor visibility contribute to the collision?
- Were alcohol or other drugs involved?
- Is there an absence of skid marks? If so, what happened to prevent the driver from braking?

Examine the vehicle interior, which is the region most likely struck by the moving occupant.

- Does the windshield show evidence of impact by the victim's head?
  - Is it bloody or broken in the characteristic spider web or star shape?
  - Did the patient's head penetrate the glass?
- Is the steering wheel deformed or collapsed?
- Is the dashboard indented from passenger contact?
- Is there significant passenger compartment intrusion?
- Were seat and shoulder belts worn? Did any SRS deploy? Was the head rest up?

Answers to such questions can complement the mechanism of injury analysis and help to develop accurate indices of suspicion.

Motorcycle Collisions

In addition to auto collisions, paramedics frequently respond to motorcycle collisions. Because motorcycles lack a protective vehicle structure, motorcycle collisions often result in serious trauma—even at lower speeds. The rider, rather than structural steel, tends to absorb much of the crash energy (Figure 2-10). Injuries from motorcycle collisions can be severe, with a high incidence of head trauma.

Table 2-3 Motor Vehicle Fatalities

Incidence by Body Area	
Head	47.7%
Internal (chest/abdominal/pelvic)	37.3%
Spinal and chest fracture	8.3%
Fractures to the extremities	2.0%
All other	4.7%

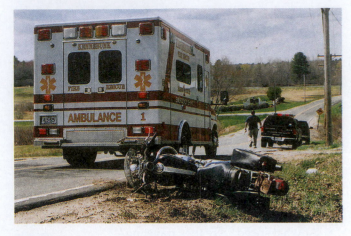

FIGURE 2-10 Motorcycle crashes result in serious trauma because the cycle provides little protection for its rider.

(© Daniel Limmer)

The types of motorcycle impacts differ somewhat from those of an auto collision. The four major types of motorcycle impacts are frontal, angular, sliding, and ejection.

FRONTAL In a frontal, or head-on, impact, the bike front dips downward, propelling the rider upward and forward. The handlebars can catch the rider's lower abdomen or pelvis, causing abdominal and/or pelvic injury. Occasionally, the rider travels through a higher trajectory. In such cases, the handlebars can trap the legs, often resulting in fractures. Frontal impact often results in rider ejection.

ANGULAR An angular impact occurs when the bike strikes an object at an oblique angle. The rider's lower extremity is often trapped between the object struck and the bike. This may fracture or crush the foot, leg, or thigh. Open wounds often result.

SLIDING Sliding impact occurs when an experienced rider, facing an imminent collision, "lays the bike down." The rider will slide the bike sideways into the object so that the bike hits the object first, absorbing much of the energy. Laying the bike down also reduces the chances of ejection. However, there is a resultant increase in lacerations, abrasions, and minor fractures, with a decrease in more serious injuries.

EJECTION Ejection is common and usually results in serious injury. It may occur with any of the mechanisms previously described, and results in the following impacts:

- Initial bike/object collision
- Rider/object impact
- Rider/ground impact

Likely injuries include head injury, spinal injuries, internal injuries, and extremity fractures.

Protective equipment plays a significant role in motorcycle crashes and affects injury patterns. Helmets reduce head injury incidence and severity in many cases. Helmet use, however, neither increases nor decreases the incidence or severity of spinal trauma. Leather clothing and boots protect the rider against open soft-tissue injury, but they can also hide underlying contusions, fractures, and internal injuries.[8]

Pedestrian Collisions

Pedestrians who are struck by autos are often severely injured because of their lack of protection and because of the vehicle's mass and speed. Adults and children suffer different injuries because of differing anatomic size and differing responses to an impending collision. Recognizing these differences helps to anticipate pedestrian injuries and better provide the needed care.

Most auto–pedestrian collisions injure the pedestrian's lower extremities. With a standard-sized vehicle, the bumper will usually strike the leg first—often the tibia, the fibula, or both. Knee injuries are also common. Further vehicle impact forces the lower extremities forward, causing the upper body to crash into the hood. This collision is likely to produce multiple injuries.

With the increasing popularity of sport utility vehicles and large pickup trucks, pedestrian injury patterns are changing. Pedestrian contact with these vehicles tends to be anatomically higher on the body (e.g., thigh, pelvis, abdomen) because the bumper and hood are higher from the ground. Examine the front of the vehicle to help determine what part or parts probably struck the patient. This will aid in determining likely resulting injuries.

Children and adults of short stature may fall below the vehicle when struck and may be run over by the vehicle. In this group, injuries may be higher on the body (e.g., abdomen, chest, head). Some, because of their size and low center of gravity, may be struck and thrown away from the vehicle, causing secondary injury as they contact the pavement or other items on scene. If a child is thrown upward and onto the hood and windshield, the injury patterns are similar to those of an adult.

When evaluating injuries associated with an auto-versus-pedestrian collision, look carefully at the scene. Try to determine the vehicle's speed at impact and the distance the pedestrian was thrown, if any. This information will be useful to emergency department personnel as they look for injuries and determine injury severity.

Off-Road Vehicle Collisions

Off-road vehicle use has increased and so has the incidence of related trauma. Off-road vehicle collisions often cause injuries similar to those associated with auto collisions.

However, most off-road vehicles afford the operator and passengers considerably less protection than automobiles and trucks. In addition, because they travel off-road, an emergency response can be complicated by delays in detecting the incident and, often, difficulty in reaching and retrieving victims. The major vehicle types most often involved in off-road vehicle collisions are snowmobiles, watercraft, and all-terrain vehicles (ATVs).

Snowmobile collisions can be very violent because their speeds can approach those of autos. In addition, snowmobiles offer very limited crumple zones for impact absorption. These collisions commonly result in passenger ejection and crush injuries secondary to roll-over, as well as glancing blows against obstructions in the snow. Riders can also experience severe head and neck injuries from collisions with other vehicles, including autos, other snowmobiles, or stationary objects such as trees. Snowmobile trauma sometimes includes severe neck injury when the rider runs into an unseen wire fence. The anterior neck can be deeply lacerated, possibly causing airway compromise, severe bleeding, and, in some cases, complete decapitation. Injuries to snowmobilers are frequently compounded by cold exposure and hypothermia.

Watercraft crashes commonly result from impact with other boats or obstructions, submerged or otherwise (Figure 2-11). Watercraft are not designed to absorb significant impact energy, nor are occupants typically provided with restraint systems. As a result, watercraft crashes can cause serious injuries, even though typical watercraft speeds are substantially lower than those of autos. Trauma in these crashes is further complicated by the potential for drowning if the occupants are thrown into the water or the boat sinks. In northern waters, temperatures can also rapidly cause hypothermia. (Water draws heat from the body about 20 times faster than air does.)

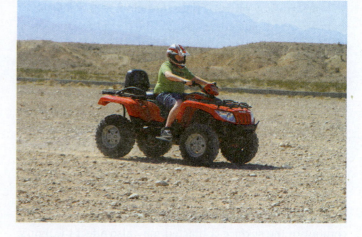

FIGURE 2-12 All-terrain vehicles (ATVs) can cause a multitude of injuries due to their speed and instability and lack of rider protection. *(© Dr. Bryan E. Bledsoe)*

The use of personal watercraft (commonly called jet skis) has increased greatly in recent years, as has the incidence of personal watercraft collisions. Jet skis are especially dangerous in the hands of inexperienced riders. The high speeds attained by jet skis often contribute to the incidence and severity of injury from crashes. Although the craft's propulsion unit is shrouded and unlikely to cause injury by itself, collision with other watercraft, as well as with objects and people in the water, can lead to blunt trauma. Drowning and hypothermia are added risks associated with personal watercraft use. Many states now require operators and passengers to wear personal flotation devices, and jet ski users often wear specialized clothing (wet suits) to protect against heat loss and hypothermia in cold water.

The all-terrain vehicle (Figure 2-12) accounts for many serious recreational injuries. In many instances, the drivers are young and, in most states, are not required to prove their driving skills or to maintain a license. The vehicle, by its very nature, travels at relatively high speeds over rough and rugged terrain. The ATV's center of gravity is relatively high, thus contributing to the likelihood of rollover during quick turns. As with snowmobiles, ATVs have a significant incidence of frontal collision. The injuries expected might include upper and lower extremity fractures, as well as head and spine injury. As with motorcycle collisions, helmet use does not protect against spine injury but can reduce the incidence of head injury.

Falls

Falls are the most common mechanism of blunt trauma, yet they result in life-threatening injury only infrequently. Those most at risk for a fall injury are the very young and the elderly. As the older population increases, the incidence of fall injuries is likely also to rise.

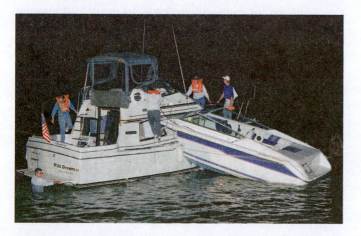

FIGURE 2-11 Watercraft crashes are common, may involve either objects on the surface or submerged, and present the risks of drowning or hypothermia.

(© Craig Jackson/In the Dark Photography)

In terms of physics, falls are simply the release of stored gravitational energy. As the height of a fall increases, so do the velocity and kinetic energy at impact and the associated energy exchange and resultant trauma. Newton's second law illustrates that the more rapid the deceleration (the shorter the stopping distance), the greater the force and resulting injury. Thus, as with auto impacts, the stopping distance may be more important than the height of the fall. A person may dive pleasurably from a 12-foot platform into deep water, which allows the body to decelerate slowly. However, a fall from a second-story window, a similar height, onto a concrete sidewalk with a virtually zero stopping distance may produce serious injury. The contour of the surface contacted may also affect the injury. An irregular surface, such as building rubble or a stairway, may increase injury severity at some body locations while sparing others.

Trauma resulting from a fall depends on the contact area and the pathway of energy transmission. For example, if a person lands feet first, energy is transmitted up the skeletal structure from the calcaneus to the leg, thigh and eventually the lumbar spine (Figure 2-13). Fractures along this skeletal pathway are common. The lumbar spine is especially prone to compression injury because it is the only skeletal component supporting the entire upper body. After the initial impact, the person may fall forward or backward. In forward falls, the victim may attempt to break the impact with an outstretched arm, resulting in wrist, shoulder, and clavicle fractures. Pelvic, thoracic, and head injury may result from a backward fall. In some cases, consequences of a fall will progress from the original straight impact.

The initial impact of a fall may involve other body surfaces with the deceleration forces transmitted from the contact point toward the body's center of mass. In diving injuries, when the patient's head strikes a lake or pool bottom, the rest of the body compresses the cervical spine between the head and shoulders. This axial loading can crush the vertebral bodies, injure the spinal cord, and paralyze the patient. This may result from even a very shallow dive, as from poolside or from within the water.

If a victim falls on an outstretched arm, the impact energy is transmitted along the skeletal system from the hand and wrist to the forearm, elbow, arm, and shoulder (metacarpals, radius and ulna, humerus, scapula and clavicle). The clavicle is often fractured in these types of impacts because it is the smallest weight-bearing bone along the transmission pathway. With collapse of the upper extremities, the head, neck, and shoulders may collide with the surface, experiencing energy exchange and injury.

In severe falls, when a person has dropped more than three times his height (20 feet for the adult, 10 feet for the small child), focus attention on potential internal injuries. Rapid deceleration can cause organs to be compressed, displaced, and twisted. The heart, for example, is held in the center of the thorax by the aorta, venae cavae, and *ligamentum arteriosum*. When a victim falling from a significant height contacts the ground, the heart is pulled downward with such force that it may tear away from its aortic attachments, possibly leading to immediate **exsanguination** (a draining of blood severe enough to cause death).

In evaluating the victim of a fall, try to determine the fall height, the anatomic point of impact, the suspected force of that impact, the nature of the impact surface, and a possible transmission pathway of forces along the skeleton. Then, try to anticipate possible fractures and internal injuries. During the physical assessment, pay particular attention to areas where you have determined that injuries are likely to be located.

Falls are a common injury mechanism for older patients. Body coordination decreases with age. In addition, failing eyesight and depth perception (often due to cataracts) and weakening muscle and bone strength increase the chances of a fall. The force required to break bones is often much less in geriatric patients than in younger ones. A brittle bone, like a femur, may actually break during ordinary activities such as walking down a step, resulting in a fall. In such a case the fracture causes the fall rather than the fall causing the fracture. Always try to assess the circumstances surrounding a fall—including the possibility of a medical condition (e.g., syncope) having caused the fall. Provide appropriate immobilization

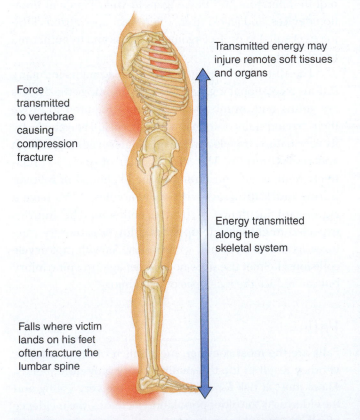

Transmitted energy may injure remote soft tissues and organs

Force transmitted to vertebrae causing compression fracture

Energy transmitted along the skeletal system

Falls where victim lands on his feet often fracture the lumbar spine

FIGURE 2-13 In falls, energy is transmitted along the skeletal system.

and gentle transport for these patients and ensure that they are comforted and reassured.

Blast Injuries

An *explosion* is a rapid increase in volume and release of energy in an extreme manner. It is often associated with the generation of high temperatures and the release of gases. Explosions can be caused by dust, as in a grain elevator; by fumes, such as from gasoline, propane, or natural gas; or by explosive compounds (combustible and **oxidizer** mixes), such as dynamite, gunpowder, and TNT. An explosion may be the result of an accidental act or an intentional one, as from terrorism or warfare. Blast magnitude may range from that of a small firecracker in the hands of a teenager to a nuclear detonation.

Explosion

An explosion occurs when an agent or environment combusts. During a conventional (non-nuclear) explosion, the fuel and oxidizing agent combine instantaneously. Chemical bonds are broken and reestablished, thus releasing a tremendous amount of energy in the form of rapidly moving molecules—better known as heat. This heat creates a great pressure differential between the exploding agent and the surrounding air. This extreme heat, and the pressure differential it produces, can create several mechanisms of injury.[9] These include a pressure wave, blast wind, projectiles, displacement of persons near the blast, and possible associated factors such as confined-space injuries, structural collapses, and burns.

Patho Pearls

Anatomy of an Explosion. Natural gas from a ruptured pipe gathers in a basement until the explosive gas–air mixture reaches the hot-water heater's pilot light. The gas–air cloud immediately ignites, and the resulting flame instantaneously heats the air in several rooms of the house by hundreds of degrees. The heated air contains molecules that are now moving at great speed. The collision of these molecules with others greatly increases the pressure within the cloud. Contained by walls and windows, the pressure builds until the windows burst and some of the walls collapse.

The Pressure Wave. As the windows collapse and allow the pressure to push outward, the rapidly moving molecules contact those of adjacent air, setting them in motion. These molecules, in turn, contact adjacent molecules and a wave of pressure moves outward at a speed just slightly faster than that of sound. The presenting surface of a person standing in the

path of this wave is impacted and compressed, then decompressed. This wave of compression/decompression progresses through the person's body, affecting organs and tissues. Solid or fluid-filled body structures transmit the energy with very limited damage, whereas air-filled structures are compressed and then decompressed violently. The lungs, auditory canals, sinuses, and bowel sustain the most significant injury. Other victims within the structure and caught by the blast experience the same compression/decompression wave and associated injuries.

Burns. People caught within the confines of the blast are affected by the explosion's great heat. Because the heat energy is released very rapidly and because people's bodies are predominantly water, primary burn injuries are generally superficial. The blast heat often produces secondary combustion of materials such as clothing and blast debris. These ignited materials can produce burns ranging from superficial to full thickness in victims.

Projectiles. Breaking glass and parts of the collapsing walls are propelled outward with the blast energy release. These materials travel at great speed and contain great kinetic energy. As a result, these projectiles may penetrate and impale themselves in victims in their path. Unless such projectiles are heavy, they do not generally penetrate deeply.

Personnel Displacement. As the explosive gases move outward from the building, they create a blast of wind that moves more slowly than the pressure wave. The blast wind and the pressure wave push victims outward from the blast center, turning them into projectiles. The victims then impact other surfaces, objects, or debris and sustain further injuries.

Structural Collapse. As the explosion tears apart the walls of the structure, the debris and the building above collapse on victims within. Trapped by debris, the victims sustain severe crush injuries. Entrapment and compression damage tissues and blood vessels and may restrict or stop circulation to a limb. Reduced blood flow results in the buildup of toxic byproducts of metabolism. When victims are released from entrapment and circulation is restored, hemorrhage from numerous damaged blood vessels and the entry of toxins into the central circulation result.

Pressure Wave

As the combustible agent ignites and burns explosively, it instantaneously superheats the surrounding air. The molecules of of the superheated air move very, very fast, thus increasing the pressure of the expanding cloud. The rapid increase in pressure compresses adjacent air. The compressed adjacent air, in turn, pushes against air that is farther out from the ignition point. As a result, a **pressure wave** begins to move away from the epicenter of the blast. This is not a gross movement of air, like wind, but rather a narrow compression wave moving rapidly outward, similar to a wave moving through water (where the wave, not the water, moves). This thin wave, called blast **overpressure**, results in a drastic but brief increase, then decrease, in air pressure as it passes. A blast overpressure wave moves outward slightly faster than the speed of sound through air (or water), and its strength decreases quickly over time and distance.

When an explosion involves a dust, aerosol, or gas cloud, the result is an area, not a single point, of detonation (i.e., the whole cloud ignites). The pressure of the exploding cloud can be extremely lethal and can involve an extensive area. If an explosion occurs in a confined space, such as within the casing of a bomb or the interior of a building, the pressure can build until the structure ruptures. The ensuing rapid pressure release enhances the peak overpressure and the potential for injury and death.

Underwater detonation can also greatly enhance the injury and death potential associated with a pressure wave. Water is a virtually noncompressible medium that transmits an overpressure wave efficiently. Any submerged portion of the victim is subject to rapid compression and then decompression as the wave passes. The lethal range of an explosion increases threefold with underwater detonation.[10]

On striking the body, an overpressure wave instantly compresses and then decompresses the body. Solid and fluid-filled organs are not adversely affected. However, the body's air-filled spaces are subject to rapid and severe compression and decompression and will sustain serious injury. This rapid compression/decompression may produce injury to the eardrum (tympanum), middle ear, sinuses, bowel, or lungs. The overpressure wave may also cause jarring of the head and, in extreme circumstances, a traumatic brain injury. Because overpressure intensity diminishes rapidly as a wave travels outward, most life-threatening compression injuries are limited to personnel in close proximity to the detonation (with the exception, as already discussed, of gas-cloud ignitions and underwater detonations).

A victim's orientation to a blast wave is also an important consideration in injury production. The greater the victim's surface that is presented to a blast wave, the greater will be the impact and damage. Personnel who are standing and facing directly toward or away from the blast tend to experience the greatest overpressure effect. People lying on the ground, with their heads away from or toward the blast, tend to experience the least pressure effects. In water, the same is true, and, in addition, the more deeply submerged a victim is, the greater the damaging effects of overpressure.

Blast Wind

Following a pressure wave, and traveling just behind it, is the **blast wind**. This is an outward movement of heated and expanding combustion gases from the explosion epicenter. Blast wind has less strength, but greater duration, than a pressure wave. It tends to cause much less direct injury, although in powerful blasts it may propel debris or displace victims, and that, in turn, will produce injuries.

Projectiles

If an explosion is contained by a casing, as with military **ordnance** or a pipe bomb, or by a structure, as with the walls of a garage filled with gas fumes, the container holds the explosive force until the container breaks apart. Following that, the container fragments can become high-speed projectiles—behaving much like bullets and bound by the same laws of physics—although these fragments are not as fast as bullets and they lack sound aerodynamic properties. Thus, these fragments can cause serious injury well beyond the injury zone of the blast's pressure wave and blast wind.

Some military ordnance contains arrow-shaped missiles called **flechettes**. Their design gives the flechette a greater following surface and aligns the missile in flight, reducing its wind resistance, thus increasing its range and penetrating ability. Conventional explosives used by a terrorist may also contain nails, screws, ball bearings, or other materials to enhance the weapon's effective range and lethality. In past terrorist incidents, projectiles have been coated with agents to increase hemorrhage, toxins to interfere with wound healing, and, in suicide bombings, there is the danger of human tissue becoming projectiles and a source of scene and patient injury contamination.

There is also an increasing risk that a conventional explosive will be used to distribute radioactive material. This "dirty bomb" contaminates the area surrounding a blast with dangerous, but difficult to detect, energy-emitting particles (radiation). Whenever an explosion is of suspicious origin, suspect possible radioactive contamination and have the proper authorities evaluate the incident. Otherwise, do not enter the scene. Remain uphill and upwind from the scene.

If the victim is very close to a strong blast, the casing and debris may move forcefully enough to tear off limbs or cause serious open wounds. The blast debris—glass fragments, building materials, or casing elements—may also become impaled in the skin and soft tissue. Although the wounds caused by blast debris are normally small, fragments that are large and heavy can deeply penetrate into victims, causing serious tissue damage and hemorrhage.

Personnel Displacement

The overpressure wave and blast wind may be strong enough to physically propel victims away from the blast's epicenter. Those victims then become projectiles and subsequently impact the ground, nearby objects, debris, or other personnel, causing blunt or, in some cases, penetrating trauma. Although the effects of this mechanism of injury are limited when compared to those produced by overpressure or projectiles, significant injuries can result.

Confined-Space Explosions and Structural Collapses

Explosive device effects are usually limited in range because the pressure wave and debris radiate outward in all directions from a central point. This rapidly reduces overpressure and projectile concentration and, to a lesser degree, projectile velocity. When an explosion occurs in a confined space, however, the pressure wave maintains its energy longer. There is also a danger of structural collapse and of debris from the confining structure increasing the blast's projectile content. Blast overpressure can also bounce off the walls and, where reflected pressure waves meet, increase the blast overpressure. The result can be an extremely deadly overpressure event. The most lethal blasts are those that cause structural collapses, the next most lethal being those that involve confined spaces.

Structural collapse can cause severe crush injuries. The collapse may also make it difficult to locate victims and, once they are found, difficult to extricate them because of the weight of the material entrapping them. Damage to nearby structures may present further hazards to both rescuers and victims. These include the possibility of additional collapse, electrocution, fire, and/or a secondary explosion due to leaking gas or fuel.

Burns

An explosion creates tremendous heat that may cause flash burns to those very close to the detonation. These injuries are generally only superficial or partial thickness burns because of the short duration of blast energy release. However, additional burns can be caused as the blast heat ignites combustible materials such as clothing, debris, other munitions, or fuel. These secondary burns can be deep and extensive. Burn injuries can also occur in conjunction with other blast-related trauma.

Some military and terrorist devices are designed to induce damage and injury through combustion. Napalm, for example, is a highly **incendiary**, jellylike substance that clings to victims or structures when spread by a blast. Other ordnance types use materials, such as phosphorus, that spontaneously combust when exposed to air. Such agents can produce severe or fatal full-thickness burns. These burns may occur at a distance from the epicenter.

Blast Injury Types

Injuries produced by explosions are usually classified into four blast injury types: primary, secondary, tertiary, and quaternary (Figure 2-14).

PRIMARY BLAST INJURIES Primary blast injuries are those caused by the heat of the explosion and the overpressure wave. Pressure injuries tend to be the most serious and life-threatening injuries associated with explosions. They generally damage air-filled body spaces such as the middle ear, sinuses, bowel, and lungs. Burn injuries are generally limited unless caused by secondary combustion.

SECONDARY BLAST INJURIES Secondary blast injuries include trauma caused by projectiles. These injuries may be as severe as or more severe than the primary blast injuries. Projectiles from an explosive blast do have the ability to extend the range of injury beyond that caused by the blast wave and wind. High concentrations of projectiles may also create multiple penetrations and impalements over large areas of a person's body. The resulting injuries may produce severe bleeding.

TERTIARY BLAST INJURIES Tertiary blast injuries include those that can result from personnel displacement and structural collapse. Blast victims may be thrown against walls, the ground, or other surfaces and suffer blunt and/or penetrating trauma. When the blast results in a structural collapse, crush injuries may also result. These injuries can be extensive.

QUATERNARY BLAST INJURIES Quaternary blast injuries include any other injuries caused by the explosion mechanism and include crush injuries, burns, asphyxia, toxic exposures, and any exacerbations of preexisting or chronic illness.

Blast Injury Assessment

Determine, if possible, whether the blast was a result of terrorist action. If terrorism is involved or suspected, be suspicious about possible secondary explosive devices that may have been set to injure rescuers. Also be concerned about the potential for radioactive contamination. Ensure that police and bomb squad personnel sweep for additional explosive devices and radiation contamination and declare the area safe before entry.

Carefully evaluate the scene for secondary hazards. Look for such things as gas leaks, disrupted electrical wiring, sharp debris, and possible further structural collapse. During scene size-up, try to determine the blast epicenter location. There will be greater destruction and injury toward the epicenter. When closer, your index of suspicion for serious injuries should increase. When an explosion occurs in a confined space, remember that bouncing pressure waves may concentrate energy and cause areas of increased mortality at a further distance than expected from the epicenter.

CONTENT REVIEW

➤ Blast Injury Types
- Primary—caused by heat of explosion and overpressure wave
- Secondary—caused by blast projectiles
- Tertiary—caused by personnel displacement and structural collapse
- Quarternary—other injuries associated with or exacerbated by a blast

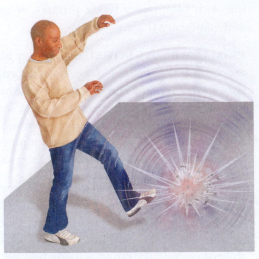

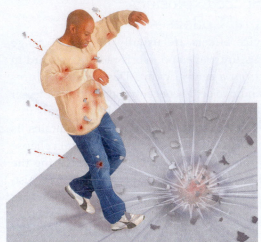

(A) Pressure Wave/Primary Injury
Air molecules slam into one another, creating a pressure wave moving outward from the blast center, causing pressure injuries.

(B) Blast Wave/Secondary Injury
Instantaneous combustion of the explosive agent creates superheated gases. The resulting pressure blows the bomb casing apart. Pieces of the bomb projectiles can cause secondary injuries by striking the patient.

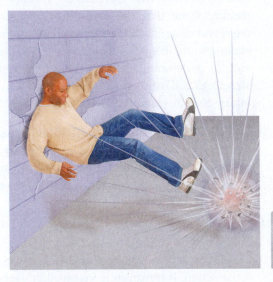

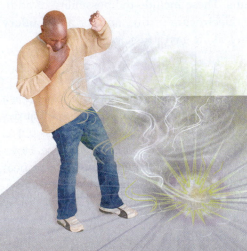

(C) Patient Displacement/Tertiary Injury
The blast wind may propel the patient to the ground or against objects, causing further injuries.

(D) Patient Exposed to Hazardous Material or Structural Collapse/Quaternary Injury
The patient may also be exposed to harmful chemicals or toxins or may be injured by structural collapse.

FIGURE 2-14 Types of blast injuries.

Blast injury mechanisms can produce extreme trauma in those who are closest to the blast epicenter. Blasts in densely populated areas may also involve a large number of victims. The role of the paramedic is to survey and size up the scene and do what is possible to secure it for further EMS operations. This normally involves implementing and ensuring overall scene management (Incident Management System). Once the Incident Management System is established and operational, begin caring for patients by applying normal assessment priorities (the ABCs of the primary assessment) and then focusing care on the most

seriously injured blast victims. If the number of patients exceeds your EMS system's immediate capabilities, employ disaster triage strategies.

The most common life-threatening trauma associated with explosions is pulmonary injury. Pulmonary injury may not manifest immediately. Thus, it should be anticipated in anyone with any other significant sign or symptom of blast trauma. Suspect pulmonary injury if anyone displays hearing loss or nosebleed (**epistaxis**). Evaluate respirations and breath sounds frequently, carefully watching and listening for any developing dyspnea and crackles or other signs of respiratory congestion. At the first sign of respiratory problems and/or falling oxygen saturations, consider supplemental oxygen (guided by the SpO_2), early airway protection, and rapid transport.

Some blast victims may suffer hearing loss from the pressure wave. After the emotional impact of the blast itself, this injury can produce extreme anxiety. Do your best to calm and reassure these patients. Remember that they will find it difficult to understand what you and others are saying and may not be able to follow spoken commands.

Blast Injury Care

Powerful explosions can produce lung, bowel, and ear injuries that require special care considerations. Otherwise, care for blunt trauma, punctures/penetrations, and burns as if these injuries if they were produced by other mechanisms.

LUNGS Pulmonary blast trauma, as already noted, is the most frequent life-threatening pressure injury associated with an explosion. The blast-induced pressure wave rapidly and forcefully compresses, distorts, and then decompresses the chest cavity, individual air passages, and alveoli. During compression/decompression, the air pressure in these body areas does not have time to equalize, as with normal respiration. The extreme pressure can damage or rupture the thin and delicate alveolar walls, resulting in inflammation, fluid accumulation, hemorrhage, and possibly even air entry directly into the bloodstream from the alveoli. Fluid accumulation (pulmonary edema) can make the lungs less elastic and air movement more difficult. The patient finds it more difficult and energy-consuming to breathe. Alveolar wall rupture releases blood into the alveoli and may allow air to enter the capillaries. The patient may spit or cough up blood or a frothy mixture of fluids, blood, and air. If air enters the bloodstream, it may then travel through the pulmonary circulation to the heart and from there to other critical organs, like the brain, causing small obstructions called **emboli** to circulate. These emboli may cause stroke or stroke-like episodes, myocardial infarction, or even death.

A patient with a history of detonation exposure should raise suspicions for lung injury. Because lung injury occurs frequently and is usually more serious than other blast-pressure injuries, carefully assess the respiratory system for signs and symptoms of pulmonary injury in patients with any signs of abdominal and ear injuries. Patients with lung injury may have progressively worsening crackles and/or difficulty breathing (**dyspnea**), and, in extreme cases, may cough up blood or blood-tinged sputum (**hemoptysis**). Patients occasionally experience an altered level of consciousness or small, stroke-like episodes. If there is any reason to suspect lung injury from a blast, immediately transport the victim to the closest trauma center or other appropriate facility.

If it becomes necessary to ventilate a patient with a blast injury, do so with the awareness that it may result in complications. The mechanism of injury may have damaged the alveolar–capillary walls and opened small blood vessels to the alveolar space. Positive-pressure ventilations may push small air bubbles into the vascular system and create emboli. These emboli may quickly travel to the heart and brain, where they can cause further injury or death. Positive ventilation pressure may also induce **pneumothorax** by pushing air past blast-induced lung defects and into the pleural space. When administering ventilations, if possible, place a patient in the left lateral recumbent position with the head somewhat down. This positioning discourages emboli from traveling up the carotid arteries and toward the brain.

Despite the risks associated with ventilating blast injury patients, always provide positive-pressure ventilations to any casualty with serious dyspnea. Use only the pressure needed to obtain moderate chest rise and adequate respiratory volumes. Supplemental oxygen may be helpful because the bloodstream absorbs small oxygen bubbles more easily than ones with the high percentage of nitrogen found in room air.

ABDOMEN The blast wave's sudden compression/decompression may also damage any air-filled bowel. Violent bowel wall movement may cause hemorrhage and possible wall rupture. Intestinal rupture may release the bowel contents into the abdominal cavity, leading to severe irritation and infection (peritonitis). Sudden abdominal compression may also push abdominal contents through wounds caused by penetrating objects, resulting in abdominal evisceration.

Abdominal blast injuries require no special attention in the early stages of care. The impact of associated injuries—bowel hemorrhage and spillage of bowel contents—on the patient's overall condition takes time to develop and is not usually apparent at the emergency scene. The only exceptions are when the blast is extremely powerful or the patient was very close to the detonation. In these cases, always be alert for signs and symptoms of developing shock and provide rapid transport and fluid resuscitation as needed.

EARS The ears are often affected from the blast wave forces associated with ordnance explosion, artillery fire, and even repeated small-arms fire at close range. The middle ear is an air-filled cavity containing the organs of hearing (cochlea and other structures) and of positional sense (semicircular canals). The pinna (the external portion of the ear) focuses and directs pressure waves (normally, sound waves) through the external auditory canal to the eardrum. The eardrum (tympanic membrane) transmits sound waves to the bones of the middle ear but prevents air from entering the middle ear. The eustachian tube provides an outlet for equalizing small and gradual changes in atmospheric pressure between the middle ear and the outside atmosphere. During blast overpressure, however, the eustachian tube cannot equalize the rapid pressure changes. Pressure on the tympanic membrane becomes so great that the membrane stretches or ruptures, resulting in acute hearing loss. The pressure change may be so great as to fracture the delicate bones of hearing, also causing acute hearing loss. Hearing losses associated with blasts are frequently temporary but may be permanent.

Often, ear injuries, even with as much as a third of the eardrum torn, will resolve over time without much attention. Provide supporting care to the victim and ensure that the ear canal remains uncontaminated.

PENETRATING WOUNDS Care for blast-generated penetrating wounds is the same as for any serious open wound. Remove as much contaminating material associated with a blast mechanism as is practical, and cover the site with a sterile dressing. If you encounter a large embedded or impaled object, stabilize it by securing gauze pads around it or cover it with a non-Styrofoam paper cup to prevent movement during transport. Large areas of damaged tissue are prone to infection, so keep the wound as clean as possible. Care of penetrating trauma is discussed at greater length elsewhere in this chapter.

BURNS Blasts can also cause extensive burn injuries, either from the explosions themselves or from the ignition of other munitions or fuels or of debris or clothing. Care for burn injuries is discussed in detail in the "Burns" chapter.

Sports Injuries

Sports medicine is an extensive and rapidly growing field and one that certainly cannot be covered in detail in this chapter or text. However, understanding some basic principles of sports medicine may help better understand and care for an injured athlete.

Sports injuries are most commonly produced by extreme exertion, by fatigue, or by direct trauma. Injuries can be secondary to acceleration, deceleration, compression, rotation, hyperextension, or hyperflexion. These forces can cause soft-tissue damage to the skin and muscle, connective tissue injury to tendons and ligaments, skeletal trauma to long bones or the spinal column, and internal damage to either hollow or solid organs.[11]

When a debilitating sports-related injury occurs, transport the athlete to an emergency department for a complete examination before allowing further participation in the sport. Injuries that present with minimal pain may be significantly worsened by the stress of further competition.

Such stress can cause additional injury and increase the potential for permanent disability.

In some contact sports, athletes may experience head trauma. If a collision leads to any period of unconsciousness, neurologic deficit, or altered mental status, ensure that the patient is subsequently evaluated in the emergency department. There is often a strong desire by coaches and players alike for an injured athlete to return to the game. Until significant injury can be safely excluded, discourage such action.

Protective gear can reduce the incidence of injuries. That same gear, however, can sometimes be a contributing factor in sports injuries. In major contact sports, for example, shoes are designed to give maximum traction by using cleats to lock the foot firmly in position. In football or soccer, a player might be struck, thus forcing the body to pivot on an immobile foot. Ligaments in the knee may tear, causing a severe and disabling leg injury. In other cases, protective gear may hinder complete assessment and patient stabilization.

Newer helmet designs for high-school contact sports use specially fitted padding to immobilize the head within the device. This padding is usually adequate to stabilize the head within a helmet in cases of suspected spinal injuries. Although it is difficult to stabilize a spherical helmet to the flat surface on which the patient may be lying, it may be preferable to attempting helmet removal. Consider leaving the shoulder pads in place to help maintain the head and neck in a neutral position (see the chapter titled "Head, Neck, and Spinal Trauma).

Crush Injuries

Crush injuries are a common type of trauma. They can result from mechanisms such as structural collapse, an industrial or agricultural incident in which a limb is caught in machinery, or an instance when a limb is caught under or between vehicles. These mechanisms of injury often result from significant crushing forces on soft tissues and bones and can cause serious, and even limb-threatening, injuries.

Crush injuries may be further compounded if the pressure remains in place for an extended period. The pressure can disrupt blood flow in the limb, resulting in anaerobic metabolism and tissue necrosis. This can cause accumulation of toxic substances in the crushed limb. If blood flow returns to the limb, the blood may carry these toxic substances to the central circulation, possibly resulting in cardiac arrhythmias and kidney injury. Another consequence of the release of the crushing pressure can be severe and difficult-to-control hemorrhage. Blood vessels within the limb can be severely damaged, with bleeding in locations that are difficult to identify. With severe and prolonged crush injury entrapment, prehospital care may include the administration of fluids and sodium bicarbonate to combat the effects of acidosis, limit tissue damage, and preserve kidney function.

Compartment Syndrome

Compartment syndrome is a form of blunt trauma sometimes often associated with a crush injury. The extremities contain various muscles and muscle groups in anatomic compartments. These compartments are separated by fibrous fascia. There are four compartments in the lower leg: the anterior compartment, superficial posterior compartment, deep posterior compartment, and lateral compartment. There are four compartments in the foot. The thigh contains three compartments, although these rarely develop compartment syndrome. There are numerous compartments in the forearm and hand, although these also rarely develop compartment syndrome. Blunt trauma to an extremity can cause the tissues to bleed and swell, leading to an increase in the pressure within the compartment. As the pressure increases, additional muscle is damaged. When pressures get too high, blood flow into and out of the compartment or compartments can be compromised, worsening tissue injury. If the pressure remains elevated, it may cause permanent and debilitating injury.

It is unlikely that compartment syndrome will be recognized in the field.[12,13] However, it is important to describe any mechanism of injury that might have caused it to emergency department personnel. Compartment syndrome is a frequent cause of post-blunt trauma disability that, without a clear description of the mechanism of injury, is difficult to recognize and correct. A patient may complain of intense muscle pain well after the injury, which is suggestive of this pathology.

Penetrating Trauma

Most trauma cases you will encounter will be due to blunt trauma mechanisms such as falls, motor vehicle collisions, and similar events. However, you will certainly also encounter patients who have sustained penetrating trauma. Penetrating trauma is an injury or injuries that occur when an object pierces the skin and enters the body. **Perforating trauma**, a form of penetrating trauma, occurs when an object enters and exits the body. Both can have devastating consequences.

Overview and Incidence

The most common causes of penetrating trauma in the United States are gunshots and stabbings. However, penetrating trauma can also occur with motor vehicle collisions, falls, industrial injuries, and similar events. Penetrating

trauma is relatively less common than one might expect.[14] However, the United States leads all economically developed countries in firearms-related deaths.[15] In a recent study of 157,045 trauma patients treated at 125 U.S. trauma centers, researchers found the incidence of penetrating trauma to be significantly less than that of blunt trauma. Only 6.4 percent of all injuries were gunshots, whereas only 1.5 percent were stab wounds.[16] However, there are significant geographic variations and racial differences in the incidence of penetrating trauma. In a Los Angeles study of 12,254 trauma patients, 24 percent of patients treated had sustained penetrating trauma. In a similar Los Angeles study, penetrating trauma accounted for 20.4 percent of trauma cases, yet resulted in 50 percent of overall trauma deaths—most of which were due to gunshot wounds.[17,18]

Because of the higher mortality seen with penetrating trauma, EMS personnel must be quick to identify these injuries and deliver the patient rapidly to the closest appropriate trauma center.

There are three levels of penetrating trauma: low-, medium-, and high-velocity. Low-velocity penetrating trauma is generally inflicted by mechanisms such as blades and pointed objects such as knives, swords, ice picks, and similar objects that enter the victim. Medium-velocity penetrating trauma is typically caused by handgun bullets, whereas high-velocity trauma results from rifle bullets.

Injury from low-velocity penetrating trauma is generally limited to the tissue actually contacted by the object during the object's path of travel. By contrast, medium- and high-velocity penetrating wounds usually involve dramatic energy exchanges and more extensive injury paths. The kinematics of penetrating trauma help to explain how and why these injuries occur.

Legal Considerations

Crime, Terrorism, and You. Unfortunately, with the exception of war, the increased incidence of penetrating trauma in the world has been due primarily to an increase in crime, terrorism, and the availability of weapons. Any scene where there is a reported case of penetrating trauma should heighten your awareness of scene hazards and safety. Never approach a scene until law enforcement personnel tell you it is safe to do so. Likewise, if you are providing care to a victim of penetrating trauma and you feel that the scene is becoming unsafe, you should retreat immediately to a safe distance—even if that requires you to leave the patient.

Our world is much different than it was 100 years ago, or even 50 years ago. Crime and terrorism pose real threats to both the public and EMS personnel. *Always* put personal safety and scene safety above all other priorities. Live to see another day.

Kinetics of Penetrating Trauma

The principles of physics detailed earlier in this chapter as related to blunt trauma also apply to penetrating trauma. When a **projectile**, such as a bullet, strikes a target, it exchanges its kinetic energy (energy of motion) with the object struck. As you will recall from earlier in the chapter when we discussed blunt trauma, the kinetic energy of an object (in this case, a penetrating object) is equal to its mass times the square of its velocity, all divided by 2:

$$\text{Kinetic Energy} = \frac{\text{Mass (Weight)} \times \text{Velocity (Speed)}^2}{2}$$

This formula demonstrates that the greater the mass *or* speed of an object, the greater its kinetic energy. The relationship of *mass* to energy is *direct*. If you double an object's mass, it has twice the kinetic energy (if the velocity remains the same). If you triple its mass, kinetic energy triples as well, and so on. However, the relationship of *velocity* to energy is *squared*. If you double an object's speed, its kinetic energy increases fourfold (if the mass remains the same). If speed triples, kinetic energy increases ninefold, and so on.

Applying these concepts now to penetrating trauma, the relationship between mass and velocity explains why even very small and relatively light bullets traveling very fast have a potential to do great harm. It also makes clear why different weights of bullets, traveling at different velocities, can cause varying degrees of damage. For example, handguns, shotguns, and low-powered (.22 caliber—non-magnum round) rifles are considered to be medium-energy/medium-velocity weapons. They deliver bullets, slugs, and pellets much faster than low-energy/low-velocity objects like knives and arrows can be wielded, but they are still slower than bullets fired by high-energy/high-velocity weapons such as hunting and assault rifles. For example, a handgun bullet is generally lighter and much slower (200 to 400 meters per second) than a rifle bullet. Civilian and military rifles, however, commonly fire heavier bullets, at speeds of 600 to 900 meters per second. Hence, a high-energy rifle bullet's kinetic energy is three to nine times that of a medium-energy handgun bullet and can be expected to do significantly more damage. In the urban warfare experience of Northern Ireland (where handguns and rifles were used in about equal proportions), rifle bullets proved to be two to four times more lethal than handgun bullets.

The law of conservation of energy (energy can be neither created nor destroyed—only changed from one form to another) explains why a projectile's kinetic energy is transformed into damage as it slows. If a projectile, such as a bullet, remains within the object it strikes, then all of its kinetic energy is transferred to the object. If a projectile

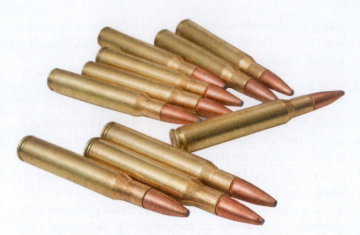

FIGURE 2-15 Examples of common bullets. Some bullets are designed to mushroom on impact, thus increasing their profile, energy exchange rate, and damage potential.

passes completely through an object, the energy transferred to the object is equal to the kinetic energy just prior to entry minus the projectile's remaining energy as it exits the object. The kinetic energy lost by the bullet as it passes through is transformed into tissue displacement, which is converted to physical tissue damage and a small amount of heat.

A final consideration regarding injury caused by penetrating objects is the deceleration rate. The forces causing trauma are related to the force formula: force = mass × acceleration (or deceleration). The more quickly an object slows, the more rapidly it gives up its kinetic energy. This plays a very important role in the study of how a bullet behaves (ballistics) and the damage it causes within human tissue (the biomechanics of penetrating trauma).

Ballistics

The study of projectiles in motion and their effects on objects they impact is called **ballistics** (Figure 2-15).

Patho Pearls

The Bullet's Travel. When a gun's firing pin strikes the shell casing primer, the resulting flash ignites the powder charge. When the charge ignites, it exerts tremendous force in all directions. Because the barrel prevents any expansion to the side, the only expansion possible occurs as the bullet moves down the barrel. The force of the exploding charge accelerates the bullet rapidly over the length of the barrel. This force gives the bullet great velocity (and kinetic energy to do great damage) as it leaves the end of the barrel. The force that pushes the bullet down the barrel also pushes the rifle in the opposite direction. The energy of the bullet's acceleration down the rifle barrel is exactly matched by the rifle's acceleration in the opposite direction (recoil). Note, however, that the rifle weighs much more than the bullet. It moves only inches, whereas the bullet accelerates over the full length of the barrel.

The rapidly burning powder pressurizes the space behind the bullet and pushes the bullet forward. The gun barrel, which is slightly smaller than the bullet, resists its movement, while the explosive pressure behind the bullet grows. As the bullet travels down the barrel, its velocity rapidly increases. The bullet also begins to spin, following the small lands and grooves, called *rifling*, in the gun's barrel. As it leaves the end of the gun barrel, the bullet is spinning rapidly and is pushed on by the barrel exhaust, often resulting in a slight wobble. For the first several inches beyond the mouth of the barrel, the bullet is followed by the very hot exhaust gases that drove the bullet down the gun barrel and by the residue of the spent explosive charge.

The bullet's spin, induced by the rifling, causes it to track very straight and generally prevents serious wobble, or yaw, during flight. The bullet's speed slows gradually as it meets resistance from the air it must push out of its way. The bullet is also accelerated toward Earth by gravity, dropping faster and faster with time. This effect gives a bullet's trajectory a curved shape. The trajectory of a very fast bullet is flatter, or much less curved, than that of a slower projectile.

As the bullet impacts its target, it exchanges its energy of motion by deforming the target and creating a shock wave within it. This kinetic energy transfer causes the damage associated with projectile injury.

Trajectory, Drag, and Cavitation

One aspect of ballistics is **trajectory**. Trajectory is the curved path that a bullet follows after it is fired from a gun. Once a bullet leaves a gun, it is pulled downward by gravity. The speed of the bullet and the distance of travel affect trajectory. The farther a bullet travels, the greater will be the effect of gravity on the trajectory. The shorter the path of travel, the straighter will be the trajectory. When a bullet is fired at close range, gravity has little time to pull it down, and it has a rather flat trajectory. The longer the distance between a gun and the object struck and/or the slower the bullet (from a handgun or lower powered rifle), the more the trajectory curves.

A second, more significant, aspect of projectile travel is the energy exchange between a bullet and the object it strikes. In addition to velocity, factors that affect this energy exchange include drag, cavitation, profile, shape, stability, expansion, and fragmentation, as well as secondary impacts.

As a bullet travels through the air, it meets air resistance, or **drag**. The faster it travels, the greater the drag and the greater the slowing effect. As a result, the damage caused by a bullet fired at close range is typically more severe than the damage from one fired at a distance that has been slowed by drag. Once the bullet strikes the target, of course, drag increases dramatically, as the density of the object struck is much greater than the density of air.

Objects traveling slowly and without much kinetic energy, such as knives or arrows, tend to damage only tissues they contact. By contrast, medium- or high-velocity projectiles, such as handgun or rifle bullets, set a portion of the semifluid body tissue in motion, creating a shock wave and a temporary cavity. This process is known as **cavitation** and its extent is determined by a bullet's velocity and rate of energy exchange. The rate of energy exchange is related to the size of the projectile's contact surface, which, in turn, is determined by its profile and shape.

Profile

Profile is the portion of the bullet you would see if it traveled straight toward you. That is, it is the cross section of the bullet along its direction of travel. The larger this surface profile, the greater the energy exchange rate, the more quickly the bullet slows, and the more extensive the damage to surrounding tissue. For bullets that remain stable during their travel and do not deform or tumble, the profile is the bullet's actual diameter, or **caliber**. To increase the energy exchange rate, however, bullets are designed to become unstable in their travel as they pass from air into another medium or to deform through expansion or fragmentation.

Shape

In addition to profile, other aspects of a bullet's shape affect the energy exchange rate and resulting damage. Handgun ammunition is rather blunt and is thus more resistant to travel through human tissue and releases kinetic energy more quickly. Rifle bullets are more pointed and cut through soft tissue more efficiently. However, if a rifle bullet tumbles (as it often does), it may exchange energy more rapidly because of an increased presenting profile.

Stability

The location of a bullet's center of mass affects its stability both during its flight and when it contacts a semisolid object such as human tissue. The longer a bullet, the farther its center of mass is from its leading edge. If a bullet is deflected from straight flight—for example, by barrel exhaust or by a gust of wind—lift created by the projectile's tip passing through air at an angle causes the bullet to tumble. If it continues to tumble, the bullet slows rapidly and its accuracy is diminished. To prevent tumbling, bullets are sent spinning through air by gun barrel rifling. This rotation gives a bullet gyroscopic stability like a spinning top. If a spinning bullet is slightly deflected, it wobbles, or **yaws**, then slowly returns to straight flight.

CONTENT REVIEW
➤ Factors Affecting Energy Exchange between a Projectile and Body Tissue
 • Velocity
 • Profile
 • Shape
 • Stability
 • Expansion
 • Fragmentation
 • Secondary impacts

When a bullet impacts a dense substance, such as human tissue, several things subsequently occur. If the projectile already has a yaw during travel, this yaw greatly increases as the bullet begins its penetration. This occurs as the bullet's mass tries to overrun its leading edge. Second, the gyroscopic spin designed for stability in air becomes insufficient. A bullet needs to spin at a rate 30 times greater in soft tissue than in air to maintain the same stability. The result may be tumbling and a great increase in the bullet's presenting profile.

A handgun bullet's center of mass is not far back from the leading edge and is rather stable. Its side profile is slightly greater than its frontal profile and will do only slightly more damage if it tumbles. Because a rifle bullet is generally longer than a handgun bullet and has its center of mass farther back from the leading edge, it is more likely to tumble when it hits body tissue. A rifle bullet's side profile is much greater than its frontal profile. With tumbling and a larger presenting profile, a rifle bullet's kinetic energy exchange rate increases, as does its potential for causing damage. In human tissue, a rifle bullet generally rotates 180 degrees and then continues its travel, base first.

Expansion and Fragmentation

Projectiles also may increase their profile and energy exchange rate by deforming when they strike a medium that is denser than air. As a bullet's tip contacts the target, it is slowed and then compressed by the weight of the bullet behind it. The bullet's tip mushrooms outward as its rear pushes into it, increasing the projectile's diameter, its profile. In some cases, the initial impact forces are so great that a bullet separates into several pieces, or fragments. This fragmentation increases the impact energy exchange rate, because the total fragment surface area is much greater than the original bullet's profile.

Handgun bullets are made of relatively soft lead, so their velocity, and thus their kinetic energy, are generally insufficient to cause significant bullet deformity. However, some bullets (e.g., hollow points) are specifically designed to mushroom and/or fragment on impact and cause increased damage. Rifle bullets have much higher velocities than handgun bullets and thus much more kinetic energy. They are more prone to deform or fragment when contacting human tissue, especially bullets intended for big-game hunting. Most military ammunition is fully jacketed with impact-resistant metal jackets that are resistant to deformity with soft tissue collision. Various international military conventions, such as the Hague Convention of 1899 and the Geneva Convention of 1949, forbid the use of expandable bullets in war. However, expandable bullets are widely available in the civilian sector and used in hunting, security, and similar endeavors.

If a bullet fragments, the irregular shape of the fragments and the increase in the profile area means that the projectile expends its energy more rapidly through more and erratic pathways than a handgun or rifle bullet that remains intact.

Secondary Impacts

The amount of energy exchanged between a projectile and the tissue it strikes is also affected by any other object the projectile strikes. Branches, window glass, or articles of clothing may all deflect a bullet and induce yaw and tumble. They may also affect bullet deformity and thereby increase the energy exchange rate once the bullet impacts the victim.

A special type of secondary impact occurs when a bullet collides with body armor. Kevlar™ and other synthetic fabrics can effectively absorb the kinetic energy of medium-velocity projectiles. The energy absorbed by the armor is then distributed to the victim over a relatively large surface area in much the same way that a gun's handgrip or shoulder stock helps distribute the force of recoil to the shooter. A bullet's impact with body armor may produce blunt trauma to the person hit (for example, chest contusions, rib fractures, and/or blunt cardiac injury), but such injury is generally much less severe than the injury caused by bullet penetration. High-energy projectiles may pass through body armor, but in doing so they dissipate much of their kinetic energy, causing more blunt trauma but thereby reducing the penetrating energy when the bullet strikes body tissue. Bullet deformity caused by body armor may increase the energy exchange rate, but the reduction in bullet velocity and lost kinetic energy reduces the overall injury potential. Ceramic or metal inserts for body armor will stop most rifle bullets but permit significant, but less lethal, blunt trauma.

Characteristics of Specific Weapons

Weapons that commonly cause wounds encountered by paramedics include handguns, rifles, shotguns, blades (knives and swords), and arrows. Each weapon type has certain characteristics associated with the injuries it produces.

Handgun

The handgun (Figure 2-16) is often a relatively short-barreled, medium-velocity weapon with limited accuracy. It is most effective at close range. Because a handgun does not typically fire a high-velocity, high-energy projectile (as does a rifle), its potential for causing damage can be limited (depending on the caliber and type of ammunition used). A blunt bullet shape and, less frequently, softer composition and associated mushrooming and fragmentation help to dissipate a bullet's energy more rapidly. Even so, the expected damage is less than that of the higher-energy rifle bullet. Injury severity is usually determined by which

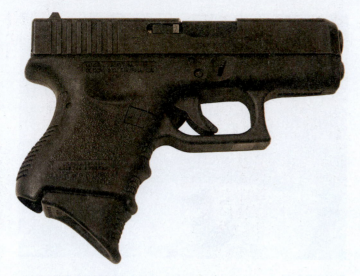

FIGURE 2-16 Handgun: Glock 09 mm.

organs, vessels, and other structures have been directly injured by the bullet's passage.

Some handguns can fire automatically (machine pistols). They continue to discharge bullets until the trigger is released or the magazine is empty. Although each projectile's energy remains the same, damage potential associated with fully automatic weapons is increased because of an increased likelihood of multiple impacts and/or multiple victims.

Rifle

The rifle (Figure 2-17) fires a heavier projectile than a handgun through a much longer barrel and with much greater final muzzle velocity. Rifles are either manually loaded, single-shot weapons with some mechanical loading mechanism to advance the next shell into the chamber, or semiautomatic weapons in which the next shell is fed into the chamber by energy resulting from the gun's recoil or exhaust gases. However, no more than one bullet is expelled with each squeeze of the semiautomatic rifle's trigger.

Generally speaking, high-energy rifle bullets travel much farther, have greater accuracy, and retain much more of their kinetic energy than do handgun projectiles. As a result of the rifle bullet's high speed and energy, it

transfers greater damaging energy to its target. Thus, rifle fire often results in extensive wounds with injuries that extend beyond the projectile's immediate track. Rifle ammunition is especially lethal. It is often designed to expand dramatically on impact, thus significantly increasing the energy delivery rate and the subsequent extent of resultant injuries.

Military-style rifles differ from hunting rifles in that they generally have a larger magazine capacity and fire in both the semiautomatic and automatic modes. Examples of these weapons include the M16, M4, FN SCAR, and AK47, among others. Resulting injuries are similar to those produced by civilian rifles, although multiple wounds and casualties can be expected. Military ammunition is fully jacketed and specifically designed not to expand. Though still very deadly, energy delivery is not as severe as with civilian hunting ammunition. The number and presence of military weapons in civilian settings are now more common—often involving gangs and drug cartels. In addition, many police departments now routinely carry military-style weapons to combat the increasing presence of similar weapons in civilian society. A civilian paramedic may actually encounter a victim of gunfire from a military weapon. This greatly increases the injury potential.

Shotgun

Shotguns can fire a single projectile (slug) or numerous spheres (pellets or shot) at medium velocity. A shell is loaded with a slug or a particular size of lead shot, varying from 00 (about 1/3 inch in diameter) to #9 shot (about the size of a pinhead). The projectile compartment size is approximately the same regardless of the size of the shot. This means that the larger the shot, the fewer the projectiles. Each projectile shares a portion of the total muzzle energy and, free of the gun's barrel, adds to total drag as they move through air.

A slug will cause a single entrance wound very similar to that caused by a rifle bullet. Large shot (e.g., buckshot) (Figure 2-18) will create multiple wounds that may be deep at a moderate range. Very small shot will cause numerous wounds at close range, but the wound depth decreases very quickly over distance. Many shotguns are equipped with a choke that reduces the exhaust leaving the barrel following the projectiles. This reduces the spreading effect of the exhaust on the shot and keeps the projectiles closer together as they travel toward the target. At very close range, the shot will create an entrance wound that appears as a single bullet wound. Farther out, there may be small entry wounds usually surrounding a central and larger wound. Beyond 20 to 30 yards, there may be just a pattern of small entry wounds.

In addition to the metal projectiles expelled by a shotgun, there will be wadding, material designed to help the

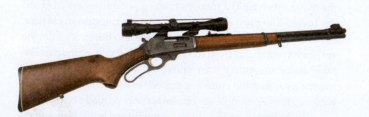

FIGURE 2-17 Rifle Remington: Model marlin 336 in 35 caliber.

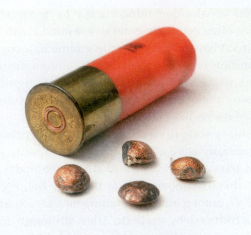

FIGURE 2-18 A shotgun propels small projectiles with limited velocity, such as the buckshot shown here. However, because of the large number of projectiles, the weapon can be extremely damaging at close range.

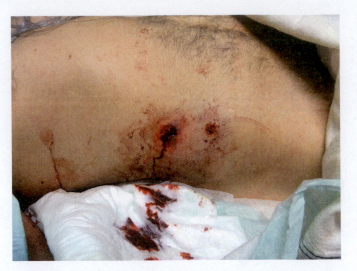

FIGURE 2-19 An impaled penetrating object can provide numerous challenges for prehospital personnel.

(© Dr. Bryan E. Bledsoe)

shotgun blast propel the shot. This plastic or fiber material may penetrate the wound and contribute to wound contamination. A shotgun is limited in range and accuracy. However, injuries sustained at close range can be severe or lethal.

Blades and Arrows

In contrast to high- or medium-velocity projectiles such as rifle or handgun bullets, objects such as knives, swords, arrows, and other slow-moving, penetrating objects cause low-velocity, low-energy wounds. Because low-velocity objects typically do not produce either a pressure wave or a cavity, damage is usually limited to the physical injury caused by direct contact between the blade or object and the victim's tissue. The penetration can result in serious internal hemorrhage or injury to individual or multiple body organs.

Hunting tips designed for arrows can be especially damaging. These feature three razor-tipped, pointed barbs that are intended to cut tissue smoothly. These tips penetrate deeply and produce severe internal hemorrhage. Also, any movement of the arrow while it is impaled in the victim increases both tissue damage and hemorrhage rate.

Other Penetrating Wound Mechanisms

Penetrating wounds can also be caused by mechanisms such as a piece of wire thrown by a lawn mower, a nail stepped on by a child, an air-powered gun firing a nail into a roofer's hand rather than the roof, or a worker falling on an exposed concrete reinforcing rod. Injuries such as these are generally low-velocity, low-energy wounds with injury confined to the actual object path of entry and penetration. Injury severity is related to the depth of penetration and the organs, blood vessels, and other structures affected. The penetrating object may introduce foreign and potentially infectious material into the wound. Some penetrating objects can complicate transport if the object remains impaled (as with the worker who falls on a reinforcing rod) (Figure 2-19).

Biomechanics of Penetrating Trauma

A high-velocity projectile results in a damage pathway that is related to three injury processes: direct injury, a pressure wave, and cavitation (the creation of a temporary cavity). These three injury processes can also create a permanent cavity and a zone of injury.

CONTENT REVIEW

➤ Factors Associated with the Damage Pathway of a Projectile Wound
- Direct injury
- Pressure shock wave
- Cavitation
  - Temporary cavity
  - Permanent cavity
  - Zone of injury

Patho Pearls

When a Projectile Enters the Body (Biomechanics of Penetrating Trauma). A spinning bullet contacts a semifluid target (such as human tissue) with great speed and kinetic energy. The tip of the bullet impacts tissue, pushing the tissue forward and to the side along the pathway of its travel. This tissue collides with adjacent tissue, ultimately creating a shock wave of pressure moving forward and lateral to the projectile. This shock wave continues to move perpendicular to the bullet's path as it passes. The rapid compression of tissue laterally and the stretching of the tissue as it moves outward from the bullet path crushes and tears the tissue structure. The motion creates a pocket, or cavity, behind the bullet. The pressure within this cavity is reduced, creating suction. This suction draws air and debris into the cavity from the entrance wound and from the exit wound, if one is present. The body tissue's elasticity then draws the sides of the cavity back together, causing the entrance wound, exit wound, and wound pathway to close completely or remain only partially open.

The bullet's exchange of energy with the body leaves various tissues disrupted and injured. Tissue in the direct pathway of the bullet suffers most. It is severely contused and likely to have been torn from its attachments. In addition to the directly injured tissue, other debris, blood, and air are found along the bullet's pathway. The cavitational wave stretches and tears adjacent tissue, damaging cell membranes and small blood vessels. The adjacent tissue is injured, but will likely regain its normal function slowly. Larger blood vessels torn by the bullet and the cavitational wave bleed heavily into the damage pathway. Over time, this pathway, because of the disruption in circulation and the introduction of infectious material with the drawing-in of debris, may develop severe infection, which will delay the healing process.

Direct Injury

Direct injury is the damage done when a penetrating object strikes tissue, contuses and tears that tissue, and pushes it out of the way. The direct injury pathway is limited to the projectile's profile as it moves through the body or the profiles of the resulting fragments as the projectile breaks apart. With the exception of magnum rounds (generating particularly high energies), handgun bullet damage is generally limited to direct injury.

Pressure Wave

When a high-velocity, high-energy projectile strikes human tissue, it creates a pressure wave (Figure 2-20). Because most human tissue is semiliquid and elastic, decelerating projectiles transmit the energy of motion forward and outward through these tissues very quickly. Tissues in front of the bullet are pushed forward and to the side at great speed. They, in turn, push adjacent tissues forward and outward, creating a moving wave of pressure and tissue in front of and to the side of a bullet. This effect increases with faster and blunter (or larger) bullets. With high-velocity rifle bullets, pressures are extreme, approaching 100 times normal atmospheric pressure or more.

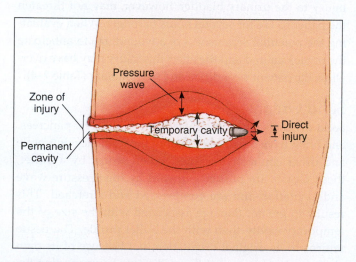

FIGURE 2-20 As a projectile passes through tissue, it creates a pressure wave and temporary cavity, with results that include direct injury, a permanent cavity, and a zone of injury.

The pressure wave travels well through liquids, such as blood, and may subsequently injure blood vessels distant from the projectile pathway. Air-filled cavities, such as the alveoli, compress very easily and absorb the pressure quickly limiting the shock wave and resulting temporary cavity. Solid organs, such as the liver and spleen, can be significantly injured because their dense structure transmits the pressure wave efficiently while it stretches and tears their inelastic structures. This pressure wave transmission can produce serious internal hemorrhage and, in extreme cases, organ disruption. Muscle tissue is also fairly dense but very elastic in nature. It tends to sustain less damage with bullet passage than do solid organs.

Temporary Cavity

The temporary cavity is a space created behind a high-energy bullet as tissue moves rapidly away from a bullet's path of travel. Creation of this temporary cavity is called *cavitation*. The cavity size depends on the amount of energy transferred during bullet passage. With rifle bullets, the temporary cavity may be as much as 12 times larger than the projectile's profile. After a bullet's passage, tissue elasticity causes the temporary cavity to close.

Cavitation also produces a subatmospheric pressure wave within the cavity as it expands. This means that air is drawn in from the entrance wound and the exit wound (if one exists). Because of this, debris and contamination can enter the cavity with the inflow of air, thus adding to infection risk.

Permanent Cavity

Physical contact with the bullet and its movement creates a temporary cavity that crushes, stretches, and tears the affected tissues. These processes can seriously injure the tissues along and adjacent to a bullet's path and may also affect resultant tissue elasticity. As a result, some tissues may not return to their normal form, thus resulting in a permanent cavity that, in some cases, may be larger than the bullet's diameter. This cavity is not a true void but is filled with the injured disrupted tissues, some air, blood and other fluids, and debris.

Zone of Injury

Associated with most projectile wounds is a **zone of injury** that extends beyond the permanent cavity. This zone contains crushed, torn, and contused tissue that does not function normally and may be slow to heal because of cell and tissue damage, disrupted blood flow, and the likelihood of infection.

Heat Injury

A bullet is heated both by the burning of the bullet's propellant and by friction as it is pushed down the gun barrel. As this takes only milliseconds, the bullet's temperature rises only slightly. Some kinetic energy is converted to heat as the bullet impacts the target. However, the bullet's temperature will reach, at most, about 300 degrees Fahrenheit. Generally, burn injury from a gunshot is typically minimal and associated mostly with the final resting location of the bullet, if at all.

Low-Velocity Wounds

As already noted, penetrating objects such as knives, swords, ice picks, arrows, or flying objects such as blast debris, ski poles in a skiing injury mechanism, nails from a nail gun, or wires thrown by a lawn mower can cause low-velocity penetrating trauma. The object's relatively slow speed limits the kinetic energy exchange rate as it enters a victim's body. Consider, for example, a victim stabbed by a 150-lb (68 kg) attacker who strikes with a knife moving at about 3 meters per second. Although the mass behind the knife blade's penetration is significantly greater than a rifle bullet's mass, the knife's velocity is vastly less. This means that injury is usually restricted to tissue the knife actually contacts (Figure 2-21).

Although injury is limited to a penetrating object's path, the object may be twisted, moved about, or inserted at an oblique angle. As a result, the entrance wound may not reflect the object's depth of penetration, extent of its motion within the body, or actual organs and tissues it contacts and injures.

Attacker and victim characteristics are important to consider during assessment of low-velocity, penetrating trauma victims. Knife-wielding men, for example, most often strike with a forward, outward, or crosswise stroke and carry the knife with the blade protruding from the thumb side of the hand. Women usually strike with an overhand and downward stroke, with the blade protruding from the little-finger side of the hand. Attack victims initially attempt to protect themselves by using their hands

and arms.[3] This means that they often receive deep upper-extremity wounds (commonly called defense wounds). If an attack continues, injuries are often then directed to the chest, abdomen, face, neck, or back.

Penetrating Injuries to Specific Tissues and Organs

Damage caused by a projectile varies with the tissue type it encounters. Organ density affects how efficiently a projectile's energy is transmitted to surrounding tissues. The tissue's connective strength and elasticity, called **resiliency**, also influence how much tissue damage occurs with kinetic energy transfer. Structures and tissues within the body that behave differently during projectile passage include connective tissue, solid organs, hollow organs, lungs, and bone.

Connective Tissue

Muscles, tendons, ligaments, skin, and other connective tissues are dense and elastic, and hold together very well. When exposed to cavitational wave pressure and stretching, these connective tissues characteristically stretch and absorb energy while limiting tissue damage. The wound track closes rapidly because of this tissue's resiliency and elastic nature, and serious injury is frequently limited to the projectile's path.

Organs

Another factor with profound effects on the victim's potential for survival is the particular organ or organs involved in a penetrating injury. Some organs, such as the heart and brain, are critical to life, and serious injury to these may cause immediate death. When large blood vessels are injured, hemorrhage can be rapid and severe. A penetrating injury to the urinary bladder, however, may not threaten the patient's life for several hours or longer. When evaluating the potential seriousness of a wound, try to anticipate the organs injured and the effect this injury may have overall on the patient's condition and survivability (Table 2–4).

Solid Organs

Solid organs such as the liver, spleen, kidneys, pancreas, and brain have the density but not the resiliency of muscle and other connective tissues. When struck by a bullet, these tissues are pushed outward by the pressure wave and cavitation and are compressed and stretched. This results in greater damage associated with the size of the temporary cavity than with the bullet profile. The tissue returns to its original orientation, not because of its own elasticity, but because of the resiliency of surrounding tissues or the organ capsule. Hemorrhage associated with solid organ projectile damage is often significant.

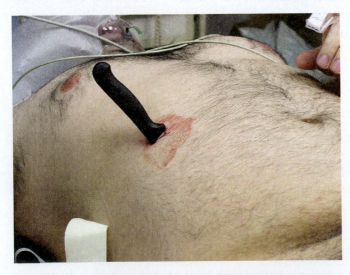

FIGURE 2-21 Damage caused by a low-velocity wounding process, such as that caused by a knife, is limited to the object's path of travel.

(© Dr. Michael Casey, MD)

Table 2-4 Abdominal Organs Injured, by Mechanism

Injury Type	Organ Injured	Percentage (%)
Gunshot wounds	Small intestine	50
	Colon	40
	Liver	30
	Abdominal vasculature	25
Stab wounds	Liver	40
	Small intestine	30
	Diaphragm	20
	Colon	15

Hollow Organs

Hollow organs such as the intestines, stomach, urinary bladder, and heart are muscular containers holding liquid or semiliquids. Liquid within these organs is generally noncompressible and rapidly transmits the energy outward. If the container is filled and distended at impact time, the energy release can cause the organ to rupture and leak its contents. (Large blood vessels can respond to projectile passage much like hollow, fluid-distended organs.) If the container is not distended or filled with air, it is much more tolerant of the cavitational forces. Slower and smaller projectiles may produce small holes in a hollow organ, resulting in slow leakage of contents. If this occurs with the heart, it may produce **pericardial tamponade** (blood filling the pericardial sac, thus limiting heart function) or life-threatening hemorrhage. Leakage of bowel contents can be particularly problematic because the contents of this organ contain bacteria that can contaminate the wound and surrounding areas. If a hollow organ, such as the bowel or stomach, contains air, the air can compress with passage of the pressure wave and attenuate (partially limit) the resulting injury.

Lungs

The lungs contain millions of air-filled alveoli. As a projectile and its associated pressure wave pass, air within these sacs is compressed, thus slowing and limiting the resulting cavitational wave. Injury to lung tissue in penetrating trauma is generally less extensive than penetrating injury to other body tissues. However, if the projectile strikes the central portions of the lung that contain the major blood vessels and bronchi or bronchioles, the injury can be devastating.

A bullet may open the chest wall and/or disrupt the larger airways, permitting air to escape into the thorax (pneumothorax) or may create a valvelike defect in the chest wall that results in accumulation of pressure within the chest (tension pneumothorax). Bullet wounds rarely cause an open pneumothorax (sucking chest wound) because the entrance wound diameter is usually limited to the bullet caliber. Close-range shotgun blasts and explosive exit wounds of high-powered rifles, however, may be large and cause significant disruption of chest wall integrity. In these cases, a sucking chest wound is a possible outcome.

Bone

In contrast to lung tissue, bone is the body's densest, most rigid, and nonelastic tissue. When struck by a projectile or its associated pressure wave, bone resists displacement until it fractures—often into numerous pieces. These bone fragments may then distribute the impact energy to surrounding tissues. A projectile's contact with bone may also significantly alter its path through the body and/or cause projectile deformity or fragmentation.[19]

Pathophysiology of Penetrating Trauma

Penetrating trauma can affect all body regions, cavities and structures. These can include the head, neck, chest, abdomen and pelvis, and the extremities (Figure 2-22).

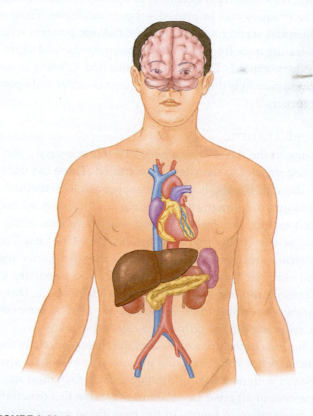

FIGURE 2-22 Critical structures in which the seriousness of a bullet's impact is increased include the brain, great vessels, heart, liver, kidneys, and pancreas.

Head Trauma

Penetrating head trauma has high morbidity and mortality rates. It has been estimated that 50 percent of all trauma deaths are due to traumatic brain injury. Gunshot wounds to the head account for approximately 35 percent of these deaths. In the civilian sector, gunshot wounds account for the vast majority of penetrating head injuries. These may be accidental, self-inflicted (suicidal), or due to homicide or assault. Penetrating head trauma by suicide is associated with a higher rate of mortality than other types of penetrating brain injury. In the military sector, penetrating head injuries from shrapnel, shell fragments, and debris are more common.[20]

Neck Trauma

Penetrating neck injuries occur in approximately 5 to 10 percent of all trauma cases. The incidence of penetrating neck trauma in a military setting is considerably higher because of the lack of body armor protection for the neck. Numerous high-risk structures traverse the neck, including the spinal cord and column, the carotid arteries, the jugular veins, the vertebral arteries, the trachea, the esophagus, and other significant structures. Thus, penetrating trauma to the neck can cause bleeding, respiratory problems, neurologic problems, or any combination of these.

Fortunately, the mortality rate for patients with penetrating neck trauma is declining as a result of better imaging techniques and improved surgical strategies. From a prehospital standpoint, the biggest risk for patients with penetrating neck trauma is airway compromise and significant hemorrhage. These can be controlled in many cases until the patient is delivered to the trauma center and operating room.[7]

Chest Trauma

Because of the size and location of the thoracic cavity, penetrating injuries to the chest are common. These can damage the chest wall, lungs, tracheobronchial structures, esophagus, diaphragm, great vessels, and the heart. As one would expect, penetrating injuries of the heart are highly lethal, with a fatality rate approaching 70 to 80 percent. The ventricles are most commonly affected—primarily the right ventricle, because of its larger size and proximity to the anterior thoracic wall relative to the left ventricle. These injuries often result in an immediate pericardial tamponade, reducing cardiac output and causing shock.

Injuries to the great vessels of the chest (especially the aorta, superior vena cava, and pulmonary vessels) are also common with penetrating chest trauma. In fact, more than 90 percent of all great vessel injuries are due to a penetrating mechanism of injury. In the past, these injuries were uniformly fatal. Now, however, the ability to rapidly image the thorax and the great vessels and perform rapid emergency surgical intervention has reduced the mortality rate significantly.

Lung injuries are common with thoracic penetrating trauma and can cause pneumothorax, hemothorax, or both. In addition to lung injuries, tracheobronchial injuries can also occur with penetrating trauma. These injuries are almost always associated with injuries to other thoracic structures, such as the great vessels.

Esophageal injuries are relatively rare. However, they can have significant long-term complications.

The diaphragm—the muscle separating the abdominal cavity from the thoracic cavity—is frequently injured in penetrating trauma to the trunk (chest and abdomen). Diaphragmatic injuries occur in approximately 45 percent of gunshot wounds and 15 percent of stab wounds to the trunk.[21]

Abdominal/Pelvic Trauma

The abdomen and pelvis are also quite vulnerable to penetrating trauma. These two body cavities contain numerous organs and associated structures. As with other types of penetrating trauma, most penetrating injuries to the abdomen result from gunshot wounds. The abdominal and pelvic structures that are injured in cases of penetrating trauma depend somewhat on the mechanism of injury.

The fatality rate for abdominal penetrating wounds varies significantly based on the structures injured and the magnitude of the injury. The average mortality rate for all penetrating abdominal injuries is approximately 5 percent. Intraabdominal vascular injuries have a higher mortality rate. Interestingly, most deaths from penetrating trauma occur within 6 hours of admission and often occur in the emergency department or operating room. Most deaths from blunt abdominal trauma tend to occur later (within 72 hours) and occur in the ICU setting. Factors associated with increased mortality from penetrating abdominal trauma include the presence of shock on admission to the hospital, massive hemorrhage, a long interval of time between the injury and subsequent surgery, female gender, and coexisting brain injury.[9]

The organs and structures of the pelvis are relatively well protected from penetrating trauma. However, projectiles that enter the pelvis can certainly damage genitourinary and reproductive structures. This is particularly prevalent in pregnant patients, where the gravid uterus fills the pelvic cavity and the lower portions of the abdomen. External structures, such as the penis and scrotum, can also be injured with penetrating trauma.

Extremity Trauma

Penetrating injuries to the extremities are common. The mechanism differs somewhat between the civilian and military experience. The widespread use of body armor in the Iraqi and Afghan conflicts resulted in an increased relative incidence of extremity trauma. Although the torso is well protected from injury with body armor, the extremities are vulnerable. Any of the anatomic structures within the extremity—bone, muscle, tendon, ligament, nerve, or blood vessel—can be affected. Most extremity injuries are non–life-threatening. However, injuries to the vascular structures of the extremities can be both life threatening and limb threatening. Injuries to nerves and tendons of the extremities can result in lifelong disabilities. Gunshots and stab wounds figure often in penetrating extremity trauma, but there are other causes. These include nails and similar sharp objects, liquids under pressure (such as grease), and lacerations and punctures from various tools (e.g., saws and drills). Again, the energy with which these are applied correlates to the severity of the resulting trauma.

Entrance Wound

Often, entrance wounds are no larger than the bullet's profile. At this point, when the bullet has just impacted the body, cavitational wave energy has not had time to develop and enlarge the wound (Figure 2-23). The situation is different, however, with bullets that deform or tumble during flight. With these projectiles, the initial impact can be especially violent, producing a much larger and more disrupted entry wound than bullet caliber alone would suggest.

Bullet entry wounds sustained at close range—a few feet or less—display special characteristics. Such wounds may be marked by elements of the barrel exhaust and bullet passage. Tattooing from propellant residue may form a darkened circle or an oval (if the gun is held at an angle) around the entry wound and contaminate the wound itself. At the wound site, you may notice a small (usually 1- to 2-mm) ridge of discoloration around the entrance caused by the bullet as it stretches the skin before it tears it. If the

gun barrel is held very close to or against the skin as the weapon is fired, it may push barrel exhaust into the wound, producing subcutaneous emphysema (air within the skin's tissue) and crepitus to the touch. If the barrel is held a few inches from the skin, you may notice some burns caused by the hot gases of the barrel exhaust.

Exit Wound

Exit wounds are caused by physical damage both from the passage of the bullet and from the resulting cavitational wave. Because the pressure wave that causes cavitation moves forward and outward, the exit wound may have a "blown out" appearance. The exit wound may appear stellate, referring to tears radiating outward in a starlike fashion. (Be aware that some entrance wounds may be stellate as well.) Because the cavitational wave has had time to develop by the time the bullet leaves the body, exit wounds may more accurately reflect the probable internal damage than entrance wounds do. If a bullet expends all its kinetic energy before it can exit the body, there is no exit wound and the bullet remains within the body. If the bullet does exit, kinetic energy expended within the body is equal to the kinetic energy of the bullet before impact minus the energy that remains in the bullet as it leaves the body. A bullet may be deflected as it travels through the body (as from contact with bone), so there may not be a direct route of travel between entrance wound and exit wound.

When you consider entrance and exit wounds, it is important to keep the focus on the medical aspects of any differences in appearance. Whether a wound is an exit or an entrance wound has important implications for crime investigation, but only a thorough forensic examination by a qualified expert can determine with certainty whether a given wound represents a projectile's entrance or exit. Therefore, avoid making assured statements or annotations in the prehospital care report about whether a wound is an exit or entrance wound. Instead, describe the wound and allow investigators to use your description and other evidence in making a valid determination.

Special Concerns with Penetrating Trauma
Scene Size-Up

Scene size-up for a shooting or stabbing can involve special concerns not usually associated with most other emergency care situations. The very nature of these injuries should suggest possible danger from further violence and potential injury to you and your crew. Do not approach a shooting or stabbing scene unless and until law enforcement personnel arrive and secure it and direct you to enter and provide care. If law enforcement personnel are not yet

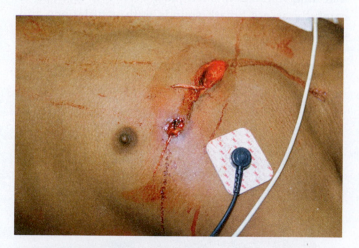

FIGURE 2-23 The entrance wound is often the same size as the projectile's profile. A bullet's exit wound often has a "blown outward" appearance. Both an entrance and an exit wound are visible on this patient.

(© Edward T. Dickinson, MD)

on scene when you arrive, stage your vehicle at a safe distance from the scene. After police or other law enforcement personnel arrive, on their direction, bring your vehicle closer to the scene but keep the police and their vehicles between you and any shooting or stabbing site. Wait there for the police to indicate that it is safe to approach the patient.

Once you reach the patient, carefully survey the area to ensure that there are no weapons within the patient's reach. Consider the possibility that a victim (the patient) may be carrying a knife or other weapon. If you have any doubts, request that police search the victim for weapons before you begin patient assessment and care.

As you carefully survey a shooting scene, try to reconstruct the event. Attempt to determine the victim's original position and angle to and distance from the shooter. This helps to determine the angle at which a bullet entered the patient (which may not otherwise be revealed by an entrance wound) and whether a wound was received at close range or from a distance. Also try to determine the weapon caliber and type—handgun, rifle, or shotgun.

If the call involves a knife or similar penetrating weapon injury, attempt to determine the blade length. (You will not be able to determine wound's depth, but the length of the weapon will likely identify the maximum possible depth of insertion.) This information will help the emergency physician determine wound severity.

During patient assessment, do all you can to preserve the crime scene while providing essential patient care. Disturb only the materials around the patient that you must move in order to render care. Cut around, not through, any bullet or knife holes in clothing, and give any clothing you have removed or cut away to police for use as evidence. If there is ever any doubt about what to do, err on the side of providing patient care. (See the chapter titled "Crime Scene Awareness.") If a victim is obviously dead, use your jurisdiction's protocols for handling the body, but try to do so without disturbing evidence that may be crucial in determining what happened.

Penetrating Wound Assessment

When assessing a penetrating trauma victim, try to determine the penetrating object's path and the organs that the object may have affected. Anticipate the potential for organ injury and use this to help set priorities for on-scene care or rapid transport. Remember, however, that a bullet may not travel in a straight line between the entrance and exit wounds. Often, a very small shift in a bullet's path may mean the difference between tearing open a large blood vessel or missing critical organs completely. The human body is also a dynamic environment. The diaphragm moves the abdominal contents during respiration. Thus, it is difficult to determine what organs may have been injured, as this depends in part on the phase of respiration during which the injury occurs.

It is often hard to estimate the magnitude of a projectile wound. Injuries to the great vessels, heart, and brain may be rapidly fatal, whereas injuries to solid organs (liver, pancreas, kidneys, or spleen) may also be deadly but take more time for the signs and symptoms to manifest. Consequently, always anticipate the worst with bullet wounds that involve the head, chest, abdomen, or pelvis. Provide rapid transport in these cases, and treat shock aggressively. Appreciate that gunshot wounds account for less than 1 percent of EMS responses, but they account for more than 15 percent of trauma mortality. Assume that any gunshot wound is serious if it involves any area of the body other than the distal extremities.

Penetrating Wound Care

Certain penetrating wounds require special attention. These include wounds to the face and chest and those involving impaled objects. Their care is described in the following sections; care for other penetrating injuries and shock is discussed in other chapters.[6,7]

Facial Wounds

Facial gunshot wounds may endanger the airway and destroy many airway landmarks (Figure 2-24). With wounds such as these, endotracheal intubation may be essential, yet is extremely difficult to perform. Some paramedics find it helpful to visualize the larynx with a laryngoscope while another rescuer gently presses on the chest. Look for any bubbling during the chest compression, and try to pass the endotracheal tube through the bubbling tissue. Then, very carefully ensure that the endotracheal tube is properly placed in the trachea and that lung ventilation is adequate. Here it is essential to carefully assess breath sounds with ventilations and capnography.

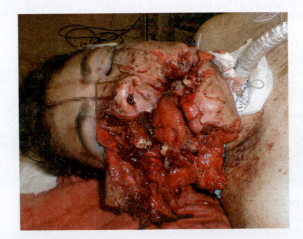

FIGURE 2-24 Facial wounds may distort or destroy airway landmarks.

(Collection of Robert Porter)

If this approach is ineffective, an invasive technique may be essential to restore the airway, at least long enough for the patient to reach more definitive care. This technique is the **percutaneous cricothyrotomy**, in which access is achieved via needle or other approved puncture device (not surgically, as with the use of a scalpel). This emergency airway procedure perforates the membrane between the thyroid and cricoid cartilages, providing a route for ventilation directly into the lower airway. (Percutaneous cricothyrotomy is discussed in detail in the chapter "Airway Management and Ventilation.")

Chest Wounds

The chest wall is rather thick and resilient. It requires a large wound to create an opening big enough to permit free air movement through the chest wall—an open pneumothorax. Wounds caused by small-caliber handguns usually result in no air movement, whereas wounds caused by shotgun blasts and exiting high-velocity bullets more commonly cause such injuries. If frothy blood is associated with a chest wound, be alert for a possible tension pneumothorax, in which air builds up under pressure within the thorax. Remember, it takes pressure to push air through the wound and froth blood. Completely sealing the chest wound may stop any outward airflow. This can increase both the speed of tension pneumothorax development and its severity. Instead, cover any open chest wound with an occlusive dressing sealed on three sides to allow airflow through the unsealed side (Figure 2-25). If dyspnea is significant, assess for tension pneumothorax and release any occlusive dressings. If this does not relieve the pressure, perform needle decompression as indicated (see the "Chest Trauma").

Always consider the possibility of heart and great vessel damage with a penetrating chest wound. These injuries may cause severe internal hemorrhage and death. Another serious complication of penetrating chest trauma is pericardial tamponade. This condition occurs when an object or projectile perforates the heart and permits blood to leak into the pericardial sac. As blood accumulates in the sac, the heart no longer fully fills with blood and circulation slows. If pericardial tamponade is uncorrected, a patient's prognosis is very poor. However, a needle introduced into the pericardial space (pericardiocentesis), a procedure

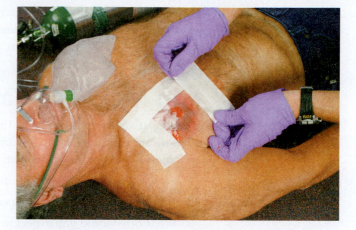

FIGURE 2-25 Seal open chest wounds and ensure adequate respirations.

available at the emergency department, can quickly alleviate the life threat.

Therefore, if the patient has a penetrating injury to the central chest, suspect and look for this condition and arrange for rapid transport. (Pericardial tamponade assessment is discussed in the "Chest Trauma" chapter.)

Impaled Objects

If an object that causes a low-velocity wound lodges in the body, removal may be dangerous for the patient. If an object bent as it hit a bone on entry, attempts at removal may cause further injury. If an object is held firmly by soft tissue, it may lie against a severed blood vessel, thereby restricting blood loss; moving or removing the object may then increase hemorrhage.

Immobilize impaled objects in place—where and as they are found—and transport the patient. Use bulky dressings and splinting materials to stabilize the object. Remove only impaled objects that are lodged in the cheek, neck, or trachea that interfere with the airway or those that must be removed to provide CPR. When a patient has fallen on an object that results in impalement, such as a concrete reinforcing rod, carefully cut the object to permit patient transport. If an object is too large to transport with the patient, cut it without subjecting the patient to unnecessary movement, or, if using a cutting torch, without causing any burn injury.

Summary

Trauma is a major cause of death and disability. Trauma is typically classified as being either blunt or penetrating with many patients having some component of both. Trauma, at its most fundamental level, is a surgical disease. Patients who have sustained trauma tend to experience less death and disability when they are treated by experienced personnel in an accredited trauma center. The modern EMS system should ensure that trauma patients are always taken to the closest trauma center, as designated by the system, that can appropriately treat the patient's injury or injuries.

You Make the Call

Arriving at an intersection that is the scene of a vehicle collision, you notice an auto that received a significant lateral impact to the driver's side. The door is pushed into the vehicle about 12 inches and the side window is broken out.

1. What scene hazards would you expect on this call?
2. What injuries would you suspect?
3. What care would you expect to provide?

See Suggested Responses at the back of this book.

Review Questions

1. In a motor vehicle collision, which organ system of the body is the first to experience the effects of trauma?
   a. Neurologic
   c. Musculoskeletal
   b. Integumentary
   d. Cardiovascular

2. Which of the following is the most common cause of blunt trauma?
   a. Altercations
   b. Motor vehicle crashes
   c. Sports injuries
   d. Falls

3. An energy transfer from an object or surface to the skin and into the body's interior describes which mechanism of injury?
   a. Blunt trauma
   b. Penetrating trauma
   c. Multisystem trauma
   d. External trauma

4. Regarding the mechanism of injury, when the speed of an object that is about to strike a body is doubled, its ability to cause trauma is _____
   a. reduced by one-half.
   b. doubled.
   c. tripled.
   d. quadrupled.

5. In determining the potential for trauma caused by an object, you need to examine _____
   a. the object's speed.
   b. the object's weight.
   c. the object's shape.
   d. all of the above.

6. Which organ in a female patient can transmit the pressure wave of a bullet very efficiently because of its dense structure?
   a. Spleen
   b. Stomach
   c. Small intestine
   d. Uterus

7. Which organ is most likely to be injured by the ligamentum teres during a rapid deceleration?
   a. Heart
   c. Lungs
   b. Liver
   d. Bladder

8. Your trauma patient who was involved in a motor vehicle collision has an injury to the head from a "secondary collision." The injury was probably from _____
   a. an organ collision.
   b. body collision.
   c. a loose item in the car that struck the patient.
   d. the seat belt.

9. Front dashboard and steering wheel air bags work much differently than seat belts and are extremely effective for what type of vehicular collisions?
   a. Frontal
   c. Rollover
   b. Rear-end
   d. Rotational

10. The child's _____ make(s) protection in vehicle crashes difficult.
    a. age
    b. size characteristics
    c. height
    d. weight

11. During a frontal impact in a motor vehicle collision, injuries sustained in the down-and-under pathway most commonly initiate with _____

    a. skull fractures.

    b. hip fractures.

    c. diaphragm ruptures.

    d. hollow organ ruptures.

12. The _____ pathway accounts for roughly 25 percent of the deaths in vehicular crashes.

    a. ejection   c. up-and-over

    b. restrained   d. down-and-under

13. When a(n) _____ impact occurs, the index of suspicion for serious and life-threatening internal injuries must be higher than vehicle damage alone suggests.

    a. frontal   c. lateral

    b. rear-end   d. oblique

14. The anatomic region most commonly injured in a rear-end impact is the _____

    a. head.   c. chest.

    b. neck.   d. extremities.

15. During an explosion, the pressure wave of the blast will likely cause injury to what structures of the body?

    a. muscles   c. hollow organs

    b. solid organs   d. bones

16. In an explosion, the fragments of the container that held the material that exploded can become _____

    a. projectiles that can enter the body.

    b. structures that limit the amount of damage to the body.

    c. structures that inhibit a secondary fire from the blast.

    d. projectiles that ascend primarily upward, not outward, from the explosion epicenter.

17. Which mechanism of injury to the thorax carries with it a 70 to 80 percent fatality rate?

    a. Penetration injury to the heart

    b. Blunt injury to the lateral thorax

    c. Deceleration injury to the lungs

    d. Acceleration injury to the lungs

18. In significant crush injuries, toxins released into the central circulation after pressure is released can lead to what additional complication?

    a. Increased liver function

    b. Cardiac arrhythmias

    c. Increased kidney output

    d. Severe alkalosis

See Answers to Review Questions at the end of this book.

References

1. National Center for Injury Prevention and Control. "Guidelines for Field Triage of Injured Patients." 2011. (Available at www.cdc.gov/fieldtriage.)

2. Lerner, E. B., et al. "Does Mechanism of Injury Predict Trauma Center Need?" *Prehosp Emerg Care* 15(4) (Oct 2011): 518–525.

3. Centers for Disease Control and Prevention. "Injury Prevention & Control: Motor Vehicle Safety. " (Available at http://www.cdc.gov/motorvehiclesafety/.)

4. Mulholland, S. A., et al. "Prehospital Prediction of the Severity of Blunt Anatomic Injury." *J Trauma* 64(3) (Mar 2008): 754–760.

5. Staff, T., et al. "A Field Evaluation of Real-Life Motor Vehicle Accidents: Presence of Unrestrained Objects and Their Association with Distribution and Severity of Patients." *Accid Anal Prev.* 45(2) (Mar 2012); 529–538.

6. Emory, J. "Hybrid Vehicles: Separating Fact from Fiction." *Fire Engineering*, V162, 7/2009.

7. Tefft, B. C. "Prevalence of Motor Vehicle Crashes Involving Drowsy Drivers, United States 1999–2008." *Accid Anal Prev* 45(2) (Mar 2012): 180–186.

8. De Rome, L., et al. "Motorcycle Protective Clothing: Protection from Injury or Just the Weather?" *Accid Anal Prev* 43(6) (Nov 2011): 1893–1900.

9. Wightman, J. and S. Gladish. "Explosions and Blast Injuries." *Ann Emerg Med* 37(6) (2001): 664–678.

10. Leibovici, D., et al. "Blast Injuries: Bus versus Open-Air Bombings—a Comparative Study of Injuries in Survivors of Open-Air versus Confined Space-Explosions." *J Trauma* 41(6) (Dec 1996): 1030–1035.

11. Laraque, D., B. Barlow, and M. Durkin. "Prevention of Youth Injuries." *J Nat Med Assoc* 91(10) (1999): 557–571.

12. Badhe, S., et al."The 'Silent' Compartment Syndrome." *Injury* 2009 Feb; 40(2): 220-222.

13. Oprel, P.P., et al. "The Acute Compartment Syndrome of the Lower Leg: A Difficult Diagnosis?" *Open Orthop J* 4 (2010): 115–119.

14. Glantz, L. H., and G. J. Annas. "Handguns, Health, and the Second Amendment." *N Engl J Med* 360 (2009): 2360–2365.

15. Richardson, E. G., and D. Hemenway. "Homicide, Suicide, and Unintentional Firearm Fatality: Comparing the United States with Other High-Income Countries, 2003." *J Trauma* 70 (2011): 238–243.

16. Glance, L. G., T. M. Osler, A. W. Dick, D. B. Mukamel, and W. Meredith. "The Survival Measurement and Reporting Trial for Trauma (SMARTT): Background and Study Design." *J Trauma* 68 (2010): 1491–1497.

17. Demetriades, D., B. Kimbrell, A. Salim, et al. "Trauma Deaths in a Mature Urban Trauma System: Is 'Trimodal' Distribution a Valid Concept?" *J Am Coll Surg* 201 (2005): 343–348.

18. Demetriades, D., M. Martin, A. Salim, P. Rhee, C. Brown, and L. Chan. "The Effect of Trauma Center Designation and Trauma Volume on Outcome in Specific Severe Injuries." *Ann Surg* 242 (2005): 512–517.

19. Dougherty, P. J., D. Sherman, N. Dau, and C. Bir. "Ballistic Fractures: Indirect Fractures to Bone." *J Trauma* 71(5) (Nov 2011): 1381–1384.

20. Glapa, M., et al. "Gunshot Wounds to the Head in Civilian Practice." *Am Surg* 75(3) (Mar 2009): 233–236.

21. Mabry, R. and J. G. McManus. "Prehospital Advances in the Management of Severe Penetrating Trauma." *Crit Care Med* 36 (2008): S258–S266.

Further Reading

American College of Surgeons, Committee on Trauma. *Advanced Trauma Life Support Course: Student Manual*. 9th ed. Chicago: American College of Surgeons, 2012.

American College of Surgeons, Committee on Trauma. *Resources for Optimal Care of the Injured Patient*. Chicago: American College of Surgeons, 2006.

Campbell, John E. *International Trauma Life Support for Prehospital Care Providers*. 7th ed. Upper Saddle River, NJ: Pearson/Prentice Hall, 2016.

De Lorenzo, Robert A., and Robert S. Porter. *Tactical Emergency Care: Military and Operational Out-of-Hospital Medicine*. Upper Saddle River, NJ: Pearson/Prentice Hall, 1999.

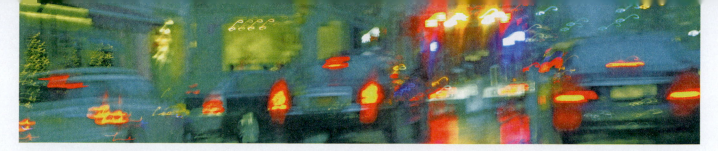

Chapter 3
Hemorrhage and Shock

Bryan E. Bledsoe, DO, FACEP, FAAEM, EMT-P

Robert S. Porter, MA, EMT-P

STANDARD
Trauma (Bleeding)

COMPETENCY
Integrates assessment findings with principles of epidemiology and pathophysiology to formulate a field impression to implement a comprehensive treatment/disposition plan for an acutely injured patient.

⌄ Learning Objectives

Terminal Performance Objective: After reading this chapter, you should be able to apply understanding of the pathophysiology of hemorrhage and shock to the assessment and management of trauma patients.

Enabling Objectives: To accomplish the terminal performance objective, you should be able to:

1. Define key terms introduced in this chapter.

2. Review the anatomy and basic physiology of the cardiovascular system and determinants of blood pressure.

3. Describe the characteristics and concerns associated with venous, arterial, and capillary bleeding.

4. Discuss the disruption of homeostasis that occurs due to hemorrhage and the body's compensatory mechanisms attempting to maintain homeostasis.

5. Describe the process of hemostasis and factors that can affect it.

6. Define internal and external hemorrhage and discuss appropriate progressive

measures for managing it, to include tourniquets, TXA administration, and topical hemostatic agents.

7. Identify what constitutes an internal hemorrhage, and if present, develop appropriate patient management plans.

8. Describe the pathophysiology and findings associated with the four classes of hemorrhage.

9. Describe the effects of hemorrhage on categories of special patients, such as pregnant women, athletes, obese patients, children, and the elderly.

10. Define and discuss the compensated, decompensated, and irreversible stages of shock.

11. Identify and discuss the phases of assessment as they relate to a patient suffering from blood loss.

12. Briefly describe the underlying pathophysiology of hypovolemic, distributive, neurogenic, obstructive, cardiogenic and respiratory causes of shock.

13. Demonstrate assessments that can identify patients with hemorrhage and shock.

14. Given various scenarios, discuss the management of patients with hemorrhage and shock to include the use of oxygen, intravenous therapy, pharmacology, and temperature regulation.

KEY TERMS

afterload, p. 60

aggregate, p. 62

anaerobic, p. 64

anaphylactic shock, p. 70

arteriole, p. 60

artery, p. 60

capillary, p. 61

cardiac contractility, p. 60

cardiogenic shock, p. 70

catecholamine, p. 67

clotting factors, p. 62

coagulation phase, p. 62

coagulopathy, p. 65

compensated shock, p. 69

decompensated shock, p. 69

direct pressure, p. 64

epistaxis, p. 65

erythrocyte, p. 61

extrinsic pathway, p. 62

fascia, p. 65

fibrin, p. 63

hematemesis, p. 66

hematochezia, p. 66

hematocrit, p. 61

hematoma, p. 65

hemoglobin, p. 61

hemoptysis, p. 66

hemorrhage, p. 59

hemostasis, p. 62

homeostasis, p. 59

hydrostatic pressure, p. 61

hypovolemic shock, p. 70

interstitial space, p. 61

intrinsic pathway, p. 63

irreversible shock, p. 69

lactic acid, p. 64

melena, p. 66

microcirculation, p. 60

neurogenic shock, p. 70

oncotic pressure, p. 61

orthostatic hypotension, p. 74

peripheral vascular resistance, p. 60

platelet, p. 62

platelet phase, p. 62

preload, p. 60

pulse pressure, p. 66

septic shock, p. 70

shock, p. 59

stroke volume, p. 60

tilt test, p. 74

tourniquet, p. 64

tranexamic acid (TXA), p. 65

vascular phase, p. 62

vein, p. 61

Case Study

City Ambulance 1 receives a mutual aid alert: a Basic Life Support ambulance needs assistance in a neighboring community. A bulldozer has overturned, trapping a 39-year-old man.

On arrival at the scene, paramedic Dave Felby and his junior partner, Ed Rouche, take a report from the two EMTs regarding a male patient named Ken. They then assess the patient themselves and find him alert and oriented. Ken's airway and breathing appear normal, as do his pulse rate and strength. His pelvis and lower extremities are pinned beneath the side of the bulldozer. The extrication team informs Dave and Ed

that it will be at least 15 minutes until they can lift and remove the bulldozer. Dave concludes the primary assessment and detects no signs of problems with airway, breathing, or circulation. Dave and Ed place Ken in the potentially unstable category for further care and transport.

Next, Dave provides a rapid trauma assessment as part of the secondary assessment. Ken's breath sounds are good, but he cannot feel his feet. From looking at the positions of the bulldozer and patient, Dave strongly suspects a pelvic fracture and expects increased internal and external hemorrhage when the heavy machine is lifted. Ed reports vital sign findings of blood pressure 110/68 mmHg, pulse 90 and strong, respirations 24, and an oxygen saturation of 99 percent. Ed continues to monitor the oxygen saturation (which remains at 99 percent), and is prepared to administer supplemental oxygen if the saturation drops below 96 percent.

Dave then quickly establishes two IVs of normal saline with large-bore catheters, both infusing at a to-keep-open rate. Ed prepares a scoop stretcher and a pelvic sling for the anticipated pelvic injury. Dave attaches the 12-lead ECG to monitor for cardiac changes that might occur with the lift of the bulldozer and release into the bloodstream of accumulating toxins. As lifting equipment is readied, the paramedics talk with Ken, explaining the various steps of the operation. Ed rechecks vital signs every 5 minutes, and Dave documents that the vital signs and oxygen saturation remain stable.

The extrication team slowly begins to lift the bulldozer. Dave and Ed rush to position Ken on the prepared scoop stretcher. It quickly becomes apparent that Ken has suffered fractures of the pelvis, both femurs, and the left tibia, and very little external hemorrhage is noted. Ed applies a pelvic binder to stabilize the pelvis.

Ken reports an increase in pain, becomes restless, and attempts to get up. He then becomes lethargic. The pulse oximeter reveals that oxygen saturation has dropped to 94 percent and then reads erratically. Ken's pulse rate is rapid and weak at about 160 beats per minute, and his systolic blood pressure is now 80 mmHg, as determined by palpation. Both IVs are set to run wide open to administer 1,000 mL of fluid before the next blood pressure assessment. With time, Ken's level of consciousness improves, but his pulse rate remains elevated.

On arrival at the hospital, Ken's systolic blood pressure remains around 80 mmHg and his heart rate is 140. A repeat rapid infusion of 500 mL of fluid is administered and his systolic blood pressure is reevaluated. It now reads 82 and the pulse rate is 116. While carefully monitoring Ken's vital signs, ECG monitor, and urine output, the emergency physician repeats 20 mL/kg normal saline boluses to mitigate the uncompensated (hypotensive) shock and prevent the effects of hyperkalemia and acidemia from the crush injury. Type-specific blood is administered because of the presumed large blood loss in the pelvis and lower extremities. CT scanning on the lower body confirms the multiple fractures and suggests that an operation to stabilize the unstable pelvis fracture will be needed.

Because of Ken's good physical condition and excellent prehospital, emergency department, and in-hospital care, he comes through the surgery well. Because of the multiple fractures, however, his rehabilitation will continue for more than a year.

Introduction to Hemorrhage and Shock

Shock, at the most fundamental level, can be defined as a state of inadequate tissue perfusion. Beyond this simple definition, however, shock is a complicated transitional stage between normal life (**homeostasis**) and death. It is the ultimate killer of all trauma and medical patients and often presents with limited signs and symptoms until it reaches a point at which the body can no longer compensate for the injury or disease and death occurs. Because of this, it is important that paramedics understand the shock process, learn to recognize early signs and symptoms, and intervene quickly and aggressively.

The most common form of shock associated with trauma is hemorrhagic shock (a form of hypovolemic shock—see "Etiology of Shock" later in the chapter). It results from blood loss (either internal or external) from the vascular container. This blood loss is called **hemorrhage**. Hemorrhage may be very minor and stop on its own, or may be massive and continue until the heart no longer has enough blood to pump to the body's cells. Hemorrhage is a frequent complication of trauma and a common cause of shock and death in trauma patients.

Although all people are subject to the effects of trauma, shock, and traumatic death, the population most at risk for trauma and trauma death is young adult males. Risk-taking behavior and a diminished regard for safety result in this group accounting for about 75 percent of trauma deaths. In this group, behavior modification and education plays a major role in helping to reduce trauma-related death and disability.

This chapter provides a brief review of the cardiovascular system as it relates to hemorrhage and shock. It then describes how to recognize and care for life-threatening hemorrhage and shock.

The Circulatory System

The three basic components of the circulatory system are the *heart*, the *blood vessels*, and the *blood*. These three elements contribute to homeostasis (the body's ability to maintain a stable and steady state) and generally play a key role in the development of shock.

The Heart

Blood flow through the circulatory system depends on a properly functioning heart (pump). The volume of blood ejected from the heart with each beat is called **stroke volume** and is determined by the blood flowing to the heart (**preload**), the strength of contraction (**cardiac contractility**), and the resistance to blood flow out of the heart (**afterload** or peripheral vascular resistance) (Figure 3-1).

The heart maintains an efficient pumping function through a rate range of 50 to 180 beats per minute (BPM). Below 50 BPM, cardiac output becomes insufficient (except in well-conditioned athletes). Above 180 BPM, the blood volume returning to the heart begins to decrease, resulting in decreased ventricular filling, stroke volume, and cardiac output. The normal heart, at rest, beats about 70 times per minute and moves about 70 mL of blood with each beat. Normal cardiac output is about 5 L/minute (70 mL of blood × 70 BPM = 4.9 L).

The Vascular System

The vascular system consists of three types of vessels: *arteries*, *capillaries*, and *veins*. The smallest arteries and veins, which are very muscular, are called *arterioles* and

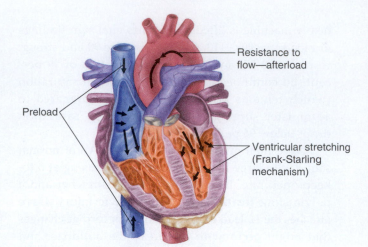

FIGURE 3-1 Factors affecting stroke volume.

venules, respectively. The smaller vessels (arterioles, capillaries, and venules) are referred to as the **microcirculation** (Figure 3-2).

ARTERIES   **Arteries** contain about 13 percent of total blood volume and have a thick external layer (tunica adventitia) that helps determine the artery's maximum diameter. The largest arteries distribute blood, at pressure, to the various regions of the body. The smaller arteries (**arterioles**) have a significant ability to vary their lumen size and control blood flow to the organs they supply and are the major determinants of **peripheral vascular resistance**.

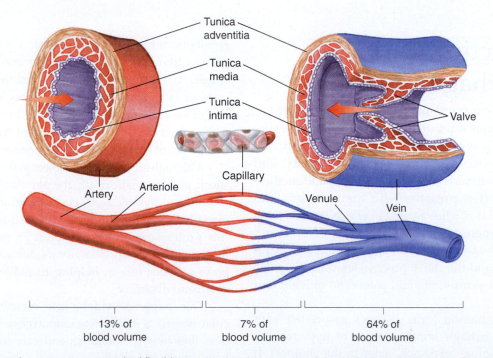

FIGURE 3-2 The vascular system is a network of flexible continuous tubing running from the heart to the body's tissues and back. Arteries distribute oxygenated blood, capillaries are the sites of oxygen–nutrient/waste product exchange, and veins return blood to the heart.

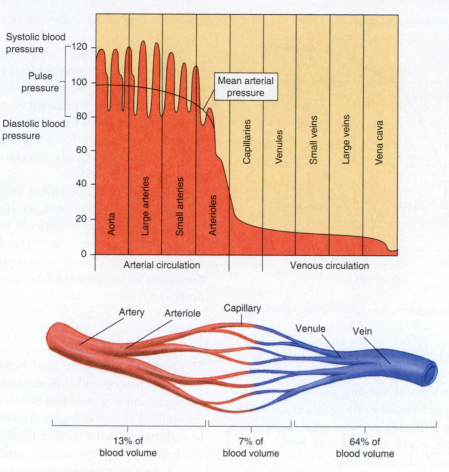

FIGURE 3-3 Vascular distribution and control of circulation.

Mean arterial pressure (MAP), which is the measure of peripheral vascular resistance, is estimated as follows:

$$MAP = \frac{(\text{Diastolic Pressure} + \text{Diastolic Pressure} + \text{Systolic Pressure})}{3}$$

Mean arterial pressure is well maintained through the arteries as they distribute blood to the arterioles. As blood moves from arterioles to capillaries, MAP drops from 80 mmHg to about 30 mmHg and continues to drop significantly as blood travels through the capillaries. Blood enters the venous system at a pressure of about 18 mmHg. As blood returns to the heart, the vascular pressure continues to drop to well below 10 mmHg (Figure 3-3).

CAPILLARIES   **Capillaries** are microscopic vessels only large enough for red blood cells to pass through in single file. They are found in close proximity to all body cells, and contain 7 percent of the vascular volume. Their walls are typically one cell thick, thus allowing efficient gas and metabolic substrate movement into and out of the **interstitial spaces.** Capillaries are not solid tubes, but have small spaces between the cells of their walls. As blood flows into the capillaries, **hydrostatic pressure** pushes intracapillary fluid (with oxygen and nutrients) into the interstitial space. As blood moves to the capillaries' distal end, the hydro-

static pressure drops significantly and the pressure exerted by protein materials in the plasma (**oncotic pressure**) pulls fluids (with carbon dioxide and waste products) back into the capillary. This fluid movement in and out of the capillary is called net filtration.

VEINS   Veins contain about 64 percent of the blood volume (and are thus called *capacitance vessels*). They contain a small amount of both connective tissue (tunica adventitia) and musculature (tunica media) in their walls. Although venous musculature is limited, any constriction significantly reduces venous vascular volume and can return up to 1 liter (about 20 percent of circulating blood volume) to the active circulation. This venous constriction is very effective in maintaining venous return (preload) in the early stages of hypovolemic (low volume) shock.

The Blood

Blood is a mixture of water, cells, proteins, and other suspended elements. Plasma, the fluid portion of blood, accounts for about 55 percent of blood volume and consists mostly of water, some dissolved salts, proteins, and other necessary materials. Red blood cells (**erythrocytes**) make up most of the remaining 45 percent of the blood volume (**hematocrit**). Erythrocytes contain **hemoglobin**, which is

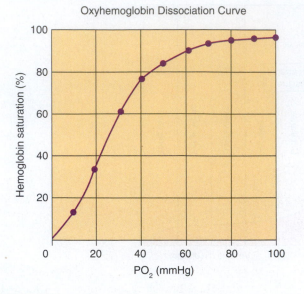

Oxyhemoglobin Dissociation Curve

FIGURE 3-4 The oxyhemoglobin dissociation curve.

responsible for oxygen transport from the alveoli to the cells. The relationship between the ability of hemoglobin to bind and release oxygen at varying partial pressures is described by the oxyhemoglobin dissociation curve (Figure 3-4). Most carbon dioxide is transported as bicarbonate, but hemoglobin plays a minor role in the carbon dioxide transport from cells to the lungs.

The second most frequent blood cell type is the **platelet**, a small, irregularly shaped cytoplasm fragment that is important for clotting and blood vessel repair.

Types of Hemorrhage

Hemorrhage is blood loss from the vascular space, usually resulting from blood vessel injury. It is the loss of whole blood—plasma and red blood cells—and can be lost either to the surface of the body (externally) or within the body (internally). The type of vessel injured usually classifies hemorrhage: arterial, venous, or capillary.

Capillary hemorrhage generally oozes from the wound. It is often caused by an abrasion or similar minor injury and stops quickly. Capillary blood is often bright red because it is well oxygenated.

Venous hemorrhage flows more quickly, though it tends to stop in a few minutes. Venous hemorrhage is generally dark because most of the oxygen has been depleted after passage though the capillary beds. Venous hemorrhage can sometimes be extensive, depending on the size and number of the vessels involved.

Arterial hemorrhage flows very rapidly—often spurting from the wound. Arterial blood is well oxygenated and appears bright red. Blood volume lost through arterial hemorrhage can be significant because of the associated pressure and the vessel size. Arterial hemorrhage also continues to bleed longer than either capillary or venous hemorrhage and is commonly associated with a greater rate and volume of blood loss.

Although it is convenient to try and determine the type of hemorrhage present, the depth and nature of the wound often make it difficult to differentiate heavy venous bleeding from arterial bleeding. Obviously, internal hemorrhage cannot be classified by type with the diagnostic techniques available to paramedics providing prehospital care.

Hemostasis

The body's response to local hemorrhage is a complex three-step process called **hemostasis**. As a blood vessel is damaged and begins to lose blood, smooth muscle within the walls of the vessel begins to contract, causing the vessel to withdraw into the wound, thicken the wall, and reduce the lumen size. These actions serve to reduce the rate of flow and volume through the vessel and out of the wound. This is called the **vascular phase** of hemostasis.

At the same time, injury also disrupts the vessel's smooth interior lining (tunica intima), causing turbulent blood flow. Turbulent blood flow, in addition to the various substances released by the injured blood vessel wall, causes the platelets to become adherent. These adherent platelets stick to each other and to collagen (protein) fibers that are exposed by the injury to the vessel. Nearby blood vessel walls also become adherent and, if the vessel is small enough (such as capillaries, arterioles, or venules), the walls may stick together, further impeding blood flow. As platelets **aggregate**, or collect and adhere, this **platelet phase** of hemostasis serves to slow the hemorrhage from capillaries and other small vessels. Although this second phase of the hemostasis is a rapid method of hemorrhage control, the resulting clot is often unstable.

With time, the third and final step of hemostasis, the **coagulation phase**, occurs. With coagulation, various **clotting factors** are activated and released into the bloodstream, initiating a complex cascade of events. These clotting factors (specific proteins) come from the damaged blood vessel walls and surrounding tissue (the **extrinsic pathway**) and from platelets damaged by turbulence

CONTENT REVIEW

➤ Types of Hemorrhage
  • Capillary
  • Venous
  • Arterial
➤ It may be hard to differentiate between heavy venous and arterial bleeding in the field; likewise, paramedics cannot classify internal hemorrhage by type when providing prehospital care.

CONTENT REVIEW

➤ Phases of Hemostasis
  • Vascular phase
  • Platelet phase
  • Coagulation phase

and aggregation (the **intrinsic pathway**). The release of these clotting factors triggers a series of chemical reactions that cause formation of strong protein fibers called **fibrin**. Individual fibrin strands adhere forming a strong protein mesh that entraps red blood cells, thus forming a stronger, more durable clot. Coagulation normally takes from 7 to 10 minutes depending on the patient's overall condition. Over time, fibers and the cells trapped in the clot's protein matrix slowly contract, closing the wound opening and the injured blood vessel walls.

The wound type affects hemostasis and clot formation. When a wound lacerates a vessel cleanly, the muscles in the vascular wall contract. This draws the torn vessel into the surrounding tissues and thickens the tunica media. This thickening further reduces the vessel's lumen, reduces blood flow, and assists in hemostasis. If the blood vessel is lacerated longitudinally rather than transversely, the vascular smooth muscle contraction can actually open the vessel, causing heavier and prolonged bleeding (Figure 3-5). If severe hemorrhage continues and hypotension occurs, the reduced blood pressure at the hemorrhage site subsequently limits blood flow, the rate of hemorrhage, and enhances clot development. Thus, systemic hypotension may be beneficial in controlling serious internal hemorrhage.

Factors Affecting Hemostasis

Numerous factors can affect hemostasis. For example, manipulation and movement of tissues around the wound can slow hemostasis and clot formation. Thus, early bandaging and splinting can aid hemostasis.

Aggressive fluid therapy, which in the past was used to treat severe hemorrhage, may adversely affect hemostasis. Large volumes of crystalloid IV fluids can increase blood pressure, which, in turn, increases the intravascular pressure (blood pressure) placing pressure on developing clots. In addition, infusing large volumes of IV fluids tends to dilute the needed clotting factors and platelets, further inhibiting the hemostasis. It is important to remember that fluid resuscitation with non-blood infusions do not replace the lost red blood cells needed for oxygen transport, thus decreasing the oxygen-carrying capacity of the blood. Thus, there is a delicate balance between providing sufficient and timely fluid in the prehospital phase of resuscitation to maintain an acceptable blood pressure while avoiding the potential consequences of hemodilution and overhydration with crystalloid.[1]

The patient's body temperature can also affect hemostasis. As the body temperature falls below normal, as often occurs in shock, hemostasis is generally slower and less effective. Thus, it is extremely important to avoid hypothermia in patients with severe hemorrhage.

Certain medications taken to prevent or limit heart attack or stroke, by definition, slow clot formation and

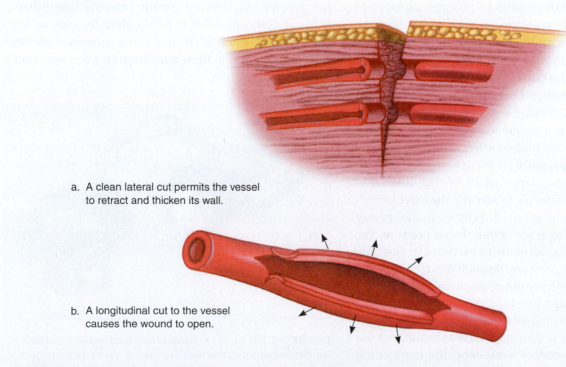

a. A clean lateral cut permits the vessel to retract and thicken its wall.

b. A longitudinal cut to the vessel causes the wound to open.

FIGURE 3-5 The type of blood vessel injury often affects the nature of the hemorrhage.

places these patients at increased risk for hemorrhage. For example, aspirin, a common drug used to prevent and treat heart attacks and strokes, inhibits platelet aggregation, thus slowing and preventing clot formation. Nonsteroidal anti-inflammatory drugs (NSAIDs), such as ibuprofen, can have effects similar to aspirin. Clopidogrel (Plavix), a commonly used platelet aggregation inhibitor, can also slow and affect the hemostasis. Anticoagulant medications, such as heparin, enoxaparin (Lovenox), warfarin (Coumadin), and dabigatran (Pradaxa), slow and interfere with hemostasis through direct effect on the coagulation cascade. These medications are effective in the prevention of clot formation and subsequent thrombosis and embolism in patients with known heart and vascular disease. However, they may also prolong or worsen hemorrhage in injured patients. Thus, it is important to try and determine whether trauma patients are taking these types of medications as these can slow hemostasis and worsen hemorrhage (both internal and external).

Hemorrhage Control

As detailed earlier, hemorrhage may be either internal or external. Although there are a number of steps that can be taken to control external hemorrhage in the field, prehospital care of internal hemorrhage is limited to early recognition, shock care, and rapid transport.

External Hemorrhage

Most external hemorrhage is relatively easy to recognize and control. However, it is important to note that serious blood loss can be hidden from view by clothing or body position. Always look for severe and continuing external hemorrhage during the primary assessment.

Capillary and venous bleeding from small vessels can almost always be controlled by firmly placing a bandage and dressing over the wound. The dressing quickly slows the blood flow and assists the natural clotting mechanisms. With hemorrhage from large veins and smaller arteries, blood volume flowing from the wound, and the pressure behind it, are somewhat higher. Minimize blood flow by applying firm **direct pressure** on the dressing and wound. If the wound involves a large artery or it is difficult to apply pressure to the site, try to identify the exact hemorrhage site and apply pressure directly to it. The power behind arterial bleeding is the systolic blood pressure. The systolic pressure can be can easily be exceeded by carefully applying direct finger pressure, through the dressing, onto the leaking vessel. With careful application of direct pressure, most hemorrhage can be controlled. In very rare cases, if ever, will a tourniquet be required.

If **tourniquet** use is considered, be judicious and use the device only to control persistent, life-threatening hemorrhage that cannot be otherwise controlled by direct pressure and elevation. Although tourniquets were once used infrequently, the use of tourniquets in civilian practice has increased. Much of this is due to experience in the tactical and military settings and to the development of commercial tourniquets that are easy to apply and remove. If you use a tourniquet, always try to apply it at a pressure adequate to stop arterial hemorrhage—but not more. If a tourniquet is effective in stopping all blood flow to the limb, blood loss stops. However, so does needed circulation to the affected extremity. During this absence of perfusion, **lactic acid**, potassium, and other **anaerobic** metabolites and acids tend to accumulate in the stagnant blood. When the tourniquet is released and blood flow resumes, these toxic products of metabolism move into the central circulation, potentially worsening the patient's condition (Figure 3-6). Once a tourniquet has been applied, allow it to remain in places until the patient arrives at the emergency department or a similar facility where blood replacement is available and the negative effects of reperfusion can be addressed. Tourniquets have been applied for hours during elective surgery with no adverse impact on a distal limb.

If a tourniquet is required, try to use a commercial tourniquet. Alternatively, use a wide cravat or belt or a blood pressure cuff. A thin or narrow tourniquet may damage underlying soft tissue and arteries and nerves beneath the tourniquet. Despite the risks of soft tissue damage and continued hemorrhage, a tourniquet may be required to control life-threatening arterial hemorrhage. Military experience with the tourniquet demonstrates its value in a battlefield environment (where there is extreme danger to the care provider while trying to control external hemorrhage). It has also shown value in severe limb injuries, as from high-velocity gunshot wounds and amputations from explosive devices. In these circumstances, moving rapidly

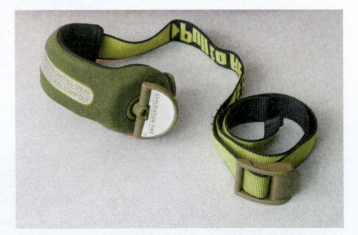

FIGURE 3-6 Release of a tourniquet may send accumulated toxins into the central circulation with devastating results for the patient.

to a tourniquet for bleeding control has been shown to improve outcomes. This has led to new developments in tourniquet technology, but the need for tourniquet use as a first-line care procedure in routine civilian practice has yet to be demonstrated. However, in the multi- or mass-casualty circumstance, tourniquet use may allow medical personnel care to quickly control serious arterial hemorrhage when they cannot afford to spend time caring for individual patients.

Internal Hemorrhage

Internal hemorrhage is associated with almost all forms of serious blunt and penetrating trauma. As with external hemorrhage, internal hemorrhage can involve capillary, venous, or arterial blood loss. Blood can accumulate in the interstitial spaces, resulting in a contusion or can be forced between tissue layers (**fascia**) forming a pocket of blood called a **hematoma**. With most internal hemorrhage, blood loss is self-limited because the pressure within the tissue or fascia ultimately controls the blood loss. However, large contusions, massive soft-tissue injuries, and large hematomas, especially those affecting large muscle masses such as the thighs or buttocks, can account for a moderate loss of blood. Long bone (e.g., humerus, radius, ulna, tibia, and fibula) fractures can cause up to 500 to 750 mL of blood loss, whereas femur fractures can cause up to 1,500 mL of blood loss. Pelvic fractures may account for even more significant hemorrhage.

Resistance to continuing blood loss generally does not occur in large body cavities such as the chest, abdomen (and retroperitoneum), and pelvis. Blood loss may continue unabated until it is halted by the normal clotting process, a significant drop in blood pressure, exsanguination, or surgical intervention.

The best indicators of significant internal hemorrhage are localized signs and symptoms and early signs and symptoms of blood loss and shock. If a patient has sustained significant trauma to the chest, abdomen, or pelvis, be alert for significant, continuing, and uncontrolled blood loss. Such patients require careful assessment and rapid transport to a trauma center or hospital for possible surgical treatment of their injuries. Recent evidence suggests that the mechanism of injury (MOI) may not be as good an injury severity predictor as was once thought. MOI is best used to help identify possible injuries and to guide assessment of specific injuries. MOI should be used in conjunction with careful evaluation of vital signs and the Glasgow Coma Score evaluation to determine a patient's transport priority.

There are some prehospital measures that can be used to attenuate internal hemorrhage. These include effective immobilization of injured extremities (including the pelvis). If the patient is a victim of serious or multisystem trauma (polytrauma), do not spend significant scene time performing comprehensive immobilization. Instead, quickly immobilize the patient to a long spine board and begin transport. Provide individual limb splinting, only if time permits, during transport.

The drug **tranexamic acid (TXA)** appears to play a beneficial role in the management of trauma and hemorrhagic shock. TXA is an antifibrinolytic, meaning that it inhibits fibrinolysis (the breakdown of blood clots).[2] Most patients with significant trauma will develop **coagulopathy**. Coagulopathy is a condition in which the blood's ability to clot is impaired. Several factors cause coagulopathy, including hypothermia, acidosis, and hemodilution (from IV fluid therapy). When fibrinolysis develops, the bleeding may increase. Studies have demonstrated that administration of TXA can reduce trauma mortality by mitigating fibrinolysis. Many EMS systems, especially those with a long transport time to a trauma center, have added TXA to their prehospital formulary (Figure 3-7).

Evidence of internal hemorrhage may present at any of the body orifices. This may be frank blood or blood modified by digestion, in addition to the physical signs and symptoms of hypovolemia. These signs can help to identify the type and location of the internal blood loss.

For example, the nasal cavity is lined with a rich supply of capillaries to warm and humidify inhaled air. Hypertension, a strong sneeze, or direct trauma may rupture vessels supplying these capillary beds and produce mild to moderate hemorrhage called **epistaxis**, commonly called nosebleed. Prolonged epistaxis can cause hypovolemia, and blood flowing into the posterior nasal cavity, down the esophagus, and into the stomach may result in nausea and vomiting. Trauma to the oral cavity may likewise result in serious hemorrhage, followed by ingestion of blood, resulting in nausea and then emesis. If blood is vomited shortly

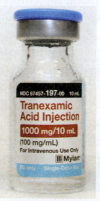

FIGURE 3-7 Several studies have shown that administration of tranexamic acid (TXA) to victims of significant trauma can mitigate bleeding by inhibiting fibrinolysis.

(© Edward T. Dickinson, MD)

after ingestion, it will often be bright red in color. If blood remains in the gastrointestinal tract for a long time, the body will begin to digest the blood and emesis can resemble coffee grounds in both color and consistency. Severe bleeding from epistaxis or the oral cavity can potentially obstruct the airway or cause aspiration in the supine patient because the natural protective mechanisms are less effective when supine. If possible, allow such patients to sit up or place them in the recovery position to promote a clear airway.

Lower respiratory injuries such as those caused by chest trauma can cause rupture of pulmonary vessels leading to hemorrhage into the lower airways including the alveoli. The patient may then cough up bright red blood (**hemoptysis**). The blood may mix with fluid and air in the lungs and subsequently be coughed out as pink, frothy sputum.

Injury to the upper digestive system may cause blood to accumulate in the stomach. This blood acts as a gastric irritant and can induce vomiting, with the emesis containing blood (**hematemesis**). As mentioned earlier, the longer blood remains in the stomach, the more it will resemble coffee grounds in both color and consistency.

Trauma to the small or large bowel can cause frank rectal bleeding, blood mixed with stool (**hematochezia**), or blood that remains in the bowel for some time and appear as a black and tarry stool (**melena**). Rectal injuries can occur in conjunction with pelvic fractures or direct trauma and may cause severe bright red hemorrhage. Vaginal hemorrhage may also be associated with trauma (although rare). Urethral hemorrhage is generally minor and may reflect damage to the prostate or urethra. Blood in the urine may indicate injury to the genitourinary tract.

Classes of Hemorrhage

Fluid accounts for about 60 percent of the body's weight and is distributed among the intracellular, interstitial, and intravascular spaces. The cells contain about approximately 62 percent of the total fluid volume (intracellular volume), whereas the interstitial space (nonvascular space between the cells) holds approximately 26 percent. Four to five percent of body fluid is found in other spaces, such as

the ventricles of the brain, chambers of the eyes, and meninges (cerebrospinal fluid). The remaining 7 percent of fluid volume resides in the intravascular space or compartment. Fluid in the vascular space is distributed among the heart, arteries, veins, and capillaries and accounts for about 5 liters (10 units) of blood volume in the healthy 70-kg adult male.

Hemorrhage is typically categorized into four classes. These classes relate to blood volume lost in acute hemorrhage and result in "classic" signs and symptoms of hemorrhage and shock. Remember, however, that the actual rate of blood loss may vary as an individual's response to blood volume loss may vary. Use these hemorrhage classes to help determine the relative loss and the need for intervention.[3] It is also important to identify the time elapsed since the injury, the class of hemorrhage suspected on initial patient contact, and the rate at which shock appears to be worsening (Table 3-1).

- *Class I hemorrhage* is a blood loss of up to 15 percent of the circulating blood volume. In a 70-kg male, that is up to 750 mL of blood, slightly more than you might give during a blood drive. The healthy patient can easily compensate for such a blood volume loss by constricting the vascular beds, especially on the venous side. In this class, the blood pressure remains constant, as do **pulse pressure**, respiratory rate, and urine

Table 3-1 Patient Signs Associated with Stages of Hemorrhage

Stage	Blood Loss	Vasoconstriction	Pulse Rate	Pulse (Pressure) Strength	Blood Pressure	Respiratory Rate	Respiratory Volume
1	<15 percent	↑	↑	→	→	→	→
2	15–30 percent	↑↑	↑↑	↓	→	↑	↑
3	30–40 percent	↑↑↑	↑↑↑	↓↓	↓	↑↑	↓
4	>40 percent	↓↓	Variable	↓↓↓	↓↓↓	↓	↓↓

output. Central venous pressure may drop slightly but quickly returns to normal. The pulse rate increases slightly, and the patient may display some signs of **catecholamine** (epinephrine and norepinephrine) release, notably nervousness and marginally cool skin with a slight pallor.

- *Class II hemorrhage* occurs as 15 to 30 percent (750 to 1,500 mL in an adult) of the circulating blood volume is lost. The body's first-line compensatory responses can no longer maintain perfusion and secondary mechanisms are now employed. Tachycardia occurs, the pulse pressure narrows, and the pulse strength diminishes. A strong catecholamine release serves to increase peripheral vascular resistance. This helps to maintain the systolic blood pressure but results in signs and symptoms of peripheral vasoconstriction (e.g., cool, clammy skin). Anxiety increases, and the patient may begin to display restlessness and thirst. Thirst is present as fluid leaves the intracellular and interstitial spaces and the blood's osmotic pressure begins to change. Renal output remains normal, but the respiratory rate increases.

- *Class III hemorrhage* occurs when blood loss reaches 30 to 40 percent of blood volume (1,500 to 2,000 mL in an adult). The body's compensatory mechanisms are unable to cope with the loss, and classic signs of shock appear. Tachycardia is more pronounced as the blood pressure begins to fall. The pulse is barely palpable and the pulse pressure becomes even narrower. The patient may display dyspnea and tachypnea. Anxiety, restlessness, and thirst become more pronounced. Mental status may be altered and the patient will become pale, cool, and diaphoretic. Urinary output declines. Patents with this class of shock are still compensating for the blood loss, but the process is rapidly becoming more difficult for the body to sustain (compensation is becoming more and more ineffective).

- *Class IV hemorrhage* occurs with a blood loss of more than 40 percent of the body's total blood supply (greater than 2,000 mL). The patient's pulse is barely palpable in the central arteries, if one can be found at all. Respirations are very rapid, shallow, and ineffective. The patient is very lethargic and confused, moving rapidly toward unconsciousness and unresponsiveness. The skin is very cool, clammy, and extremely pale. Urinary output ceases. Even with aggressive fluid resuscitation and blood transfusions, patient survival is unlikely.

These descriptions of the classes of hemorrhage presume that the patient is a normally healthy adult. Any preexisting condition (e.g., hydration status, medication usage, age) can affect the volume of blood loss and speed the transition from one hemorrhage class to another.

The rate of blood loss also has a profound effect on how quickly a patient transitions from class I to class IV. If the blood loss is very rapid, compensatory mechanisms may not have time to work effectively. However, a small wound bleeding uncontrolled but very slowly for days may not move the patient from class I to class II, even with a loss much greater than 750 mL.

Certain patient categories—pregnant women, athletes, obese patients, children, those with alcohol intoxication, and the elderly—react differently to blood loss. The blood volume of a woman in late pregnancy is around 50 percent greater than a normal nonpregnant female. She may lose greater blood volumes before moving through progressive hemorrhage classes. Although the expectant mother is somewhat protected from the effects of serious hemorrhage, the fetus may be deprived of adequate circulation early in the blood loss and is more susceptible to harm.

A well-conditioned athlete often has greater cardiac reserves and a more robust cardiovascular system than a typical patient. Therefore, the athlete may move more slowly through the early classes of hemorrhage with greater loss percentages needed to transition from one class to another.

Obese patients have a blood volume close to 7 percent of their ideal body weight, not their actual weight. Their total blood volume, as a percentage of actual body weight, is lower than for non-obese patients. This means that what appears to be only a small blood loss may have a more serious effect in such patients.

Infants and young children have blood volumes approximately 8 to 9 percent of their body weight. This represents a blood volume about 20 percent greater than for an adult. However, infant and child compensatory mechanisms are neither as well developed nor as effective. These young patients may not demonstrate early signs and symptoms of hemorrhage compensation as clearly as with adults. They may instead show few signs of blood loss until they move quickly into shock's later stages. Always remember to consider the possibility of shock in pediatric trauma patients and be prepared to treat blood loss aggressively.

Alcohol may increase the likelihood of injury and may also negatively affect the body's systems as they attempt to compensate for hemorrhage and shock. As a central nervous system depressant and a dilator of peripheral vessels, alcohol slows the speed and effectiveness of compensation and may limit the degree of the body's shock responses.

The elderly are likewise more adversely affected by blood loss than average adults. They have lower fluid reserve volumes and their compensatory systems are less responsive to fluid losses. These patients may also be on medications such as beta-blockers and anticoagulants that further reduce the body's response to blood loss. Often, elderly patients do not experience the tachycardia associated with blood loss, and their blood pressures drop before those of healthy adults. Signs of blood loss and shock may

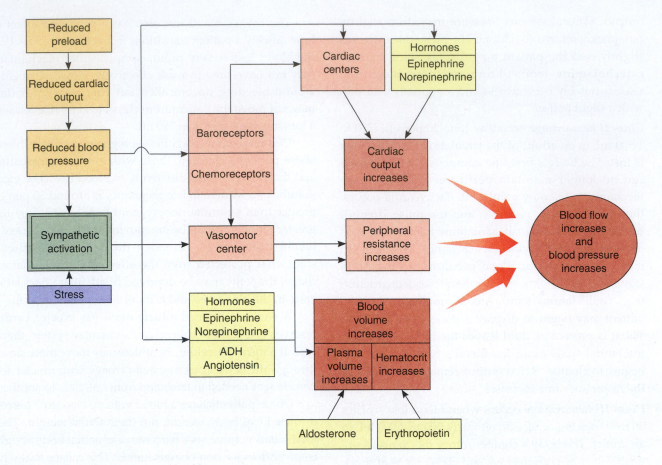

FIGURE 3-8 The body's response to blood loss.

be masked by reduced pain perception in the elderly and by lowered levels of mental acuity resulting from disease. The elderly also do not tolerate periods of inadequate tissue perfusion well because of chronic cardiovascular inefficiency. Lastly, the elderly patient is more prone to hypothermia (possibly chronic), which interferes with clotting mechanisms.

Hemorrhage, whether internal or external, can lead to shock. This type of shock is called *hemorrhagic shock*, a subclass of hypovolemic shock, and is commonly associated with trauma. That said, shock in trauma can sometimes caused by other mechanisms and may be due to multiple factors (Figure 3-8).

Stages of Shock

The shock process, as previously described, can be divided into three stages based on the body's ability to compensate and the presenting signs and symptoms. These stages are progressively more serious, and include compensated, decompensated, and irreversible shock (Table 3-2).

CONTENT REVIEW

➤ Stages of Shock
  • Compensated
  • Decompensated
  • Irreversible

Table 3-2 The Stages of Shock

Compensated Shock

Initial stage of shock in which the body progressively compensates for continuing blood loss.

- Pulse rate increases.
- Pulse strength decreases.
- Skin becomes cool and clammy.
- Progressing anxiety, restlessness, combativeness.
- Thirst, weakness, eventual air hunger.

Decompensated Shock

Begins when the body's compensatory mechanisms can no longer maintain preload.

- Pulse becomes unpalpable.
- Blood pressure drops precipitously.
- Patient becomes unconscious.
- Respirations slow or cease.

Irreversible Shock

Shortly after the patient enters decompensated shock, the lack of circulation begins to have profound effects on body cells. As they are irreversibly damaged, the cells die, tissues dysfunction, organs dysfunction, and the patient dies.

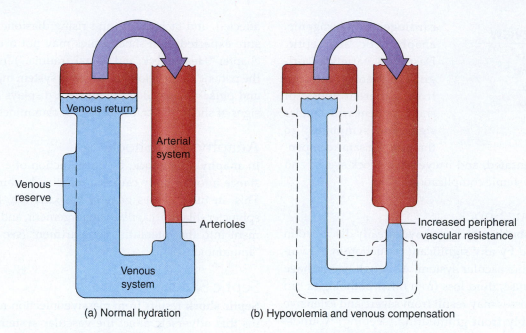

(a) Normal hydration   (b) Hypovolemia and venous compensation

FIGURE 3-9 In compensated shock, the body reduces venous capacitance in response to blood loss.

Compensated Shock

Compensated shock is the initial shock state. In this stage, the body is capable of meeting its critical metabolic needs through a series of progressive compensating actions (Figure 3-9). This progressive compensation creates a series of signs and symptoms that range from subtle to obvious. Compensated shock ends with a precipitous drop in blood pressure. This is the shock stage in which prehospital interventions and rapid transport are most likely to be successful.

A patient's first recognizable response to serious blood loss is an increase in pulse rate. However, this may be difficult to differentiate from tachycardia caused by pain, excitement, and the autonomic sympathetic response. The first sign reliably attributable to shock is a narrowing pulse pressure, as cardiac output drops and peripheral vascular resistance increases to maintain circulation. The pulse weakens and the rate increases. During the initial hypovolemic state, the patient may complain of thirst. As blood loss continues and becomes more serious, vasoconstriction will cause the patient's skin to become pale, cyanotic, or ashen as blood is directed away from skin and toward more critical organs. The skin also becomes cool and moist (clammy) and capillary refill times increase. The respiratory rate increases slowly and becomes more labored (increased minute volume). As compensation continues, the patient may become anxious, restless, or even combative. Patients often complain of increasing thirst and weakness. Near the end of the compensated shock stage, the patient may experience dyspnea and tachypnea.

Decompensated Shock

Decompensated shock begins as compensatory mechanisms become unable to compensate for continuing blood loss. The hallmark of decompensated shock is the inability to maintain a normal blood pressure. As compensatory mechanisms fail, venous return becomes inadequate and blood return to the heart is inadequate to maintain an adequate cardiac output. In this case, even extreme tachycardia produces little additional cardiac output. No amount of vascular resistance can continue to maintain blood pressure and circulation. Even the most critical organs of the body are now hypoperfused. The heart, already hypoxic because of poor perfusion and the increased oxygen demands created by tachycardia and increased contractility, begins to fail. In this stage, the brain is extremely hypoxic, causing a rapidly declining level of responsiveness. The brain's control over bodily functions, including respiration, diminishes, and the body takes on a deathlike appearance.

Irreversible Shock

Irreversible shock exists when the body's cells are so badly injured and die in such quantities that organs no longer are able to function normally. Although aggressive resuscitation may restore blood pressure and a pulse, organ failure ultimately results in death. The transition between decompensated and irreversible shock is a clinical one and impossible to differentiate using signs or symptoms. Clearly, the longer a patient is in decompensated shock, the more likely it is that he will develop irreversible shock.

Etiology of Shock

The shock discussion to this point has focused on blood loss and its effects on the cardiovascular system. However, shock can have many causes, and a common way of classifying types of shock is based on its origins: hypovolemic, cardiogenic, neurogenic, anaphylactic, and septic. Despite a variety of origins, patients suffering from different types of shock present with similar signs and symptoms; go through the same compensated, decompensated, and irreversible shock stages; and suffer similar systemic complications.

Hypovolemic Shock

Hypovolemic shock, which we have already discussed in detail, is caused by any significant reduction in the volume of the cardiovascular system. Although hemorrhage is a common cause, fluid loss from other pathologies can occur. Plasma losses may result from severe and extensive burns or possibly from granulating (seeping) wounds. Fluid and electrolyte losses, such as those that occur with protracted vomiting, diarrhea, sweating, and urination, also diminish the body's vascular fluids and may result in hypovolemia. Hypovolemic shock may also result from "third space" losses such as fluid shifts into various body compartments, as occurs in severe pancreatitis. Hemorrhagic shock is a specific subset of hypovolemia caused by blood loss.

Cardiogenic Shock

Cardiogenic shock results from cardiac insufficiency. Because of the heart's essential function, any cardiac pathology has a profound impact on circulation. If cardiac artery blockage deprives a portion of the heart muscle of oxygenated circulation, it becomes hypoxic, then ischemic, and then necrotic. During infarct evolution, cardiac electrical system disturbances, cardiac valve failure, cardiac rupture, or reduced cardiac pumping action may occur. Any of these problems reduces cardiac output, which cannot be compensated for by some other body system. If cardiac output falls below what the body requires, cardiogenic shock ensues. Cardiogenic shock may present with the signs and symptoms of myocardial infarction or pulmonary edema and with the classic signs and symptoms of shock. The prognosis for cardiogenic shock is very poor, with an 80 percent mortality rate.

Neurogenic Shock

Neurogenic shock results from an interruption in the communication pathway between the central nervous system and the body. A spinal injury or, in some cases, a head injury, either temporary or permanent, disrupts nervous (generally sympathetic nervous) system control over vasculature distal to the injury. Arterioles dilate, the vascular container expands, and fluid is driven into the interstitial space. The body's compensatory mechanisms are often affected, and tachycardia and rising diastolic blood pressure expected with shock states may not occur. (See the chapter "Head, Neck, and Spinal Trauma.") In these cases, the patient's skin below the nervous system injury is warm and pink, whereas the skin above it displays more classic signs of shock: pallor, coolness, and clamminess.

Anaphylactic Shock

In **anaphylactic shock**, the introduction of a foreign substance into the body causes a massive histamine release. This, in turn, causes general vasodilation, precapillary sphincter dilation, capillary engorgement, and fluid movement into the interstitial compartment (see the chapter "Immunology").

Septic Shock

Septic shock results from massive infection releasing toxins that adversely affect the vascular system's ability to control blood vessels and distribute blood.

Assessment of the Patient with Hemorrhage and Shock

Assessment of the patient with hemorrhage and shock follows the same priorities as for other conditions. However, it is more focused, based on the need to quickly determine the need for more comprehensive care. In trauma, minimizing out-of-hospital time can improve patient outcomes and decrease morbidity and mortality.

Scene Size-Up

Remember that Standard Precautions are essential during trauma patient assessment. Standard Precautions protect you from possible disease transmission from the patient, but they also protect the patient from any diseases or you may have (or carry). In fact, the risk of your transmitting disease or infection to patients with open wounds or burns is much greater than the risk that they will transmit disease or infection to you. For these reasons, use Standard Precautions with all trauma patients. These precautions include using gloves and a mask when you inspect or palpate any injured area, especially one with open wounds.

Always look for other scene hazards, such as traffic, downed electrical wires, sharp objects, fire and explosives, hot objects, hazardous materials, confined spaces, structural instability, hazardous terrain, environmental extremes, and violence. If these hazards cannot be excluded and the scene rendered safe, do not enter. Also, ensure the safety of fellow rescuers, the patient (or patients), and bystanders.

Always evaluate weather conditions on scene, as these will affect patient assessment and care. Remember that extremes of temperature can provide additional stress to the patient who is in shock. Overall, be sure to keep the hemorrhage and shock patient warm.

When scene hazards have been addressed, continue with scene size-up. Evaluate the mechanism of injury (MOI) to anticipate external and internal hemorrhage so you can begin to plan treatment and transport.

When evaluating the MOI, also attempt to determine the time elapsed between the injury and assessment. Knowing this time interval is important in determining the amount and rate of blood loss. For example, if a patient is losing about 150 mL of blood per minute and you arrive on a scene 3 minutes after an injury, the patient will have lost 450 mL of blood. Thus, you would not expect this patient to display signs and symptoms of Class I hemorrhage. If, however, you arrive 10 minutes after the incident, the same patient, losing blood at the same rate, will have lost 1,500 mL of blood and is likely to have reached Class III hemorrhage and to display frank signs of shock. In both these cases, the patient is suffering serious, life-threatening hemorrhage. Good assessment techniques and early hemorrhage severity recognition will help ensure the proper course of care.

Finally, complete the remaining elements of the scene size-up. Be sure to identify and locate all possible patients and determine what effect, if any, environmental conditions will have on patient assessment, care, and transport. Last, ensure that there is scene oversight. In a limited event, assign roles to the members of your team. In a large event or one in which there are several or many services involved, employ a more involved system of incident management.

Primary Assessment

The primary assessment addresses immediate threats to life. As the primary assessment begins, try to develop a general patient impression of injury severity. Always assess the patient's initial mental status to determine alertness, orientation, and responsiveness. Be alert for any signs of anxiety, confusion, or combativeness. Any change in mental status may be secondary to hemorrhage, hypovolemia, and shock, so be suspicious. Also look for facial expression and any signs of fear that might suggest how the patient perceives his condition. Carefully observe the patient's body surface and consider the possible presence of shock, either as a causative or contributing factor to the patient's overall condition. Look at the patient's general skin condition. It should be warm, pink, and dry. If it is cyanotic, gray, ashen, pale, and cool and moist (clammy), suspect peripheral vasoconstriction—an early sign of shock. Using this information, formulate a preliminary patient impression that continues to evolve during all aspects of assessment and

care. If the patient is in cardiac arrest, begin the CAB of CPR, in which circulatory support (compressions) precedes airway and breathing care. Otherwise, continue with the ABC approach to primary assessment and care, as well as secondary assessment and trauma care.

If spinal injury cannot be excluded, provide spinal precautions. (Apply manual stabilization but delay cervical collar application until after assessment of the neck during the rapid trauma assessment.)

Assess the airway for patency and breathing adequacy. Assess oxygenation and provide supplemental oxygen if the patient is hypoxic (based on the SpO_2). Ensure that injuries do not interfere with airway control and that the patient is fully able to protect his airway. If the airway cannot be maintained, endotracheal intubation or an extraglottic airway should be considered.

Carefully visualize the chest and observe the patient's respiratory effort and chest excursion. Watch for tachypnea and air hunger, which are late signs of shock. Continue to monitor oxygen saturation and keep it at least 96 percent, if possible. If it falls below 90 percent, consider ventilating the patient.

Capnography is a valuable assessment tool during trauma patient care and is now a standard of care. Waveform capnography analysis helps ensure proper initial and continuing endotracheal tube placement and guides artificial ventilation. It can also provide information regarding the severity of shock (acidosis). Falling capnography readings indicate a worsening patient condition. Increased CO_2 levels indicate hypoventilation, respiratory depression, or hyperthermia. $ETCO_2$ readings above 40 mmHg suggest the need for increased ventilatory support. Readings below 30 mmHg suggest hyperventilation or the need for circulatory support. Capnography may not signal intubation of a mainstem bronchus, so ensure that breath sounds are bilaterally equal while an endotracheal tube is in place.

Capnography is especially important in head-injured patients who are intubated, as abnormally low alveolar CO_2 levels (hyperventilation) may produce cerebral vasoconstriction. Normal expiratory CO_2 levels are between 35 and 40 mmHg and should not drop below 30 mmHg, especially in head trauma patients. An expiratory CO_2 level above 40 mmHg suggests hypoventilation and the need for improved ventilations.

When assessing circulation, note heart rate and pulse strength. A heart rate above 100 in an adult (tachycardia) suggests hypovolemia or excitement. An increase of 20 beats per minute above any of these rates suggests a significant blood loss. Pay special attention to the pulse pressure. Remember that it narrows well before systolic pressure begins to drop. A fast—and especially a fast, weak (thready)—pulse may be the first noticeable sign of serious internal blood loss, hypovolemia, and shock. Also note skin color and condition. As the body begins its compensation for blood loss, it constricts the peripheral arterioles and reduces blood flow to and through the skin. Pale or mottled skin is an early sign of shock, as is cool and clammy skin.

Complete the primary assessment by establishing patient priorities, using the CUPS acronym. A patient who, because of serious and life-threatening injury, does not make it out of the primary assessment (you cannot stabilize the airway, breathing, or circulation) is considered critical (C). Otherwise, categorize the patient as unstable (U), potentially unstable (P), or stable (S). Decide, based on your findings to this point, whether the patient is to receive a rapid trauma assessment, quick care, and rapid transport (the unstable and potentially unstable patient) or a focused trauma assessment (the stable patient) and more traditional care and transport. If any sign or symptom suggests serious internal hemorrhage or uncontrolled external hemorrhage and/or shock, ensure rapid trauma assessment and then immediate patient transport.

Secondary Assessment

Critical trauma patients should not receive a secondary assessment on scene because, by definition, if it is difficult or impossible to stabilize the airway, breathing, and/or circulation during the primary assessment of a critical patient. For the critical patient, always continue primary assessment and the associated interventions. Unstable and potentially unstable patients receive a rapid trauma assessment and transport. Stable patients (and, generally, ones with a single isolated injury) receive a focused trauma assessment with delayed transport.

Rapid Trauma Assessment

For trauma patients with serious injury and/or a significant MOI, perform a rapid trauma assessment, quickly inspecting and palpating the patient from head to toe. Pay particular attention to areas where serious injuries may have occurred and areas where the MOI suggests forces were applied. Immediately control any significant hemorrhage. Quickly place a dressing and bandage over the wound and apply direct pressure. Provide more complete hemorrhage control after the secondary assessment is finished and attend to any injuries that have a higher priority for care.

Carefully and quickly inspect the head for serious bleeding. Remember,

internal head injuries rarely account for the classic signs of shock (except in very young patients). However, the scalp can bleed profusely because vessels there are large and lack ability to constrict (at least as well as other peripheral vessels can). If any external bleeding appears serious, try to control it immediately. Look at the patient's face to determine whether an injury is present that might compromise the airway or be a source of serious hemorrhage.

Next, examine the neck. In the supine, normovolemic patient, the jugular veins should be fully distended. If they are flat, suspect hypovolemia. The carotid arteries and jugular veins are large blood vessels located close to the anterior and lateral surfaces of the neck. Injury to these can result in rapid and fatal exsanguination. An added danger is the aspiration of air directly into an open jugular vein and the venous circulation. At times, jugular venous pressure, as a result of gravity and deep inspiration, may be less than atmospheric pressure. Air may then be drawn into the vein through an open wound, traveling to the heart and forming air (gas) emboli, which then may lodge in the pulmonary circulation. Quickly control any serious hemorrhage from neck wounds with a sterile occlusive dressing. If spinal injury is suspected, apply a rigid cervical collar when neck assessment is complete, but maintain manual spinal immobilization until the patient is secured to an immobilization device.

Inspect the anterior and lateral chest and abdomen (assuming the patient is supine) for any serious external hemorrhage, although such external bleeding is uncommon in these locations. Examine the abdomen for signs of soft-tissue injury, contusions, abrasions, rigidity, guarding, and tenderness that suggest internal injury. Remember that the dramatic discoloration of a contusion is unlikely to develop by the time of

CONTENT REVIEW

➤ Injuries That Can Cause Significant Blood Loss
- Fractured pelvis (2,000 mL)
- Fractured femur (1,500 mL)
- Fractured tibia (750 mL)
- Fractured humerus (750 mL)
- Large contusion (500 mL)

CONTENT REVIEW

➤ Signs and Symptoms of Internal Hemorrhage

Early
- Pain, tenderness, swelling, or discoloration of suspected injury site
- Bleeding from mouth, rectum, vagina, or other orifice
- Vomiting of bright red blood
- Tender, rigid, and/or distended abdomen

Late
- Anxiety, restlessness, combativeness, or altered mental status
- Weakness, faintness, or dizziness
- Vomiting of blood the color of dark coffee grounds
- Thirst
- Melena
- Shallow, rapid breathing
- Rapid, weak pulse
- Pale, cool, clammy skin
- Capillary refill greater than 2 seconds (most reliable in infants and children under age 6)
- Dropping blood pressure
- Dilated pupils sluggish in responding to light
- Nausea and vomiting

your arrival. Simple erythema (skin reddening) may be the only early indicator of serious blunt trauma to either the chest or abdomen.

During the rapid trauma assessment, consider the possibility of obstructive shock. Assess the chest for possible tension pneumothorax. Look for dyspnea, a hyperinflated chest, asymmetrical chest movement, distended jugular veins, hyperresonant percussion, diminished or absent breath sounds on the affected side, tracheal shift to the opposite side (a late sign), and any subcutaneous emphysema. Consider pleural decompression if the signs suggest tension pneumothorax (see the chapter "Chest Trauma"). Also consider the possibility of pericardial tamponade with penetrating central chest trauma. Look for distended jugular veins, muffled or distant heart tones, tachycardia, and progressive and extreme hypotension. Pericardial tamponade is treated with IV fluids in the field and requires immediate and rapid transport to a trauma center. If the patient received significant anterior chest trauma, consider the possibility of myocardial contusion. Apply an ECG monitor and analyze the cardiac rhythm. ST-segment changes and arrhythmias can be seen with myocardial contusions.

Quickly examine the pelvic and groin region. Test pelvic ring integrity by pressing gently on the iliac crests. If a pelvic fracture is suspected, do not compress the iliac crests or otherwise manipulate the pelvis. Remember that pelvic fractures can account for blood loss of more than 2,000 mL. Lacerations to the male genitalia may also account for serious external hemorrhage.

Assess the extremities for the presence of femur, tibia/fibula, radius/ulna, or humerus fractures. Keep in mind that a femur fracture can account for up to 1,500 mL of blood loss, whereas each tibia/fibula or humerus fracture may contribute an additional 500 to 750 mL of blood loss. Hematomas and large contusions may account for up to 500 mL of blood loss in the larger muscle masses. Check distal pulse strength, capillary refill, muscle tone, and sensation in each extremity, comparing these findings to the opposite extremity.

Be sure to carefully examine body areas where the mechanism of injury and index of suspicion suggest serious injury. Examine these areas carefully because signs and symptoms of serious internal injury may be difficult to recognize. Remember, minor skin reddening may be the only sign of a developing contusion and serious internal injury. Remember also that classic signs of shock take time to develop.

Finally, sweep all body regions hidden from view for external hemorrhage that may have gone unnoticed during the examination up to this point. Remember to assess these areas as they become accessible during patient movement or further patient care.

During assessment, be alert for problems other than hemorrhagic shock. Medical conditions such as stroke, seizures, or heart attack can lead to auto crashes and other trauma events. Always consider the possibility of cardiogenic shock by questioning the patient about chest pain and looking for pulmonary edema, jugular vein distention, and cardiac arrhythmias (see the chapter "Cardiology"). Also suspect and check for neurogenic shock (see the chapter "Head, Neck, and Spinal Trauma"). Ask about neck or back pain and evaluate for tenderness along the spine or any numbness or tingling sensations. Look for the presence of pink and warm skin below a nervous system injury while the skin above the injury is pale, cool, and clammy. Other shock states such as anaphylactic, septic, and diabetic shock are not likely unless the patient history suggests them.

At the end of the rapid trauma assessment, assess patient vital signs, determine a Glasgow Coma Score, complete a patient medical history as time permits, and inventory injuries found that may contribute to shock. Revise the patient's priority for transport and for injury care, as necessary. If any sign or symptom suggests serious internal or uncontrolled external hemorrhage, consider rapid transport. Try to estimate the probable volume of blood lost to fractures, large contusions, and hematomas. Also note the probable sources of internal hemorrhage and attempt to approximate blood loss from them. Identify all significant injuries and assign each a priority for care. There may not be time to care for all injuries. Thus, set priorities to ensure that critical injuries—those most likely to contribute to patient hypovolemia and shock—are rapidly addressed. As more and more signs of shock compensation are noted, increase the patient's priority for transport and care. Be sure to record the assessment results carefully. Compare these results with signs and symptoms discovered during reassessments to identify trends in the patient's condition.

Focused Trauma Assessment

Employ a focused trauma assessment for patients without signs or symptoms of serious injury or blood loss—for example, a patient who has lacerated her finger with a knife. Hemorrhage can be controlled on the scene when the MOI and primary assessment do not suggest additional problems (CUPS—stable patient). With patients such as this, focus on the injured area. Inspect and palpate the area thoroughly, looking for additional injuries beyond the one initially seen. Obtain baseline vital signs and a patient history, and prepare and transport the patient.

In some cases, it may be prudent to perform a rapid trauma assessment even though the patient does not have significant signs of injury. This would be the case, for example, if you suspect that a patient has more serious injuries than he complains of, his general condition appears worse than the noted injuries would typically cause, the presence of abnormal vital sounds is found, or the patient's condition suddenly begins to deteriorate.

Additional Assessment Considerations

In trauma or medical patients with signs and symptoms of blood loss and shock, it is important to search for evidence of internal hemorrhage. This evidence may be frank blood or other material suggestive of blood loss. Bright red blood from the mouth, nose, rectum, or other orifice suggests direct and active bleeding. Coffee-grounds–appearing emesis is often associated with slow hemorrhage into the stomach. Stool with frank blood in it (hematochezia) reflects active bleeding in the colon or rectum. A black, tarry stool (melena) suggests that blood has remained in the bowel for some time. During the rapid trauma assessment, be sure to examine all body openings for signs of hemorrhage.

In patients with nonspecific complaints—general ill feeling, anxiousness, restlessness—or a lowered level of responsiveness, suspect and look for other signs of internal hemorrhage. Watch the patient for an increasing pulse rate, weakening pulse strength (rising diastolic blood pressure and narrowing pulse pressure), and cool and clammy skin.

Also observe for dizziness or syncope when a patient moves from a supine to a sitting or standing position. This diagnostic sign is called **orthostatic hypotension** and suggests a blood volume loss, possibly attributable to internal hemorrhage. This phenomenon is the basis of the **tilt test** that can be used to help determine blood or fluid loss and the body's reduced ability to compensate for normal positional change. Perform this test only on patients who do not already display signs and symptoms of shock. Prepare for the test by obtaining the blood pressure and pulse rates with the patient in a supine or seated position. Then have the supine patient move to a seated position or the seated patient stand up, and obtain another blood pressure and pulse rate. If the systolic blood pressure drops more than 15 to 20 mmHg, the pulse rate rises by more than 20 beats per minute, or the patient experiences light-headedness, the test is considered positive and indicates hypovolemia.[4]

Patient Medical History

During the rapid or focused trauma assessment, question the patient regarding the chief complaint and his past medical history. Pay particular attention to any patient complaints of weakness, thirst, or nausea that may be further signs of shock. Pay close attention to any preexisting medical problems, medications, last oral intake, and other medical information to help determine how the patient may respond to the stress of blood loss and shock compensation. Aspirin and other anticoagulants (e.g., warfarin, dabigatran, and enoxaparin) can prolong or worsen hemorrhage. Beta-blockers can inhibit the tachycardia associated with reduced venous blood return and hypotension. Any significant preexisting medical condition can reduce the patient's ability to tolerate and compensate for hemorrhage and shock.

Detailed Physical Exam

Perform a detailed physical exam only on a potential shock patient and only after all priorities have been addressed and the patient is either en route to the trauma center or circumstances, such as a prolonged extrication, prevent immediate transport. If time permits, assess the patient from head to toe and look for any additional signs of injury. Remember, some signs and symptoms of trauma take time to develop. In most cases, the ecchymosis associated with injuries has not had time to develop. Therefore, carefully look for erythema and areas of local warmth suggestive of injury.

Reassessment

Perform periodic, serial reassessments after completing the primary assessment, rapid or focused trauma assessment, and all appropriate lifesaving measures. Perform these reassessments frequently—at least every 5 minutes with critical, unstable, or potentially unstable patients and every 15 minutes with stable ones. Reevaluate the patient's general impression; reassess mental status, airway, breathing, and circulation; and obtain an additional set of vital signs and Glasgow Coma Scale score. Note pulse oximetry and capnography readings.

Compare each finding with earlier ones to determine whether the patient's condition is stable, deteriorating, or improving. Pay particular attention to the pulse rate and pulse pressure. If the pulse rate is increasing and/or the pulse pressure is decreasing, suspect increasing compensation and worsening shock. Also pay particular attention to changes in the patient's other symptoms or mental status, noting any increasing confusion, anxiety, or restlessness. Perform a focused assessment for any changes in symptoms the patient reports. Also, check the adequacy and effectiveness of any interventions performed.

Management of the Patient with Hemorrhage and Shock

Hemorrhage and shock management is an integral part of trauma patient care. It begins during the primary assessment and is shaped by findings of the rapid or focused trauma assessment. A patient who is hemorrhaging may not need further shock care if bleeding can be controlled early and effectively. Otherwise, shock care will be essential. We address the care for the patient with active bleeding first and then discuss hemorrhagic shock care.

Hemorrhage Management

First, ensure that the airway is patent and breathing is adequate or establish and maintain the airway and provide the necessary ventilatory support. Administer supplemental oxygen as needed and monitor the oxygen saturation and ventilation status using pulse oximetry, capnography, and the patient's signs and symptoms to guide minute volume and rate.

During primary assessment, treat serious (arterial and heavy venous) hemorrhage immediately after addressing airway and breathing problems. Quickly apply dressings, held firmly in place using an appropriate bandage. Return to provide better hemorrhage control and bandaging after you complete the primary and rapid trauma assessments. Then set priorities for care of wound sites and other injuries discovered. If the patient displays early signs of shock, consider initiating one or two large-bore IVs as long as the procedure does not delay transport. If IV initiation is likely to delay transport of a critical or unstable patient, provide it during transport.

Once the rapid trauma assessment is complete, begin caring for injuries, including hemorrhage, in the priority order previously established. Look at each wound in an organized fashion. With each wound, inspect the site to identify the type and exact location of bleeding. This helps to apply pressure—either digitally or with dressings and bandages—to most effectively halt blood loss. Carefully describe the wound in the prehospital care report. If this information is documented and conveyed clearly to emergency department staff, it may reduce any need for others to remove the dressing (thus disrupting the clotting process) to identify the severity of the injury or bleeding.

Direct Pressure

Direct pressure controls all but the most persistent hemorrhage. Although the systolic blood pressure drives arterial hemorrhage, it often can be controlled with simple digital pressure properly applied to the bleeding source. If a wound looks as though it may pose a problem, insert a wad of dressing material over the heaviest bleeding site and apply a firm bandage over the dressing. This focuses pressure on the site and away from the surrounding area. If bleeding saturates the dressing, cover it with another dressing and apply another bandage to keep pressure on the wound. Removing the soaked bandage and dressing disrupts the clotting process and prolongs hemorrhage. If, however, the wound continues to bleed through the dressing and bandage layers, consider removing all dressing materials to visualize the exact site of bleeding. Then reapply a wad of dressing and firm direct pressure to the precise hemorrhage site. Often, when blood loss control is ineffective, direct pressure has not been applied to the hemorrhage source.

There are three anatomic sites where firm digital pressure to control bleeding must be performed with precision to avoid damaging nearby or underlying tissues. These are the head, the eye orbits, and the neck. When a head wound is associated with an open fracture and possible brain injury (e.g., brain tissue is exposed), do not place pressure directly on the fractured skull or brain, neither of which contribute much bleeding. Instead, apply digital pressure to the scalp edges. When serious bleeding arises from the eye orbits, avoid placing pressure directly on the globe of the eye, which is sensitive to pressure and may be permanently damaged if severely compressed. The neck contains many large blood vessels that can bleed profusely if lacerated. Firm digital pressure may be critical to stanching hemorrhage. However, avoid pressure on the trachea, larynx, and other airway structures, as this may lead to airway constriction and hypoxia.

Other techniques that can aid in hemorrhage control include standard limb splinting, and possibly the use of pneumatic splints. Splinting helps maintain wound site stability and does not disturb clot development. Splinting may also protect the site from movement and injury that might occur if the patient is jostled as wound assessment and care are provided, or during extrication and transport. Pneumatic splints immobilize and apply direct pressure, circumferentially, to the injured limb.

Elevation and Pressure Points

Elevation and pressure point application have been used in the past to augment direct pressure and hemorrhage control. Research has put into question just how effective these techniques are, however. Elevation also causes movement of the patient's injured limb, and pressure point application requires a care provider to maintain the pressure once applied (limiting any additional care the provider is able to apply). Consult your instructor, protocols, and system medical director about using elevation and pressure points in your EMS system.

If direct pressure alone does not halt minor-to-moderate extremity hemorrhage, though, consider elevation. Elevation reduces the systolic blood pressure because the heart has to push the blood against gravity and up the limb. Use elevation only when there is an isolated bleeding wound on a limb and movement will not aggravate any other injuries. Remember, however, that direct pressure is the most effective hemorrhage control procedure.

If bleeding still persists, find an arterial pulse point proximal to the wound and apply firm pressure there. This further reduces blood pressure within the limb and may reduce the hemorrhage rate. Keep in mind that such pressure must be maintained once applied.

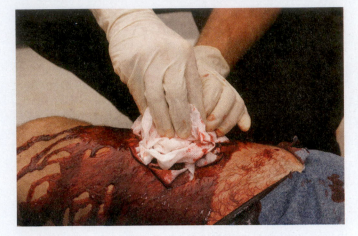

FIGURE 3-10 Hemostatic agents can play a role in hemorrhage control.

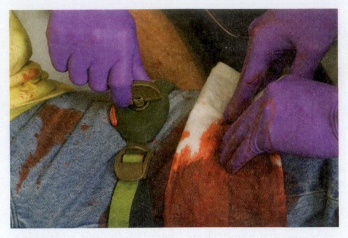

FIGURE 3-11 Use a tourniquet as a last resort when hemorrhage is prolonged and persistent.

Topical Hemostatic Agents

A recent development in hemorrhage care is the introduction of hemostatic dressings and agents (Figure 3-10). These materials are FDA approved and are applied directly or indirectly to active hemorrhage. They use various methods to support blood coagulation and help control further blood loss. Agents either are in dust or powder form applied directly to the wound or contained within a fabric pouch, or are impregnated into dressings that are then applied directly to the wound. Some hemostatic agents are made from the shells of shrimp, crabs, and other crustaceans (e.g., chitosan). When moistened by blood, they become adherent, collect red blood cells, and stop the hemorrhage. These agents are also somewhat antibacterial and hypoallergenic. Another class of hemostatic agents is made from chemically altered volcanic rock (e.g., zeolite). When poured on fresh blood, it reacts, creating heat (an exothermic reaction) and drawing water from the blood. The heat and dehydration concentrate the blood and enhance coagulation. A final hemostatic agent is a starch-based powder derived from plants. It is dusted over the wound with a small bellows device and causes its action by drawing up water and dehydrating the clotting blood.[5–7]

Tourniquets

Consider using a tourniquet only as a last resort when hemorrhage is prolonged and persistent (Figure 3-11). Tourniquet use may be necessary in crush injuries when it is very hard to locate the exact location of bleeding. Deep and penetrating wounds can make hemorrhage difficult to control. However, as mentioned earlier, there are hazards associated with tourniquet use. Apply a commercial tourniquet just proximal to the hemorrhage site and secure it firmly. If you use a blood pressure cuff, inflate it to a pressure of 20 to 30 mmHg greater than the systolic blood pressure. Ensure that bleeding does not continue after application of the tourniquet. If hemorrhage does continue, increase the pressure in the blood pressure cuff or tighten the commercial tourniquet. Be sure that emergency department personnel are aware of the use of a tourniquet.[8–10]

With the increasing incidence of gunshot wounds and acts of terrorism, care under fire in emergency medical services is becoming a reality. The use of both hemostatic agents and tourniquets provides quick solutions to hemorrhage control and may be indicated when the patient's and your life are in danger during patient care.

Specific Wound Considerations

Several wound types require special attention for hemorrhage control. They include head wounds, neck wounds, large gaping wounds, and crush injuries.

Head injuries raise some special concerns regarding hemorrhage control. These include controlling hemorrhage associated with a skull fracture, bleeding or fluids leaking from the ears and nose, and facial injuries threatening the airway. Head wounds may be associated with both severe hemorrhage and loss of skull integrity (fracture). Attempts at applying direct pressure to control hemorrhage may risk displacing unstable skull fracture fragments into the brain tissue. Always control bleeding carefully when you suspect such a wound, using direct pressure on the scalp and around the wound site and against the stable skull.

Fluid drainage from the ears and nose may be secondary to skull fracture. Cerebrospinal fluid, as it escapes the cranial vault, helps to relieve any increasing intracranial pressure. Stopping fluid flow would end this relief mechanism and compound any increasing intracranial pressure, and is generally impossible. In addition, stopping the flow may provide an easier pathway for pathogens to enter the meninges and cause serious infection (meningitis). Cerebrospinal fluid will quickly regenerate as the injury heals. Thus, if there is hemorrhage from either the nose or ear canal, simply cover the area with a soft, porous dressing (such as a 4 × 4 gauze), bandage it loosely in place, and permit some blood to flow from the wound.

Wounds associated with the orbits can be controlled with digital pressure. However, avoid compressing the globe because it is sensitive to pressure and may be damaged by prolonged or high pressure. If ruptured, the globe can lose irreplaceable vitreous contents even if compressed only gently. Apply pressure only to the intact and stable bony orbital rim.

Neck wounds carry the risk of air being drawn into the venous circulation, with life-threatening consequences. Cover any open neck wound with an occlusive dressing, covered by a soft dressing and held firmly in place with bandaging. Do not employ circumferential bandages to create direct pressure with neck wounds. Digital pressure controls most, if not all, neck bleeding. Avoid compressing the trachea, larynx, and other structures, as this may cause airway compromise. It may be necessary to apply and maintain continuous manual pressure during the patient's prehospital care and transport.

Gaping wounds often present hemorrhage control problems. With such wounds, bleeding originates from multiple sites and their open nature prevents application of uniform direct pressure. To manage bleeding from such a wound, create a mass of dressing material approximating the volume and shape of the wound. Place the material with the sterile, nonadherent side down into the wound and bandage it firmly in place.

Controlling hemorrhage associated with crush injuries can be particularly challenging. Frequently, the source of bleeding is difficult to locate and the nature of vessel damage prevents the clotting mechanisms from being effective. In this case, place a dressing around and over the crushed tissue, place a pneumatic splint over the dressing, and inflate to a pressure that holds the dressing firmly in place and controls the bleeding. If bleeding is heavy and persistent, consider using a tourniquet, but keep in mind the precautions associated with its use.

Transport Considerations

Consider rapid transport for any patient with serious hemorrhage that cannot be controlled and for any patient with suspected internal hemorrhage. Be vigilant for any signs and symptoms of blood loss compensation and early shock. Monitor the patient's mental status, Glasgow Coma Score, pulse rate, respiratory rate, and blood pressure (for narrowing pulse pressure). When in doubt, transport.

Understand that serious hemorrhage can have a significant psychological impact on patients. Stress triggers the fight-or-flight response, increases heart rate and blood pressure, increases the body's metabolic demands, complicates the body's hemorrhage control mechanisms, and contributes to the development of shock. Do what you can to ease the patient's anxiety. Communicate often with him and explain what care measures are being provided and why. Be especially alert to the patient's comfort needs and address them as appropriate. If possible, keep these patients from seeing their injuries or the serious injuries affecting friends and other event victims.

Shock Management

The management of hemorrhage and of hypovolemic (hemorrhagic) shock go hand in hand, with similar priorities and goals.

Airway and Breathing Management

Management of the shock patient begins with the corrective actions taken during the primary assessment. One of the primary principles of shock care is to ensure the best possible chances for adequate tissue oxygenation and carbon dioxide removal. This can be accomplished by ensuring or providing a secure and patent airway and good ventilations with supplemental oxygen, if needed (as guided by pulse oximetry) to maintain a saturation of at least 96 percent.

As necessary, protect the airway as needed. Shock patients frequently vomit, and gastric aspiration is an untoward, possibly fatal, consequence. If endotracheal intubation is chosen, capnography should be used to ensure proper tube placement and to guide ventilation. Rapid sequence intubation (RSI) may be considered if allowed in the system where you work.

If the patient is moving air ineffectively (at a breathing rate less than 8/minute or with inadequate respiratory volume), provide positive-pressure ventilations.[11] Ensure that the ventilations provide both a good tidal volume (500 mL) and an adequate respiratory rate (at 10 to 12 per minute). Two techniques to improve ventilation are positive end-expiratory pressure (PEEP) and continuous positive airway pressure (CPAP). PEEP uses a restrictive valve on an endotracheal tube or mask of the bag-valve unit. Thus, for PEEP to be effective, the patient must be intubated. CPAP uses special ventilation equipment to increase pressure during both inspiration and expiration. This keeps the airway open during more of the respiratory cycle, improves ventilation, increases the partial pressure of oxygen, and may push fluid (in cases of pulmonary edema) back into the capillary circulation (Figure 3-12).[12]

If there is any sign of tension pneumothorax, confirm it and provide pleural decompression at the second intercostal space, midclavicular line (see the chapter "Chest Trauma"). Continue to monitor the patient, because it is common for the catheter to clog and tension pneumothorax to reappear. Insert another needle close to the first to relieve any subsequent pressure buildup.

Ensure that an unconscious and unresponsive patient has a palpable carotid pulse. If not, initiate CPR, attach a

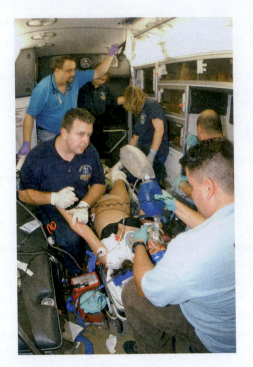

FIGURE 3-12 Ensure that the potential shock patient receives adequate ventilation.

(© Craig Jackson/In the Dark Photography)

monitor–defibrillator, and employ advanced life support measures. Consider possible pericardial tamponade and tension pneumothorax as possible causes of cardiac dysfunction. Understand that traumatic cardiac arrest carries an extremely poor prognosis, especially when it is due to hypovolemia. When resources are scarce, your efforts may be better utilized in caring for other seriously injured but salvageable patients.

Hemorrhage Control

Provide rapid control of any significant external hemorrhage, as explained earlier in this chapter.

Fluid Resuscitation

The field treatment of choice for significant blood loss in trauma is whole blood. It has red blood cells to carry oxygen, contains clotting factors and platelets to assist in hemostasis, and remains in the bloodstream once it is infused. Whole blood, however, is almost never available in blood banks or hospitals. Most banked blood is fractionated and known as packed red blood cells. It must be refrigerated, typed, and cross-matched. (O-negative blood may be given in emergency circumstances.) Blood also has a short shelf life, is costly, and is impractical for field use. The most practical fluid for prehospital administration is an isotonic crystalloid like normal saline. (Lactated Ringer's solution may be used in some systems.)

Hypertonic and synthetic solutions may have some applications for fluid resuscitation. None of these, however, has demonstrated superiority to isotonic electrolyte solutions for use in the civilian prehospital setting. Hypertonic crystalloid solutions decrease the interstitial and intracellular fluid volumes to replace lost intravascular volume but, like other crystalloids, they are not able to carry either the oxygen or the clotting factors essential for hemorrhage control. The advantage of hypertonic solutions is their low volume and weight—an advantage in wilderness and military applications. Synthetic agents that can carry oxygen are being tested. These agents, however, have not yet proven their efficacy in the emergency department or prehospital setting.

ISOTONIC FLUID ADMINISTRATION   Isotonic fluid administration is indicated for the patient with the classic signs and symptoms of shock and isolated but controlled external hemorrhage. Employ aggressive fluid resuscitation, using normal saline via one line running wide open. Remember, the goal of fluid resuscitation is to restore organ perfusion and not blood pressure. The continued infusion of large volumes of isotonic fluids actually dilutes the clotting elements, decreases the hematocrit, and worsens patient outcomes. Generally, most adult trauma patients will require 1 to 2 L of fluid (20 mL/kg for children) to restore organ perfusion. This, of course, will vary from patient to patient. Different patients will respond differently to a rapid bolus of intravenous fluid. By observing how a patient responds to the initial fluid bolus, we can identify patients whose blood loss may be greater than initially estimated and help to identify those with continued blood loss. It is important to try differentiate, if possible, between patients who are "hemodynamically stable" from those who are "hemodynamically normal." The hemodynamically stable patient may have tachycardia, tachypnea, and decreased urine output and still be in shock. On the other hand, hemodynamically normal patients do not have signs of inadequate tissue perfusion. Stated another way, the difference between the hemodynamically stable patient and hemodynamically normal patient is the same as the difference between the patient with relatively normal vital signs and no shock and the one with relatively normal vitals or minimally abnormal vital signs (compensated shock) and signs of inadequate tissue perfusion.

Patients in hypovolemic shock will respond to intravenous fluids in one of three ways: rapid response, transient response, and minimal or no response (Table 3-3).

The first class, referred to as *rapid responders*, will respond quickly to the initial bolus of intravenous fluids and remain hemodynamically normal after the initial fluid bolus. Following the initial fluid bolus, most of these patients can be managed with maintenance IV fluids. Generally, rapid responders typically have less than 20 percent loss of the total blood volume.

Table 3-3 Response to Initial Fluid Resuscitation (2 L of isotonic crystalloids in adults; 20 mL/kg in children)

	Rapid Response	Transient Response	Minimal or no Response
Estimated blood loss	Minimal (10–20%)	Moderate and ongoing (20–40%)	Severe (>40%)
Vital signs	Return to normal	Transient improvement followed by recurrence of abnormal findings	Remain abnormal
Need for more crystalloids	Low	High	High
Need for blood	Low	Moderate to high	Immediate
Need for surgery	Possibly	Likely	Highly likely

The second class of patients is referred to as *transient responders*. These patients will respond favorably to the initial fluid bolus. However, once the initial fluid bolus has been administered, they will begin to show deterioration in perfusion, indicating either ongoing blood loss and/or inadequate fluid resuscitation. Most patients who were transient responders have lost between 20 and 40 percent of their total blood volume.

The third class of responders is those who have a *minimal or no response* to either intravenous crystalloid and/or blood administration. These patients often have ongoing uncontrolled hemorrhage. In some cases, although rare, the failure to respond to the intravenous fluids may be due to an obstructive process such as myocardial contusion, pericardial tamponade, or a tension pneumothorax.

Use large-bore catheters (14 or 16 gauge) connected to trauma or blood tubing to ensure unimpeded flow and a non–flow-restrictive saline lock if your system so requires. If the patient has continuing (internal or uncontrolled external) hemorrhage with absent peripheral pulses or a systolic blood pressure below 80 mmHg, infuse the fluids wide open until 250 to 500 mL of solution is infused. Then evaluate for the return of peripheral pulses or a rise in the systolic blood pressure to just less than 80 mmHg—sometimes referred to as *permissive hypotension*. If the patient's condition or blood pressure does not improve, consider repeating the fluid bolus.[13]

Traumatic brain injury patients (Glasgow Coma Score [GCS] of 8 or less) may require a slightly higher systolic blood pressure (100 mmHg) to ensure cerebral perfusion. Even brief periods of hypotension are detrimental to good outcomes in traumatic brain injury. Note, however, that prehospital fluid resuscitation is an area of much research and controversy. Consult with your medical director and local protocols to determine your system's parameters for prehospital fluid resuscitation of the shock patient with head injury.

In children, infuse 20 mL/kg of body weight rapidly if there are any signs and symptoms of shock. Administer a second fluid bolus if the vital signs do not improve after the first bolus or if, at some later time, the patient again begins to deteriorate. The objective of fluid resuscitation in the field is not the return of normal vital signs, but the stabilization of vital signs until the patient reaches the trauma center.

When preparing to administer large volumes of fluid to a trauma patient, consider the internal lumen size of both the catheter and the administration set. Fluid flow is proportional to the fourth power of the internal diameter. This means that as the lumen's diameter is doubled, the same fluid under the same pressure will flow 16 times more quickly. Use the largest catheter you can place into the patient's vein and use a large-bore trauma or blood administration set.

Catheter length and fluid pressure also influence fluid flow. The longer the catheter, the greater the resistance to fluid flow. The ideal catheter for the shock patient is relatively short: 1.5 inches or shorter. Likewise, an increase in fluid pressure increases flow. This means that the higher the bag is positioned or the greater the pressure differential between the solution and the venous system, the faster the fluid will flow. If the fluid bag cannot be elevated (as in a helicopter), place it under the patient with some of his weight on it or place it in a pressure infuser or a blood-pressure cuff inflated to 100 or 200 mmHg.

During fluid resuscitation, cautiously monitor fluid volume, remembering that your goal is maintaining organ perfusion and not restoring vital signs to normal. Increases in blood pressure can dislodge developing clots and disrupt the normal clotting processes. The result may be further hemorrhage with further dilution of clotting factors and hemoglobin. Closely monitor the patient's vital signs, and administer lactated Ringer's solution or normal saline to keep the patient's mental status and pulse pressure steady. Maintain the blood pressure at a steady level once it has dropped below 80 mmHg. Do not let the pressure drop below 50 mmHg or below 100 mmHg for head injury patients with a GCS of 8 or less.

Temperature Control

Trauma and blood loss deal serious blows to the mechanisms that normally adjust the body's core temperature. Reduced body activity reduces heat production to subnormal levels.

Cutaneous vasoconstriction decreases the skin's ability to act as part of the body's temperature control system. The result is a patient highly susceptible to fluctuations in body temperature. In cases of trauma, patients commonly lose heat more rapidly than normal and heat production is low. At the same time, the heat-generating reflexes, like shivering, are ineffective and, in fact, are counterproductive to the shock care process. Shivering will consume oxygen and glucose when the body needs these materials to keep other cells alive. Hypothermia also reduces the effectiveness of the clotting mechanism and can worsen and prolong hemorrhage.

In all except the warmest environments, help conserve body temperature by covering the patient with a blanket and keeping the patient compartment of the ambulance very warm. If you infuse fluids, ensure that they are well above room temperature—ideally at body temperature or slightly above (but no more than 104°F). Use fluid warmers or keep IV solutions in a compartment that is warmer than the rest of the ambulance. Be very sensitive to any patient complaints about being cold, and provide whatever assistance you can to ensure that heat loss is limited.

Pharmacological Intervention

In shock, pharmacological interventions (with the exception of tranexamic acid) are of generally limited use, especially in hypovolemic patients. The sympathetic nervous system efficiently compensates for low volume, and no agent has been shown effective in the prehospital setting, other than intravenous fluid and, in some cases, blood and blood products. For cardiogenic shock, fluid challenge, vasopressors like dopamine, and the other cardiac drugs are indicated (see the chapter "Cardiology"). For spinal and obstructive shock, consider intravenous fluids like normal saline and lactated Ringer's solution. For distributive shock, consider IV fluids or a vasopressor.

The patient who has experienced trauma sufficient to induce hemorrhage and hypovolemia will be anxious and bewildered. As the care provider on scene, it is your responsibility to be calm and reassuring, thus helping to counteract the natural fight-or-flight response. By acting in this manner, you not only help your patient deal with the event's emotional trauma but also combat some of the negative effects of sympathetic stimulation.

Summary

Significant hemorrhage and its serious consequence, shock, are genuine threats to the trauma patient's life. The signs of these threats are often subtle or hidden, especially if bleeding is internal. Only through careful analysis of the mechanism of injury during the scene size-up and careful evaluation of the patient during the assessment process can you recognize and then treat these life-threatening problems. Treatment often involves rapidly bringing the patient to the services of a trauma center and, while doing so, providing aggressive care aimed at maintaining organ perfusion, not necessarily improving vital signs to normal. With this approach, you can provide your patient with the best chances for survival.

You Make the Call

A teenager working in a high school wood shop slips and runs his forearm into the running blade of a table saw. The blade cuts deeply into an artery, resulting in serious hemorrhage. On your arrival, you find the teenager to be very agitated and anxious. Your assessment reveals a blood pressure of 130/86 mmHg, a pulse of 110, normal respirations at 24 breaths per minute, and skin that is cool and moist.

1. What signs suggest hypovolemia and early shock?

2. Does the blood pressure suggest shock? Why or why not?

3. What progressive steps would you take to control the hemorrhage?

4. What supportive care measures would you employ?

See Suggested Responses at the back of this book.

Review Questions

1. Signs and symptoms of a patient in compensated shock may include all of the following *except* _____

   a. unconsciousness.
   c. combativeness.
   b. thirst.
   d. weakness.

2. You and your crew respond to a motor vehicle collision in which a 20-year-old female patient has received several cuts over her body. You determine that her airway is patent and she is breathing adequately. Her blood pressure is maintaining at a stable level, and you estimate that she has lost approximately 10 percent of her circulating blood volume. She is alert and oriented but seems a bit nervous. From these findings, you determine that your patient is in _____ hemorrhage.

   a. class I
   c. class III
   b. class II
   d. class IV

3. In a patient with no suspected trauma, and signs and symptoms of shock, you can perform the tilt test. This test is performed to determine whether which finding is present?

   a. Cardiogenic shock
   b. Septic shock
   c. Orthostatic hypertension
   d. Orthostatic hypotension

4. What is the name of the sensory structures located in the aortic arch and carotid bodies that are responsible for monitoring blood pressure?

   a. Chemoreceptors
   b. Baroreceptors
   c. Cardioinhibitory centers
   d. Cardioacceleratory centers

5. The release of which hormone(s) from the body results in the most immediate response to the effects of hypoperfusion?

   a. Angiotensin II
   b. Glucocorticoids
   c. Antidiuretic hormone
   d. Catecholamines

6. You are called to a scene where a man responds only to deep painful stimuli. You note an absence of peripheral pulses and a rapidly dropping blood pressure. Based on these assessment findings, you conclude that the patient is most likely progressing into which stage of shock?

   a. Neurogenic shock
   b. Irreversible shock
   c. Decompensated shock
   d. Compensated shock

7. Rapid transport to a trauma facility is *most* indicated in which of the following patients?

   a. A patient in class I hemorrhage
   b. A patient with suspected serious internal hemorrhage
   c. A patient who is vomiting coffee-grounds material
   d. A patient with external hemorrhage that is controlled on the scene

8. Which if the following controls all but the most persistent hemorrhage?

   a. Elevation
   c. Occlusive dressing
   b. Direct pressure
   d. Pressure dressing

9. Your patient is determined to be in a hypoperfusive state. Your standing orders indicate that you should initiate an IV line to administer a fluid bolus. The most practical fluid for prehospital administration is _____

   a. D_5W.
   b. 3% normal saline.
   c. lactated Ringer's.
   d. D_5W in half normal saline.

10. The development of what metabolic process leads to overwhelming acidosis in the hypotensive, hyperperfusing trauma patient?

    a. Anabolic
    c. Catabolic
    b. Aerobic
    d. Anaerobic

See Answers to Review Questions at the end of this book.

References

1. Haut, E. R., et al. "Prehospital Intravenous Fluid Administration Is Associated with Higher Mortality in Trauma Patients: A National Trauma Data Bank Analysis." *Ann Surg* 253(2) (Feb 2011): 371–377.

2. Napolitano, L.M., G. M. Cohen, B.A. Cotton, et al. "Tranexemic Acid in Trauma: How Should We Use It?" *J Trauma Acute Care Surg* 74(6) (2013): 1575–1586.

3. Frank, M., et al. "Proper Estimation of Blood Loss on Scene of Trauma: Tool or Tale?" *J Trauma* 69(5) (Nov 2010): 1191–1195.

4. Bates, B. and P. G. Szilagyi. *A Guide to Physical Examination and History Taking.* 9th ed. Philadelphia: J.B. Lippincott, 2007.

5. Alam, H. B., et al. "Hemorrhage Control in the Battlefield: Role of the New Hemostatic Agents." *Mil Med* 170 (2005): 63–69.

6. Clay, J. G., J. K. Grayson, and D. Zierold. "Comparative Testing of New Hemostatic Agents in a Swine Model of Extremity Arterial and Venous Hemorrhage." *Mil Med* 175(4) (Apr 2010): 280–284.

7. Ran, Y., et al. "QuikClit Combat Gauze Use for Hemorrhage Control in Military Trauma: January 2009 Israel Defense Force Experience in the Gaza Strip—a Preliminary Report of 14 Cases." *Prehosp Emerg Care* 25(6) (Nov–Dec 2010): 584–588.

8. Taylor, D. M., G. M. Vater, and P. J. Parker. "An Evaluation of Two Tourniquet Systems for the Control of Prehospital Lower Limb Hemorrhage." *J Trauma* 71(3) (Sept 2011): 591–595.

9. Kragh, J. F., Jr., et al. "Survival with Emergency Tourniquet Use to Stop Bleeding in Major Limb Trauma." *Ann Surg* 249(1) (Jan 2009): 1–7.

10. Kragh, J. F., et al. "Battle Casualty Survival with Emergency Tourniquet Use to Stop Limb Bleeding." *J Emerg Med* 41(6) (Dec 2011): 590–597.

11. Stockinger, Z. T. and N. E. McSwain. "Prehospital Endotracheal Intubation for Trauma Does Not Improve Survival over Bag-Valve-Mask Ventilation." *J Trauma* 56(3) (2004): 531–536.

12. Stockinger, Z. T. and N. E. McSwain. "Prehospital Supplemental Oxygen in Trauma Patients." *Mil Med* 169 (Aug 2004): 609–612.

13. Merlin, M. A., et al. "Study of Placing a Second Intravenous Line in Trauma." *Prehosp Emerg Care* 15(2) (Apr–Jun 2011): 208–213.

Further Reading

Bickley, L. *Bates' Guide to Physical Examination and History Taking.* 11th ed. Philadelphia: Wolters-Kluwer, 2012.

Bledsoe, B. E., and D. Clayden. *Prehospital Emergency Pharmacology.* 7th ed. Upper Saddle River, NJ: Pearson/Prentice Hall, 2011.

Bledsoe, B. E., B. J. Colbert, and J. E. Ankney. *Essentials of A & P for Emergency Care.* Upper Saddle River, NJ: Pearson/Prentice Hall, 2010.

Martini, Frederic. *Fundamentals of Anatomy and Physiology.* 7th ed. San Francisco: Benjamin Cummings, 2007.

Rosen, P., and R. Barkin, eds. *Emergency Medicine: Concepts and Clinical Practice.* 7th ed. St. Louis: Mosby, 2009.

Tintinelli, J. E., ed. *Emergency Medicine: A Comprehensive Study Guide.* 7th ed. New York: McGraw-Hill, 2011.

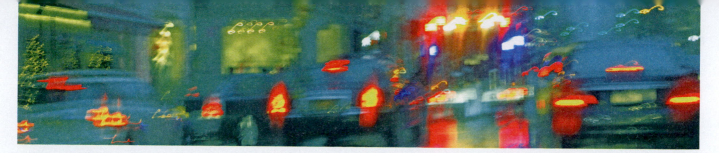

Chapter 4
Soft Tissue Trauma

Bryan E. Bledsoe, DO, FACEP, FAAEM, EMT-P

Robert S. Porter, MA, EMT-P

STANDARD
Trauma (Soft Tissue Trauma)

COMPETENCY
Integrates assessment findings with principles of epidemiology and pathophysiology to formulate a field impression to implement a comprehensive treatment/disposition plan for an acutely injured patient.

Learning Objectives

Terminal Performance Objective: After reading this chapter you should be able to assess and manage patients with soft tissue injuries.

Enabling Objectives: To accomplish the terminal performance objective, you should be able to:

1. Define key terms introduced in this chapter.

2. Describe the epidemiology of soft tissue injuries.

3. Describe the anatomy and physiology of the skin and associated soft tissues.

4. Discuss the pathophysiology of open and closed soft tissue injuries.

5. Describe the process and phases of wound healing.

6. Discuss soft tissue injury complications, including infection, impaired hemostasis, delayed healing, compartment syndrome, scarring, pressure injuries, crush syndrome, and injection injuries.

7. Describe and differentiate between the use of different dressings and bandaging materials, given various scenarios requiring management.

8. Discuss the phases and process of assessment as they relate to the assessment and management of a patient with a soft tissue injury.

9. Reassess patients with soft tissue injuries for complications of bandaging.

10. Describe special considerations in the management of the injuries such as amputations, impalements, crush and compartment syndromes, and injuries to the face, neck, thorax, and abdomen.

11. Describe considerations in decisions to transport or treat and release patients with soft tissue injuries.

KEY TERMS

abrasion, p. 89

amputation, p. 91

avulsion, p. 91

chemotactic factors, p. 93

collagen, p. 94

compartment syndrome, p. 96

contusion, p. 88

crush injury, p. 89

crush syndrome, p. 89

degloving injury, p. 91

dermis, p. 87

ecchymosis, p. 89

epidermis, p. 86

epithelialization, p. 94

erythema, p. 89

fascia, p. 88

fibroblasts, p. 94

gangrene, p. 95

granulocytes, p. 93

hematoma, p. 89

hemostasis, p. 92

hyperemia, p. 93

impaled object, p. 90

incision, p. 90

infection, p. 94

inflammation, p. 93

integumentary system, p. 85

keloid, p. 97

laceration, p. 90

lumen, p. 92

lymphangitis, p. 94

lymphatic system, p. 87

lymphocyte, p. 87

macrophage, p. 87

necrosis, p. 98

neovascularization, p. 94

phagocytosis, p. 93

puncture, p. 90

remodeling, p. 94

rhabdomyolysis, p. 98

sebaceous glands, p. 87

sebum, p. 86

serous fluid, p. 96

skeletal muscle, p. 87

subcutaneous tissue, p. 87

sudoriferous glands, p. 87

tendons, p. 87

tension lines, p. 88

tetanus, p. 95

Case Study

Maria Gonza and Jon O'Sullivan, paramedics with University Medic 151, respond to an "axe injury." On arrival, they find an adult male standing next to a wood pile with a bloody axe at his feet. The man is holding a blood-soaked rag against his arm. Maria quickly ascertains from the patient and several bystanders that the wound is accidental and occurred while the patient was chopping wood. No other victims are present.

Maria and Jon proceed to help, donning disposable gloves and splash protection as they approach the patient. Primary assessment reveals the patient to be a healthy 42-year-old man, named Walter, who lacerated his left upper arm when an axe blade slipped during a chopping stroke. Walter states the wound is "deep" and there was "lots of blood" initially, but that he stopped the bleeding fairly easily by "putting this rag on it." Walter reports no other injuries or complaints. He is alert and oriented, standing upright, and shows no apparent distress. His airway is obviously open and his breathing is adequate, his skin is slightly pale, and his pulse rate is somewhat rapid.

Because Walter has an isolated injury and no significant mechanism of injury, Maria and Jon proceed with the focused trauma assessment at the scene. They perform an evaluation of the upper extremity, which reveals a large open and deep wound to the central upper arm just over the biceps muscle. Close inspection of the wound is not yet possible because the patient is holding a folded rag over the wound in an effort to control bleeding. Despite these efforts, a trickle of dark blood continues to flow. A small stain of dark blood is visible on the ground. Distal pulses and capillary refill are both present and equal to those in the opposite extremity. The patient can move all his fingers and his wrist, but cannot flex his elbow. Sensation appears intact, although Walter reports some vague tingling in the fingers.

To control the bleeding and better visualize the wound, Maria will need to remove the rag and inspect the wound. To prepare for this, she and Jon gather several bulky sterile dressings and have them ready. They then position Walter in a seated position on the stretcher. In a coordinated fashion, they remove the rag (taking care to avoid dislodging clots) and simultaneously replace it with a bulky, sterile dressing. A quick look at the wound indicates that it measures approximately 8 cm long and extends deep through the skin and into subcutaneous tissue and muscle layers. There is no spurting or bright red blood, but a large amount of dark red blood flows from the uncovered wound. The new dressings and direct pressure applied with a bandage easily bring the bleeding under control.

While performing the focused assessment, the paramedics also gather a patient history. Walter reports no significant medical problems and says he takes no medications. He doesn't recall the date of his last tetanus booster. He reports no allergies and that his last meal was a large lunch 2 hours ago.

Following application of the dressings and bandage, distal pulse, motor function, sensation, and capillary refill in the extremity are unchanged. Maria and Jon then take a baseline set of vital signs: respirations, 20 per minute and adequate; pulse, 92; skin warm, moist, and slightly pale; pupils equal and reactive; blood pressure (obtained on the right arm)—134/78 mmHg.

Maria and Jon now transport Walter, with his bleeding under control, uneventfully to the hospital emergency department. In the hospital, the emergency physician examines Walter using a local anesthetic and a pneumatic limb tourniquet to obtain a bloodless field. Using a combination of inspection under powerful exam lights and careful palpation with gloved fingers, the physician determines that the wound has not damaged any bones, arteries, nerves, or tendons, and that no foreign bodies have lodged in it. The wound does, however, extend into the muscle layer of the biceps. Using layered closure, the physician sutures the wound, and Walter receives a tetanus booster. The sutures will be removed after 10 to 14 days, by which time Walter should be well on his way to recovery.

Introduction to Soft Tissue Trauma

The skin is one of the largest and most important organs of the human body, accounting for 16 percent of total body weight. It provides a protective barrier to invading pathogens while containing body substances and fluids. It is also a key organ of sensation and a radiator of excess body heat in warm weather and a conservator of heat in cold conditions. Even as it accomplishes these various functions, the skin remains a remarkably durable, pliable, accommodating, and self-repairing tissue.

Known as the **integumentary system**, the skin is often the first body tissue to experience the effects of trauma. Because skin covers the entire body surface, any penetrating injury or the kinetic forces of blunt injury must pass through it before impacting on other vital organs. Often, the signs of this energy transmission can be recognized only with very careful examination of the skin. Therefore, the skin is of great significance at all stages of the patient assessment process.

Trauma to the skin may present as open injuries—abrasions, lacerations, incisions, punctures, avulsions, and amputations—or as closed injuries—contusions, hematomas, and crush injuries. Although such injuries only infrequently pose direct threats to life, they may endanger blood vessels, nerves, connective tissue, and other important internal structures. Uncontrolled bleeding may lead to hypovolemia and shock. In addition, the wound may provide a pathway for infection.

Epidemiology

Soft tissue injuries are by far the most common form of trauma. More than 10 million patients present to emergency departments annually with soft tissue wounds, many of which require closure. Most, but not all, open wounds require only simple care. A significant minority, however, damage arteries, nerves, or tendons and can lead to permanent disability. Uncontrolled external hemorrhage of an otherwise uncomplicated open wound is a very rare—but completely preventable—situation that sometimes occurs with this type of injury and can result in death. Of the open wounds presenting to emergency departments, up to 6.5 percent will eventually become infected, resulting in significant morbidity.

Closed wounds share a similar epidemiology, except that they are probably even more common than open injuries. Most minor "bumps and bruises" are treated without EMS and medial care. Despite their frequency and usually minor nature, closed injuries *can* result in significant pain, suffering, and morbidity. Infection, however, is not usually a complication with closed wounds.

Risk factors for soft tissue wounds include age (school-age children and the elderly are most prone), alcohol or drug abuse, and occupation. Laborers, machine operators, and others whose hands and body parts are exposed to heavy objects, machines, or tools are at greater risk.

Simple measures can reduce risks and prevent soft tissue injuries. For example, locating playgrounds on grass, sand, gravel, or other forgiving surfaces and padding the equipment in them can cut injury rates among children. In factories, machine guards, fail-safe switches, and similar engineering controls can reduce injuries. Protective clothing such as steel-toed boots and leather gloves also provide simple methods of reducing the incidence and severity of soft tissue injuries. In EMS, we need to establish a culture of safety: carefully ensuring scene safety, not entering an unsafe scene, wearing the appropriate protective clothing, properly disposing of sharps, carefully using patient movement devices to protect against pinch and back injuries, using restraint systems when in the ambulance, and driving responsibly, to just name a few.

Anatomy and Physiology of Soft Tissue Injury

The skin is a complex structure. Understanding the anatomy and physiology will help paramedics appreciate the importance of soft tissue injuries and the value of proper care.

Layers of the Skin

The epidermis, dermis, and subcutaneous tissue layers constitute what is commonly known as the skin (Figure 4-1). Each of these layers performs functions essential to helping the body maintain homeostasis (maintenance of a stable, steady, and normal state), and each plays an important role in the wound repair process.

Epidermis

The outermost skin layer is the **epidermis**, generated by a layer of cells just above the dermis (stratum germinativum). These cells divide rapidly and there is a constant movement of cells upward toward the epidermal surface, where they are sloughed off. Because the epidermis contains no vasculature, the farther these cells are pushed away from the dermis, the less circulation they receive, and they eventually die. As they die, they flatten and interlock, providing a firm and secure barrier (stratum corneum) around the body. These cells contain a high percentage of a protein called *keratin*, the same substance that makes nails hard and hair strong and flexible. The outermost cells are eventually abraded or washed away and then replaced, allowing the epidermis to constantly refresh and maintain its thickness. It normally takes two weeks for a cell to move from the dermal border to the epidermis surface and another two to four weeks until it is abraded away. This outward movement of cells helps the body resist bacterial invasion.

A waxy substance called **sebum** lubricates the surface of the epidermis. This lubrication acts much like oil on leather. It keeps the outer skin layers flexible, strong, and resistant to penetration by water. The epidermis is also responsible for pigmentation that protects the skin from harmful effects of ultraviolet radiation. The epidermal thickness varies greatly, depending on the amount of daily abrasion and pressure it receives. For example, the skin on the soles of the feet and the back is very thick and strong, whereas the skin over the eyelid is very thin and delicate.

CONTENT REVIEW

➤ Layers of the Skin
  • Epidermis
  • Dermis
  • Subcutaneous tissue

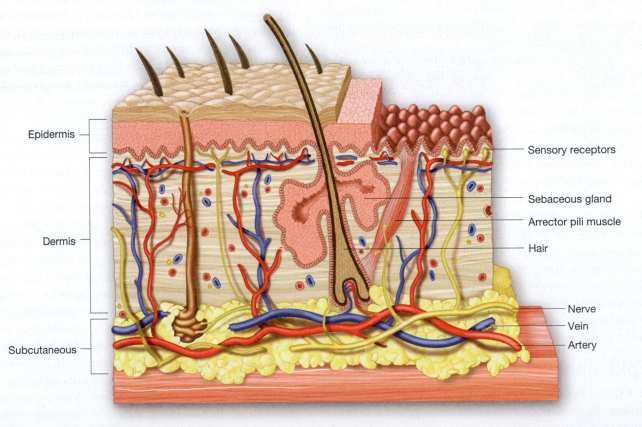

Epidermis

Dermis

Subcutaneous

Sensory receptors

Sebaceous gland

Arrector pili muscle

Hair

Nerve

Vein

Artery

FIGURE 4-1 Layers and major structures of the skin.

Dermis

Directly beneath the epidermis is the **dermis**, a connective tissue that helps contain the body and supports the functions of the epidermis. The upper dermal layer is the papillary layer, consisting of loose connective tissue, capillaries, and nerves supplying the epidermis. The reticular layer is the deeper dermal layer and is made up of strong connective tissue that integrates the dermis firmly with the subcutaneous layer below. The connective tissue in the dermis is rich in the protein collagen—the same fibers that give tendons and ligaments their great strength and flexibility.

The dermis contains blood vessels, nerve endings, glands, and other structures. Located here are the **sebaceous glands** that produce sebum and secrete it directly onto the skin's surface or into hair follicles. **Sudoriferous glands** secrete sweat to help transfer heat out of and away from the body through evaporation. Hair follicles produce hair that helps to reduce surface abrasion, friction, and conserve heat. The connective tissue within the dermis bonds it strongly to the subcutaneous tissue beneath and to the epidermis above. This tissue also holds the skin firmly around the body and permits stretching and flexibility necessary for articulation.

The dermis contains several body cell types responsible for initiating the attack on invading organisms, foreign materials, and damaged cells, and for beginning the repair of damaged tissue. The **macrophages** and **lymphocytes** begin the inflammatory response by killing invading bodies and triggering a call for other, similar cells. Mast cells control the microcirculation to tissues and respond to the initial invasion, increasing capillary flow and permeability. Fibroblasts lay down and repair protein strands (collagen, mostly) to strengthen the wound site and begin restoring the skin's integrity.

Subcutaneous Tissue

Subcutaneous tissue is the body layer beneath the dermis. It is rich in fatty or adipose tissue, which helps it absorb the forces of trauma, protecting tissues and vital organs beneath. Because of its fatty content, heat moves through the subcutaneous tissue three times more slowly than through muscles or other layers of the skin. Thus, it is of great value in conserving body temperature. The body directs blood below the subcutaneous tissue to conserve heat and above it through the dermis when it is necessary to radiate heat.

Blood Vessels

An important medium that moves through the dermis and subcutaneous layers of the skin is blood. Blood consists of water, electrolytes, proteins, and cells traveling through arteries, arterioles, capillaries, venules, and veins. Any soft tissue wound can affect this blood flow; therefore, it is

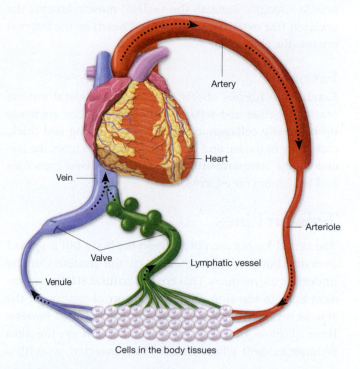

FIGURE 4-2 Lymphatic vessels (shown in green) pick up excess tissue fluid and purify it within lymph nodes before returning it to the circulatory system.

important to review the basic structure of blood vessels and actions the body takes once they are injured (as were introduced in the chapter "Hemorrhage and Shock").

The Lymphatic System

Not all fluids brought to the body cells are returned to the bloodstream directly. Some fluid is instead returned to the major veins by a system of channels and tissues called the **lymphatic system**. This system is especially important in carrying byproducts of pathogen destruction to nodes where macrophages further break down the material. Lymph fluid is then directed to ducts just above the superior vena cava, where it is mixed with returning venous blood (Figure 4-2).

Muscles

Beneath the skin layers are the **skeletal muscles** that provide the power for movement and give the body its shape. They also produce much of the heat necessary to maintain body temperature. Muscles are strong contractile tissue and their bulk helps protect vital organs, blood vessels, and nerves underneath. The muscle layer can be quite thick, as in the upper arms, shoulders, thighs and legs, and buttocks; or thin, as in the forehead and hands. Muscles are connected to the skeleton by **tendons**, providing the movement of the system of levers that moves the body and its appendages. Tendons are made up of almost pure collagen fibers arranged in a parallel fashion that gives them great tensile strength. Beneath the skeletal muscle layer is the skeleton (the extremities, chest, and head) or the internal organs (the abdomen).

Fasciae

Fasciae are fibrous sheets that bundle skeletal muscle masses together and separate them. The fasciae are made up of mostly collagen and can be very strong and thick, especially in the leg and upper arm. Within a limb, the fasciae define compartments with relatively fixed capacities and little room for expansion.

Tension Lines

The skin does not merely hang on the body but is spread over the body and attached to fit the contours of the underlying structures. This creates natural stretch or tension lines in the skin. The orientation of tension in the skin is revealed in characteristic patterns called **tension lines** (Figure 4-3). The effects of tension on the skin become evident when the skin is transected, as with a laceration. Lacerations cutting across tension lines have a tendency to be pulled apart and thus spread widely or gape. Lacerations parallel to tension lines tend to gape very little. An example of this is seen in the forehead, where tension lines run across the forehead in a transverse direction. Here, a vertically oriented laceration gapes widely, whereas a horizontal laceration gapes less so. Wounds that spread widely tend to bleed more than those with minimal gaping. Large gaping wounds heal more slowly and are more likely to leave noticeable scars than wounds that spread less.

Tension represented by skin tension lines can be either static or dynamic. Static tension is noted in areas with limited movement of the tissue and structures beneath, as in the anterior abdomen or between joints in the extremities. Dynamic tension lines occur in areas subject to great movement, such as in the skin over joints such as the elbow, wrist, or knee. The increased motion in areas with dynamic skin tension lines means that clotting and tissue repair processes in these areas are more frequently interrupted, disrupting and complicating skin repair. It also explains why immobilizing a joint involved in a significant laceration can reduce blood loss and improve the formation of a clot.

Pathophysiology of Soft Tissue Injury

Although the functions of the skin are often taken for granted, soft tissue injuries can seriously affect health by causing severe blood and fluid loss, infection, hypothermia, and other problems. Therefore, paramedics need to become familiar with the pathophysiology of soft tissue injuries.

Trauma is a violent transfer of energy that produces an open or closed wound to the skin and possible injury to the structures underneath. Wounds can be either blunt or penetrating. All penetrating wounds are open, but blunt trauma can, on occasion, also create open wounds. Common soft tissue injuries include closed wounds—contusions, hematomas, and crush injuries—and open wounds—abrasions, lacerations, incisions, punctures, avulsions, and amputations. Each type of wound is different and deserves special consideration.

Closed Wounds

Contusions

Contusions are blunt, non-penetrating injuries that crush and damage small blood vessels (Figure 4-4).

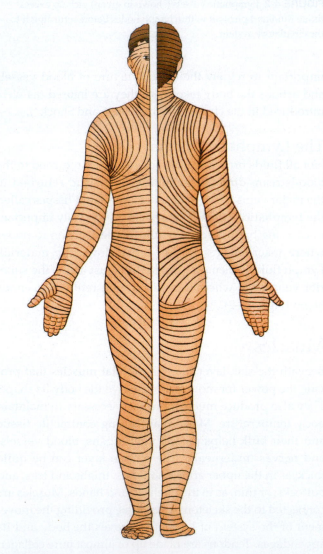

FIGURE 4-3 Tension lines of the skin.

CONTENT REVIEW
➤ Types of Closed Wounds
• Contusions
• Hematomas
• Crush injuries

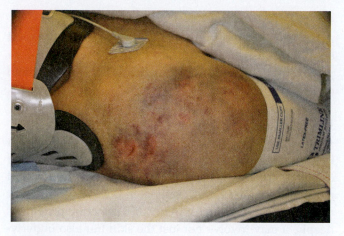

FIGURE 4-4 A contusion. Note that the discoloration of a contusion is a delayed sign.

(© Edward T. Dickinson, MD)

Blood is drawn to the inflamed tissue, causing a reddening called **erythema**. Blood also leaks into the surrounding interstitial spaces through damaged vessels. As hemoglobin within the blood that flows into the interstitial space loses its oxygen, it becomes dark red and then bluish, resulting in the black-and-blue discoloration called **ecchymosis**. Because the development of ecchymosis is a progressive process, the discoloration may not be evident during prehospital care.

Contusions are more pronounced in areas where the mechanism causing the injury (for example, a steering wheel) and skeletal structures (such as the ribs or skull) trap the skin. Occasionally, a chest injury displays an erythematous or ecchymotic outline of the ribs and sternum, reflecting an impact with the auto dashboard or some other blunt object. The same effect can occasionally be seen when a hard object such as a belt buckle strikes the skin, with the resulting outline of the object visible as an ecchymotic pattern in the skin. Early signs of these injuries may be difficult to identify. However, they will become more evident as time passes and discoloration increases.

Hematomas

Soft tissue bleeding can occur within tissue and at times can be quite significant. When the injury involves a larger blood vessel, most commonly an artery, blood can actually separate tissue and pool in a pocket. Such a trapped pocket of blood is called a **hematoma**. These injuries are easily visible in cases of head trauma because of the hard skull below. Hematomas tend to be less pronounced in other body areas, even though they can contain significant hemorrhage. If the hematoma is deep, it can be difficult to distinguish from the ordinary swelling and edema that occurs from blunt force injury. Severe hematomas to the thigh, leg, or arm may contribute to hypovolemia. A

hematoma in the thigh, for example, can contain a massive amount of blood before swelling becomes obvious.[1]

Crush Injuries

The term **crush injury** describes a collection of traumatic insults that

includes both crush injury itself and crush syndrome. In crush injury, a body part that is compressed, possibly by a heavy object, sustains deep injury to the muscles, blood vessels, bones, and other internal structures (Figure 4-5). Damage can be massive, despite minimal signs on the skin. **Crush syndrome** is the term used to describe the systemic effects of a large crush injury. If the pressure that causes a crush injury remains in place for several hours, the resulting destruction of skeletal muscle cells leads to the accumulation of large quantities of myoglobin, potassium, lactic acid, and other toxins. When the pressure is released, these products enter the bloodstream. They circulate, causing a severe metabolic acidosis. These materials are also toxic to the kidneys and heart. Crush syndrome is thus a potentially life-threatening trauma event. It is discussed in more detail later in this chapter.

Open Wounds

Abrasions

Abrasions are typically the most minor of injuries that violate the protective barrier of the skin. They involve a scraping or abrasive action that removes layers of the epidermis and the upper reaches of the dermis (Figure 4-6). Bleeding from an abrasion can be persistent but is usually limited because the injury involves only superficial

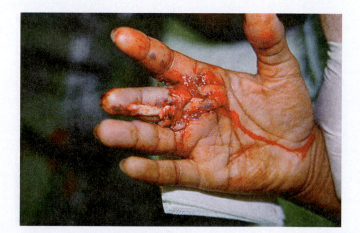

FIGURE 4-5 A crush injury.

(© Edward T. Dickinson, MD)

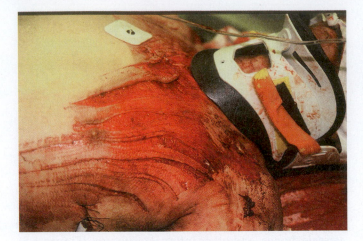

FIGURE 4-6 Abrasions.

(© Edward T. Dickinson, MD)

arterioles, venules, and capillaries. If the injury compromises a large area of the epidermis, it carries a danger of serious infection.

Lacerations

A **laceration** is an open wound that penetrates more deeply into the dermis than an abrasion (Figure 4-7). A laceration tends to involve a smaller surface area, being limited to the tissue immediately surrounding the penetration. It endangers deeper and more significant vasculature—arteries, arterioles, venules, and veins—as well as nerves, muscles, tendons, ligaments, and perhaps some underlying organs. As with an abrasion, the injury breaks the skin's protective barrier and provides a pathway for infection. Always try to note a laceration's orientation to the skin tension lines during patient assessment. If the orientation parallels those lines, the wound may remain closed. If it is perpendicular to them, the wound may gape open.

Incisions

An **incision** is a surgically smooth laceration, often caused by a sharp instrument such as a knife, straight razor, or piece of glass. Such a wound tends to bleed freely. In all other ways, it is a laceration.

Punctures

Another special type of laceration is the **puncture**. It involves a small entrance wound with damage that extends into the body's interior (Figure 4-8). The wound normally seals itself and presents in a way that does not reflect the actual extent of injury. If a puncture penetrates deeply, it may involve not just the skin but also underlying muscles, nerves, bones, and organs. A puncture additionally carries an increased danger of infection. A penetrating object introduces bacteria and other pathogens deep into a wound. There, the injured tissue and blood vessels, along with reduced oxygen levels, create a warm and moist environment that is ideal for the colonization of bacteria.

Impaled Objects

An **impaled object** is not a wound itself, but rather a wound complication often associated with a puncture or laceration. Impaled objects are important for the damage they may cause if withdrawn. Frequently, embedded objects are irregular in shape and may become entangled

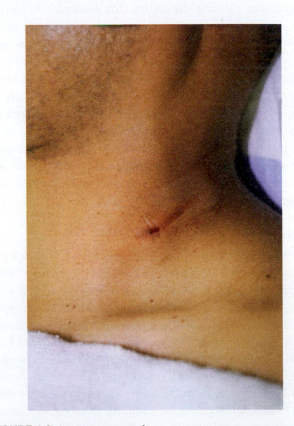

FIGURE 4-8 A puncture wound.

(© Edward T. Dickinson, MD)

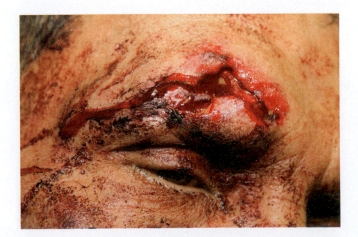

FIGURE 4-7 Lacerations.

(© Dr. Bryan E. Bledsoe)

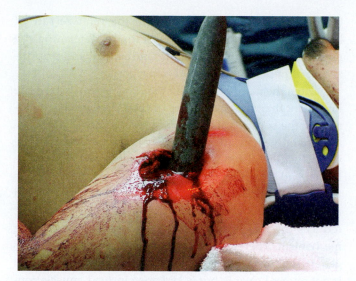

FIGURE 4-9 An impaled object.

(© Michael Casey, MD)

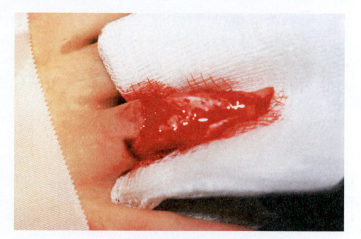

FIGURE 4-11 A ring-type degloving injury.

in important structures such as arteries, nerves, or tendons (Figure 4-9). Removal of impaled objects in the field can cause additional damage. More importantly, the embedded object may have lacerated a large blood vessel and the object's presence temporarily blocks, or tamponades, the blood loss. Removal of the object then may cause uncontrollable hemorrhage. This situation is particularly dangerous when the object is impaled in the neck or trunk, where effective direct pressure application is difficult or impossible.

Avulsions

Avulsion occurs when a flap of skin, though torn or cut, is not torn completely loose from the body (Figure 4-10). Avulsion is frequently seen with blunt trauma to the head, where the scalp is torn and folds back. It may also occur with animal bites and machinery injuries. The seriousness of an avulsion depends on the area involved, the condition

of the circulation to (and distal to) the injury site, and the degree of contamination.

A special type of avulsion is the **degloving injury**. In this wound, the mechanism of injury tears the skin off the underlying muscle, connective tissue, blood vessels, and bone. It is a particularly gruesome injury, occurring occasionally with farm and industrial machinery. The device pulls the skin off with great force as the skeletal tissue underneath is held stationary. The wound exposes a large area of tissue and is often severely contaminated. The injury carries with it a poor prognosis. If, however, the vasculature and innervation remain intact, there may be some hope for future use of the digit or extremity.

A variation of the degloving process is the ring injury (Figure 4-11). As a person jumps or falls, the ring is caught, pulling the skin of the finger against the victim's weight. The force may tear the upper layers of tissue away from the finger exposing the tendons, nerves, and blood vessels. Although the ring injury involves a smaller area, it is otherwise a degloving injury. The potential for degloving injuries is a reason for paramedics to not wear rings and other jewelry while on duty.

Amputations

The partial or complete severance of a digit or limb is an **amputation** (Figure 4-12). It often results in the complete loss of the limb at the site of the severance. The hemorrhage associated with the amputation may be limited if the limb or digit is cut cleanly or may be severe and continuing if the wound is a jagged or crushing one. Surgeons may attempt to replant the amputated part or use the tissues and skin for grafting as the remaining limb is repaired. If this skin is unavailable, the surgeon may have to cut the bone and musculature back further to close the wound. This reduces the limb length as well as its future usefulness. When amputation is encountered, use great care to ensure that the stump will be as functional as possible and suitable for prosthetic devices.

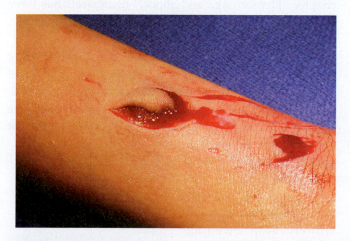

FIGURE 4-10 An avulsion.

(© Dr. Bryan E. Bledsoe)

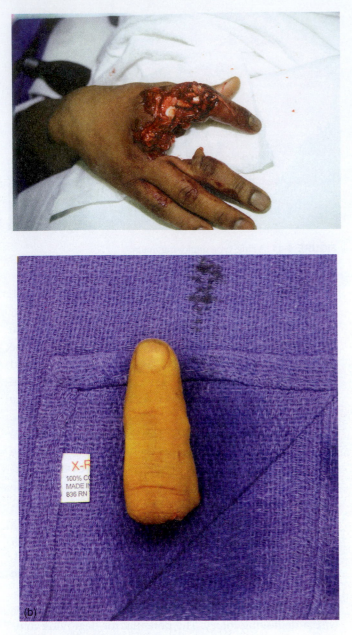

(b)

FIGURE 4-12 An amputated finger.

(© Edward T. Dickinson, MD)

Hemorrhage

Soft tissue injuries frequently cause blood loss, ranging in severity from inconsequential to life threatening. The loss can be arterial, venous, or capillary. Bleeding can be easy or almost impossible to control. Hemorrhage is usually dark red with venous injury, red with capillary injury, and bright red with arterial injury. The rate of hemorrhage also varies from oozing capillary, to flowing venous, to pulsing arterial bleeding. In practice, it may be hard to differentiate among the types and origins of hemorrhage. Research has proven that it is very difficult to approximate the volume of blood loss at the scene. However, the relative amount of blood visible and the

time since the injury may suggest the relative rate of hemorrhage. This information helps to determine the most effective means of hemorrhage control and prioritization of patient for care and transport.

Often the nature of the soft tissue wound may be more important than the size or type of vessel involved in determining the severity of the blood vessel injury. If a moderately sized vein or artery is cleanly cut, the muscles in the vessel wall will tend to contract, thus constricting the **lumen** and retracting the severed vessel into the tissue. As the muscle is withdrawn from the wound, it thickens and further restricts the lumen. This restricts blood flow, reduces the rate of hemorrhage, and assists the clotting mechanism. Therefore, clean lacerations and amputations generally may not bleed profusely. If, however, the vessel is not severed cleanly but is laid open instead, muscle contraction opens the wound, thereby increasing and prolonging blood loss.

Wound Healing

Wound healing is a complex process that begins immediately following injury and can take many months to complete. Wound healing is an essential component of homeostasis, the process whereby the body maintains a uniform environment for itself. Although it is useful to divide the wound healing process into stages or parts, it is important to note that these phases overlap considerably and are intertwined physiologically (Figure 4-13).

Hemostasis

Arguably the most important aspect of wound healing is the body's ability to stop most bleeding on its own. This process is called **hemostasis**. Without hemostasis, even the most trivial nicks and scratches would continue to bleed, leading to life-threatening hemorrhage. As discussed in the chapter "Hemorrhage and Shock," hemostasis has three major components: the vascular phase, the platelet phase, and the coagulation phase.

Hemostasis begins almost immediately following injury with the vascular phase. Arteries, arterioles, and some veins are endowed with a muscular layer that reflexively constricts the vessel in response to local injury. The longitudinal muscles, too, play a role by retracting the cut ends of larger vessels back into the contracted muscle, thus reducing flow. This immediate response usually reduces but does not entirely stop bleeding. Capillaries, which do not have a muscle layer, cannot

> **CONTENT REVIEW**
>
> ➤ Stages of Wound Healing
> - Hemostasis
> - Inflammation
> - Epithelialization
> - Neovascularization
> - Collagen synthesis

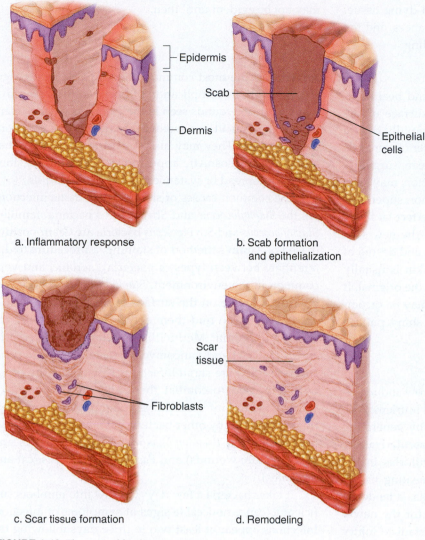

a. Inflammatory response

b. Scab formation
and epithelialization

c. Scar tissue formation

d. Remodeling

FIGURE 4-13 The wound healing process.

is no longer required, it is ultimately resorbed by the body. Any superficial scab merely drops off.

Inflammation

Shortly after hemostasis begins, the body sets in motion a very complex process of healing called **inflammation**. The inflammatory process involves a host of elements, including various kinds of white blood cells, proteins involved in immunity, and hormone-like chemicals that signal other cells to mobilize.

Cells damaged by direct trauma or by invading pathogens release a number of proteins and chemicals into the surrounding tissue and blood. These agents, called **chemotactic factors**, recruit cells responsible for consuming cellular debris, invading bacteria, or other foreign or damaged cells and for beginning the inflammatory process. The first cells to arrive are specialized white blood cells called **granulocytes** and macrophages. These cells (also called phagocytes) are capable of engulfing bacteria, debris, and foreign material, digesting them and then releasing the byproducts in a process called **phagocytosis**. Other white blood cells, called *lymphocytes*, in combination with immunoglobulins or immune proteins, are also mobilized. Lymphocytes attack invading pathogens directly or through an antibody response.

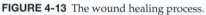

contract and will continue to bleed. This explains the continuing but minor bleeding associated with capillary wounds such as paper cuts and minor abrasions.

Platelets initiate the clotting process (the platelet phase of hemostasis). The damaged vessel wall becomes "sticky," as do the platelets in the turbulent flow of the disrupted vessel. Platelets adhere to the vessel wall and other platelets, forming a platelet plug and reducing blood flow or, in small vessels, stopping it altogether.

When a blood vessel is injured, the disrupted tunica intima exposes collagen and other structural proteins to the blood. In the coagulation phase of hemostasis, these proteins activate a complicated series of enzyme reactions that change certain blood proteins into long fibrin strands. These strands then entrap erythrocytes and produce a gelatinous mass that further occludes the bleeding vessel. This complex process, called *coagulation*, stops all but the most severe and persistent hemorrhage. With time, the clot shrinks or contracts, bringing the wound margins closer together, further facilitating wound healing. When the clot

The injury process, the material released from injured cells, and the debris released as the phagocytes destroy invading cells cause mast cells to release histamine. Histamine dilates precapillary blood vessels, increases capillary permeability, and increases blood flow into and through the injured or infected tissue. This is called **hyperemia** and is responsible for the reddish skin color, or erythema, associated with inflammation. The increased blood flow, along with increased capillary permeability, results in the transfer of protein and electrolyte-rich fluid into the surrounding tissues that is called *edema*. When edema is significant, it is manifest as swelling of the area. Hyperemia brings much-needed oxygen and more phagocytes to the injured area and draws away the byproducts of cell destruction and repair. The increasing blood flow and local tissue metabolism also increase tissue temperature, which may, in turn, denature pathogen membranes. Overall, this response produces a swollen, reddened, and warm region, characteristic of inflammation in response to local infection or injury. The result of the inflammation stage is the accumulation of fluid, heat, and immune and repair cells that enables the clearing away of dead and dying tissue, removal of bacteria and other foreign substances, and the preparation of the damaged area for rebuilding.

Epithelialization

Epithelialization is an early stage in wound healing in which epithelial cells migrate over the surface of the wound. The stratum germinativum cells rapidly divide and regenerate, thus restoring a uniform layer of skin cells along the edges of the healing wound. In clean, surgically prepared wounds, complete epithelialization may take place in as little as 48 hours. Except in minor, superficial wounds, the new epithelial layer is not a perfect facsimile of the original, undamaged skin. Instead, the new skin layer may be thinner, pigmented differently, and devoid of normal hair follicles. However, the new skin is usually quite functional and cosmetically similar to the original. If the wound is very large, epithelialization may be incomplete, and collagen will show through as a shiny, pinkish line of tissue called a *scar*.

Neovascularization

For healing to take place, new tissue must grow and regenerate. This requires blood rich in oxygen and nutrients. The body responds to this increased demand by generating new blood vessels in a process called **neovascularization**. These vessels bud from undamaged capillaries in the wound margins and then grow into the healing tissue. Neovascularized tissue is very fragile and has a tendency to bleed easily. It takes weeks to months for the newly formed blood vessels to become fully resistant to injury and for the surrounding tissue to strengthen enough to protect the new and delicate circulation.

Collagen Synthesis

Collagen is the body's main structural protein. It is a strong, tough fiber forming part of the hair, bones, and connective tissue. Scar tissue, cartilage, and tendons are almost entirely collagen. Specialized cells called **fibroblasts** are brought to the wound area and synthesize collagen as an important step in rebuilding damaged tissues. Collagen binds the wound margins together and strengthens the healing wound. It is important to note that as the wound heals, it is not "as good as new." Regenerated skin has only about 60 percent of the tensile strength of undamaged skin at four months, when the scar is fully mature. This accounts for the occasional reinjury and reopening of wounds weeks or months after healing. The fibroblasts continue to reshape scar tissue and shrink the wound for months after the scab falls off. This **remodeling** involves reorganizing collagen fibers into neat, parallel bands, strengthening the healing tissue still more. Remodeling can continue for up to 6 to 12 months after the initial injury, so the final cosmetic outcome of the healing process may not be evident until then.

Infection

Infection is the most common and, next to hemorrhage, the most serious complication of open wounds. Approximately 1 in 15 wounds seen at the emergency department (6.5 percent) result in a wound infection. These infections delay healing. They may also spread to adjacent tissues and endanger cosmetic appearances. Occasionally, they cause widespread or systemic infection, called *sepsis*.

The common causes of skin and soft tissue infections are the *Staphylococcus* and *Streptococcus* bacterial families. *Staphylococcus* and *Streptococcus* bacteria are Gram-positive (based on Gram's method of staining, a procedure to differentiate between types of bacteria), aerobic, and very common in the environment. *Staphylococcus* bacteria frequently colonize on the surface of normal skin, so it is not surprising to find them driven into wounds by the forces of trauma. Methicillin-resistant *Staphylococcus aureus* (MRSA) and vancomycin-resistant *Staphylococcus aureus* (VRSA) are staph infections resistant to the drugs normally used to combat them and are now a major cause of wound infections. Less commonly, wound infections are caused by other bacteria such as Gram-negative rods, including *Pseudomonas aeruginosa* (diabetics and foot puncture wounds) and *Pasteurella multocida* (cat and dog bites).

It takes bacteria a few days to grow into numbers sufficient to cause noticeable signs or symptoms of infection. Infections appear at least two to three days following the initial wound and commonly present with pain, tenderness, erythema, and warmth. Infection earlier than that is very unusual. Pus, a collection of white blood cells, cellular debris, and dead bacteria, may be visible draining from the wound. The pus is usually thick, pale yellowish to greenish in color, and has a foul smell. Visible red streaks, or **lymphangitis**, may extend from the wound margins up the affected extremity proximally. These streaks represent lymph channel inflammation as a result of the infection. The patient may also complain of fever and malaise, especially if the infection has begun to spread systemically.

Infection Risk Factors

Risk factors for wound infections are related to the host's health, the wound type and location, any associated contamination, and the treatment provided. Diabetics, the infirm, the elderly, and individuals with serious chronic diseases such as chronic obstructive pulmonary disease are at greater risk for infection and heal more slowly and less efficiently than healthy individuals. Patients with any significant disease or preexisting medical problem such as cancer, anemia, hepatic failure, or cardiovascular disease have difficulty mobilizing the immune and tissue-repair response necessary for good wound healing. HIV and AIDS attack the body's immune system and seriously impair its ability to ward off infection, increasing risk significantly. Smoking constricts blood vessels and robs healing tissues of needed oxygen and nutrients, also increasing infection risk, especially to the distal extremities.

Several drugs detract from the body's ability to fight infection. Persons on immunosuppressant medications such as prednisone or cortisone (corticosteroids) are also at increased risk for serious infection. Nonsteroidal anti-inflammatory drugs (NSAIDs), such as ibuprofen, also reduce the body's inflammation response. Chemotherapy agents used to combat rapidly reproducing cells in cancer patients (as well as for other conditions) can also slow repair and cell regeneration at the injury site.

The wound type strongly affects the likelihood of a wound infection. A puncture wound can trap contamination deep within tissue, where there is a perfect environment for bacterial growth. Avulsion tears away blood vessels and supporting structures, interrupting the blood supply—a critical factor in preventing or reducing infection. Crush injuries and other wounds that produce large areas of injured or dead (devitalized) tissue provide an excellent environment for bacterial growth and are at great risk for wound infection.

In a similar fashion, certain wound locations influence infection risk. Well-vascularized areas such as the face and scalp are very resistant to infection. Distal extremities—the feet in particular—are at greater risk.

Clean objects, such as uncontaminated sheet metal or a clean knife, usually leave only small amounts of bacteria in a wound and, consequently, do not often cause infections. However, objects contaminated with organic matter and bacteria, such as a nail on a barnyard floor, a knife used to clean raw meat, or a piece of wood, pose much greater risks of infection. The infection risk associated with bites caused by mammals, and carnivores in particular, is very great. Bites by humans, cats, and dogs are among the most common and most serious types of bites.[2]

The type of treatment provided for a wound affects the risk of infection. Use of sterile dressings and clean examination gloves minimizes wound contamination during prehospital treatment. Gloves protect not only the rescuer but also the patient from contaminants on the rescuer's hands. Wound irrigation with sterile saline using a pressurized stream device has been shown to reduce bacterial loads and reduce infection rates. Closing wounds (with sutures or staples, for example) increases infection risks as compared to leaving wounds open. However, the risks associated with wound closure are frequently accepted in order to achieve the best possible cosmetic outcome and more rapid healing.

In most cases, routine use of antibiotics with wounds does not help reduce infection rates and, in fact, may increase the likelihood of infection with antibiotic-resistant microorganisms. Antibiotics may be helpful if given within the first hour or so after deep major wounds, such as those from gunshots or stabbings, puncture wounds to the feet, and wounds where retention of a foreign body is suspected.

GANGRENE Gangrene is tissue decomposition by bacteria resulting from loss of blood supply, crush injury, or infection. It is one of the rarest and most feared wound complications. Gangrene is a deep-space infection usually caused by the anaerobic bacterium *Clostridium perfringens*. These bacteria characteristically produce a gas deep within a wound, causing subcutaneous emphysema and a foul smell whenever the gas escapes. Once they have become established, the bacteria are particularly prolific and can rapidly involve an entire extremity. Left unchecked, gangrene frequently leads to sepsis and death. In the days before antibiotics, amputation was frequently necessary to stop the spread of the disease. Modern treatment with a combination of antibiotics, surgery, and hyperbaric oxygenation effectively arrests most cases of gangrene if caught early in their course.

TETANUS Another highly feared but, fortunately, rare complication of wound infections is **tetanus**, or lockjaw. Tetanus is caused by the bacterium *Clostridium tetani*, and, like its cousin *Clostridium perfringens*, it is anaerobic. Tetanus presents with few signs or symptoms at the local wound site, but the bacteria produce a potent toxin that causes widespread, painful, involuntary muscle contractions. Early observers noted mandibular trismus, or jaw clenching ("lockjaw"). There is an antidote for the tetanus toxin, but it neutralizes only circulating toxin molecules, not those already bound to the motor endplates. Thus, treatment is slow and recovery prolonged.

Fortunately, tetanus is preventable through immunization. Widespread immunization has reduced incidence to a very few cases. The standard immunization is a series of three shots in childhood, with boosters every ten years thereafter. It is common practice in emergency departments to provide boosters to wound patients if they have not been immunized in the past five years. Immigrants from undeveloped countries often have never completed a tetanus vaccine series. In these cases, it is prudent to administer tetanus immune globulin (TIG) in addition to the tetanus vaccine to prevent development of the disease while the body gears up to make new antibodies.

Other Wound Complications

Several circumstances or conditions can interfere with normal wound healing processes. These conditions include impaired hemostasis, rebleeding, and delayed healing.

Impaired Hemostasis

Several medications can interfere with hemostasis and the clotting process. Aspirin and clopidogrel (Plavix) are powerful inhibitors of platelet aggregation, and are used clinically to help prevent clot formation in the coronary and cerebral arteries of patients at risk for myocardial infarction or stroke. Thus, a side effect of aspirin or clopidogrel use is a prolongation of clotting time, an important consideration in a patient who has sustained significant trauma or is undergoing major surgery. Likewise, anticoagulants, such as warfarin (Coumadin) and heparin, and fibrinolytics, such as rtPA and streptokinase, interfere with or break down the protein fibers that form clots and are used to prevent or destroy obstructions at critical locations. Additionally, abnormalities in proteins involved in the fibrin formation cascade may result in delayed clotting, as is the case in hemophiliacs.

Rebleeding

Despite treatment that provides adequate initial bleeding control, rebleeding is possible from any wound. Movement of underlying structures, such as muscles or bones, or of the bandage or dressing material may dislodge clots and reinstitute hemorrhage.

In addition, hemorrhage that appears to have been stopped may actually be bleeding into an oversized dressing until it saturates the dressing and pushes through it. Monitor dressings and bandages frequently to ensure that blood loss is not continuing.

Partially healed wounds are also at risk for rebleeding. Postoperative wounds, in particular, can rebleed—sometimes with life-threatening results. Because patients are being discharged from hospitals more quickly than in the past, be wary of this potential complication.

Delayed Healing

In some patients, the wound repair process may be delayed or even arrested, resulting in incomplete wound healing. Persons at greatest risk for this complication are diabetics, the elderly, the chronically ill, and the malnourished. Nutrition must be adequate for wound healing to occur. Patients with multiple injuries often require significantly more calories during the healing phase than normal. Seriously or chronically infected wounds and wounds in locations with limited blood flow (distal extremities) are also at risk for incomplete healing. Incompletely healed wounds remain tender and are easily reinjured. A pale yellow or blood-tinged **serous fluid** may drain from them. Out-of-hospital treatment of incompletely healed wounds includes frequent changes of sterile, nonadherent dressings, and protection of the wound.

Compartment Syndrome

Compartment syndrome is a complication most commonly associated with closed injuries to the extremities, most commonly a fracture or crushing-type injury. In the extremities, major muscle groups are contained in compartments formed by strong and inelastic fascia (Figure 4-14).

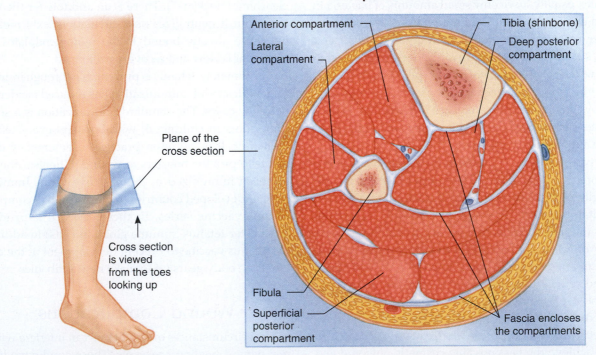

Compartments of the Leg

Anterior compartment
Lateral compartment
Plane of the cross section
Cross section is viewed from the toes looking up
Fibula
Superficial posterior compartment
Tibia (shinbone)
Deep posterior compartment
Fascia encloses the compartments

FIGURE 4-14 Musculoskeletal compartments segregated by fasciae.

injury is accidentally discharging the device with the tip in proximity to the skin. This causes a small superficial skin wound. However, tissues below the wound can sustain serious injury from the grease or fluid, the pressure, or a combination of the two. These wounds often cause serious infections and loss of function if not surgically explored and adequately treated. If the injury involves the hand (as is common), the pressure may inject materials into the forearm and even as far as the arm or shoulder. The grease or other foreign substance tends to follow the fascial planes of the hand and forearm and can become embedded within the muscle sheaths. The injury generally presents with a small open wound with some contamination, but its nature is generally far worse than the wound's physical signs and symptoms suggest.

Contaminants introduced deep into the wound exist in an environment with limited air and circulation (anaerobic state). However, the area is warm and moist, providing any bacteria introduced into the wound an ideal environment to proliferate. Hydraulic fluid and grease are toxic to the internal tissues and cause cell injury and death. Because of the depth and extent of contamination, surgical debridement is extremely difficult and may, itself, cause significant and extensive tissue injury. Whenever a patient presents with this type of injury, recognize the likelihood of extensive limb involvement and seek the services of the trauma center.

Dressing and Bandage Materials

Several types of dressings and bandages are effective in prehospital care. A *dressing* is material placed directly on the wound to control bleeding and maintain wound cleanliness.[3] A *bandage* is material used to hold a dressing in place and to apply direct pressure to control hemorrhage. Dressings and bandages have various designs and are used for a variety of purposes in emergency care.

CONTENT REVIEW

➤ Types of Bandaging and Dressing Materials

Dressings
- Sterile/nonsterile
- Occlusive/nonocclusive
- Adherent/nonadherent
- Absorbent/nonabsorbent
- Wet/dry
- Hemostatic

Bandages
- Self-adherent roller
- Gauze
- Adhesive
- Elastic
- Triangular

Dressings

Sterile/Nonsterile Dressings

Sterile dressings are cotton or other fiber pads that have been specially prepared to be without microorganisms. They are usually packaged individually and remain sterile for as long as the package is intact. Once the packaging is opened, sterile dressings become contaminated by airborne dust and particles that harbor bacteria and other microorganisms. Sterile dressings are designed to be applied in direct contact with wounds.

Nonsterile dressings are clean—that is, free of gross contamination—but are not free of microscopic contamination and microorganisms. Nonsterile dressings are not intended to be applied directly to a wound, but rather to be placed over a sterile dressing to add bulk or absorptive power.

Occlusive/Nonocclusive Dressings

Some dressings, such as sterilized plastic wrap and petroleum-impregnated gauze, are designed to prevent the movement of fluid and air through them. These dressings are called *occlusive* and are helpful in preventing air aspiration into chest wounds (open pneumothorax) and open neck wounds (air emboli into the jugular vein). Most dressing material is nonocclusive.

Adherent/Nonadherent Dressings

Adherent dressings are untreated cotton or other fiber pads that will stick to drying blood and fluid that has leaked from open wounds. Adherent dressings have the advantage of promoting clot formation and thus reducing hemorrhage, but their removal from wounds can be quite painful. Removal or disturbance of an adherent dressing is also likely to break the clot and cause rebleeding. Nonadherent dressings are specially treated with chemicals such as polymers to prevent the wound fluids and clotting materials from adhering to the dressing. Nonadherent dressings are preferred for most uncomplicated wounds.

Absorbent/Nonabsorbent Dressings

Absorbent dressings readily soak up blood and other fluids, much as a sponge soaks up water. This property is helpful in many bleeding situations. Nonabsorbent dressings absorb little or no fluid and are used when a barrier to leaking is desired. The clear membrane dressings frequently placed over intravenous puncture sites are good examples of nonabsorbent dressings. Most other dressings used in prehospital care are absorbent dressings.

Wet/Dry Dressings

Wet dressings are sometimes applied to special types of wounds, such as burns. They are also used in the hospital to effect healing in some complicated postoperative wounds. Sterile normal saline is the usual fluid used to wet dressings. Wet dressings provide a medium for the movement of infectious material into wounds, however, and are not commonly used in prehospital care, except with injuries such as abdominal eviscerations or burns involving only a limited body surface area. Dry dressings are the type most often employed for wounds in prehospital care.

Hemostatic Dressings

A new development in wound care is the topical hemostatic agents (Figure 4-17). These products, approved by the FDA, can be applied directly to a bleeding wound and will help to slow or stop the bleeding. There are several products on the market. These include the following:

- *Celox*™ is a granular powder placed immediately on a bleeding wound to control or stop bleeding. The principal ingredient is chitosan, a polysaccharide that is derived from the shells of crustaceans (e.g., shrimp, crabs). When chitosan becomes moistened with blood, it becomes extremely adherent and stops bleeding. Chitosan has antibacterial properties and is hypoallergenic. Celox has a shelf life of three years.

- *HemCon* bandages are dressings impregnated with chitosan. They are supplied in 2″ × 2″, 2″ × 4″, and 4″ × 4″ dressings. They have been widely used in battlefield care.

- *QuickClot*® is hemostatic agent that is made from zeolite. Zeolite is a proprietary substance derived from volcanic rock. It is supplied in 3.5-ounce packets that can be poured directly on the wound. QuickClot quickly absorbs water, thus concentrating the blood and promoting clot formation. The reaction can generate heat (exothermic reaction), however. Temperatures up to 143°C and burn injuries have been reported. The company has modified the formulation to reduce the severity of the exothermic reaction. The shelf life is three years.

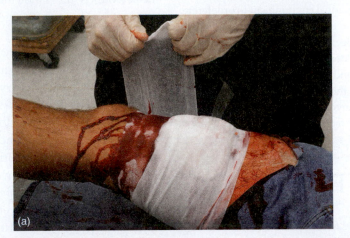

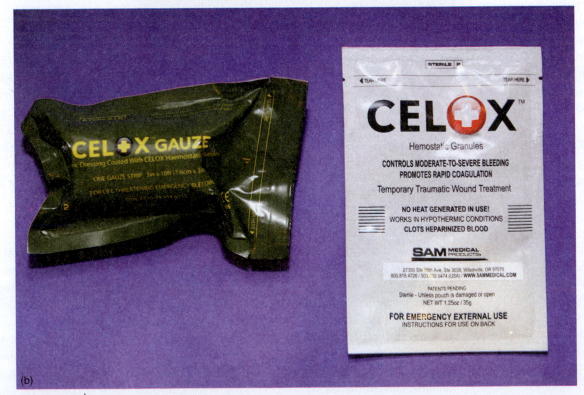

FIGURE 4-17 (a) A hemostatic dressing applied to a large wound. (b) Hemostatic agents are available as dressings or granules.

(Photo b: Dr. Bryan E. Bledsoe)

- *TraumaDEX*™ is a starch-based powder derived from plants. It is supplied in a bellows and applied directly to the wound. The hemostatic effects are derived from the absorption of the water from blood, which promotes clot formation.

Bandages

Self-Adherent Roller Bandages

The most common and convenient bandage material is the soft, self-adherent, roller bandage (Kling or Kerlix). It has limited stretch and resists unraveling as it is rolled over itself. It conforms well to body contours and is quick and easy to use. This bandage is most appropriate for injuries located where it can be wrapped circumferentially. It comes in rolls from 1 to 6 inches wide.

Gauze Bandages

Like soft, self-adherent bandages, gauze bandages are a convenient material for securing dressings. They do not stretch, however, and thus do not conform as well to body contours as the self-adherent material, but they are otherwise functional for bandaging. Because gauze bandages do not stretch, they may increase the pressure associated with tissue swelling at injury sites. Gauze usually comes in rolls from 0.5 to 2 inches wide.

Adhesive Bandages

An adhesive bandage (or adhesive tape) is a strong plastic, paper, or fabric material with adhesive applied to one side. It can effectively secure a small dressing to a location where circumferential wrapping is impractical. When used circumferentially, an adhesive bandage does not allow for any swelling and permits pressure to accumulate in tissues beneath it. Adhesive bandages usually come in widths that range from 0.25 to 3 inches.

Elastic (Ace) Bandages

Elastic bandages stretch easily and conform to body contours. Elastic bandages provide stability and support for minor musculoskeletal injuries, but they are not commonly used in prehospital care. When using these bandages, however, remember that it is very easy to apply too much pressure with them. Each consecutive wrap applied will contain and add to pressure on the wound site. Swelling associated with the wound may increase the pressure until blood flow through and out of the affected limb is reduced or stopped.

Triangular Bandages

Triangular bandages, or cravats, are large triangles of cotton or linen fabric. They are strong, nonelastic bandages commonly used to make slings and swathes and, in some cases, to affix splints. They can also be used to hold dressings in place, but they do not conform as well to body contours as soft, self-adherent bandages and do not maintain pressure or immobilize wound dressings very well.

Assessment of Soft Tissue Injuries

Careful observation of the skin is an essential element of trauma assessment. Not only is the skin the first body organ to experience the effects of trauma, but it is also the first and often the only organ to display them. Therefore, assessment of the skin must be deliberate, careful, and complete. Although the processes that cause soft-tissue injuries and the manifestations of those injuries vary, prehospital assessment is a simple, well-structured process. Follow the assessment process carefully and completely to establish the nature and extent of each injury. Doing so enables you to assign soft tissue injuries, and other injuries associated with them, the appropriate priorities for care.

Assessment of patients with soft tissue wounds follows the same general progression as the assessment of other trauma patients. First, size up the scene, ruling out potential hazards. Then, try to determine the mechanism of injury. Look for any environmental conditions that may affect extrication, assessment, patient packaging, patient care, and transport. Determine the need for additional medical and rescue resources in coordination with scene oversight (incident command). Next, perform a quick primary assessment and identify and care for any immediately life-threatening injuries. For the patient with a mechanism of injury or signs and symptoms that suggest serious trauma, perform a rapid trauma assessment and use trauma triage criteria to determine the need for rapid transport. For a patient with no significant mechanism of injury and no indication from the primary assessment of a serious injury or life threat, perform a focused trauma assessment and gather vital signs and patient history at the scene. Perform a detailed physical exam only if conditions warrant and time permits. Provide serial reassessments to track the patient's response to his injuries and care.

Scene Size-Up

During the scene size-up, look for evidence that will help determine the mechanism of injury and anticipate the likely injuries and their severity. Although soft tissue injuries are not usually life threatening, they can suggest other, serious problems. Identify where injury is likely and be prepared to carefully examine the skin for evidence that suggests internal injury. Consider mechanisms of injury that could cause entrapment and either crush injury or crush syndrome.

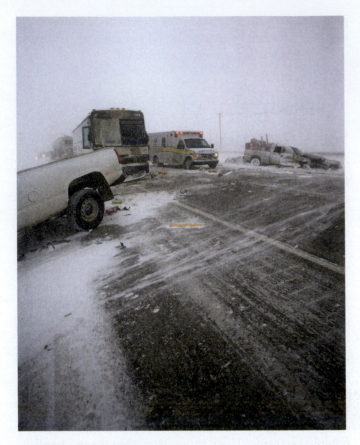

FIGURE 4-18 During the scene size-up, rule out hazards, don gloves, and analyze the mechanism of injury.

(© Kevin Link/Science Source)

Be alert, because any mechanisms that injured the patient may still be present and pose threats to rescuers. Rule out or eliminate any hazards before entering the scene (Figure 4-18).

Primary Assessment

Begin the primary assessment by forming a general patient impression. Be sure to maintain spinal stabilization as directed in your local protocols if significant head or spine injury is suspected. Determine the patient's level of consciousness and assess the airway, breathing, and circulation. Assess perfusion by noting skin color, temperature, and condition and by assessing capillary refill.

During this assessment, pay particular attention to the location and types of visible wounds to gain further understanding of the mechanism of injury and whether it produced blunt or penetrating trauma. If responsive, the patient may be able to provide critical information about how the wound occurred. If the patient is unable to speak, first responders or bystanders may be able to provide this information. Correct any immediate threats to the patient's life when discovered and prioritize the patient for care and transport.

Secondary Assessment

Use the information gathered through the primary assessment to determine how to proceed in the secondary assessment process. Patients with serious trauma, suggested by a significant mechanism of injury or the findings of the primary assessment, should receive a rapid trauma assessment. All other patients will receive a focused trauma assessment.

Significant Mechanism of Injury— Rapid Trauma Assessment

In the rapid trauma assessment, perform a swift evaluation of the patient's head, neck, chest, abdomen, pelvis, extremities, and posterior body. Examine these areas for signs of internal or life-endangering injuries. Quickly investigate any discolorations, deformities, temperature variations, abnormal muscle tone, or open wounds.

Ensure that any detected wounds or any injuries suggested beneath them do not involve or endanger the airway or breathing or contribute significantly to blood loss. Focus immediate care during the rapid trauma assessment on continuing to support the patient's airway and breathing and then on controlling severe blood loss.

Inspect and palpate areas where the mechanism of injury suggests serious injuries may exist. Again, look for discoloration, temperature variation, abnormal muscle tone, and deformity suggestive of trauma (Figure 4-19). If the mechanism of injury suggests open wounds, sweep body areas hidden from sight with gloved hands. This will rule out the possibility of unseen blood loss and pooling. Control moderate to severe hemorrhage immediately. Hemorrhage control need not be definitive, but should stop continuing significant blood loss. Once more serious injuries are cared for, return and dress and bandage wounds more carefully.

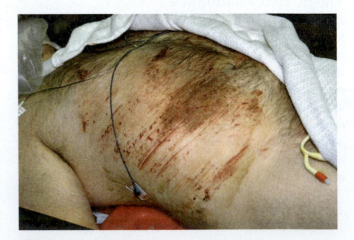

FIGURE 4-19 Often, the only signs of serious internal injury are external soft tissue injuries.

(© Edward T. Dickinson, MD)

Survey all bleeding wounds to determine the type of hemorrhage—arterial, venous, or capillary. Attempt to approximate the relative rate of blood lost since the time of the incident.

Carry out the exam using the methods described in "Assessment Techniques" later in this chapter. Apply a cervical collar or cervical stabilization per local protocols once rapid assessment of the head and neck has been completed, if indicated.

When the rapid trauma assessment is complete, obtain a set of baseline vital signs, Glasgow Coma Score, and a patient history. Be sure to maintain spinal stabilization as directed in your local protocols, if indicated, while the signs and history are being gathered. If there are enough personnel, the vital signs, Glasgow Coma Score, and history may be obtained simultaneously as the rapid trauma assessment is performed.

When obtaining the history, be sure to question the patient about medications, especially those that may have some direct relevance to soft tissue injuries. For example, the patient's tetanus history is important with any trauma that breaks the skin. Determine whether the patient has had a tetanus booster, and how long ago it was given. Note that a patient's routine use of aspirin, clopidogrel, or blood thinners—for example, heparin or warfarin for stroke or MI risk—may affect the body's ability to halt even minimal hemorrhage. Ask about the use of anti-inflammatory medications, such as prednisone, because these medications reduce the inflammatory response and slow the normal healing process. Question the patient about any preexisting diseases. Certain diseases, especially AIDS, hepatitis C, and hemophilia, increase the risks of infection and the problems of hemorrhage control.

At the conclusion of the rapid trauma assessment, confirm the decision either to transport the patient immediately with further care provided en route to the hospital or to remain at the scene and complete treatment of non–life-threatening injuries. Consider the rate and volume of any blood loss and any uncontrollable bleeding in this decision.

If the patient's condition merits care at the scene, prioritize the identified soft tissue to establish the order of care to follow. The few moments taken to sort out injuries and to plan the management process may save valuable time in the field. They also ensure that the needed care for injuries with the highest priority is provided.

No Significant Mechanism of Injury—Focused Trauma Assessment

When a patient has a soft tissue injury but neither a significant mechanism of injury nor an indication of a serious problem from the primary assessment—for example, a cut finger or a knee abrasion from a fall—the sequence of assessment steps is different from that for a patient with a significant injury mechanism. Begin this phase of the assessment with a focused trauma assessment, which is an exam directed at the injury site—the finger or the knee in the examples previously noted. A full head-to-toe rapid trauma assessment is not necessary in most such cases.

Direct the focused assessment at the chief complaint and any area of injury suggested by the mechanism of injury. Use the examination techniques of inquiry, inspection, and palpation (described in the following sections) to evaluate the injury and the surrounding area. In the case of a wound to an extremity, be sure to check the distal extremity for pulses, capillary refill, color, and temperature. Then, obtain a set of baseline vital signs and a history from the patient. If any of the findings suggest that the patient has more serious injuries, perform a rapid trauma assessment and consider rapid transport.

Depending on the nature of the injury, the decision must be made to provide transport or to release/refer the patient. When treating an isolated injury, such as a cut finger, your system's protocols may determine whether to release/refer the patient or transport the patient. Increasingly, EMS systems are employing release/referral protocols to improve system efficiency. If transport is indicated, provide ongoing assessment.

Detailed Physical Exam

Once the rapid or focused trauma assessment has been completed, vital signs and history have been gathered, and necessary emergency care steps have been taken, perform a detailed physical exam. Like the rapid trauma assessment, this head-to-toe evaluation of the skin (and the rest of the body) involves the techniques of inquiry, observation, and palpation. The detailed exam should follow a planned and comprehensive process, ideally progressing from head to toe, although the order is not critical. The main purpose of the detailed assessment is to detect any additional information regarding the patient's condition and to search for any unsuspected or subtle injuries. Manage any additional injuries discovered during the examination. The detailed physical exam is usually performed during transport or on scene if transport has been delayed. Never delay transport to perform it and perform it only if the patient's condition permits.

Assessment Techniques

The assessment techniques that follow can be used during both the rapid trauma assessment and the detailed physical exam.

Inquiry

Question the patient about the mechanism of injury, any pain, pain on touch or movement, and any loss of function or unusual sensation specific to an area. Additionally, attempt to determine the exact nature of the pain or sensory or motor loss by using elements of the OPQRST mnemonic (see the chapter "Patient Assessment in the Field"). Question the patient about signs and symptoms before touching an area.

Inspection

Continue the exam by carefully observing a particular body region. Identify any discolorations, deformities, or open wounds in those regions.

Determine if any discoloration is local, distal, or systemic, reflecting local injury, circulation compromise, or systemic complications such as shock. Contusions, blood vessel injuries, dislocations, and fractures may cause local discoloration, including erythema or ecchymosis. Distal discoloration may present as a pale, cyanotic, or ashen-colored limb distal to the point of circulation loss. Look for systemic discoloration, such as pale, ashen, or grayish skin in all limbs, suggestive of hypovolemia and shock.

Examine any deformities found to determine their cause. Is the deformity due to a developing hematoma, to the normal swelling associated with the inflammatory process, or to underlying injuries?

Inspect any wounds in detail. Examine the wound to determine the depth and evaluate the potential for damage to underlying muscles, nerves, blood vessels, organs, or bones. If possible, identify the object that caused the wound and determine the amount of force transmitted by it to the body's interior. Ascertain whether there are any foreign bodies, contamination, or impaled objects in the wound. Finally, identify the nature and location of any hemorrhage.

Observe each wound carefully in order to describe it to the attending physician. This information will help the emergency department staff prioritize the patient. Careful observation will also aid in preparation of the prehospital care report. Adequate lighting is crucial for evaluating wounds. If necessary, defer this portion of the detailed physical exam until better lighting is available, as in the back of the ambulance.

If a patient's limb or digit has been amputated, have other rescuers conduct a brief but thorough search for the amputated part. If the part cannot be located immediately or remains entrapped, do not delay transport. Instead, leave someone on scene to continue the search. Ensure that once the body part is found and retrieved, it is properly handled, packaged, and brought to the same hospital as the patient.

Palpation

In addition to questioning the patient and inspecting the body regions, palpate the body's entire surface. Be alert for any deformity, asymmetry, temperature variation, unexpected mass, or localized loss of skin or muscle tone. Gently palpate all apparent closed wounds for evidence of tenderness, swelling, crepitus, and subcutaneous emphysema. Avoid palpating the interior of open wounds, which may introduce contamination and disturb the clotting process. Ascertain the presence or absence of distal pulses and capillary refill time with any extremity injury. Also, check motor and sensory function distal to any extremity wound and compare findings with those from the opposite limb.

Reassessment

During transport, provide periodic reassessments, reexamining the patient's mental status, airway, breathing, and circulation. Obtain additional sets of vital signs and evaluate the patient's injuries. Also inspect any interventions performed. Provide a reassessment at least every 5 minutes with unstable patients and every 15 minutes with stable patients. If any change in the patient's condition is noted, modify the patient's priority for transport and care accordingly.

Management of Soft Tissue Injuries

Once patient assessment is completed, take steps to manage the soft tissue injury. Control of hemorrhage, prevention of shock, and decontamination of affected areas take priority. The following sections describe some of the most important of these care steps.

Unless extensive bleeding is detected, wound management by dressing and bandaging is a late priority in the care of trauma patients. Dress and bandage wounds whose bleeding does not represent a life threat only after treating higher priority injuries.

Objectives of Wound Dressing and Bandaging

The dressing and bandaging of a wound has three basic objectives: to control all hemorrhaging, to keep the wound as clean as possible, and to immobilize the wound. The appearance of the final dressing and bandage is not as critical as the achievement of these three objectives.

Hemorrhage Control

The primary method of controlling hemorrhage associated with soft tissue injury—and the most effective one—is direct pressure. In cases of serious hemorrhage flowing from a wound with some force, place a small dressing directly over the site of the bleeding and apply pressure directly to it with a finger. When the bleeding is the more commonly encountered slow-to-moderate type, use a dressing that has been sized to cover and pad the wound. Then simply wrap the dressing with a soft, self-adherent bandage using moderate pressure to hold the dressing in place and halt the blood loss. Monitor the wound frequently to ensure that bleeding has stopped.

Occasionally, bleeding from a soft tissue injury can be difficult to control. If the bleeding continues despite the use of direct pressure, reassess the wound and ensure that direct pressure is properly applied to the bleeding site. If the dressing and bandage are ineffective, reapply direct digital pressure to the precise bleeding point. Often, hemorrhage continues because the bandaging technique distributes pressure over the entire wound site rather than focusing it directly on the bleeding source. The force driving hemorrhage is the patient's systolic blood pressure. Properly applied digital pressure can exceed this to compress the vessel slowing or controlling any blood loss.

In certain circumstances, direct pressure may not control hemorrhage. Crush injuries, amputations, and some penetrating trauma are situations in which normal bleeding control measures may be ineffective. With these injuries, several blood vessels are jaggedly torn, confounding the body's normal hemorrhage control mechanisms and making it difficult to pinpoint the bleeding source. Even if the source of bleeding can be found, applying firm direct pressure to it may be difficult. In such cases, the application of a tourniquet may be useful. Although the tourniquet should be considered the last option for controlling hemorrhage, its use should never be delayed when indicated. If properly applied, the tourniquet will stop the flow of life-threatening hemorrhage. However, its use has serious associated risks.[4] Keep the following precautions in mind whenever considering using a tourniquet:

1. If the pressure applied is insufficient, the tourniquet may stop venous return while permitting continued arterial blood flow into the extremity, thus increasing the rate and volume of blood loss and swelling.

2. When the tourniquet is applied properly, the entire limb distal to the device is without circulation. Hypoxia, ischemia, and necrosis may permanently damage the tissue distal to the tourniquet.

3. A tourniquet should be tightened only enough to stop the blood flow. Overtightening may result in crush injury to the body part directly beneath the tourniquet.

4. When circulation is restored, the blood flows and pools in the extremity, adding to any hypovolemia. In addition, any blood that returns to the central circulation may be highly hypoxic, acidic, and toxic. This blood can cause shock, lethal arrhythmias, renal failure, and death. The return of circulation may also restart hemorrhage and introduce emboli into the central circulation.

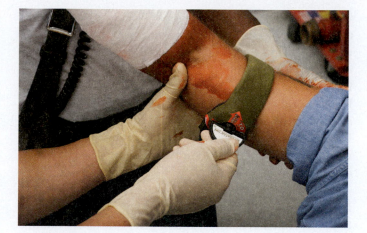

FIGURE 4-20 A commercial tourniquet.

Use a tourniquet when severe bleeding cannot be controlled by any other means. Place it just proximal to the wound site, but stay away from the elbow or knee joints (Figure 4-20). Apply the tourniquet in a way that will not injure the tissue beneath. For example, do not use very narrow material, like rope or wire, for a tourniquet; applying great pressure to a limb with such material may cause serious injury in the compressed tissue. Instead, select a 2-inch or wider band for compression.

Commercial tourniquets now available are very effective in hemorrhage control, easy to apply, and their design reduces any chance of associated injury. If a commercial tourniquet is not at hand, a readily available tourniquet is the sphygmomanometer (regular for the upper extremity and thigh for the lower). It is wide, simple to apply, rapid to inflate, and easy to monitor. Inflate it to a pressure 20 to 30 mmHg above the patient's systolic blood pressure and beyond the pressure at which the patient's hemorrhage ceases. Once applied—because sphygmomanometers tend to leak air—it is essential to record the initial pressure within the cuff and monitor it frequently to ensure the pressure does not diminish.

Once a tourniquet is applied, leave it in place until the patient arrives at the emergency department. Monitor the tourniquet during transport to ensure that it does not lose pressure, and watch for signs of renewed bleeding. If bleeding starts again, increase the tourniquet pressure. Alert the hospital staff to the tourniquet during transport as well as on arrival. Make sure the receiving physician is aware that a tourniquet has been applied.

In general, a tourniquet is released only when the patient arrives at a facility with blood transfusion and surgical capability.[4] Do not release a tourniquet in the field except under exceptional circumstances, and then only during consultation with medical direction. Be prepared to provide vigorous fluid resuscitation, ECG monitoring, arrhythmia treatment, and rapid transport if a tourniquet release is attempted.

Cleanliness

Once severe bleeding has been controlled, try to keep the wound as clean as possible. Under field conditions, sterility is impossible, but any contamination can make healing more difficult. With very small open wounds, like an IV start or a small laceration, consider the application of an antibacterial ointment to help with infection control. However, the effectiveness of such ointments on larger wounds is limited and ointments are not generally applied to these wounds.

Under normal conditions, do not cleanse the wound. If a wound is grossly contaminated and there is a longer transport time, consider irrigating it with normal saline solution. A 1,000-mL bag of saline, connected to a macrodrip administration set and pressurized by squeezing the bag under your arm, may allow rapid and gentle wound cleansing. Try to move any contamination from the center of the wound outward. Carefully remove larger particles—glass, gravel, debris, and so forth—if this can be accomplished quickly without inducing further injury.

Apply a bandage to make the dressing appear as neat as time and conditions allow. Often, this is as easy as covering the entire dressing with wraps of soft, self-adherent roller bandage. The neat appearance calms and reassures the patient while the bandaging reduces contamination and the chances of post-injury infection.

Immobilization

The final objective of bandaging is immobilization. Stability of the wound site helps the natural clotting mechanisms operate and reduces patient discomfort. This is especially true of wounds in or near a joint where motion is most likely to cause the wound to gape, dislodge clots, and bleed more profusely.

Maintaining gentle pressure with the bandage may reduce pain and local swelling as well. Immobilize the limb with bandaging material to the patient's body or to a rigid surface such as a padded board or ladder splint. When immobilizing a limb, do not use elastic bandaging material or apply the bandage too tightly. The edema that develops rapidly with an injury puts increasing pressure on underlying tissue. This pressure may quickly reduce or halt circulation. (See more about controlling pain and edema in the next section.)

Frequently monitor any limb that was bandaged circumferentially to ensure that the distal pulse and capillary refill remain adequate and that the distal extremity maintains good color and does not swell. If a distal pulse cannot be detected, monitor capillary refill, skin color, and temperature. If signs or symptoms suggest that the distal circulation is compromised, elevate the extremity, if possible, and consider loosening or reapplying the bandage.

Pain and Edema Control

Treat painful soft tissue injuries or those likely to cause large debilitating edema with the application of cold packs and moderate-pressure bandages. Cold reduces inflammatory response and local edema. It also dulls the pain associated with soft tissue trauma. Use a commercial cold pack or ice in a plastic bag wrapped in a dry towel and apply it to the wound. Do not use a cold pack directly against the skin, as it cools beyond any therapeutic value. Direct application of a cold pack may also cause tissue freezing, especially in areas with reduced circulation. A mnemonic used by sports medicine (regarding blunt muscle injury)—RICE—stands for **R**est, **I**ce, **C**ompression, and **E**levation. Mild compression reduces the edema associated with injury, and elevation enhances venous return and also reduced edema.

Gentle pressure over the wound area may also help reduce pain and wound edema.[3] If the patient reports severe pain, consider use of morphine sulfate, fentanyl, or other analgesics for patient comfort. Avoid aspirin or NSAIDs (e.g., ibuprofen [Motrin, Advil], naproxen [Aleve]), as they may reduce clotting.

Anatomic Considerations for Bandaging

Each area of the body has specific anatomic characteristics. Application of bandages and dressings should take these characteristics into account to provide effective prehospital wound care.

Scalp

The scalp has a rich supply of vessels that can bleed heavily when injured. It is commonly said that internal head injuries rarely account for hypovolemic shock, but scalp hemorrhage can be severe and difficult to control and can lead to the loss of moderate to large volumes of blood.

In scalp hemorrhage uncomplicated by skull fracture, direct pressure against the skull is effective in the control of bleeding. To hold a dressing in place and maintain pressure, wrap a bandage around the head, capturing the occiput or brow or, in some cases, passing the bandage under the chin (while still allowing for jaw movement and mouth opening).

If a head wound is complicated by fracture, be very careful in your application of pressure. Apply gentle digital pressure around the wound and attempt to locate the small scalp arteries that feed it to use as pressure points. Then simply hold a dressing on the wound without much pressure.

Face

Facial wounds are frequently gruesome and bleed heavily. Gentle direct pressure to these wounds can effectively control hemorrhage. Maintain pressure by wrapping a bandage around the head. Be careful to ensure a clear airway and use the bandaging to splint any facial instability.

Remember, blood is a gastric irritant and swallowed blood may cause vomiting. Be ready to provide suctioning in patients with oral or nasal hemorrhage because unexpected emesis may compromise the airway.

Ear or Mastoid

Wounds to the ear region can be easily bandaged by wrapping the head circumferentially. Use open gauze to collect, not stop, any bleeding or fluids flowing from the ear canal. These materials may contain cerebrospinal fluid, and stopping flow may add to any increasing intracranial pressure.

Neck

Minor neck wounds may be taped to hold dressings in place. If bleeding is moderate to severe, however, direct manual pressure may be necessary because the amount of pressure applied by circumferential wrapping may compromise both the airway and circulation to and from the head. In cases of large wounds or moderate to severe bleeding, also consider using an occlusive dressing to prevent aspiration of air into a jugular vein. In any neck wound, careful monitoring of the airway is required as continued bleeding, tissue swelling, or hematoma formation may all obstruct the airway.

Shoulder

The shoulder is an easy area to bandage, as soft, self-adherent roller bandages readily conform to body contours. Use the axilla, arm, and neck as points of fixation, but be careful not to put pressure on the anterior neck and trachea.

Trunk

For minor trunk wounds, adhesive tape may be sufficient to hold dressings in place. With larger wounds, bandaging can be more difficult because it may be necessary to wrap the patient's body circumferentially to apply direct pressure to a wound. Be aware that applying a circumferential bandage to the thorax may impede the normal chest wall excursion during breathing. Monitor the respiratory rate and depth and the pulse oximeter in such cases. Applying a bandage circumferentially may also require moving the patient and risk causing or worsening an injury. Consider instead using a formable SAM splint that is negotiated beneath the patient's torso and molded to the patient's torso to serve as an anchor for bandaging (Figure 4-21).

Groin and Hip

The groin and the hip are easy places to affix a dressing. Bandage by following the contours of the upper thighs and waist, similar to the technique of bandaging a shoulder. Be

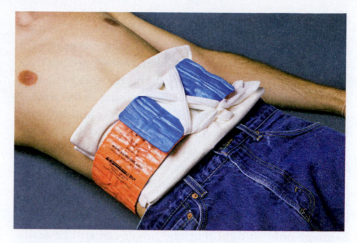

FIGURE 4-21 Using a formable SAM splint as an anchor may help in circumferential bandaging of a wound to the trunk.

careful here, though. Any patient movement is likely to affect bandage tightness and the amount of pressure over the dressing. With these injuries, therefore, bandage after the patient is in the final position for transport.

Elbow and Knee

Joints, especially the elbow and knee, are difficult to bandage. Bandage using circumferential wraps and then splint the area to ensure that the bandage does not loosen with movement. If possible, place the joint in a position halfway between flexion and extension. This position, called the *position of function*, relaxes the muscles controlling the joint and the skin tension lines, and is most comfortable for the patient during long transports or periods of immobilization.

Hand and Finger

Hand and finger injuries are easy to bandage by simple circumferential wrapping. Again, consider placing the hand or digit in the position of function, halfway between flexion and extension. Accomplish this by placing a large, bulky dressing in the palm of the patient's hand and then wrapping around it. Use a malleable finger splint to obtain the position of function and then wrap circumferentially to splint the finger. If possible, before bandaging, carefully remove any jewelry from the wrist and fingers, as swelling may restrict distal circulation and also make it difficult to remove the jewelry later.

Ankle and Foot

Ankle and foot wounds are also easy to bandage by wrapping circumferentially and by using the natural body contours. If strong direct pressure is needed to maintain hemorrhage control, start wrapping from the toes and work proximally. This ensures that the bandaging pressure does not form a venous tourniquet and compromise circulation to this very distal injury.

Complications of Bandaging

Bandaging can lead to some complications, although such occurrences are infrequent. If a bandage—particularly a circumferential bandage—is too tight, the area beneath it may continue to swell, increasing pressure in the wound area. This can lead to decreased blood flow and ischemia distal to the bandage. Pressure can build to such an extreme that the bandage acts like a tourniquet. Pain, pallor, tingling, a loss of pulses, and prolonged capillary refill time are typical signs of developing pressure and ischemia. Avoid this complication by making bandages snug, but not too tight. A useful technique is to wrap a bandage only so tight that one finger can still be easily slipped beneath it.

Bandages and dressings left on too long can become soaked with blood and body fluids and then serve as incubators for infection. This problem usually takes at least two to three days to develop, though, and is not a common concern in most prehospital settings.

The size of the dressing is an important consideration in bandaging. An unnecessarily large and bulky dressing can prevent proper inspection of a wound and hide contamination and continued serious bleeding. Too small a dressing can become lost in a wound and become, in effect, a foreign body. This is most frequently a problem with large, gaping wounds and deep wounds that penetrate the thoracic or abdominal body cavities. When dressing a wound, choose a dressing just larger than the wound yet not so small as to become lost in it.

Care of Specific Wounds

Some circumstances—amputations, impaled objects, and crush syndrome cases—deserve special attention during the patient management process. These injuries can challenge even the seasoned paramedic to provide the most appropriate care.

Amputations

Amputations may bleed either heavily or minimally. Attempt to control hemorrhage with direct pressure by applying a large, bulky dressing to the wound. If this fails to control hemorrhage, consider using a tourniquet just above the point of severance. If there is a crushing wound associated with the limb loss, apply the tourniquet just above the crushed area. Do not delay patient transport while locating or extricating the amputated body part. Transport the patient immediately, and then have other personnel transport the part once it is located or released from entrapment.

Current recommendations for managing separated body parts include moist cooling (Figure 4-22a) and rapid transport. For transport, place the amputated part in a plastic bag with the part wrapped in gauze moistened with lactated Ringer's solution or normal saline, and immerse

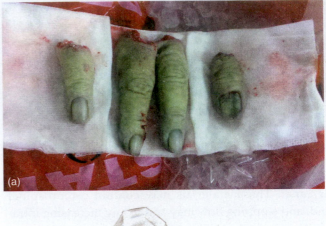

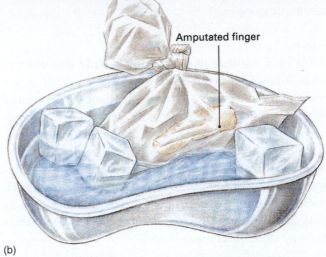

FIGURE 4-22 (a) Amputated parts should be cooled without direct contact between ice and the amputated part. (b) For transport, put the amputated part in a dry, sealed bag and place it in cool water that contains a few ice cubes.

(Photo a: Dr. Bryan E. Bledsoe)

the bag in cold water (Figure 4-22b). The water may have a few ice cubes in it, but avoid direct contact between the ice and the amputated part. Even if the amputated part cannot be totally reattached, skin from it may be used to cover the stump (Figure 4-23).

Impaled Objects

When possible, immobilize all impaled objects in place. Position bulky dressings around the object to stabilize it, and tape over the dressings to hold them in place. Try to make patient movement to the ambulance and transport to the emergency department as smooth and non-jarring as possible. Remember that any movement of an impaled object may cause continued internal bleeding and additional tissue damage.

If the impaled object is too large to transport or is affixed to something that cannot be moved, such as a reinforcing rod set in concrete, consider cutting it. Use appropriate techniques and tools depending on the circumstances of the impalement. A hand or power saw, an acetylene

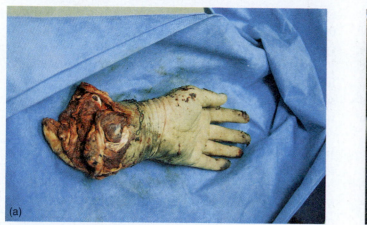

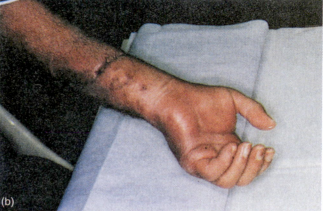

FIGURE 4-23 Amputated parts should be located and transported with the patient to the hospital for possible replantation. (a) An amputated hand. (b) A successfully replanted hand.

(© Dr. Bryan E. Bledsoe)

torch, or bolt cutters might be employed. Whatever tools and techniques are used, be sure to take steps to limit the heat, vibration, or jolting transmitted to the patient. Provide the best possible support for both the object and the patient during the cutting procedure.

In some special circumstances, an impaled object should be removed. For example, it may be necessary to remove an object impaled in the cheek if removal is required to maintain a patent airway. In this case, be prepared to apply direct pressure to the wound both from inside the cheek (intraorally) and externally.

Another object that would require removal is one impaled in the central chest of a patient who needs CPR. In such a circumstance, the risk associated with not performing resuscitation outweighs the risk of removing the object. Be aware, however, that a trauma patient who needs CPR has a very poor prognosis.

Another complication associated with an impaled object occurs when a patient is impaled on an object that cannot be cut or moved. In such a case, contact medical direction for advice and guidance. If the object is impaled in a limb, bleeding may be controllable. If it has entered the head, neck, chest, or abdomen, it may not be.

Crush Syndrome

The key to successful prehospital management of a crush syndrome patient is anticipation of the problem and prevention of its effects. Because, by definition, all crush syndrome patients are victims of prolonged entrapment, cases can be identified before extrication is complete. The focus of prehospital crush injury care is on rapid transport, adequate fluid resuscitation, diuresis, and—possibly—systemic alkalinization with sodium bicarbonate.

The prehospital approach to crush syndrome is similar to that with other trauma patients. Ensuring scene safety is particularly important in these cases. Crush syndrome

victims are often buried in heavy rubble or other large debris, and access may be difficult. Assistance may be needed from specialized personnel and their equipment—urban search and rescue teams, or trench, heavy, or confined space rescue teams. Never place rescuers in unreasonable danger when providing care or attempting a rescue.

Once the scene is safe and the patient has been accessed, conduct the primary assessment. Remove debris from around the head, neck, and thorax to minimize airway obstruction and restriction of ventilation. Control any reachable and obvious bleeding. Perform as much of the primary and rapid trauma assessment as possible, keeping in mind that portions of the patient's body may be inaccessible as a result of the entrapment. The dark, dusty, and cramped conditions of many confined-space rescues may force you to improvise. Be alert for signs and symptoms of associated injuries such as dust inhalation, dehydration, and hypothermia.

Remember that the greater the body area compressed and the longer the time of entrapment, the greater the risk of crush syndrome. Initially, a trapped patient will complain only of entrapment symptoms: pain, lack of motor function, tingling, or loss of sensation in the affected limb. The patient may also experience flaccid paralysis and sensory loss in the limb unrelated to the normal distribution of peripheral nerve control and sensation.

As long as the body part remains entrapped and the metabolic byproducts of the crush injury are confined to the entrapped part, the patient will not experience the full effects of crush syndrome. With extrication, however, toxic byproducts are released into the circulation, and the patient may rapidly develop shock and die. If the patient survives the initial release of the byproducts, he remains at great risk of developing renal failure with serious morbidity or delayed death. Note, too, that a crush injury may also induce compartment syndrome (explained earlier and in the next section), especially with prolonged entrapment.

Once the patient's ABCs (airway, breathing, and circulation) have been ensured, turn attention to obtaining IV access. Intravenous fluids and selected medications are important in treating crush syndrome. Initiate a large-bore IV, if possible. Because of the entrapment, it may be necessary to consider alternative IV sites such as the external jugular vein, sternal or humoral (IO), or the veins of a lower extremity. Avoid any site distal to a crush injury.

When crush syndrome is encountered, consider contact with the trauma center for medical direction and communicate, on-line, with the attending physician. Expect to provide frequent vital sign and patient updates and be prepared to administer large fluid volumes and, possibly, alkalizing agents.

Alkalization of the blood and urine is a consideration for preventing and treating crush syndrome. In combination with fluid resuscitation, alkalinization can reverse acidosis, help prevent renal failure, and help correct hyperkalemia. Administer sodium bicarbonate as directed by local protocols.

Consider applying a tourniquet before the entrapping pressure is released if you have been unable to medicate the patient and provide fluid resuscitation. The tourniquet will sequester the toxins and prevent reperfusion injury. Tourniquet use, however, will continue crush injury development and worsen its effects.

If the entrapping object may not be moved for many hours or days, medical direction may consider field amputation. This operation will likely be performed by a physician responding to the scene but, in dire circumstances, may be performed by a paramedic under direction of a physician.

Cardiac (ECG) monitoring is important with all crush syndrome patients. Arrhythmias may develop at any time but are most likely to occur immediately following the release of pressure on extrication. This is because both potassium and lactate are released with the pressure release and travel with the blood to the heart. Sudden cardiac arrest should be treated in the usual fashion with defibrillation and cardiac drugs as appropriate. Consider 500 mg calcium chloride IV push (in addition to the sodium bicarbonate) to counteract life-threatening arrhythmias induced by hyperkalemia. Watch for the tenting, or peaking, of the T-wave, a prolonged P–R interval, and S–T segment depression. Severely elevated blood levels of potassium may induce a widening of the QRS complex that quickly leads to refractory ventricular fibrillation. Be sure to flush the IV line between infusions or to use different lines because calcium chloride and sodium bicarbonate precipitate.

Once the patient is freed from entrapment, be prepared to treat rapidly progressing shock. Continue the normal saline infusions at 30 mL/kg/hr and provide additional boluses of sodium bicarbonate as needed.

Rapidly transport the patient to an appropriate hospital (usually a trauma center) for all cases of suspected crush syndrome.

Prehospital care of the crushed limb or body parts requires no special techniques. Cover open wounds and splint fractures, keeping in mind that progressive swelling will necessitate reassessment, with monitoring of distal circulation and the tightness of bandages, straps, and splints. Handle all crushed limbs gently because ischemic tissue is prone to injury.

Care at the hospital for crush injury is aggressive and may use techniques such as debridement and hyperbaric oxygenation. During hyperbaric oxygenation, the patient is placed in a chamber with artificially high concentrations of oxygen under several atmospheres of pressure. This drives oxygen into poorly oxygenated tissue to help with the destruction of anaerobic bacteria and to increase tissue oxygenation for repair and regeneration, ultimately reducing tissue necrosis and edema. Hyperbaric oxygenation is most effective when provided early in the course of care.

Compartment Syndrome

The most prominent symptom of compartment syndrome is severe pain, often out of proportion to the physical findings. Other signs are often subtle or absent, or they may be overshadowed by the original injury, such as a fracture or contusion. Some people suggest using the six Ps—pain, pallor, paralysis, paresthesia, pressure (feeling of tension within the extremity), and pulses (diminished or absent distally)—plus a seventh P sometimes cited, poikilothermia, referring to a limb that is cool to the touch. However, many of these signs are not dependable, or they appear very late in the course of the injury.

Motor and sensory functions are usually normal with compartment syndrome, as are distal pulses. Even capillary refill shows little or no change. It is important to note that compartment syndrome rarely occurs within the first 4 hours after an acute injury. It is more likely to appear 6 to 8 hours (or as much as a day or more) after the initial injury. Recognition of compartment syndrome can be challenging and requires a healthy suspicion for the problem.

The first step in prehospital treatment for compartment syndrome is care of the underlying injury. Splint and immobilize all suspected fractures, and use traction as appropriate for femur fractures. Apply cold packs to severe contusions. Elevation of the affected extremity is the single most effective prehospital treatment for compartment syndrome. This reduces edema, increases venous return, lowers compartment pressure, and helps prevent ischemia. In the hospital, compartment syndrome is diagnosed by inserting a hollow needle into the affected compartment to directly obtain a pressure reading. Severe cases are treated surgically, through a procedure called a fasciotomy that incises the restrictive fascia.

Special Anatomic Sites

Several anatomic sites provide challenges to the care of soft tissue injuries. These include the face and neck, the thorax, and the abdomen.

Face and Neck

Soft tissue injuries to the face and neck present potential challenges, owing to the anatomic relationships of the airway and great vessels. Injuries to the face may result in blood and tissue debris in the airway, posing risks of airway obstruction, asphyxia, and aspiration. Pooled secretions and tissue edema may add to airway problems. Trauma to the face or neck may also distort the anatomic structures of the upper airway, leading to airway compromise and complicating attempts at endotracheal intubation (Figure 4-24).

Emergency treatment of face and neck injuries can be challenging. First, gain control of the airway. Open the airway using manual maneuvers. If spinal injury is suspected, maintain spinal stabilization as directed in your local protocols, if indicated. Aggressively suction blood, saliva, and debris from the pharynx to maintain the airway, but limit the depth of suction catheter insertion to that which is necessary to maintain the airway, to avoid stimulating the gag reflex. Insert a basic airway as needed.

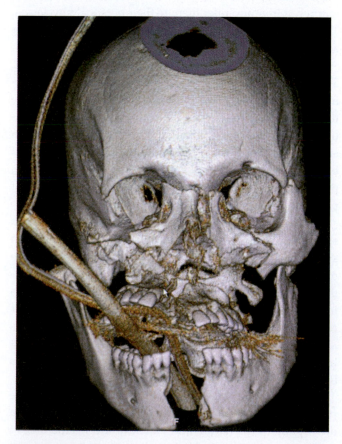

FIGURE 4-24 Severe facial injuries may interfere with airway control and distort landmarks used for intubation.

(© Dr. Bryan E. Bledsoe)

Direct visualization of the endotracheal tube passing through the cords is the gold standard for securing the airway, but achieving it is fraught with complications in cases of face and neck trauma. Secretions and blood may prevent adequate visualization, even with aggressive suctioning. Airway edema can distort the anatomy beyond recognition, and even prevent passage of the ET tube. Extraglottic airways, such as the newer LMAs and King airways, may be very effective when injury to the airway is noted. In all cases, meticulous and absolute confirmation of tube placement is mandatory to avoid fatal hypoxia. Continuous waveform capnography is essential to ensure initial and ongoing proper endotracheal tube placement.

In desperate circumstances, cricothyrotomy may be lifesaving. Avoid placing the device through neck hematomas to avoid life-threatening bleeding.

Once the airway is secured, focus attention on any serious facial or neck bleeding. Direct pressure is usually successful for bleeding control. Be certain to avoid compressing or occluding the airway. A tourniquet should not be used because of the risks of cerebral ischemia and strangulation. In a similar fashion, as noted earlier, circumferential neck bandaging carries the same risk and should be meticulously monitored if used. Open neck wounds also carry the danger of air aspiration and emboli. Cover any open neck wound with an occlusive dressing, which should then be held or bandaged firmly in place. Because of the neck's anatomy, digital pressure may need to be maintained throughout the course of prehospital care to ensure effective bleeding control.

Thorax

Superficial soft tissue injury to the thorax may suggest more serious intrathoracic injuries. The pleural space extends superiorly to the supraclavicular fossa and inferiorly to include the entire rib cage both anteriorly and posteriorly. Small "lacerations" may actually be deep, penetrating stab or gunshot wounds with resultant hemothorax, pneumothorax, pericardial tamponade, penetrating heart trauma, or injury to the great vessels, esophagus, bronchi, or diaphragm. A seemingly minor "rib bruise" may be the only visible sign of serious lung or cardiac contusions beneath.

Perform a thorough physical examination to detect any signs of internal bleeding, pulmonary edema, arrhythmias, or shock. However, never explore a thoracic wound beyond the skin edges. Probing deeper can convert a minor wound to a pneumothorax or a bleeding disaster. Consider all thoracic wounds to be potentially life threatening until evidence proves otherwise. (See the "Chest Trauma" chapter for detailed care procedures.)

Dress all open thoracic wounds with sterile dressings in the usual fashion. As noted earlier, if a circumferential bandage is applied to the thorax, be aware of the risk of impeding the normal chest wall excursion during breathing.

Monitor the respiratory rate and depth and the pulse oximeter in such cases. Be alert for the presence of air bubbling, subcutaneous emphysema, crepitus, or other hints of open pneumothorax.

Be extremely cautious about making an airtight seal on any thoracic wound, because doing so can rapidly convert a simple pneumothorax to a tension pneumothorax and death. Instead, use an occlusive dressing sealed on three sides and be prepared to assist ventilations. Watch the occlusive dressing so it does not seal with blood against the chest wall and convert a simple pneumothorax into a tension pneumothorax. If indicated by deteriorating vital signs, completely unseal an occlusive dressing (even one that was prepared with an opening and sealed on only three sides) to ensure that the dressing is not contributing to the development of tension pneumothorax. Auscultate the chest and monitor vital signs frequently.

Abdomen

The peritoneal cavity extends approximately from the symphysis pubis inferiorly to the diaphragm superiorly. Because the diaphragm rises and falls with respiration, so, too, does the border between the abdominal and thoracic cavities. It is impossible to know the diaphragm's exact position at the time the injury occurred, so suspect associated injuries to both abdominal and thoracic organs if the soft tissue injury involves the region between the rib margin and the fifth rib anteriorly, the seventh rib laterally, and the ninth rib posteriorly.

Some abdominal organs are located posterior to the peritoneum and are called *retroperitoneal*. These include the kidneys, ureters, adrenal glands, most of the pancreas, and the abdominal aorta and inferior vena cava. The retroperitoneal space does not restrict the blood loss as well as the peritoneal space and has a reduced pain response to free blood in this space.

Blunt or penetrating trauma to the abdomen can injure both hollow and solid organs, penetrate or rupture the diaphragm, and cause serious internal bleeding. Anteriorly and just underlying the rib margin are the liver on the right and the spleen on the left. Posteriorly, the kidneys (not true abdominal organs, as they lie retroperitoneally) are located in the costovertebral angle region. Hollow organs—the bowel, stomach, and urinary bladder—may rupture. In addition to bleeding copiously, these organs may release their contents and inflame the peritoneum.

Consider any soft tissue wound in the abdominal region as potentially damaging to the underlying organs. Signs and symptoms of internal damage can be subtle, particularly early on. Eviscerations and other massive injuries are obvious, but other internal injuries that are just as serious may not be apparent. Prehospital treatment is primarily supportive and includes ensuring adequate oxygenation (based on SpO_2), preventing shock, dressing open wounds,

and rapid transport (see the chapter "Abdominal and Pelvic Trauma"). Be aware that bulky abdominal dressings, especially if they are secured with circumferential bandages, may restrict movement of the abdominal contents during the excursion of the diaphragm. This, in turn, may compromise breathing. Monitor the rate and depth of breathing and the pulse oximeter in such cases.

Wounds Requiring Transport

Transport any patient with a wound that involves a structure beneath the skin for emergency department evaluation. This includes wounds involving, or possibly involving, nerves, blood vessels, ligaments, tendons, or muscles. Transport any patient with a significantly contaminated wound, a wound involving an impaled object, or a wound that was received in a particularly unclean environment. In addition, transport any patient with a wound with likely cosmetic implications, such as facial wounds or large gaping wounds.

Soft Tissue Treatment and Release/Refer

In some EMS systems, paramedics are permitted to treat and release patients with minor and superficial soft tissue injuries or treat and refer them to their personal physicians. This generally occurs under on-line medical direction or according to strict protocols.

In such circumstances, evaluate and dress the wound. Then explain to the patient the steps to follow for continuing care of the injury. Tell the patient of the need to change the dressing and to monitor the injury site for further hemorrhage or developing infection. Provide the patient with simple written instructions (approved and/or published by medical direction) explaining wound care, monitoring, protection, dressing change, cleansing, and the signs of problems such as infection or hemorrhage.

Instruct the patient to contact a physician if certain signs and symptoms appear, and describe those signs and symptoms thoroughly. Ensure that the patient has the means to obtain physician or health care provider follow-up, and again stress the circumstances in which such follow-up care should be sought. During any referral or release, if the patient's tetanus immunization history is unclear or it has been longer than five years since the last immunization, instruct the patient to obtain a tetanus booster as soon as possible (generally within 72 hours).

Document all release/refer incidents carefully in the prehospital care report. The report should include a description of the nature and extent of the wound and of the care provided for it. Note in the report all instructions and materials provided to the patient and any medical direction received.

Summary

Soft tissue injury may compromise the skin—the envelope that protects and contains the human body. Any damage to the skin may interfere with its ability to contain water and blood and to prevent damaging agents from entering. For these reasons, the assessment and care of soft tissue injuries are important parts of prehospital care.

Assess wounds carefully, because they may provide the only overt signs of serious internal injury. Realize that discoloration and swelling take time to develop and may not be as apparent in the field as they are when the patient arrives at the emergency department. Look carefully for the early signs of wounds and use the mechanism of injury to locate potential injury sites. When caring for soft tissue injuries, keep in mind the basic goals: controlling hemorrhage, keeping the wound as clean as possible, and immobilizing the injury site. Although soft tissue injuries are not often assigned a high priority in prehospital care, they do account for a large number of patient injuries and are significant to the overall assessment and care of trauma victims.

You Make the Call

You arrive at the scene of a "foot injury" to find a young child lying on the lawn, surrounded by his parents. As you begin to question his father about what happened, he explains, "My son stepped on a board with a nail in it." After donning gloves, you carefully remove the boy's shoe to discover an almost invisible penetration to the sole of the foot. The child is now resting quietly, without much pain.

1. What type of wound is this, and what significance does it have for infection?

2. What elements of history and specifically vaccinations will be important in assessing this patient?

3. What direction would you give this patient if his parents do not wish to have him transported to the local emergency department?

See Suggested Responses at the back of this book.

Review Questions

1. How does the integumentary system prevent pathogens from attacking the body?

   a. The skin provides a pathway out of the body for pathogens.

   b. Leukocytes in the skin attack pathogens.

   c. Antibodies in the skin attack and destroy pathogens.

   d. The skin provides a protective physical barrier against pathogens.

2. Your patient with soft tissue trauma, following being struck accidentally by a baseball bat during a family reunion, has an area of the upper arm that is purplish in color and painful. Distal motor/sensory function is normal. This type of injury is most likely a(n) _____

   a. hematoma.

   b. contusion.

   c. stellate laceration.

   d. bone fracture.

3. Glands within the dermis that secrete sweat are properly called _____

   a. diaphoresis glands.

   b. sebaceous glands.

   c. sudoriferous glands.

   d. lymphocyte glands.

4. When an artery is ruptured but the skin is not broken, blood can separate the tissues and pool in a pocket. This pocket of blood is known as what type of injury?

   a. Contusion

   b. Abrasion

   c. Hematoma

   d. Crush injury

5. Which injuries are typically the most superficial of injuries that violate the protective barrier of the skin?

    a. Incisions
    b. Avulsions
    c. Abrasions
    d. Lacerations

6. Specialized white blood cells capable of engulfing bacteria are known as _____

    a. granulocytes.
    b. macrophages.
    c. phagocytes.
    d. all of the above.

7. The anaerobic bacterium *Clostridium perfringens* causes a deep space infection called _____.

    a. gangrene.
    b. tetanus.
    c. collagen.
    d. cholera

8. You have been called to a construction scene where a patient has caught one of his legs between two pieces of machinery. As the leg is removed from the machinery, you see that there is no break in the continuity of the skin, but the leg is deformed and the patient has pain. You should suspect the internal injuries to be _____

    a. extensive.
    b. unimportant.
    c. absent.
    d. minimally significant.

9. Which type of dressing is designed to be placed over a wound as a barrier to leaking?

    a. Adherent
    b. Nonabsorbent
    c. Absorbent
    d. Nonadherent

10. As you begin to bandage a soft tissue injury, you should continue to check distal pulses to ensure proper tissue perfusion. This is done primarily to detect _____

    a. shrinking of the bandage.
    b. development of shock.
    c. toxins entering central circulation.
    d. swelling of the damaged tissue.

11. When bandaging the foot and ankle to create pressure and maintain hemorrhage control, wrap in a _____

    a. distal-to-proximal fashion to avoid forming a venous tourniquet.
    b. proximal-to-distal fashion to avoid forming a venous tourniquet.
    c. proximal-to-distal fashion to help maintain gentle traction.
    d. distal-to-proximal fashion to help maintain gentle traction.

12. The ability of the body to stop bleeding on its own is known as _____

    a. inflammation.
    b. hemostasis.
    c. epithelialization.
    d. neovascularization.

13. Which of the following drugs a traumatized patient is taking will be *least* likely to render the patient more susceptible to infection following soft tissue trauma?

    a. Ibuprofen
    b. Chemotherapy
    c. Prednisone
    d. Nitroglycerin

14. You are treating a patient who was shot in the chest following an argument. During your assessment and treatment of this patient, what type of dressing will you apply initially to the open chest wound?

    a. Absorbent
    b. Occlusive
    c. Nonadherent
    d. Porous

15. Your patient has a penetration injury to the lower arm, and you apply a dressing that helps to form a clot. This type of dressing is known as a _____

    a. hemostatic dressing.
    b. hemogenetic dressing.
    c. hemoporous dressing.
    d. hemolytic dressing.

See Answers to Review Questions at the end of this book.

References

1. Lieurance, R., J. B. Benjamin, and W. D. Rappaport. "Blood Loss and Transfusion in Patients with Isolated Femur Fractures." *J Orthop Trauma* 6(2) (1992): 175–179.

2. Horswell, B. B. and C. J. Chahine. "Dog Bites of the Face, Head, and Neck in Children." *W V Med J* 107(6) (Nov–Dec 2011): 24–27.

3. Jones, A. P., K. Allison, H. Wright, and K. Porter. "Use of Prehospital Dressings in Soft Tissue Trauma: Is There Any Conformity or Plan?" *Emerg Med J* 26(7) (Jul 2009): 532–534.

4. Kragh, J. F., Jr., et al. "Survival with Emergency Tourniquet Use to Stop Bleeding in Major Limb Trauma." *Ann Surg* 249(1) (Jan 2009): 1–7.

Further Reading

Bickley, L. *Bates' Guide to Physical Examination and History Taking.* 11th ed. Philadelphia: Wolters-Kluwer, 2012..

Bledsoe, B. E., and D. Clayden. *Prehospital Emergency Pharmacology.* 7th ed. Upper Saddle River, NJ: Pearson/ Prentice Hall, 2011.

Bledsoe, B. E., B. J. Colbert, and J. E. Ankney. *Essentials of A & P for Emergency Care.* Upper Saddle River, NJ: Pearson/Prentice Hall, 2010.

Martini, Frederic. *Fundamentals of Anatomy and Physiology.* 10th ed. San Francisco: Pearson, 2014.

Marx, J., R. Hockberger, and R. Walls. *Emergency Medicine: Concepts and Clinical Practice.* 8th ed. St. Louis: Mosby, 2013.

Tintinelli, J. E., ed. *Emergency Medicine: A Comprehensive Study Guide.* 7th ed. New York: McGraw-Hill, 2008.

Trott, A. T. *Wounds and Lacerations: Emergency Care and Closure.* 4th ed. St. Louis, Saunders 2012.

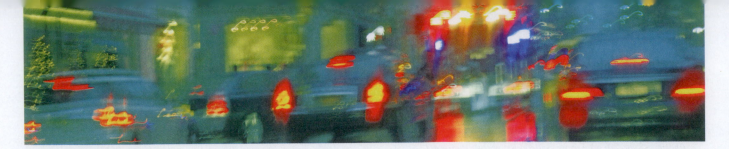

Chapter 5
Burns

Bryan E. Bledsoe, DO, FACEP, FAAEM, EMT-P

Robert S. Porter, MA, EMT-P

STANDARD
Trauma (Soft Tissue Trauma)

COMPETENCY
Integrates assessment findings with principles of epidemiology and pathophysiology to formulate a field impression to implement a comprehensive treatment/disposition plan for an acutely injured patient.

∨ Learning Objectives

Terminal Performance Objective: After reading this chapter you should be able to integrate knowledge of anatomy, physiology, pathophysiology, and treatment principles to assess and provide prehospital management for patients with burns.

Enabling Objectives: To accomplish the terminal performance objective, you should be able to:

1. Define key terms introduced in this chapter.

2. Describe the epidemiology of burn injuries.

3. Describe the anatomy and physiology of the skin.

4. Describe the basic pathophysiology of thermal, electrical, chemical, radiation, and inhalation burns.

5. Delineate among the various depths of burns, including superficial, partial thickness, and full thickness.

6. Identify basic assessment principles for burn injuries, including the determination of burn depth and extent of body surface area involved.

7. Discuss the systemic complications of burns and how these may be managed.

8. Identify and describe the phases of patient assessment for a patient with a burn injury.

9. Identify patients whose burns are considered minor, moderate, and critical.

10. Given a variety of scenarios, develop management plans for patients with burns resulting from thermal, inhalation, electrical, chemical, and radiation burn mechanisms.

KEY TERMS

Case Study

Ben and Ronnie, Fire Rescue paramedics, respond with trucks 23 and 56 to a working structural fire. On arrival, they find two fire units already deployed, with firefighters engaging a wood frame home fully engulfed in flames. As Ronnie positions their vehicle, she and Ben see the structure's south exterior wall collapsing on a firefighter. Within minutes, other firefighters extinguish the burning wall and free the firefighter. They also douse their comrade with water to extinguish any smoldering embers in contact with him and stop the burn process.

When firefighters have secured the scene, Ben and Ronnie proceed to the patient and begin their primary assessment. The patient is a man who is lying supine with his turnout gear burned and charred in places, indicating that he has received serious burns. Because of the wall's collapse onto the firefighter, they provide cervical stabilization while proceeding with assessment. The downed firefighter's respirations appear adequate, although he is coughing up sooty sputum and is slightly hoarse. The firefighter, who gives his name as Karl, is conscious and alert. His airway seems clear except for the hoarseness. However, the sooty sputum and hoarseness indicate possible airway burns, making Karl a priority for rapid transport.

Ben proceeds to perform the rapid trauma assessment. On removal of Karl's turnout gear, Ben exposes dark, discolored burns to the patient's posterior thorax and lower back as well as circumferential burns of the left upper extremity. Despite the burn severity, Karl denies much pain. Ben also finds angulation, false motion, and pain to the right forearm. Vital signs reveal normal breathing in terms of volume and rate and a strong, regular pulse at a rate of about 100. Distal pulses are also strong, and capillary refill is timed at 2 seconds. Karl is fully conscious and oriented and is joking about the incident.

The rescue crew now takes some initial care steps. Ben cuts away Karl's clothing and then covers the burn site with a dry, clean sheet and starts an IV line, running normal saline at a to-keep-open rate. Ronnie applies oxygen via a nonrebreather mask and observes an oximetry reading of 97 percent. They package Karl and quickly load him into the ambulance for rapid transport. En route to the hospital, Ben checks Karl's blood pressure (120/88 mmHg) and respirations (30 and shallow), noting that he displays increasing respiratory effort.

While Ronnie is splinting the right upper limb, Karl begins to cough deeply and experiences severe dyspnea. The dyspnea progresses, and Karl's level of consciousness drops. Oxygen saturation falls to 86 percent. Ben begins to provide supplemental oxygen via a bag-valve mask, while Ronnie prepares intubation equipment.

Medical direction orders the crew to intubate, and they attempt to do so during transport. The airway is edematous, and vocal cord visualization is difficult. After the first attempt, Ronnie withdraws the tube when auscultation of breath sounds, failure to obtain chest rise, absent end-tidal CO_2 levels, and a dropping oxygen saturation indicate esophageal placement. Ben reventilates Karl using a bag-valve-mask device while Ronnie prepares for another intubation attempt. She is again unsuccessful.

As they withdraw the tube, the ambulance arrives at the emergency department. The ED physician quickly views the airway and finds it severely swollen. She then decides to insert a Quick-trach into the cricothyroid membrane and attempts ventilation. The technique is successful. Karl begins spontaneous respirations and maintains a strong pulse. His level of consciousness does not improve, however, and the hospital staff transfers him to the burn unit for definitive care.

Introduction to Burn Trauma

The incidence of burn injuries in the United States and other developed countries has been declining for several decades. Despite this decline, an estimated 450,000 Americans are treated for burns annually and 45,000 are hospitalized. Some 3 to 5 percent of these burns are considered life threatening. Persons at greatest risk for serious burns include the very young and old, the infirm, and workers (e.g., firefighters, metal smelters, and chemical workers) who are exposed to occupational combustion and chemical sources. Burn injuries remain the second leading cause of death in children under 12 years of age and the fourth overall cause of trauma death after vehicular crashes, penetrating trauma, and falls. Males account for 70 percent of burn mortality.

Much of the national decline in burn mortality is attributed to improved building codes, safer construction techniques, sprinkler systems, and smoke detector use. Smaller but still important effects are attributed to educational campaigns aimed primarily at schoolchildren. Other simple and inexpensive measures that have helped prevent burns include keeping cigarette lighters and matches away from children and reducing household hot-water temperatures to below scalding levels. Half of all tap-water burns occur in children under five years old. Merely adjusting the hot-water temperature to below 48.9°C (120°F) can prevent most scalding burns.

Burns are a specific subset of soft-tissue injuries with a specific pathologic process. Although the term "burn" suggests combustion, the actual process producing burn injuries is much different. The human body is predominantly water and does not support combustion. Instead, body tissues change chemically, evaporating water and denaturing proteins that make up cell membranes. The result can be widespread damage to the skin, also known as the integumentary system.

To effectively assess and treat burns, paramedics must have a good understanding of the structures and functions of the integumentary system, as well as of thermal, chemical, electrical, and radiologic pathologies that may affect it. This understanding ensures provision of the best possible assessment and care for patients who sustain burns.

Anatomy and Physiology of the Skin

The skin is one of the largest, most important, and least appreciated human organs. Covering the entire body, the skin protects it from fluid loss and bacterial invasion. The skin also provides a massive surface for sensation and is a natural radiator for dissipating excess body heat. With all these functions, the skin still remains durable, flexible, and very able to repair itself.

Layers of the Skin

Skin comprises three layers of tissue: the epidermis, dermis, and subcutaneous tissue. Together they form the body's outermost shell. Following is a review of the information on skin layers introduced in the chapter "Soft Tissue Trauma."

Epidermis
The first and outermost skin layer is the epidermis. It is an area of dying and dead cells being pushed outward by new cells growing from beneath. As these cells reach the surface, they are abraded away during everyday activity. The constant movement outward provides a barrier that is difficult for bacteria and other pathogens to penetrate.

Glands beneath the epidermis secrete an oil called sebum. This oil coats the outer skin layers and makes the epidermis pliable. In addition, sebum provides a barrier to water and other fluid flow through the skin.

Dermis
Directly below the epidermis is a tissue layer called the dermis. It contains many structures, including

> **CONTENT REVIEW**
> ➤ Layers of the Skin
> - Epidermis (outermost layer)
> - Dermis (layer beneath the epidermis)
> - Subcutaneous tissue (fatty layer beneath the dermis)

blood vessels, glands, and nerve endings. It is in this layer that sebaceous glands produce sebum and secrete it directly onto the skin's surface and into hair follicles. Sudoriferous glands in the dermis secrete sweat and direct it to the skin's surface. As water in sweat evaporates, passing air carries the vapor and associated heat energy away with it. The change of a fluid to a vapor (evaporation) is an efficient method of skin cooling. This process helps the body maintain a normal temperature even when ambient temperatures are greater than 100°F (as long as evaporation is possible). The primary mechanism for maintaining body temperature uses the skin as a radiator of excess body heat. Warm blood from the body's core travels either through blood vessels in the dermis (close to the skin surface) or through the subcutaneous tissues, from which radiation of the blood's heat into the atmosphere can occur.

Subcutaneous Tissue

Subcutaneous tissue, which is composed of adipose (fat) and connective tissues, serves as a stratum of insulation against both trauma and heat loss. As just noted, when warm core blood is directed to the dermis, skin temperature increases, resulting in increased heat loss and cooling of the body. By contrast, heat moves two to three times more slowly through adipose tissue than through muscle or through the dermis. Therefore, when blood is directed to, and beneath, subcutaneous tissues, it takes longer for heat to move to the skin, the skin's surface cools, and heat loss slows. This allows the body to retain warmth.

Underlying Structures

It is important to identify the structures underneath the skin, even though they are not part of the skin. These structures include the muscles and their thick, fibrous capsules of fascia as well as nerves, tendons, bones, and, of course, the vital organs such as the heart, lungs, and brain. Each of these structures is sensitive to the effects of thermal, chemical, electrical, and radiation injury.

Functions of the Skin

The skin varies in thickness from almost a centimeter on the heel of the foot to microscopic dimensions on the surface of the eye. As a durable container for the human body, the skin performs a number of valuable functions:

- Skin protects the body from infection by bacteria and other microorganisms.
- Skin functions as an organ of sensation, perceiving temperature, pressure (touch), and pain.
- Skin contains vital body fluids and controls their loss to the environment as well as the movement of fluids into the body when it is exposed to water or other fluids.

- Skin aids in temperature regulation through secretion of sweat and shunting of blood.
- Skin provides insulation from trauma.
- Skin is flexible to accommodate free body movement.

The skin and its functions are often taken for granted, but burn injury can lead to severe fluid loss, infection, hypothermia, and death. Therefore, paramedics must be familiar with burn pathophysiology.

Burn Pathophysiology

Burns result from protein disruption in the cell membranes. Burns can be caused by several different mechanisms including thermal, electrical, chemical, or radiation energies, as well as a combination of these. Understanding burn mechanisms and being able to determine the degree and area of a burn helps assess the seriousness of the burn and thus guides subsequent care.

Types of Burns

Soft tissue burns can occur from thermal (heat), electrical, chemical, or radiation insults to the body. Although the resulting burns are much the same, the damage process differs with the various mechanisms. The following sections describe each of these four types of burns.

Thermal Burns

A thermal burn causes damage by increasing the rate at which the molecules within an object move and collide with each other. The degree of heat is a measure of the speed of the molecules within an object. The more rapidly molecules move and the more frequently they collide with one another, the greater the object's temperature. This phenomenon explains why, as ice is heated and the speed of the molecules increases, ice changes form to become water and then steam. At absolute zero, the molecules within a substance are stopped. As the molecules begin to move, the object's temperature rises. If an object feels cool, it is because the object has less molecular movement (and temperature) than you do. If an object feels warm, it is because its molecules have greater movement (and temperature) than you do. If you contact something hotter than you, its molecular movement (heat) is transferred rapidly to your skin, heating it, and if the transfer of molecular movement is great enough, it may cause a burn.[1]

Heat energy may also cause chemical changes. As temperature increases, substances such as gasoline

CONTENT REVIEW
➤ Basic Types of Burns
- Thermal
- Electrical
- Chemical
- Radiation

may combine with oxygen. The form of matter may change as well. Water, for example, may change into ice (with decreasing heat energy) or steam (with increasing heat energy). In addition, the chemical structure of proteins can be affected by heat. An egg changes its nature as the proteins break down, or **denature,** in a hot frying pan. This is what makes cooked eggs take on a rubbery consistency.

Similar changes also take place in burned tissue. As molecular speed increases, cell components, especially membranes and proteins, begin to break down, just as with the egg in a frying pan. The result of extreme heat exposure is progressive injury and cell death.[1]

The extent of burn injury is related to the amount of heat energy transferred to the patient's skin. The amount of that heat energy in turn depends on three components of the burning agent: its temperature, the concentration of heat energy it possesses, and the length of its contact time with the patient's skin.

Obviously, the greater an agent's temperature, the greater its potential to cause damage. However, it is also important to consider the amount of heat energy possessed by the object or substance. Receiving a blast of heated air from an oven at 350°F is much less damaging than contact with hot cooking oil at the same temperature. In general, water, oils, and other liquids tend to have a high heat energy content. This content is roughly related to the material's density. In a similar fashion, solids also usually have a high heat content. Gases, however, usually have less capacity to hold heat owing to their being less dense.

The duration of exposure to a heat source is obviously important in determining burn severity. A patient's momentary contact with hot oil would result in less damage than if the oil were poured into his shoe with his foot in it.

A burn is a progressive process, and the greater the heat energy transmitted to the body, the deeper the wound. Initially, the burn damages the epidermis through an increase in its temperature. As contact with the substance continues, heat energy penetrates deeper into body tissue. Thus, a burn may involve the epidermis, dermis, and subcutaneous tissue as well as muscles, bone, and other internal tissues.

At the local tissue level, thermal burns cause a number of effects collectively described by **Jackson's theory of thermal wounds.** This theory helps us understand the physical effects of high heat and

helps explain a number of clinical effects (Figure 5-1).

With a burn, the skin nearest the heat source suffers the most profound changes. Cell membranes rupture and are destroyed, blood coagulates, and structural proteins denature. This most-damaged area is the **zone of coagulation.** If the zone of coagulation penetrates the dermis, the resulting injury is termed a full thickness or third-degree burn. Adjacent to the zone of coagulation is a less-damaged yet still inflamed region where blood flow decreases. This burn region is called the **zone of stasis**. Even more distant from the burn source is a broader area where inflammation and changes in blood flow are limited. This is the **zone of hyperemia**; this zone accounts for the erythema (redness) associated with some burns.

Large burns have profound pathological effects on the body as a whole. In general, these effects are important in any burn that covers more than 15 to 20 percent of the patient's body surface area. To understand these effects and the resulting burn shock, it is essential to first learn a little about the progression of burns.

The body's response to burns occurs over time and can usefully be classified into four phases. The first phase

CONTENT REVIEW

➤ Effects of Heat According to Jackson's Theory of Thermal Wounds
  • Zone of coagulation—most damaged area nearest heat source; cell membranes rupture and are destroyed, blood coagulates, structural proteins denature
  • Zone of stasis—adjacent to most damaged region; inflammation present, blood flow decreased
  • Zone of hyperemia—area farthest from heat source; limited inflammation and changes in blood flow

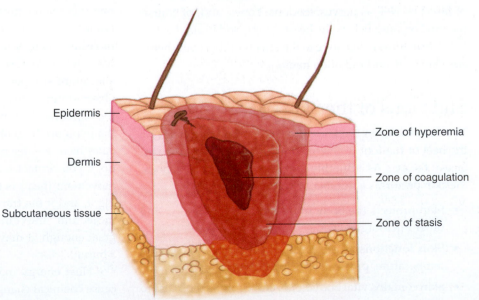

FIGURE 5-1 The zones of injury commonly caused by a thermal burn.

Epidermis

Dermis

Subcutaneous tissue

Zone of hyperemia

Zone of coagulation

Zone of stasis

occurs immediately following a burn and is called the **emergent phase**. This is the body's initial reaction to the burn. This phase includes a pain response, as well as an outpouring of catecholamines in response to the pain and the physical and emotional stress. During this stage, the patient displays tachycardia, tachypnea, mild hypertension, and mild anxiety.

The **fluid shift phase** follows the initial phase and can last up to 24 hours. It occurs in those with thermal burns larger than 15 to 20 percent total body surface area and is unlikely to occur in those with smaller burns. The fluid shift phase begins shortly after the burn and reaches its peak in 6 to 8 hours. Generally, EMS personnel are likely to see only the beginning of it in the prehospital setting. In this phase, damaged cells release agents that initiate an inflammatory response. This increases blood flow to capillaries surrounding the burn and increases capillary permeability. The response results in a large fluid shift away from the **intravascular space** into the **extravascular space** (massive edema). Note that capillaries leak plasma (water, electrolytes, and some dissolved proteins) and not blood cells. Red blood cell loss from burns uncomplicated by other trauma is usually minimal.

After the fluid shift phase comes the **hypermetabolic phase**, which may last many days or weeks, depending on burn severity. This phase is characterized by a large increase in the body's demands for nutrients as it begins the long process of repairing damaged tissue. Gradually this phase evolves into the **resolution phase**, in which scar tissue is laid down and remodeled, and the burn patient begins to rehabilitate and return to normal function.

Electrical Burns

Electricity's power is the result of an electron flow from a point of high concentration to one of low concentration. The difference between the two concentrations is called **voltage**. It is helpful to envision voltage as the "pressure" of the electric flow. The rate or amount of flow in a given time is termed **current** and is measured in **amperes**. With direct current, electrons flow in one direction, whereas alternating current reverses the flow in short intervals. Standard house current is alternating at 60 cycles per second.

Another factor affecting electricity flow is **resistance**, which is measured in **ohms**. Copper electrical wire has very little resistance and allows a free flow of electrons. Tungsten (the filament in a light bulb) is moderately resistant and heats, glows, and emits light as more and more current is applied to it.

The relationship among current (I), resistance (R), and voltage (V) is well known as **Ohm's law**:

$$V = IR \text{ or } I = V/R$$

Like tungsten, internal human tissues vary in conductivity and are moderately resistant to electron flow. Skin, however, is highly resistant to electrical flow. Moisture or sweat on the skin lowers this resistance. Nerve tissue, on the other hand, conducts electricity very easily. If the human body is subjected to voltage, tissue initially resists the flow. If the voltage is strong enough, the current begins to pass into and through the body. As it does, heat energy is created. The heat produced by the electrical current (power, or P) is equal to the product of the square of the current (I^2), the resistance of the conductor (R), and the time during which it flows, as expressed in **Joule's law**:

$$P = I^2Rt$$

The highest heat occurs at the points of greatest resistance, often at the skin. This accounts for the severe "entry" and "exit" wounds sometimes seen in electrical injuries. Dry, callused skin can have enormous resistance values, ranging from 500,000 to 1,000,000 ohms/cm. Wet skin, particularly the thin skin on the palm side of the arm or on the inner thigh, can have values as low as 300 to 10,000 ohms/cm. Mucous membranes have very low resistance (100 ohms/cm) and allow even small currents to pass. This accounts for the relative ease with which household current can cause lip and oral burns in children who accidentally bite electrical cords (Figure 5-2).

With small currents, heat energy produced is of little consequence. But if the voltage or current is high, profound damage can occur. The longer the duration of contact, the greater will be the potential for injury. Electrical burns can be particularly damaging because the burn heats the victim from the inside out, causing great damage

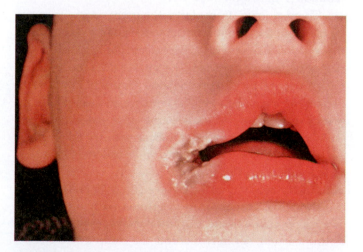

FIGURE 5-2 Electrical burns to a child's mouth caused by chewing on an electrical cord.

(Photo courtesy of Scott & White Healthcare)

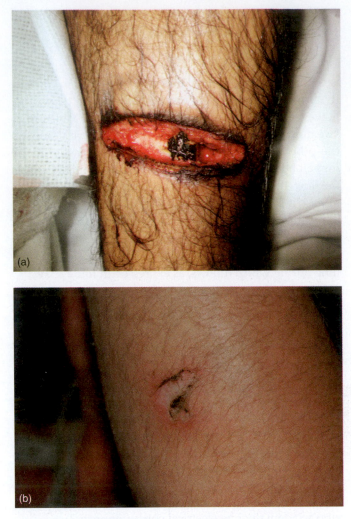

FIGURE 5-3 Injuries from electrical shock: (a) electrical entrance wound; (b) electrical exit wound.

(Photo a: © Dr. Bryan E. Bledsoe; Photo b: © Edward T. Dickinson, MD)

to internal organs and structures while possibly leaving little visible surface damage, except for the entry and exit wounds (Figure 5-3).

Thermal injury from electrical current occurs as energy travels from the point of contact to the point of exit. At both these points, the concentration of electricity is great, as is the degree of damage expected. The smaller the area of contact, the greater will be the concentration of current flow and the greater the injury. Between the entrance and exit points, the energy spreads out over a larger cross-sectional area and generally causes less injury. Electrical current may follow blood vessels and nerves because they offer less resistance than muscle and bone. This may lead to serious vascular and nervous injury deep within the involved limbs or body cavity.

Electrical contact also interferes with the nervous control of muscle tissue. Current passage, especially alternating current, severely disrupts the complicated electrochemical reactions that control muscles. If contact with a current as small as 20 to 50 milliamperes (mA) is maintained for a period of time, the muscles of respiration may

be immobilized. The result is prolonged respiratory arrest, anoxia, hypoxemia, and—eventually—death. Electrical currents greater than 50 mA may also disrupt the heart's electrical system, causing ventricular fibrillation accompanied by ineffective pumping action. Alternating electrical current such as that found in household current can also cause tetanic convulsions or uncontrolled contractions of muscles. If the victim is holding a wire at such a time, the victim may be unable to let go, thereby prolonging exposure and increasing the injury severity. This can occur with as little as 9 mA of current.

Electrical injury may also physically injure muscle and other tissue, leading to its degeneration. As the tissue dies, it releases materials toxic to the human body. These materials may damage the liver and kidneys, leading to failure.

At times, electrical energy may cause flash burns secondary to heat of current passing through adjacent air. Air is very resistant to electrical current passage. If the current is strong enough and the space through which it passes is small, the electricity arcs, producing tremendous heat. If the patient's skin is close by, heat may severely burn or vaporize tissue. In addition, heat may ignite articles of clothing or other combustibles and produce thermal burns.

Chemical Burns

Chemical burns denature the biochemical makeup of cell membranes (primarily the proteins) and destroy the cells. Such injuries are not transmitted through the tissue as are thermal injuries. Instead, a chemical burn must destroy the tissue before it can chemically burn any deeper. This fact generally limits the "burn" process unless very strong chemicals are involved (Figure 5-4). Agents that can cause chemical burns are too numerous to mention. However, the most common causes of these burns are either strong acids or alkalis (bases).

Both acids and alkalis burn by disrupting cell membranes and damaging tissues on contact. As they cause

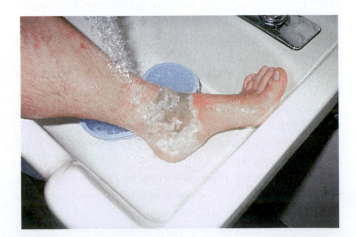

FIGURE 5-4 An acid burn to the ankle.

(© Roy Alson, PhD, MD, FACEP, FAAEM)

damage, acids usually form a thick, insoluble mass, or coagulum, at the point of contact. This process is called **coagulation necrosis** and helps to limit acid burn depth. Acid burns usually cause immediate pain. Alkalis, however, have limited pain and do not form a protective coagulum. Instead, the alkali continues to destroy cell membranes, releasing intercellular and interstitial fluid, destroying tissue in a process called **liquefaction necrosis**. Liquifaction necrosis progressively denatures proteins and collagen, dissolves fats (saponification), dehydrates tissues, and damages blood vessels. This process allows the alkali to rapidly penetrate underlying tissue, causing progressively deeper burns. For this reason, alkali burns can be quite serious. Alkalis are commonly used as oven and drain cleaners, agricultural fertilizers, and in industry.

Radiation Injury

Ionizing radiation has bombarded Earth since long before recorded time. It is a daily, natural phenomenon arising from the sun and the distant cosmos. Natural radiation also occurs from radioactive rocks and gases found throughout our planet. In most cases, this natural background radiation is inconsequential. Radiation becomes a danger when people are exposed to synthetic sources that greatly increase radiation intensity. Medicine and industry use radioactive materials for diagnostic testing and treatment and for energy production. Deaths from exposure to radiation are extremely rare, as are serious injuries, because of safety measures commonly used with the handling of nuclear materials. However, the possibility of a large risk of injury typically comes from accidents associated with improper handling, either in the on-site environment or during transport.

Radiation causes damage through a process known as **ionization**, in which a radioactive energy particle travels into a substance and changes an internal atom. In the human body, the affected cell either repairs the damage, dies, or goes on to produce damaged cells (cancer). The cells most sensitive to radiation injury are the cells that reproduce most quickly. These include those responsible for erythrocyte, leukocyte, and platelet production (bone marrow); cells lining the intestinal tract; and cells involved in human reproduction.

Four types of ionizing radiation are commonly encountered. These are:

- **Alpha radiation.** The unstable atomic nucleus releases **alpha radiation** in the form of a small helium nucleus. Alpha radiation is a very weak energy source and can travel only inches through air. Paper or clothing can easily stop alpha radiation. This radiation also cannot penetrate the epidermis. On the subatomic scale, however, alpha particles are massive and can cause great damage over the short distance they travel. Alpha radiation is a significant hazard only if the patient inhales or ingests contaminated material, thus bringing the source in proximity to sensitive respiratory and digestive tract tissue.

- **Beta radiation.** A second type of radiologic process produces **beta radiation.** Its energy is greater than that of alpha radiation. However, the beta particle is relatively lightweight, with the mass of an electron. Beta radiation can travel 6 to 10 feet through air and can penetrate a few layers of clothing. Beta particles can invade the first few millimeters of skin and thus have the potential for causing external as well as internal injury.

- **Gamma radiation. Gamma radiation**, also known as X-rays, is the most powerful type of ionizing (atom-changing) radiation. It can travel through the entire body or ionize any atom within. Its lack of mass or charge (it is pure electromagnetic energy, or photons) helps give it great penetrating power. Gamma radiation evokes the greatest concern for external exposure. It is the most dangerous and most feared type of radiation because it is difficult to protect against. Many feet of concrete or many inches of lead are needed to shield against the highest-energy gamma rays. Fortunately, exposure to high-energy gamma rays occurs only in individuals who are exposed to nuclear blasts, are near nuclear reactor cores, or are very close to highly radioactive materials. More modest amounts of concrete, steel, or lead can provide shielding from the more common and lower energy X-rays and gamma rays encountered in medicine and industry.

- *Neutron radiation.* Neutrons are small, yet moderately massive subatomic particles with no charge. Their small size and lack of charge account for their great penetrating power. Fortunately, strong **neutron radiation** is uncommon outside of nuclear reactors and bombs.

    Exposure to radiation and the effects of ionization can occur through two mechanisms. In the first, an unshielded person is directly exposed to a strong radioactive source—for example, an unstable material such as uranium. The second exposure mechanism is contamination by dust, debris, or fluids that contain very small particles of radioactive material. These contaminants give off weaker radiation than a direct radioactive source like uranium. However, the proximity of these contaminants to the body and their longer contact times with it may result in greater exposure and contamination. Note that most substances, including human tissue, do not give off radiation. The patient is not the danger in a radiologic exposure incident. Any danger comes from the radioactive source, such as the contaminated material on the patient.

Three factors are important to keep in mind whenever called to a radiation exposure incident. These include the duration of exposure; the distance from the radioactive source; and the shielding between you, the patient, and the source. Knowledge of these three factors can limit exposure and potential for injury.

- *Duration.* Radiation exposure is an accumulative danger. The longer a person remains exposed to the source, the greater the injury potential. The relationship is linear—for example, twice the exposure doubles the risk.

- *Distance.* Radiation strength diminishes quickly as distance from the source increases. The effect is similar to that of a light bulb's intensity. At a few feet, you can easily read by it, whereas at a few hundred feet the light barely casts a shadow. Mathematically, the relationship is inverse and squared. As you double your distance from a radioactive source, its strength drops to one-fourth of the original strength. As you triple the distance, its strength diminishes to one-ninth, and so on.

- *Shielding.* The more material between you and a radioactive source, the less exposure you experience. With alpha and beta radiation, shielding is very easy to provide and reasonably effective. With gamma and neutron sources, dense objects such as earth, concrete, metal, and lead are needed to provide any real protection. Shielding

CONTENT REVIEW

➤ Factors Affecting Exposure to Radiation
- Duration of exposure
- Distance from the source
- Shielding from the source

generally follows a linear relationship; for example, three times the shielding thickness yields one-third the radiation exposure.

Radiation emission, usually in units per hour, is measured with a Geiger counter, and cumulative exposure is recorded by a device called a dosimeter. Both devices record units of radiation, expressed as either the **rad** or the **Gray** (Gy), with 1 Gray equal to 100 rads.

Radiation effects vary with different tissues. As little as 0.2 Gy can cause cataracts in exposed eyes and damage blood-cell–producing bone marrow tissue. The radiation dose that is lethal to about 50 percent of exposed individuals is approximately 4.5 Gy.

With whole-body exposure, and as the radiation dose increases, signs and symptoms of exposure appear earlier and become more severe. The first signs of serious exposure are slight nausea and fatigue, occurring between 4 and 24 hours after exposure. As radiation doses move toward the lethal range, nausea severity increases and is joined by anorexia, vomiting, diarrhea, and malaise. Erythema may be present, and fatigue becomes more intense. These signs appear within 2 to 6 hours. With exposure to even higher, fatal doses, the patient displays all radiation exposure signs almost immediately and soon thereafter experiences confusion, watery diarrhea, and physical collapse. The signs and symptoms of radiation exposure and the injuries associated with it vary because individual sensitivity to radiation exposure varies greatly.

Prolonged exposure to even small radiation amounts may produce long-term and delayed problems. Infertility is a potential injury, because the cells producing eggs and sperm are very susceptible to ionization damage. Cancer is another delayed and severe side effect. It may occur years or even decades after a radiation exposure.

Inhalation Injury

The burn environment, on occasion (10 to 25 percent of the time), produces inhalation injury. This occurs most commonly if the patient is trapped or unconscious in an enclosed space, but it can occasionally occur even in an open field if the smoke is dense enough. A victim will eventually inhale gases, heated air, flames, or steam. This inhalation results in airway and respiratory injury.

When approaching a burn environment, ensure personal protection and anticipate the following inhalation conditions. Keep these in mind when surveying the scene. Always take necessary protective measures and begin patient assessment.

TOXIC INHALATION Modern residential and commercial construction uses synthetic resins and plastics that release toxic gases as they burn. Combustion of these materials can form agents such as cyanide, hydrogen sulfide, and other toxic or caustic substances. If a patient inhales these gases, they either react with the lung tissue, causing internal chemical burns, or they diffuse across the alveolar–capillary membrane, enter the bloodstream, and interfere with delivery to or the cell's use of oxygen. Signs and symptoms of these injuries may be present immediately following exposure or onset may be delayed for an hour or two after inhalation. Toxic inhalation injury occurs more frequently than thermal inhalation burns.

CARBON MONOXIDE POISONING A significant concern associated with the fire/burn environment is carbon monoxide (CO) poisoning. Carbon monoxide is the product of incomplete hydrocarbon combustion. It is a tasteless, odorless, and otherwise unrecognizable gas. There is a very small amount of carbon monoxide in ambient air, but as that concentration increases by more than 100 times, the danger of carbon monoxide poisoning begins. This poisoning risk exists with improperly ventilated open flame in a contained area (house fires, faulty fuel-fired heating units, nonelectric stoves and ovens, gas and charcoal grills and camp stoves, improperly ventilated fireplaces) and internal combustion engines (auto exhaust fumes, home generators, propane-fueled vehicles, boat exhaust fumes). Each year, as many as 6,000 people die from carbon monoxide poisoning, and it accounts for 40,000 emergency department visits yearly.

Carbon monoxide is a stable molecule consisting of one carbon and one oxygen atom firmly bonded to each other. It competes for the four oxygen-bonding sites on each hemoglobin molecule. Hemoglobin has an affinity for carbon monoxide that is more than 200 times its affinity for oxygen. Carbon monoxide bound to hemoglobin prevents oxygen from attaching and, thereby, prevents hemoglobin from transporting oxygen from the alveoli to the tissue capillaries. As carbon monoxide concentrations increase, and as the time of exposure increases, more and more hemoglobin is saturated with carbon monoxide (carboxyhemoglobin), whereas less and less hemoglobin is saturated with oxygen (oxyhemoglobin).

Carbon monoxide also attaches to myoglobin. Myoglobin is another iron-containing protein that serves as an oxygen storage site in muscles, including those of the heart. The resulting reduction in oxygen availability can induce cardiac ischemia and arrhythmias.

Recognizing carbon monoxide poisoning is a challenge, as the signs and symptoms of toxicity are very nonspecific. The victim of this poisoning presents with a general ill feeling (malaise) and CNS symptoms: headache, dizziness, blurred vision, nausea, and vomiting. As the exposure increases, the victim may present with confusion, weakness, syncope, dyspnea, tachypnea, tachycardia, and chest pain. With extreme exposure, the victim may present with hypotension, cardiac ischemia, arrhythmias, pulmonary

edema, seizures, coma, pulmonary arrest, cardiac arrest, and death. Paramedics should have a high index of suspicion for this poisoning as temperatures drop (causing heating units to function) in the late fall or early winter, and especially when a group of people who work or live together suffer flu-like symptoms.

Carbon monoxide poisoning is of special concern for the young, the elderly, patients with preexisting heart disease, and the fetuses of pregnant patients. Young pediatric patients are susceptible to CO poisoning because of alterations in their physiology. The elderly are more likely to have preexisting disease, including COPD and other respiratory problems, as well as reduced respiratory reserves. This leaves them more adversely affected by CO poisoning. Patients with cardiac problems are at special risk because the myocardium does not store oxygen, and CO poisoning reduces oxygen transport by the blood. The myocardium is then even more prone to hypoxia. Finally, fetal hemoglobin is different from normal hemoglobin and has an increased affinity for carbon monoxide. With exposure, the fetus may suffer ill effects well before they appear in the mother.

AIRWAY THERMAL BURN Another, though less frequent, injury is the airway thermal burn. Very moist mucosa lines the airway and helps insulate it against heat damage. Because of this mucosa, **supraglottic**, or upper airway, structures may absorb the heat and prevent lower airway burns. High levels of thermal energy are required to evaporate the fluid and injure cells. Inspiration of hot air or flame rarely produces enough heat to cause significant thermal burns to the lower airway.

Superheated steam has greater heat content than hot, dry air and can cause **subglottic**, or lower airway, burns. Superheated steam is created under great pressure and can have a temperature well above 212°F. A common hazard to firefighters, superheated steam develops when a stream of water strikes a hot spot and vaporizes explosively. The blast can dislodge the mask of a firefighter's self-contained breathing apparatus, exposing the firefighter to superheated steam inhalation. Steam contains enough heat energy to severely burn the upper airway. It also may damage the lower respiratory tract, although this happens less frequently.

Risk factors for inhalation injuries associated with burns include standing in the burn environment (hot gases rise), screaming or yelling there (the open glottis allows toxic gases to enter the lower airway), and being trapped in a closed burn environment.

With any thermal or smoke-related chemical burn injury to the respiratory tract, there is the danger of airway restriction, severe dyspnea, and possible respiratory arrest. The airway is a narrow tube lined with extremely vascular tissue. If damaged, this tissue swells rapidly, seriously reducing the size of the airway lumen. The patient presents with minor hoarseness, followed precipitously by dyspnea. Stridor or high-pitched "crowing" sounds on inspiration are ominous signs of impending airway obstruction. Other clues leading you to suspect potential airway burns include singed facial and nasal hair, black-tinged (carbonaceous) sputum, and facial burns. The airway injury may be so extensive that it induces complete respiratory obstruction and arrest. Accurate assessment is important because 20 to 35 percent of patients admitted to burn centers, and some 60 to 80 percent of burn patients who die, have an associated inhalation injury.

Burn Depth

After you determine the burn source and assess the possibility of associated inhalation injury, you need to assess the burn's severity. One element in determining the severity of a burn is the depth of damage it causes. Depth of burn damage is normally classified into three categories (Figure 5-5).

Superficial Burn

The **superficial burn**, also termed a *first-degree burn*, involves only the epidermis and upper dermis. It is an irritation of the living cells and nerve endings in this region and results in some pain, minor edema, and erythema. It normally heals without complication.

Partial Thickness Burn

The **partial thickness burn**, also termed a *second-degree burn*, penetrates slightly deeper than a superficial burn and produces blisters. Heat energy travels into the dermis, involving more of the tissue and resulting in greater destruction. The partial thickness burn is similar to a superficial burn in that it is reddened, painful, and edematous. You can differentiate it from the superficial burn only after blisters form. Because there are many nerve endings in the dermis, both superficial and partial thickness burns are often very painful. With both superficial and partial thickness burns, the dermis is still intact and complete skin regeneration is very likely.

Sunburn is a common, but specialized, type of burn. Ultraviolet radiation, rather than normal thermal processes, causes the burn. The radiation penetrates superficially and damages the uppermost layers of the dermis. Sunburn can present as either a superficial or partial thickness burn.

> **CONTENT REVIEW**
>
> ➤ Depth of Burn
> - Superficial (first degree)—involves only the epidermis; produces pain, minor edema, and erythema (redness)
> - Partial thickness (second degree)—involves epidermis and dermis; produces pain, edema, erythema, blisters
> - Full thickness (third degree)—involves all skin layers and possibly structures beneath; painless, but tissue is destroyed; white, brown, or charred, leatherlike appearance

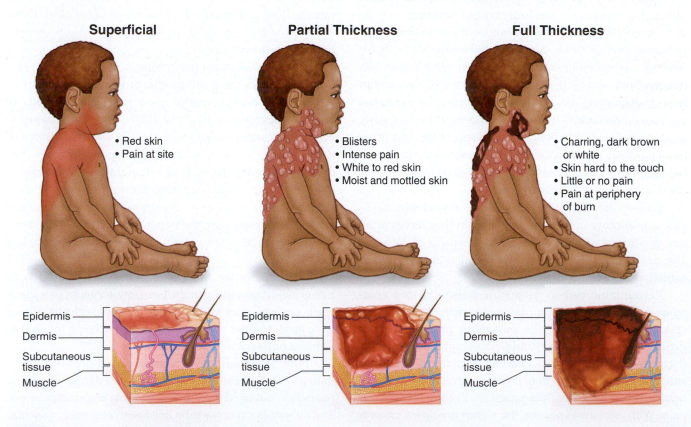

Superficial
- Red skin
- Pain at site

Partial Thickness
- Blisters
- Intense pain
- White to red skin
- Moist and mottled skin

Full Thickness
- Charring, dark brown or white
- Skin hard to the touch
- Little or no pain
- Pain at periphery of burn

Epidermis
Dermis
Subcutaneous tissue
Muscle

Epidermis
Dermis
Subcutaneous tissue
Muscle

Epidermis
Dermis
Subcutaneous tissue
Muscle

FIGURE 5-5 Classification of burns by depth.

Another similar type of burn occurs as someone watches an arc welder without proper protection. In this injury, called *ultraviolet keratitis*, the outermost parts of the eye (cornea) trap the ultraviolet radiation, causing injury to the layer. This causes delayed eye pain and, possibly, transient blindness. The injury usually heals completely within 24 hours.

Full Thickness Burn

The **full thickness burn**, or *third-degree burn*, penetrates both the epidermis and the dermis and extends into the subcutaneous layers or even deeper, into muscles, bones, and internal organs. These burns destroy the tissue's regenerative properties and the peripheral nerve endings. Injury is painless because of nerve destruction, but the margins of full thickness burns are frequently partial thickness burns, which can be quite painful. Full thickness burns take on various colorations depending on the nature of the burning agent and the damaged, dying, or dead tissue. They can be white, brown, dark red, or a charred color and typically have a dry, leatherlike appearance. Because the burn destroys the entire dermis, skin grafting is usually required.

Body Surface Area

Another factor affecting burn severity is how much of a person's **body surface area (BSA)** the burn involves. There are two approaches to estimating the BSA involved in a burn. The first, the rule of nines, is useful in estimating large burn areas. The second method, the rule of palms, is helpful in assessing smaller burns more accurately.

Rule of Nines

The **rule of nines** identifies 11 topographical adult body regions, each of which approximates 9 percent of the patient's BSA (Figure 5-6). These regions include the entire head and neck, the anterior chest, the anterior abdomen, the posterior chest, the lower back (the posterior abdomen), the anterior surface of each lower extremity, the posterior surface of each lower extremity, and the entirety of each upper extremity. The genitalia make up the remaining 1 percent of BSA.

Because infant and child anatomy differs significantly from that of adults, you must modify the rule of nines to maintain an accurate approximation of BSA. Divide the head and neck area into the anterior and posterior surface and

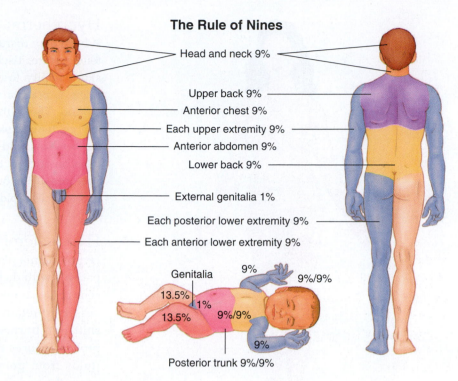

The Rule of Nines

Head and neck 9%

Upper back 9%
Anterior chest 9%
Each upper extremity 9%
Anterior abdomen 9%
Lower back 9%

External genitalia 1%

Each posterior lower extremity 9%
Each anterior lower extremity 9%

Genitalia
9%
9%/9%
13.5%
1%
13.5%
9%/9%
9%
Posterior trunk 9%/9%

FIGURE 5-6 The rule of nines.

award 9 percent for each. Reduce the surface area of each lower extremity by 4.5 percent to ensure that the total body surface area remains at 100 percent. The rule of nines is, at best, an approximation of the area burned. It is, however, an expedient and useful tool to help measure a burn's extent.

Rule of Palms

The **rule of palms** is an alternative system for approximating a burn's extent. It uses the palmar surface as a point of comparison in gauging the size of the affected body area (Figure 5-7). The patient's palm (the hand less the fingers) represents about 1 percent of the BSA, whether the patient is an adult, a child, or an infant. Visualize the palmar surface area and apply it to the burn area mentally and obtain an estimate of the total BSA affected.

The rule of palms is easier to use for local burns of up to about 10 percent BSA, whereas the rule of nines is simpler and more appropriate for larger burns. Many other burn approximation techniques exist that are both more specific to age and, in general, more accurate, such as the Lund and Browder chart (Figure 5-8). However, these techniques are more complicated and time consuming to use. Both the rule of nines and the rule of palms provide reasonable approximations of BSA when used properly in the field.

Systemic Complications

Burns cause several systemic complications. These can affect the overall severity of a burn. Typical complications include hypothermia, hypovolemia, eschar formation, and infection.

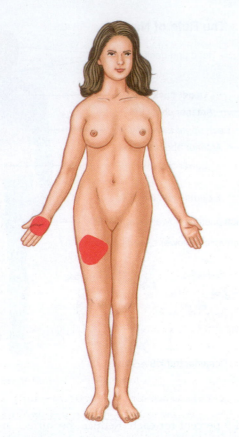

FIGURE 5-7 Using the rule of palms, the surface of the patient's palm represents approximately 1 percent of BSA and is helpful in estimating the area of small burns.

Hypothermia

A burn may disrupt the body's ability to regulate its core temperature. Tissue destruction reduces or eliminates the skin's ability to contain fluid within. The burn process releases plasma and other fluids, which seep into the wound. There, they evaporate and rapidly remove heat energy. Injured skin has increased blood flow, enhancing the heat loss, and the burn injury does not have the reflex vasoconstriction that normally protects against excessive heat loss. If the burn is extensive, uncontrolled body heat loss induces rapid and severe hypothermia.[2]

Hypovolemia

Hypovolemia also may complicate the severe burn. In patients with thermal burns over more than 15 to 20 percent of the total BSA, the inability of damaged blood vessels to retain plasma causes a fluid and electrolyte shift into burned tissue. Additionally, loss of plasma protein reduces the blood's ability, via osmosis, to draw fluids from uninjured tissues. This, in turn, compromises the body's natural response to fluid loss and may produce a profound hypovolemia. Although this is a serious and life-threatening complication of extensive burns, it takes hours to develop. Modern aggressive fluid resuscitation can effectively counteract this aspect of the burn process.

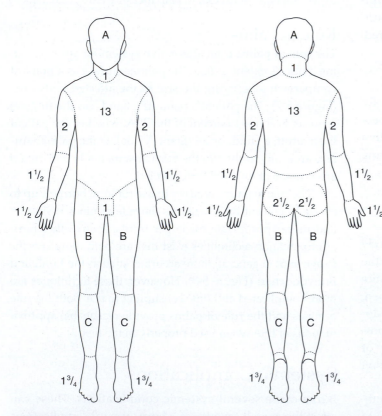

Region	Partial thickness (%) [NB1]	Full thickness (%)
head		
neck		
anterior trunk		
posterior trunk		
right arm		
left arm		
buttocks		
genitalia		
right leg		
left leg		
Total burn		

NB1: Do not include erythema

Area	Age 0	1	5	10	15	Adult
A = half of head	9½	8½	6½	5½	4½	3½
B = half of one thigh	2¾	3¼	4	4½	4½	4¾
C = half of one lower leg	2½	2½	2¾	3	3¼	3½

FIGURE 5-8 The Lund and Browder chart takes into consideration the fact that proportions of the head and lower extremities vary at different ages from infancy to adulthood and provides age-appropriate percentages for calculating the burn area of half the head, half the thigh, and half the leg. (For areas of the body other than the head, thigh, and leg, use the usual "rule of nines" percentages as shown in Figure 5-6 for an adult or child.)

A related complication is electrolyte imbalance. With the massive fluid shift to the interstitial space, the body's ability to regulate sodium, potassium, and other electrolytes becomes overwhelmed. In addition, large thermal and electrical burns can lead to massive tissue destruction, with a resultant release of breakdown products into the bloodstream. Potassium is one such breakdown product; its oversupply, or hyperkalemia, can lead to life-threatening cardiac arrhythmias. Careful ECG monitoring and appropriate fluid resuscitation can help prevent hyperkalemic complications.

Eschar

Skin denaturing further complicates full thickness thermal burns. As the burn destroys dermal cells, they become hard and leathery, producing what is known as an **eschar**. Skin as a whole constricts over the wound site, increasing the pressure of any edema beneath and restricting the flow of blood (Figure 5-9). If an extremity burn is circumferential, constriction may be severe enough to occlude all blood flow into the distal extremity. In the case of a thoracic burn, eschar may drastically reduce chest excursion and respiratory tidal volume.

Infection

Although infection is the most persistent killer of burn victims, its effects do not appear for several days following an acute injury. Pathogens invade the wound shortly after the burn occurs and continue to do so until the wound heals. These pathogens pose a hazard to life when they grow to massive numbers—a process that takes days or weeks. To reduce a patient's exposure to infectious pathogens, carefully employ Standard Precautions, use clean or sterile dressings and clean equipment, and avoid gross contamination of the burn.

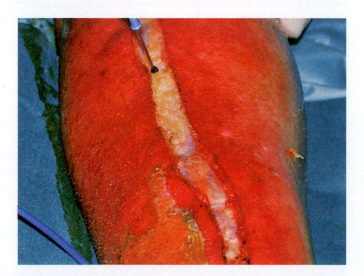

FIGURE 5-9 The constriction created by an eschar can limit chest excursion or cut off blood flow to and from a limb.

(© Michael Schurr, MD, Professor, University of Denver)

Organ Failure

As previously noted, the burn process releases material from damaged or dying body cells into the bloodstream. Myoglobin, released from the muscles in patients with severe electrical injuries, clogs the tubules of the kidneys and, with hypovolemia, may cause kidney failure. Hypovolemia and the circulating byproducts of cellular destruction may also induce liver failure. In addition, the release of cellular potassium into the bloodstream affects the heart's electrical system, causing arrhythmias and possible cardiac arrest.

Special Factors

Certain factors involving the burn patient's overall health and age will also affect the patient's response to a burn and should influence field decisions regarding treatment and transport. Geriatric and pediatric patients and patients who are already ill or otherwise injured have greater difficulty coping with burn injuries than do healthy individuals. The pediatric patient has a high ratio of BSA to body weight, which means that the fluid reserves needed for dealing with the burn effects are low. Geriatric patients have reduced mechanisms for fluid retention and lower fluid reserves. They are also less able to combat infection and more apt to have underlying diseases. Ill patients are already using body energy to fight their diseases; with burns, these patients have additional medical stresses to combat. The fluid loss that accompanies a burn also compounds the effects of blood loss in a trauma patient. This patient now must recover from two injuries.

Physical Abuse

When assessing any burn, particularly in a child or an elderly and infirm adult, be alert for any signs of potential physical abuse. Look for mechanisms of injury that don't make sense, such as stove burns on an infant who cannot yet stand or walk. Certain burn patterns should also give rise to suspicion. Multiple circular burns, each about a centimeter in diameter, may reflect intentional cigarette burns. Infants who have been dipped in scalding hot water will have characteristic circumferential burns to their buttocks as they raise their feet and legs in an attempt to avoid the burning water or "stocking" burns if their feet and legs have been dipped into the scalding water (Figure 5-10). Branding is an unusual form of abuse and is sometimes seen in ritualistic or hazing ceremonies in some cultures and organizations. In all cases of suspected abuse, document findings objectively and accurately, report them to the person assuming patient care in the emergency department, and notify the proper authorities as state and local laws require.

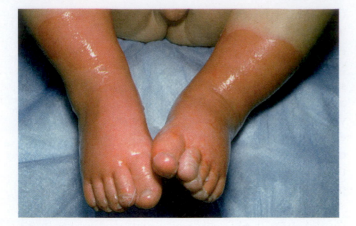

FIGURE 5-10 Burn injury from placing a child's feet and legs into hot water as punishment.

(© Roy Alson, PhD, MD, FACEP, FAAEM)

Assessment of Thermal Burns

Skin evaluation tells more about the body's condition than any other aspect of patient assessment. Not only is the skin the first body organ to experience the effects of burns, but it is also the first—and often the only—organ to display them. Therefore, assessment of the skin and associated burns must be deliberate, careful, and complete.

Burn assessment is simple and well structured. Assess burn patients carefully and completely to ensure to establish the nature and extent of each injury. This helps assign burns the appropriate priority for care.

Assessment of thermal burns follows established procedures for performing the scene size-up, the primary assessment, the rapid or focused trauma assessment, the detailed physical exam, and reassessments.

Scene Size-Up

The safety of the patient, fellow rescuers, and yourself depends on a complete and thorough scene size-up. Look around carefully on initial scene arrival to ensure that there is no continuing danger. Examine the scene to ensure that it is safe for entry. If there is any doubt, do not enter until the scene is made safe by appropriate emergency personnel.

On calls involving burn patients, be wary of entering enclosed spaces, such as a bedroom or a garage, if there is recent evidence of a fire. Even small fires can cause intense heat in small, enclosed spaces. This can rapidly lead to a near-explosive process (called flashover) in which the contents of a room rise in temperature to the point of rapid ignition. Flashover is frequently fatal to victims caught in the immediate area.

Another significant hazard at fire-ground scenes is the buildup of toxic gases. Carbon monoxide, cyanide, and hydrogen sulfide are common byproducts of combustion and can be produced in large quantities in some fires. Cyanide, in particular, can kill after as little as 15 seconds of exposure, a time short enough to fell any would-be rescuer without proper protection.

Never enter any potentially hazardous scene. Instead, ensure that the fire is thoroughly extinguished or that the patient is brought to you by persons skilled in working in hazardous environments who are using proper personal protective equipment. Ensure that the area where patient care will occur is free from dangers such as structural collapse, contamination, electricity, and any other hazards.

Once you reach the burn patient, stop the burning process so it no longer threatens you or the patient. Extinguish any overt flame using copious irrigation, if water is available. As an alternative, a heavy wool or cotton blanket (avoid most synthetics, such as nylon or polyester) will smother flames.

Quickly survey the patient for other materials he is wearing that may continue to burn. Remember that burn patients may be an actual hazard both to themselves and others. Leather articles, such as shoes, belts, or watchbands, can smolder for hours and continue to cause thermal injury. Watches, rings, and other jewelry may also hold and transmit heat or may restrict swelling tissue and occlude distal circulation. Synthetics (such as a nylon windbreaker) produce great heat as they burn and leave a hot, smoldering residue once the overt flames are out. Remove materials like these as soon as possible. Be careful when checking for and removing these items, as they can cause burns.

Once the scene is safe and no further dangers are noted, consider the burn mechanism. Always consider the possibility that the patient was unconscious during the fire or trapped within the building. If so, be ready to place a special emphasis on assessment and management of the patient's airway and breathing. Be alert for any signs of airway restriction, and be alert to possible poisoning from carbon monoxide or other toxic gases.

Also consider and examine for other mechanisms of injury associated with the burn. Remember that the victim, in attempting to escape the flames, may have fallen down a flight of stairs or jumped from a second- or third-story window. Anticipate skeletal and internal injuries. In cases of electrical burns, consider the possibility that muscle spasms caused by contact with high voltage may also have caused skeletal or spinal fractures. Be aware that associated trauma will increase the severity of the burn's impact on the patient.

Conclude the scene size-up by considering the need for other resources to manage the scene and treat the patient. Request additional EMS, police, and fire personnel and equipment as necessary. Assess for any impact the environment might have on assessment and care and integrate with scene oversight (incident command).

Primary Assessment

Start the primary assessment by forming a general impression of the patient. Try to detect any associated trauma or the possibility of head and spine injury. Evaluate the patient's level of consciousness, and, if the patient displays an altered state of consciousness, consider toxic inhalation as a cause. Assess for possible spinal injury and provide care based on your local protocols.

Next, ensure that the airway is patent. If it is not, protect it. Always give a burn patient's airway special consideration. Look for the signs of any thermal or inhalation injury during the primary airway assessment (Figure 5-11). Look carefully at facial and nasal hairs to see if they have been singed. Examine any sputum and areas around the mouth and nose for carbonaceous residue or any other evidence of inhalation burns. Listen for airway sounds, such as stridor, hoarseness, or coughing, that indicate irritation or inflammation of the mucosa. Such sounds raise the possibility of an inhalation injury and, likely, progressive airway swelling and restriction. Stridor, in particular, is a serious finding. Consider a patient with any signs of respiratory involvement as a potential acute emergency, and provide immediate care and transport.

With patients in whom respiratory involvement is suspected, provide high-concentration oxygen and prepare the equipment for endotracheal intubation. High-concentration oxygen (at levels approaching 100 percent) is especially important for burn patients because they may be suffering from carbon monoxide poisoning. Very high oxygen percentages more effectively provide oxygen to body cells and may reduce the half-life of carbon monoxide on the hemoglobin molecule by up to two-thirds.

Pulse oximetry is a very useful tool in evaluating respiratory and cardiovascular effectiveness in the burn patient. However, carbon monoxide replaces oxygen in the red blood cell and colors it much as oxygen does. This leads the oximeter to display high saturation readings when the blood actually has greatly reduced oxygen-carrying capacity. Do not rely on pulse oximetry readings alone for the patient who is suspected of suffering carbon monoxide poisoning, who has been burned in an enclosed space, or who has inhaled significant amounts of smoke.

Pulse CO-oximetry monitors are now available that monitor oxygen saturation (SpO_2) and the amount of total hemoglobin (SpHb), carboxyhemoglobin (SpCO), and methemoglobin (SpMET). Consider their use when there is any reason to suspect inhalation of smoke or the byproducts of combustion. Normal carbon monoxide levels should be less than 5 percent in nonsmokers and less than 10 percent in smokers. Consider carbon monoxide poisoning to exist when levels exceed 10 to 12 percent. Care includes supplemental oxygen, positive-pressure ventilation as needed, and rapid transport.

Cyanide poisoning is a significant risk associated with the burn environment and toxic inhalation. It is often found in combination with CO poisoning. Whenever CO poisoning is suspected, consider the administration of hydroxocobalamin (a precursor to vitamin B_{12}). Hydroxocobalamin chelates cyanide from cytochrome oxidase to form cyanocobalamin (vitamin B_{12}), a harmless compound easily excreted by the kidneys. Hydroxocobalamin is marketed as a cyanide antidote—Cyanokit®.

Burn patients may progress rapidly from mild dyspnea to total respiratory arrest. Although intubation of a respiratory burn patient may be difficult in the field, there are distinct advantages to performing it early. Edema associated with airway burns is progressive and rapidly reduces the airway lumen. If intubation is delayed until the patient becomes extremely dyspneic or goes into respiratory arrest, the airway may be so edematous that it will be difficult, if not impossible, to intubate.

If field intubation is indicated for the burn patient, perform it quickly and carefully. The airway is already narrowing, and the normal trauma associated with intubation could make matters worse. Intubation can be more complicated if the patient is conscious and fights the process. Consider using rapid sequence intubation techniques and pharmacological adjuncts, including sedatives and paralytics. Use succinylcholine (see the chapter "Airway Management and Ventilation") cautiously, if at all, as it may worsen the hyperkalemia sometimes associated with severe burns. You may also find nasotracheal intubation useful. In any case, select the crew member with the most experience to ensure that intubation is completed quickly and with the least amount of associated airway trauma.

As with all intubation, it is best to maintain an airway using the largest endotracheal tube possible. Be sure, however, to have several tubes smaller than normally used available and ready, because edema may have reduced the

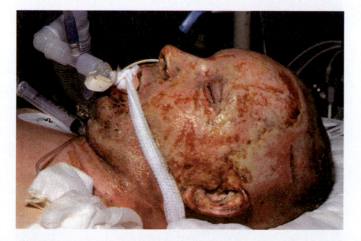

FIGURE 5-11 Facial burns or carbonaceous material around the mouth and nose suggest the potential for chemical and thermal burns to the airway.

(Edward T. Dickinson, MD)

size of the airway. Select the largest tube that you think will easily pass through the cords. In extreme cases, creation of a surgical airway by cricothyrotomy may be a lifesaving necessity. In such cases, follow local protocols or on-line medical direction. Confirm tube placement with at least three methods, including capnography.

Ensure that the patient's breathing is adequate in both volume and rate. Carefully assess tidal volume if there are circumferential chest burns, because developing eschar may restrict chest excursion. Ventilate as necessary via bag-valve mask using the reservoir and supplemental oxygen.

Secondary Assessment

Begin secondary assessment of the burn patient with either a rapid or focused trauma assessment and proceed to determining baseline vital signs, Glasgow Coma Score, and a patient history. With a burn patient, however, try to accurately approximate the burn surface area and depth. This approximation guides subsequent care and helps emergency department personnel prepare for patient arrival.

Except in cases of very localized burns, examine the patient's entire body surface—both anterior and posterior. Remove any clothing that was or could have been involved in the burn. If any of the clothing adheres to the burn or resists removal, cut around it as necessary.

Apply the rule of nines to determine the total body surface area (BSA) burned. Add 9 percent if the burn involves an entire "rule of nines" region. If it involves only a portion, add that proportion of 9 percent. For example, if 1/3 of the upper extremity is burned, the surface area approximation is 3 percent (1/3 × 9 percent = 3 percent). For small burns, use the rule of palms to approximate the affected BSA. It is helpful in burn assessment to identify the relative burn BSA that is full thickness and the relative burn BSA that is not full thickness.

Burn injury depth is also an important consideration. Identify areas of painful sensation as partial thickness burns (Figure 5-12). Consider those that present with limited or absent pain as probable full thickness burns (Figure 5-13). This differentiation is difficult because partial thickness injury and its associated pain commonly surrounds a full thickness burn (Figure 5-14). See Table 5–1 for the characteristics of the different types of burns.

A third consideration in determining the burn severity is the body area affected. The face, hands, feet, joints, genitalia, and circumferential burns deserve particular consideration. Each presents with special problems to patients and their recovery.

Assessment of facial burns to eliminate respiratory involvement should have been completed during the primary assessment. However, this area also needs special consideration for aesthetic reasons. Facial damage and scarring may be more socially debilitating than those from

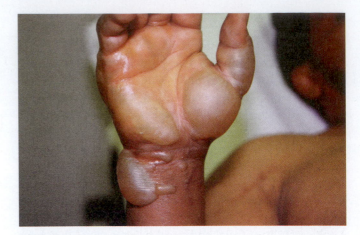

FIGURE 5-12 A partial thickness burn.

(© Edward T. Dickinson, MD)

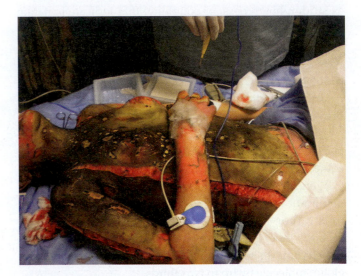

FIGURE 5-13 A deep full thickness burn.

(© Bryan E. Bledsoe)

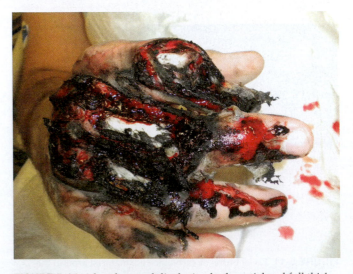

FIGURE 5-14 A hand wound displaying both partial and full thickness burns.

(© Bryan E. Bledsoe)

Table 5-1 Characteristics of Various Depths of Burns

	Superficial (First Degree)	Partial Thickness (Second Degree)	Full Thickness (Third Degree)
Cause	Sun or minor flame	Hot liquids, flame	Chemicals, electricity, hot metals, flame
Skin color	Red	Mottled red	Pearly white and/or charred, translucent, and parchment-like
Skin	Dry with no blisters	Blisters with weeping	Dry with thrombosed blood vessels
Sensation	Painful	Painful	Anesthetic
Healing	3–6 days	2–4 weeks	May require skin grafting

a joint or limb burn. Carefully assess and give a high priority to these injuries, even if airway and respiratory involvement has been excluded.

Consider full thickness burns involving feet or hands as serious. These areas are critical for much of the patient's daily activities. Serious burns and resulting scar tissue make thermal hand or foot injuries very debilitating. Assess these areas and communicate the precise injury location and the burn degree to the receiving physician. Joint burns can likewise be debilitating for patients. Scar tissue replaces skin, leading to loss of joint flexibility and mobility.

Also pay particular attention to burns that completely ring an extremity, thorax, abdomen, or neck. Because of the nature of a full thickness burn, the area underneath the burn may be drastically compressed as an eschar forms. The resulting constriction may hinder respirations, restrict distal blood flow, or cause hypoxia of the tissues beneath. Carefully assess any burn encircling a part of the body for distal circulation or other signs of vascular compromise. Once detected, perform reassessments to monitor distal circulatory status.

Finally, assign a higher priority to any burns affecting pediatric or geriatric patients or patients who are ill or otherwise injured. Serious burns cause great stress for these patients. The massive fluid and heat loss, as well as infection often associated with burns, challenge the ability of body systems to perform adequately. Consider a burn more serious whenever it is accompanied by any other serious patient problem.

Once the depth, extent, and other factors that contribute to burn severity have been determined, categorize the patient as having either minor, moderate, or severe burns. Use the criteria in Table 5–2 as a guide.

Burn severity should be increased one level with pediatric and geriatric patients and patients suffering from other trauma or acute medical problems. Also consider burns as critical with a patient who shows any signs or symptoms of respiratory involvement.

A newer scoring system for burn severity is the **Baux score**. The score takes into account the burn victim's age and the percentage of surface area burned. It also adds 17 if there is any significant respiratory involvement. The resulting score reflects seriousness/mortality, with a score of 130 to 140 generally approaching a mortality of 100 percent. The scale works well except for those very young and those over 75 years of age.

Seriously burned patients require immediate transport to a burn (or trauma) center, if possible (Table 5–3). A burn center is a hospital with a special commitment to providing

Table 5-2 Burn Severity

Minor

Superficial: BSA < 50 percent (sunburns, etc.)

Partial thickness: BSA < 10 percent

Moderate

Superficial: BSA > 50 percent

Partial thickness: BSA < 30 percent

Full thickness: BSA < 10 percent

Any partial or full thickness burns involving hands, feet, joints, face, or genitalia

Critical

Partial thickness: BSA > 30 percent

Full thickness: BSA > 10 percent

Inhalation injury

Source: American Burn Association.

Table 5-3 Injuries That Benefit from Burn Center Care

Partial thickness (second-degree) burn greater than 10 percent of BSA

Full thickness (third-degree) burn

Significant burns to the face, feet, hands, perineum, or major joints

High-voltage electrical burns

Inhalation injuries

Chemical burns

Associated significant injuries or medical conditions

Source: American Burn Association.

treatment to burn patients. That commitment includes intensive patient care focused on reducing infection risk presented by serious burns, performing skin grafting to replaced lost skin, and providing extensive rehabilitation services to help restore joint function. Immediate transport to a burn center is not as critically time dependent as transport for other seriously injured patients to a trauma center, but burn center resources can optimize a patient's recovery prospects. Review local protocols for criteria regarding patient transport to a burn center.

Conclude the rapid or focused trauma assessment by prioritizing the patient for transport. Rapidly transport any patient with full thickness burns over a large portion of the BSA. Patients with associated full thickness injuries to the face, joints, hands, feet, or genitalia are also candidates for immediate transport. Other cases needing rapid transport include patients who have experienced smoke, steam, or flame inhalation, or any geriatric, pediatric, otherwise ill, or trauma patients. Direct these patients to the nearest burn center as defined by local protocols or by online medical direction.

Reassessment

Conduct reassessments for all burn patients every 15 minutes for minor burns and every 5 minutes for moderate or critical burns. Even after the burn injury mechanism has been stopped, the nature of the burn will continue to affect the patient. In addition to monitoring vital signs, watch for early signs of hypovolemia and airway problems. Also be cautious with aggressive fluid therapy. Monitor lung sounds and respiratory effort suggestive of pulmonary

Legal Considerations

Transporting a Burn Patient. Burn patients require highly specialized care in a facility specifically designed for burn injuries. Burn centers offer a multidisciplinary approach to burn care, using plastic surgeons, general surgeons, orthopedic surgeons, rehabilitation specialists, pain management specialists, and others. In addition, burn centers provide nutritional counseling (very important to burn healing), pastoral care, and psychological care. Burn care facilities are expensive to operate and patients tend to remain in them for prolonged periods of time. The American Burn Association (ABA) has published guidelines for determining which patients might benefit from treatment in a burn center.

Most burn centers are regional facilities, and frequently patients must be transported some distance to them. Personnel who routinely transport burn patients should be familiar with burn care, including dressings, fluid therapy, and escharotomy (if required). In addition, continued adequate analgesia should be provided according to local protocols and interhospital transfer orders. Burn care should be addressed in any trauma system plan.

edema, and slow fluid resuscitation if any signs develop. Carefully monitor distal circulation and sensation with any circumferential burn. Finally, monitor the ECG to identify any abnormalities, which may be caused by electrolyte imbalances secondary to fluid movement and tissue destruction.

Management of Thermal Burns

Once you complete burn patient assessment and correct or address any immediate life threats, begin needed burn management steps, either in the field or en route to the hospital. These include preventing shock, hypothermia, and any further wound contamination.[3]

Thermal burn management can be divided into two categories: for local and minor burns and for moderate to severe burns.

Local and Minor Burns

Use local cooling to treat minor soft tissue burns involving only a partial thickness injury and a small proportion of the body surface area. Provide this care only for partial thickness burns that involve less than 15 percent of the BSA, or very small full thickness burns (less than 2 percent BSA). Cooling of larger surface areas may subject the patient to the risk of hypothermia. Cold or cool water immersion has some effect in reducing pain and may limit the depth of the burning process if applied immediately (within 1 or 2 minutes) after the burn.

If not already completed, remove any article of clothing or jewelry that might possibly act to constrain edema. As body fluids accumulate at the injury site, the site begins to swell. If the swelling encounters any constriction, it increases pressure on other tissues and may, in effect, serve as a tourniquet. This pressure may result in the loss of pulse and circulation distal to the injury. Evaluate distal circulation and sensation frequently during care and transport.

Provide a burn patient with comfort and support. Even rather minor burns can be very painful. Calm and reassure the patient. In moderate to severe cases, consider fentanyl or morphine sulfate for pain. Encourage the patient, as much as practical, to keep the burn elevated.

Standard in-hospital treatment for minor burns can vary, depending on the clinical circumstances. Therapies may include the application of topical (not systemic) antibiotic ointments and sterile dressings. Other options, such as biological dressings, may be appropriate. This is why it is important to cover burns only with a clean, nonadherent dressing or sheet until a definitive management decision has been reached. For example, the early use of silver sulfadiazine may preclude the use of biological dressings. Full thickness burns are open wounds, so any patient without an up-to-date tetanus immunization is given a booster of tetanus-diphtheria toxoid.

Moderate to Severe Burns

Use dry, clean (not necessarily sterile), nonadherent dressings or simply a clean sheet to cover partial thickness burns that involve more than 15 percent BSA or full thickness burns involving more than 5 percent of the BSA. Dressings keep air movement from the sensitive partial thickness burn to a minimum and thereby reduce pain. Bulky dressings also provide padding against minor bumping and other trauma. In full thickness burns, they provide a barrier to possible contamination.

Keep the patient warm. When burns involve large surface areas, the patient loses his ability to effectively control body temperature. If a burn begins to seep fluid, as in a full thickness burn, evaporative heat loss can be extreme. Cover such the area with dry dressings, cover the patient with a blanket, and maintain a warm environment.

When treating full thickness burns to the fingers, toes, or other locations where burned surfaces may contact each other, place soft, nonadherent dressings between the burned skin areas.

If the surface area of the burn is great, medical direction may ask to provide aggressive fluid therapy during prehospital care. Hypovolemia is not an early development after a burn, but fluid migration into the wound later during the burn evolution eventually leads to serious fluid loss. Early and aggressive fluid therapy can effectively reduce the impact of this fluid loss.

If burns cover all the normal IV access sites, place the catheter through tissue with partial thickness burns proximal to any more serious injury. (Full thickness burns usually damage blood vessels or coagulate the blood, making intravenous cannulation difficult and possibly impeding effective fluid flow.) Be careful with insertion. The skin may be leathery, but the tissue underneath is very delicate. Adhesive tape may not stick to burn tissue or may injure skin when it is removed. Try to secure the intravenous needle and lines by alternative means (as with gentle circumferential bandaging), when possible.

Establish intravenous routes in any patient with moderate to severe burns. Introduce two large-bore catheters and hang 1,000-mL bags of either normal saline or lactated Ringer's solution. Current fluid resuscitation formulas recommend 4 mL of fluid for every kilogram of patient weight multiplied by the percentage body surface area sustaining full thickness burns:

$$4 \text{ mL} \times \text{Patient weight in kg} \times \text{BSA of full thickness burns}$$
$$= \text{Amount of fluid over 24 hours}$$

Thus, for a 70-kg patient with 30 percent BSA full thickness burns, the calculation is

$$4 \times 70 \times 30 = 8,400 \text{ mL}$$

The patient needs half this amount of fluid in the first 8 hours after the burn. (Note that first degree burns are not considered when calculating fluid requirements.) This particular fluid resuscitation protocol is known as the *Parkland formula*. Other variations exist and may be in use in your local area. In most prehospital situations when transport time is short (less than 1 hour), an initial fluid bolus of 0.25 mL of fluid for every kilogram of patient weight multiplied by the percentage of BSA burned is reasonable:

$$0.25 \text{ mL} \times \text{Patient weight in kg} \times \text{BSA burned} = \text{Amount of fluid}$$

Thus, for an 80-kg patient with 20 percent BSA burned, the calculation is

$$0.25 \times 80 \times 20 = 400 \text{ mL}$$

Repeat this infusion once or twice during the first hour or so of care.

Be cautious and conservative when administering fluids to the burn patient if there is any possibility of airway or lung injury. Rapid fluid administration may worsen airway swelling or edema that accompanies toxic inhalation. Carefully monitor the airway and auscultate for breath sounds frequently whenever you administer fluid to a burn patient.[4]

Burns are quite painful, yet the pain is often paradoxical to burn severity. Less severe superficial and partial thickness (first- and second-degree) burns are very uncomfortable, whereas extensive full thickness (third-degree) burns are often almost without pain. Provide patients in severe pain with narcotic analgesia. Fentanyl or morphine should be administered as needed. Consider morphine in 2 to 5 mg IV increments every 5 minutes until suffering is relieved. Use morphine with caution, though, as it may depress the respiratory drive and increase any existing hypovolemia. With fentanyl, start with a loading dose of 25 to 50 mcg IV and administer repeat doses of 25 mcg IV as needed.

Infection is another classic and deadly problem associated with extensive soft tissue burns. This life-threatening condition does not develop until well after prehospital care is concluded. However, proper field care can significantly reduce mortality and morbidity. Providing a clean environment and dressings can lessen the bacterial load for the patient. Avoid prophylactic antibiotics because their early use has been shown to actually worsen outcomes for burn patients.

In dire circumstances, medical direction may request you to perform an emergency escharotomy. This is accomplished by incising the burned tissue through the eschar perpendicular to the constriction. Be certain to incise about

1 cm deeper than the developing eschar to ensure pressure release. If adequate respirations or distal pulses do not return after the escharotomy, consider hypovolemia as the cause. Alternatively, medical direction may request you to repeat the escharotomy a short distance from the first incision.

Emergency department personnel will continue fluid resuscitation for serious burn patients according to the Parkland or another suitable formula. They will often perform arterial blood gas evaluation to determine oxygen tension and carbon monoxide concentration. Urine output and cardiac monitoring are instituted as well. The staff will ensure adequate administration of parenteral narcotic analgesia and provide tetanus immunization if necessary. They will closely evaluate severe circumferential burns for eschar development. If the blood flow in an extremity is impaired, the physician may perform an escharotomy.

Inhalation Injury

If thermal (or chemical) airway burns are present and airway compromise is imminent, intubation can be lifesaving. Monitor the airway carefully, as swelling can quickly restrict it and result in extreme hypoxemia and, possibly, respiratory arrest. A cricothyrotomy, using a Quick-trach or similar device, may be required. Once the patient's airway has been ensured, provide high-concentration oxygen by nonrebreather mask at 15 lpm, titrated to an oxygen saturation of 96 percent. Oxygen not only counters hypoxia, but is also therapeutic in carbon monoxide poisoning.[4]

If there is reason to suspect carbon monoxide poisoning, administer 100 percent oxygen regardless of the pulse oximetry reading. A standard pulse oximeter cannot distinguish between hemoglobin carrying oxygen and hemoglobin carrying carbon monoxide. When carbon monoxide poisoning is suspected (or confirmed by a pulse CO-oximeter), oxygen will serve to reduce carbon monoxide's half-life on the hemoglobin molecule. The use of CPAP will increase this effect as the continuous airway pressure forces more oxygen into the bloodstream and displaces carbon monoxide more rapidly.[5]

In some EMS systems, protocols call for possible CO poisoning patients to be transported to facilities able to provide hyperbaric oxygen (HBO) therapy. The HBO chamber provides oxygen under the pressure of two or more atmospheres. This drives oxygen into the patient's bloodstream, carrying it directly to the body's cells. HBO also drives carbon monoxide from the hemoglobin, shortening carbon monoxide's half-life and the patient's time to recovery. HBO therapy also appears to aid with tissue ischemia. However, despite its widespread use, there is no scientific evidence that HBO benefits the patient with carbon monoxide poisoning.

Cyanide should be suspected in any environment where carbon monoxide is present. Suspect cyanide toxicity in patients with severe symptoms such as dyspnea, chest pain, altered mental status, seizures, and unconsciousness. To be effective, antidotal treatment of serious cyanide poisoning must be started early. Vapor exposures are likely to result in severe respiratory distress or apnea in addition to unconsciousness. Rapid airway intervention with endotracheal intubation and ventilatory support with a bag-valve mask are initial priorities. However, a rapid shift to antidotal therapy is essential to save the patient.[5]

There are two cyanide antidote regimens available: the older cyanide kit (amyl nitrite, sodium nitrite, and sodium thiosulfate) and the newer antidote Cyanokit® (hydroxocobalamin).

Hydroxocobalamin, marketed as Cyanokit®, is available in the United States and is much safer than the older nitrite-based cyanide kit. Hydroxocobalamin is a precursor to vitamin B_{12} (cyanocobalamin). When hydroxocobalamin is administered intravenously it binds cyanide by freeing it from the cytochrome$_{a3}$ enzyme (an enzyme necessary for oxygen processing by cells), allowing the resumption of cellular metabolism and energy processing via the electron transport chain. Cyanocobalamin is nontoxic and is excreted in the urine.

Administration of the older cyanide antidote, the cyanide kit, is a two-stage process, first using a nitrite compound, followed by a sulfur-containing compound. The nitrite acts by converting hemoglobin (the primary oxygen-carrying protein in blood) to methemoglobin. Methemoglobin then binds to cyanide, removing it from the cytochrome$_{a3}$. The sulfur-containing antidote then removes the cyanide by forming a nontoxic compound (thiocyanate), which is excreted in the urine. The administration of the cyanide antidote should be reserved for patients with a history of acute cyanide inhalation and frank signs and symptoms of serious exposure. Nitrite administration is not without risk because methemoglobin cannot carry oxygen and acts much like carbon monoxide.

If an IV is already established, administer 300 mg sodium nitrite over 2 to 4 minutes for adults. Otherwise, crush one amyl nitrite ampule and place it under an oxygen mask with high-concentration oxygen running or in the bag or oxygen reservoir of a bag-valve mask. Do not let the ampule fall into the patient's mouth or down the endotracheal tube. Always follow inhaled amyl nitrite with intravenous sodium nitrite, and do not use amyl nitrite if the patient has already received sodium nitrite. Use care in the administration of sodium nitrite or amyl nitrite, as they may induce hypotension. They also bind to the hemoglobin, reducing its ability to carry oxygen.

Following administration of IV sodium nitrite, administer 12.5 g of sodium thiosulfate for the adult. In addition to antidotal therapy, keep the patient supine and administer high-concentration oxygen.

Assessment and Management of Electrical, Chemical, and Radiation Injuries

Electrical Injuries

Be certain that the power has been shut off before you approach the scene of a suspected electrical injury. Until it is, do not allow anyone to approach the patient or the proximity of the electrical source. Remember that an energized power line need not spark or whip around to be deadly. A power line simply lying on the ground can still present a significant danger. Establish a safety zone if there is any question about the status of lines that are down. Keep vehicles and personnel at a distance from downed lines or the source pole that is greater than the distance between power poles. Also be aware that downed power lines may energize metal structures such as buildings, vehicles, or fences.

Once the scene is secure, assess the patient and prepare him for transport. Search for both an entrance and an exit wound. Look specifically for possible contact points with both the ground and the electrical source. In some circumstances, multiple entrance and exit wounds are present. Remember that electrical current passes through the body and therefore may result in significant internal burns, especially to blood vessels and nerves, even though the assessment reveals only minimal superficial findings. Rapidly progressive cardiovascular collapse can follow contact with an electrical source. Also, examine the patient for any fractures resulting from forceful muscle contractions caused by the current's passage and check distal sensation for signs of nervous system injury. Suspect spinal injury caused by muscle spasm in any significant electrical contact and provide appropriate spinal precautions.

As with thermal burns, look for smoldering shoes, belts, or other clothing items. Such items may continue the burning process well after the current is shut off. Also remove rings, watches, and any other constrictive items from the fingers, limbs, and neck.

Perform ECG monitoring for possible cardiac disturbances in victims of electrical burns. Electrical current may induce arrhythmias, including bradycardias, tachycardias, ventricular fibrillation, and asystole. Ensure that emergency department personnel examine any patient who has sustained a significant electrical shock. Damage from the current may be internal and not apparent to you or your patient during assessment. Consider any significant electrical burn or exposure patient as a high priority for immediate transport.

Lightning strikes to humans occur more than 300 times each year in the United States and result in more than 100 deaths. Strikes to people riding tractors, on open water, on golf courses, and under trees are most common, and men are the victims of 75 percent of all strikes. A lightning strike is a high-voltage (up to 100,000 volts), high-current (10,000 amperes), and high-temperature (50,000°F) event that lasts only a fraction of a second. A direct strike will impart this energy to the patient (Figure 5-15). However, the lightning will often strike a nearby object with some current traveling sideways (sideflash), or current may radiate outward in alternate pathways from the strike point, thus diminishing the voltage (step voltage).

By the time anyone reaches a victim of a lightning strike, the electricity has long since dissipated. (There will be a continued risk of further strikes, however, as long as the storm remains nearby.) There is no danger of electrical shock from touching someone who has been struck by lightning. The person's clothing, however, may continue to smolder, so remove it as necessary. Among other serious effects, lightning can produce a sudden cessation of breathing. Despite being apneic and perhaps pulseless, these patients frequently survive with prompt prehospital intervention.

Treat visible burns ("entrance" and "exit" wounds) just as any thermal burn, with cooling, if necessary, followed by the application of a dry, clean sheet or dressings. Do not focus too much on the visible burns, but instead recognize that the electricity has passed through the body, possibly causing widespread internal effects.

Treat cardiac or respiratory arrest in electrical burn patients with aggressive circulatory, ventilatory, and airway management (CAB). Patients in cardiac arrest because of contact with electrical current have a high survival rate if prehospital intervention is prompt. Check immediately for ventricular fibrillation and defibrillate if necessary. Secure the airway with an endotracheal tube and begin

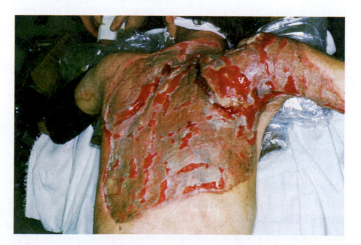

FIGURE 5-15 A lightning strike injury.

(© Wythenshawe Hospital/Wellcome Images)

ventilations and chest compressions. The usual resuscitative procedures for cardiac arrest apply equally when the cause of the arrest is electrical injury and might include the use of vasopressors and antiarrhythmics.

For serious electrical burn injuries, initiate at least two large-bore IVs and administer 1,000 mL of fluid per hour in 20 mL/kg boluses. Consider sodium bicarbonate and mannitol, usually at the discretion of medical direction, to prevent the complications of rhabdomyolysis (the destruction of muscle tissue and the release of toxic elements of that process) and hyperkalemia. The usual starting dose is 1 mEq/kg for sodium bicarbonate and 10 g for mannitol.

Chemical Burns

During the scene size-up, identify the nature of the chemical spill/contamination and, if necessary and possible, approach from uphill and upwind. Identify the chemical's location and ensure that it poses no continuing hazard to the patient, rescuers, and/or the public. Be wary of toxic fumes and cross-contamination from the patient and the surrounding environment. If necessary, have hazardous material team members evacuate and decontaminate the victim before you begin assessment and care. Seek out personnel on the scene who are familiar with the agent and consult with them regarding dangers posed by the agent and any specific medical care and patient handling procedures required with it.

During assessment and care, always wear medical examination (preferably nitrile) gloves and never presume that they protect you from the agent. Take appropriate protective action against airborne dust, toxic fumes, and splash exposure for both yourself and the patient (goggles and mask, as needed). Wear a disposable gown if there is danger of the agent contacting your clothing. Make certain the agent is isolated and no longer a danger to the patient or others. Have any of the patient's clothing that you suspect may be contaminated removed and isolate it from accidental contact. Save the clothing and ensure that it is disposed of properly. Identify the type of agent, its exact chemical name, the length of the patient's contact time with it, and the precise patient body areas affected by it.

As you begin the primary assessment, ensure that the patient is alert and fully oriented and that airway and breathing are unaffected by the contact. If there is any airway restriction or respiratory involvement, consider early intubation. As airway tissue swells, the obstruction worsens and intubation becomes more difficult. Monitor the patient's heart rate and consider ECG monitoring, because many chemicals (for example, organophosphates) may affect the heart. If the patient is stable, begin the rapid trauma assessment.

Examine any chemical burn carefully to establish the depth, extent, and nature of the injury. If you suspect phenol, dry lime, sodium, or riot agents, then treat as indicated below.

- *Phenol.* A gelatinous caustic called phenol is used as a powerful industrial cleaner. Phenol is very difficult to remove because it is sticky and relatively insoluble in water. Alcohol, which dissolves it, is frequently available in places where phenol is regularly used. Alcohol will help to dissolve and help remove the phenol; follow removal with irrigation using large volumes of cool water. In the absence of alcohol for phenol removal, use copious volumes of water to remove the agent.[6]

- *Dry lime.* Dry lime (calcium oxide) is a strong corrosive that reacts with water. It produces heat and subsequent chemical and thermal injuries. Brush dry lime off the patient gently, but as completely as possible. Then rinse the contaminated area with large volumes of cool to cold water. While the water reacts with any remaining lime, it will cool the contact area and remove any chemical residue. Rinsing with water helps to ensure that the lime reacts with that water rather than with water contained within the patient's soft tissues.

- *Sodium.* Sodium is an unstable metal that reacts destructively with many substances, including human tissue. It reacts vigorously with water, creating extreme heat, explosive hydrogen gas, and possible ignition. Sodium is normally stored submerged in oil because the metal reacts with moisture in the air. If a patient is contaminated with sodium, decontaminate him quickly by gentle brushing and then cover the wound with the oil used to store the substance.

- *Riot control agents.* These agents, which include CS (tear gas), CN (Mace), and oleoresin capsicum (OC, pepper spray), deserve special mention because people are the targets of their intended use and because that use is frequent. These agents cause intense eye, mucous membrane, and respiratory tract irritation. In general, they do not cause permanent damage when properly deployed. Patients who have contacted them typically present with eye pain, tearing, and temporary "blindness." Coughing, gagging, and vomiting are also common. Treatment is supportive and most patients recover spontaneously within 10 to 20 minutes of fresh air exposure. If necessary, irrigate the patient's eyes with normal saline if any riot agent contamination remains in the eye.

If it has not been done earlier, decontaminate the patient who has come in contact with any other chemical capable of causing tissue damage. Stop the damage by irrigating the site with large volumes of cool water. Water rinses away the offending material and dilutes any water-soluble agents. The water also reduces the heat and rate of a chemical reaction and, ultimately, the chemical's effects on the patient's skin. If contamination is widespread, douse the patient with large volumes of water. Use a garden hose or low-pressure water from a fire truck. Ensure that the water is neither warm nor too cold.

When the patient has been thoroughly rinsed for a few minutes, remove any remaining clothing. Take care that the process does not contaminate rescuers. If the agent is dangerous, save all clothing and contain the rinse water for proper disposal at a later time. Next, gently wash the burn with a mild soap (such as ordinary dish detergent) and a gentle brush or sponge. Be careful not to cause further soft tissue damage. After washing, gently irrigate the wound with a constant flow of water. Even though the pain and the burning process may appear to subside, it is important to continue irrigation until the patient arrives at the emergency department. If practical, transport the corrosive's container label or a sample of the agent (safely contained and marked) along with the patient. On arrival at the hospital, be sure to describe to emergency department personnel and enter in your prehospital care report any first aid measures given prior to your arrival.

Do not use any neutralizing agent without first gaining approval of medical direction. Neutralizing agents often react violently with the agents they neutralize and may ultimately increase the reaction heat and induce thermal burns. In some cases, the neutralizing agent is more damaging to the skin than the original contaminant.

With chemical burns, pay particular attention to the patient's eyes. Eyes are very sensitive to chemicals and can easily be damaged, even by weak agents. Prompt treatment of chemical eye injury is critical and can reduce damage and preserve eyesight. Ask the patient about chemical contact with the eyes, eye pain, vision changes, and contact lens use. Examine the eyes for eyelid spasm (**blepharospasm**), conjunctival erythema, discoloration, tearing, and other evidence of burns or irritation.

Irrigate chemical splashes that involve the eye with large volumes of water. Alkali burns are especially damaging; with these burns, you should flush the eye for at least 15 minutes. Irrigate acid burns for at least 5 minutes. Flush splashes of an unknown agent for up to 20 minutes. Do not, however, delay transport while irrigating.

A useful technique for eye irrigation is to hang a bag of normal saline (lactated Ringer's is an acceptable substitute) and use the flow regulator to control the fluid flow into the nasal corner of the eye. Turn the patient's head to the side to facilitate drainage and avoid cross-contaminating the other eye with waste fluid. Be alert for contact lenses in cases in which chemicals are splashed into the eyes. Chemicals may become trapped under the lenses, preventing adequate irrigation. Gently remove the lenses (see the chapter, "Head, Neck, and Spinal Trauma") before continuing irrigation.

Radiation Burns

An incident involving potential radiation exposure or burns must raise concern during both dispatch and response phases of an emergency call. Because radiation can be neither seen nor felt, it can endanger EMS personnel unless the hazard is anticipated and proper precautions taken. If radiation exposure is suspected, approach the scene very carefully. If the incident occurs at a power generation plant or in an industrial or a medical facility, seek out personnel knowledgeable about the radioactive substance being used. Such persons are always on staff and frequently on site at these facilities. Stay a good distance from the scene and ensure that bystanders, rescuers, and patients remain remote from the exposure source. Remember that distance and the nature of shielding materials, like concrete or earth, between you and the radiation source reduce potential exposure. If the exposure may be from dust or fire, approach from and remain upwind of the radiation source.

In radiation exposure incidents, ensure that personnel trained in radiation hazards isolate the source, contain it, and test the scene for safety. If the scene is not deemed safe, move the patient to a site remote from the radioactivity source, where you can give care without danger either to yourself or the patient. Plan the removal carefully. Use as much shielding as possible and keep exposure times to a minimum. Remember, the radiation dose received is related to three primary factors: duration, distance, and shielding.

If patient removal is required, consider using the oldest rescuers for the evacuation team. This approach is prudent because many of the radiation exposure effects become evident many years after exposure. If you use older rescuers, they are more likely to be past their reproductive years and have fewer years of life left if and when a problem does surface. This concern is especially important with pregnant women and young adults of both sexes. Remember that radiation damages the reproductive system very easily.

If there is a risk that patients are contaminated, ensure that they are properly decontaminated before assessment and care begins. If available for this task, use persons knowledgeable in decontamination and monitoring techniques who have the appropriate protective gear. If this is not possible, don goggles, a mask, gloves, and a disposable gown. Direct the evacuation team to place the patients in a decontamination area remote from your vehicle and other personnel and where any contamination can be contained. Have patients disrobe or carefully disrobe them, rinse them with large volumes of water, then wash them with a soft brush and rinse again. Ordinary dish detergent is an effective cleansing agent. Gently scrub, or closely trim (but do not shave) and then gently scrub, any areas of body hair. As in incidents of chemical contamination, save all clothing

Table 5-4 Dose-Effect Relationships to Ionizing Radiation

Whole Body Exposure Dose (RAD)	Effect
5–25	Asymptomatic. Blood studies are normal.
50–75	Asymptomatic. Minor depressions of white blood cells and platelets in a few patients.
75–125	May produce anorexia, nausea, vomiting, and fatigue in approximately 10–20 percent of patients within two days.
125–200	Possible nausea and vomiting. Diarrhea, anxiety, tachycardia. Fatal to less than 5 percent of patients.
200–600	Nausea and vomiting. Diarrhea in the first several hours. Weakness, fatigue. Fatal to approximately 50 percent of patients within 6 weeks without prompt medical attention.
600–1,000	"Burning sensation" within minutes. Nausea and vomiting within 10 minutes. Confusion, ataxia, and collapse within 1 hour. Watery diarrhea within 1 to 2 hours. Fatal to 100 percent within short time without prompt medical attention.
Localized Exposure Dose (RAD)	**Effect**
50	Asymptomatic.
500	Asymptomatic (usually). May have risk of altered function of exposed area.
2,500	Atrophy, vascular lesion, and altered pigmentation.
5,000	Chronic ulcer, risk of carcinogenesis.

and decontamination water and dispose of them safely. Perform decontamination before moving the patients to the ambulance.

Carefully document the circumstances of the radioactive exposure. If possible, identify the source and agent strength. Determine the patient's proximity to the source during the exposure, as well as the length of exposure.

Once decontaminated, treat a radiation exposure patient as any other patient. Because the human body by itself cannot be a source of ionizing radiation, a decontaminated patient poses no threat to you or your crew. Remember, however, that any contaminated material remaining on the patient or any contamination transferred to you does provide a source of radiation exposure and may contaminate you and your vehicle.

The actual assessment of a patient exposed to radiation is quite simple and usually reveals minimal signs or symptoms of injury. Only extreme exposures result in the classical presentation of nausea, vomiting, and malaise. Burns are extremely rare, although they may occur if the exposure is extremely intense. Even though a patient seems well, delayed consequences of high-dose radiation exposure can be devastating. If you note any early patient complaints, record the findings in the patient's own words and include the time the complaint was first made. This information is helpful in determining the patient's degree of radiation exposure (Table 5–4).

Treat the radiation injury patient's symptoms, make the patient as comfortable as possible, and offer psychological support. Cover any burns with sterile dressings and, if general symptoms are noticeable, provide oxygen and initiate an IV. Maintain the patient's body temperature and provide transport to the emergency department.

Reassessment

Monitor patients with inhalation, chemical, and electrical burns and radiation exposure for signs of increasing complications associated with their burn mechanisms. Also monitor blood pressure, pulse, and respirations and trend any changes. Perform these evaluations every 15 minutes in stable patients and every 5 minutes in unstable patients.

Summary

Burn injuries may compromise the skin—the protective envelope that protects and contains the human body. Burn damage to the skin may interfere with its ability to contain water within the body and to prevent damaging agents from entering. For these reasons, assessment and care of these soft tissue injuries are important.

Assess the burn to determine its depth and the body surface area it involves. Be sensitive to any respiratory, joint, hand, foot, or circumferential regions affected by the burn. Give special consideration to pediatric and geriatric burn patients and to burn patients who are also ill or otherwise injured. Consider all these factors in determining the overall burn severity. If the patient's condition warrants, institute aggressive care. Anticipate airway compromise and fluid loss. Secure the airway very early in prehospital care. Initiate IV access and begin fluid administration.

Electrical, chemical, or radiation burns require special care and assessment. An electrical burn requires careful assessment to determine the area and depth of burn involvement and should be followed by wound site dressing and cardiac monitoring. Chemical burns need rapid and effective decontamination. Radiation burns call for extreme care in removing the patient from the radiation source and in providing decontamination and supportive care.

You Make the Call

A young Boy Scout on a camping trip ignites his coat and shirt sleeve while attempting to light a campfire. By the time his scoutmaster extinguishes the flames, the arm is seriously burned. Your assessment finds the scout with a relatively painless hand and forearm with some skin discoloration. The upper arm is very painful and reddened, with its distal portion just starting to blister.

1. What severity are the burns of the forearm and hand and of the upper arm?

2. What percentage of the body surface area is burned?

3. What level of acuity would you assign this patient?

See Suggested Responses at the back of this book.

Review Questions

1. In which phase of the healing process for burns is scar tissue is laid down and remodeled, and the patient begins to rehabilitate and return to normal function?

   a. Fluid shift phase

   b. Resolution phase

   c. Emergent phase

   d. Hypermetabolic phase

2. What type of chemical burn is characterized by ongoing cell membrane destruction through liquefaction necrosis, thus allowing the chemical to penetrate underlying tissue more easily and cause deeper burns?

   a. Acids

   b. Alkalis

   c. Electrical

   d. Coagulation

3. The type of radiation that can travel through 6 to 10 feet of air, penetrate a few layers of clothing, and cause both external and internal injuries is known as _____.

   a. gamma radiation.

   b. alpha radiation.

   c. beta radiation.

   d. neutron radiation.

4. If airway edema is a major concern when dealing with inhalation injuries, as evidenced by dyspnea and stridor, what intervention should you attempt to protect the airway and help prevent deterioration?

   a. Cardiac monitoring

   b. Endotracheal intubation

   c. Intravenous cannulation

   d. Rapid fluid replacement

5. To reduce the burn patient's exposure to infectious pathogens, you must carefully _____

   a. employ Standard Precautions.

   b. use a dry, clean sheet or dressings and clean equipment.

   c. avoid gross contamination of the burn.

   d. do all of the above.

6. For pediatric or geriatric patients and patients with burns who are suffering from other trauma or medical conditions, always _____

   a. increase burn severity by one level.

   b. initiate immediate intubation.

   c. reduce administered fluids by half to prevent pulmonary edema.

   d. administer analgesics at double the standard dose.

7. Your patient is experiencing airway compromise from an inhalation injury. You elect to perform rapid sequence intubation to protect the patient's airway. Which of the following paralytics should you use with caution, if at all, because it may worsen hyperkalemia?

   a. Morphine

   b. Vecuronium

   c. Succinylcholine

   d. Pancuronium

8. Which of the following burns would be classified as a moderate burn?

   a. full thickness burn >2 percent body surface area

   b. superficial burn <50 percent body surface area

   c. partial thickness burn >30 percent body surface area

   d. partial thickness burn <30 percent body surface area

9. Which is a suitable formula for calculating an initial fluid bolus for a burn patient when transport time is less than 1 hour?

   a. 0.25 mL × patient weight in kilograms × BSA involved

   b. 1.25 mL × patient weight in pounds × BSA involved

   c. 0.75 mL × patient weight in kilograms × BSA involved

   d. 0.15 mL × patient weight in pounds × BSA involved

10. In general, how should dry lime be removed from the skin?

    a. Flush with vinegar, then with water.

    b. Brush dry lime away and then flush with cool water.

    c. Apply liberal amounts of baking soda over the lime, followed by a sterile dressing.

    d. Cover the lime with a dressing, flush with water, and transport.

11. Your 45-year-old male patient was working on his roof, came into contact with power lines, and has experienced electrocution. The patient is alert and oriented, has an irregular pulse of 124 BPM, and respirations are 22 and regular. The patient's blood pressure is 136/76 mmHg. You note both entrance and exit wounds, which have been managed properly by first responders. After starting low-flow oxygen and an IV, you elect to administer an analgesic for pain management. Which of the following drug/dose combinations is correct for this patient?

    a. Fentanyl 25 mcg   c. Morphine 25 mcg

    b. Fentanyl 25 mg   d. Morphine 25 mg

12. What should you do for the burn patient after any life threats are properly managed?

    a. Transport cautiously and slowly.

    b. Remove restrictive jewelry.

    c. Administer high-concentration oxygen.

    d. Cool the burn with water.

See Answers to Review Questions at the end of this book.

References

1. McManus, W. F. and B. A. Pruitt, Jr. "Thermal Injuries," in D. V. Feliciano, E. E. Moore, and K. L. Mattox, eds. *Trauma*. 6th ed. New York: McGraw Hill, 2008.

2. Singer, A. J., et al. "The Association between Hypothermia, Prehospital Cooling, and Mortality in Burn Victims." *Acad Emerg Med* 17(4) (Apr 2010): 456–459.

3. Monafo, W. W. "Initial Management of Burns." *New Eng J Med* 335 (1996): 1581–1586.

4. Eastman, A. L., B. A. Arnoldo, J. L. Hunt, and G. F. Purdue. "Pre-Burn Center Management of the Burned Airway: Do We Know Enough?" *J Burn Care Res* 31 (2010): 701–705.

5. Bizovi, K. E. and J. D. Leikin. "Smoke Inhalation among Firefighters." *Occup Med* 10(4) (Oct–Dec 1995): 721–733.

6. Pullin, T. G., M. N. Pinkerton, R. V. Johnson, and D. J. Kilian. "Decontamination of the Skin of Swine following Phenol Exposure: A Comparison of the Relative Efficacy of Water versus Polyethylene Glycol/Industrial Methylated Spirits." *Toxicol Appl Pharmacol* 43(1) (1978): 199–206.

Further Reading

American Burn Association National Burn Repository Advisory Committee. *National Burn Repository 2009 Report*. Worldwide 2010.

Bickley, L. *Bates' Guide to Physical Examination and History Taking*. 11th ed. Philadelphia: Wolters-Kluwer, 2012.

Bledsoe, B. E. and D. Clayden. *Prehospital Emergency Pharmacology*. 7th ed. Upper Saddle River, NJ: Pearson/Prentice Hall, 2011.

Bledsoe, B. E., B. J. Colbert, and J. E. Ankney. *Essentials of A & P for Emergency Care*. Upper Saddle River, NJ: Pearson/Prentice Hall, 2010.

Martini, F. *Fundamentals of Anatomy and Physiology*. 10th ed. San Francisco: Pearson, 2014.

Marx, J., R. Hockberger, and R. Walls. *Emergency Medicine: Concepts and Clinical Practice*. 8th ed. St. Louis: Mosby, 2013.

Tintinelli, J. E., ed. *Emergency Medicine: A Comprehensive Study Guide*. 7th ed. New York: McGraw-Hill, 2012.

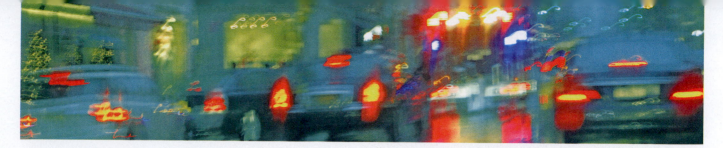

Chapter 6
Head, Neck, and Spinal Trauma

Bryan E. Bledsoe, DO, FACEP, FAAEM, EMT-P

Robert S. Porter, MA, EMT-P

STANDARD
Trauma (Head, Facial, Neck, and Spine Trauma)

COMPETENCY
Integrates assessment findings with principles of epidemiology and pathophysiology to formulate a field impression to implement a comprehensive treatment/disposition plan for an acutely injured patient.

 ## Learning Objectives

Terminal Performance Objective: After reading this chapter you should be able to integrate knowledge of anatomy, physiology, pathophysiology, and treatment principles to assess and provide prehospital management for patients with injuries of the head, face, neck, and spinal column, as well as the nervous system.

Enabling Objectives: To accomplish the terminal performance objective, you should be able to:

1. Define key terms introduced in this chapter.

2. Identify the epidemiology of injuries to the head, neck, and spinal column.

3. Describe the anatomy and physiology of the head and face, neck, and spinal column.

4. Describe the various mechanisms of injury that could cause trauma to the head, neck, and spinal cord.

5. Identify and describe the various types of brain injuries that can occur after trauma.

6. Discuss intracranial pressure, autoregulation, and the detrimental effects of increasing pressure on the brain in the adult and pediatric patient.

7. Identify the types and describe the pathophysiology of syndromes associated with spinal cord trauma.

8. Identify and discuss the types of injuries to the head, face, and neck.

9. Identify the steps and discuss the procedure for performing a comprehensive assessment of patients with head, face, neck, and spinal column injuries.

10. Given a variety of scenarios, develop treatment plans for patients with injuries to the head, face, neck, and spinal column.

KEY TERMS

Case Study

Paramedics Fred and Lisa are providing standby service at a local high school football game. Just before the end of the third quarter, they are called onto the field when a player is thrown to the ground and "can't get up."

On arrival at the player's side, they find Bill, a well-developed teenager who is oriented to person but not to time and place. He states that he was hit hard from the side and now has a burning sensation (commonly called a "stinger") in his arms and neck. On further questioning, the player complains of some localized pain just above the shoulders in his central lower neck. His medical history is unremarkable. He has no allergies and his tetanus vaccination is up to date.

The paramedics' physical exam reveals a patient clothed in protective football gear and helmet without external signs of physical injury. The patient's airway is clear, and the rate, strength, and quality of his breathing and pulse are within normal limits. Physical examination of the head is limited by the helmet, but palpation of the posterior neck reveals some localized midline tenderness at or slightly above the first thoracic vertebra. Respiratory excursion and diaphragm movement seem unaffected by the injury. The paresthesia appears to affect the entire chest, abdomen, and lower extremities, as well as the posterior surface of the upper extremities. The patient's upper extremity grip is strong, whereas the strength of foot dorsiflexion and plantar flexion appears diminished. The patient is able to maintain both bowel and bladder control.

Fred feels it will be very difficult to stabilize the player with the helmet and shoulder pads in place. He has the athletic trainer hold the helmet while he and Lisa release the air pressure in the bladder, remove the face shield, and begin its removal. Lisa stabilizes the player's head, while Fred gently and carefully negotiates the helmet around the patient's face. Once the helmet is removed, Fred assumes manual stabilization of the player's head, which is well above the surface of the playing field because the shoulder pads raise his shoulders more than an inch off the ground. Lisa proceeds to cut off the patient's shirt and the webbing that holds the pads in place and gently removes the pads. Then, a cervical collar is carefully applied. Fred, Lisa, and the athletic trainer use a scoop stretcher to secure the patient. After the torso is secured with straps, they are careful to maintain the head and neck in a neutral position.

The patient's blood pressure, pulse rate and strength, and respiratory rate and volume have all remained relatively normal during these procedures. Fred notes no differences in skin temperature or capillary refill in any extremity, which reduces the likelihood of neurogenic shock from spinal cord injury. The pulse oximeter reads 98 percent, and the ECG displays a normal sinus rhythm at 68 as the paramedics load the patient into the ambulance and begin transport to the regional trauma center.

Fred and Lisa learn from the local paper that the unfortunate player suffered a compression fracture of the seventh cervical vertebra and will miss the rest of the season. His neurologic signs and symptoms resolved. Although the injury may limit Bill's athletic career, it is not expected otherwise to affect his life.

Introduction to Head, Neck, and Spinal Trauma

Head, neck, and spinal injuries are common with major trauma.[1] Approximately 4 million people experience a significant head injury each year, with 1 in 10 requiring hospitalization. Although most of these hospitalizations are due to relatively minor injuries, severe head injury is the most frequent cause of trauma-related deaths. It is especially lethal in auto crashes and frequently produces significant long-term disability in patients who survive. Gunshot wounds to the head occur less frequently, but result in a mortality rate of about 75 to 80 percent. Sports injuries and falls account for a significant number of head, face, neck, and spinal injuries as well. Injuries to the face and neck can threaten critical airway structures, sensory organs, and the significant vasculature found in these regions. They are also suggestive of injury to the central nervous system.

The populations most at risk for serious head and spinal column injury are males between the years of 15 and 24, infants and young children, and the elderly. Educational programs promoting safe practices and the use of head protection, seat belts, and air bags have had major effects in reducing head injury morbidity and mortality.

The use of helmets for bicycling, rollerblading, and motorcycling and in contact sports such as football and hockey has also significantly reduced the incidence of serious head injury. In motorcycle crashes, for example, helmet use reduces serious head injury by more than 50 percent. Once a head injury occurs, however, time becomes a critical consideration. Intracranial hemorrhage and progressing edema can increase the intracranial pressure, hypoxia, and the internal and permanent damage done.[2]

Despite the dangers posed by these injuries, head, neck, and spinal injury severity is often difficult to recognize in the prehospital setting. As a result, subtle and unforeseen problems associated with injuries to these regions may cause a patient to quietly deteriorate while EMS personnel direct their attention toward more apparent and gruesome injuries that are not as critical. Even if a life-threatening injury is recognized, paramedics can provide important supportive field care while transporting the patient to the hospital and definitive care. To lessen the chances of death and disability, learn to recognize the signs and symptoms of head, face, neck, spinal column and central nervous system injury early in the assessment, maintain a clear airway and adequate respirations, maintain the patient's blood pressure, and provide rapid transport to a facility that can administer proper care.

Head, Face, Neck, and Spine Anatomy and Physiology

This chapter addresses injuries to four areas: the head, the face, neck, and spine. It also reviews the relevant anatomy and physiology of these four areas. A more detailed discussion of human anatomy and physiology is available in companion texts.

Anatomy and Physiology of the Head

In addition to the brain, the head is made up of three structures that cover and protect the brain: the scalp, the cranium, and the meninges. Each of these structures provides essential protection from environmental extremes and from trauma.

The Scalp

The scalp is a strong and flexible layer of skin, fascia (bands of connective tissue), and muscle tissue that is able to withstand and absorb a significant amount of kinetic energy. The scalp is also extremely vascular, to help maintain the brain at the appropriate temperature. The hair further insulates the brain from environmental temperatures and, to a lesser degree, from trauma.

The scalp is only loosely attached to the skull and is made up of the overlying skin and a number of thin muscle layers and connective tissue underneath. Directly beneath the skin and covering the most superior surface of the head is a fibrous connective tissue sheet called the **galea aponeurotica**. Connected anteriorly to it and covering the forehead is a flat sheet of muscle (the frontal muscle). Connected posteriorly and covering the posterior skull surface is the occipitalis muscle. Laterally, the auricularis muscles cover the areas above the ears and between the lateral brow ridge and occiput. A layer of loose connective tissue beneath these muscles and the galea and just above the periosteum is called the areolar tissue. It contains emissary veins that permit venous blood to flow from the dural sinuses into the venous scalp vessels. These emissary veins also exist in the upper portions of the nasal cavity. These veins become potential routes of infection in scalp wounds or nasal injuries. A helpful way to remember the layers of skin protecting the scalp is the mnemonic SCALP: S—skin; C—connective tissue; A—aponeurotica; L—layer of subaponeurotica (areolar) tissue; P—the skull's periosteum (the pericranium).

The Cranium

The bony structure supporting the head and face is the skull. It can be subdivided into two components: the vault for the brain, called the **cranium**, or *cranial vault*, and facial bones that form the skeletal base for the face (Figure 6-1). The cranium actually consists of several bones fused together at pseudojoints called **sutures**. These bony plates consist of two narrow plates of hard compact bone separated by a layer of spongy cancellous bone. The plates form a strong, light, rigid, and spherical container for the brain. The cranium is quite effective in protecting its contents from the direct effects of trauma. The cranial vault, however, provides very little space for internal swelling or hemorrhage. Any expanding lesion within the cranium will displace other contents and increase in **intracranial pressure (ICP)**. This can subsequently reduce cerebral perfusion and can severely damage brain tissue.

The Meninges

The soft tissues of the scalp and skin, as well as the skeletal components of the cranial vault and spinal column, protect the brain and the spinal cord. Beneath these structures are specialized connective tissues called the **meninges** (Figure 6-2). They are three layers of tissue that lie between the cranium and the brain and also between the spinal column and the spinal cord. The outermost meningeal layer is the **dura mater** (meaning, literally, "tough mother"). It is a strong and resilient connective tissue and actually consists of two layers. The outer dural portion is the periosteum of the cranial vault and spinal column and is attached directly and firmly to the bone. The inner dural portion is made up of tough, continuous connective tissue that extends into the cranial cavity, where it forms partial structural divisions (the falx cerebri and the tentorium cerebelli) for the brain. Above the dura mater are some of the larger arteries that provide blood flow to the brain's surface. Between the dural layers lie the dural sinuses—major venous drains for the brain.

The meningeal layer closest to the brain and spinal cord is the **pia mater** (meaning "tender mother"). It is a delicate tissue that covers all the convolutions of the brain and spinal cord. Although delicate compared to the dura mater, the pia mater is still more substantial than the brain and spinal cord tissue. The pia mater is a highly vascular tissue with large vessels that supply the superficial areas of the brain and spinal cord.

Separating the two layers of mater is a stratum of connective tissue called the **arachnoid membrane**. It covers the inner dura mater and suspends the brain in the cranial cavity with collagen and elastin fibers. The arachnoid membrane gets its name from its weblike appearance (arachnoid meaning "spiderlike"). Beneath the arachnoid membrane is the subarachnoid space, which is filled with cerebrospinal fluid. This region provides cushioning for the brain when the head is subjected to strong forces of acceleration or deceleration.

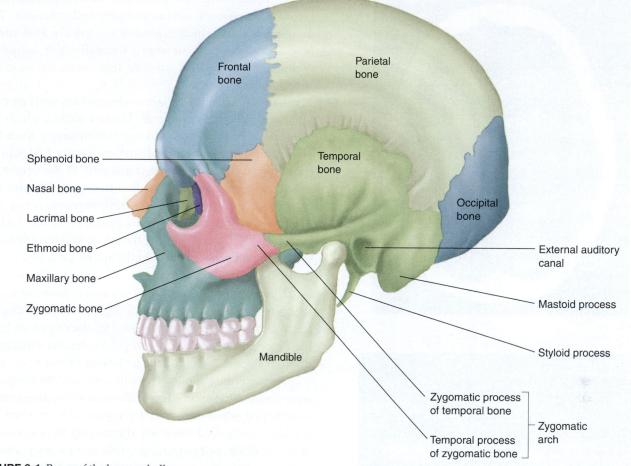

Frontal
bone

Parietal
bone

Sphenoid bone

Temporal
bone

Nasal bone

Lacrimal bone

Occipital
bone

Ethmoid bone

Maxillary bone

External auditory
canal

Zygomatic bone

Mastoid process

Styloid process

Mandible

Zygomatic process
of temporal bone

Zygomatic
arch

Temporal process
of zygomatic bone

FIGURE 6-1 Bones of the human skull.

Cerebrospinal Fluid

Cerebrospinal fluid (CSF) is a clear, colorless solution of water, proteins, and salts that surrounds the central nervous system and absorbs the shock of minor acceleration and deceleration. A structure within the ventricles of the brain, the choroid plexus, constantly generates cerebrospinal fluid in the largest two of four ventricles. The fluid

flows from the lateral ventricles to the third and fourth ventricle and then through the subarachnoid space surrounding both the brain and the spinal cord. Cerebrospinal fluid is returned to the venous circulation through arachnoid granulations and into the dural sinuses of the brain, as well as through the spinal arachnoid space to the arachnoid villi found at the end of the spinal cord (spinal cistern). Cerebrospinal fluid provides buoyancy for the brain and actually floats it in a near-weightless environment within the cranial vault. This fluid also is a medium through which nutrients and waste products, such as oxygen, proteins, glucose, salts, and carbon dioxide, are diffused into and out of the brain tissue. These functions of the CSF are especially important because the brain is insulated from many substances found in the blood by the blood–brain barrier (discussed later).

The Brain

The brain (Figure 6-3) occupies about 80 percent of the volume of the cranial vault. It is made up of three major structures essential to human function: the cerebrum, the cerebellum, and the brainstem.

The **cerebrum** is the largest nervous system element and occupies most of the cranial vault. It has an exterior

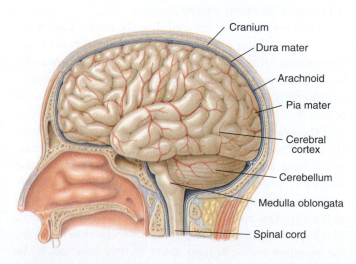

Cranium

Dura mater

Arachnoid

Pia mater

Cerebral
cortex

Cerebellum

Medulla oblongata

Spinal cord

FIGURE 6-2 The meninges and skull.

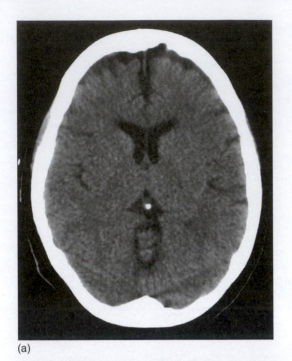

(a)

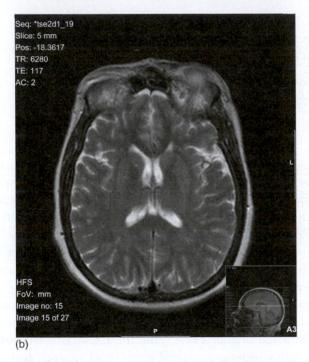

Seq: *tse2d1_19
Slice: 5 mm
Pos: -18.3617
TR: 6280
TE: 117
AC: 2

L

HFS
FoV: mm
Image no: 15
Image 15 of 27

P   A3

(b)

FIGURE 6-3 (a) Axial CT of the brain. (b) Axial MRI of the brain.

(© Dr. Bryan E. Bledsoe)

cortex consisting of gray matter (cell bodies), whereas the central cerebrum is predominantly white matter—mostly comprising communication pathways (axons). The cerebrum is the portion of the brain that performs higher functions. It is the center of consciousness, thought, personality, speech, and motor control, as well as visual, auditory, and tactile (touch) perception. The cerebrum is regionalized into lobes roughly lying beneath corresponding cranial bones (and given the same names). The frontal region is anterior and plays a role in personality. The parietal

region, which is superior and posterior, directs motor and sensory activities as well as memory and emotions. The occipital region, which is located posteriorly and inferiorly, is responsible for sight. Laterally, the temporal regions are the centers for long-term memory, hearing, speech, taste, and smell.

A structure called the falx cerebri divides the cerebrum into right and left hemispheres. The falx cerebri, which is a dural partition, extends into the cranial cavity from the interior and superior cranial surface (Figure 6-4). Corresponding to the falx cerebri is a fissure in the cerebrum called the central sulcus. This fissure physically splits the cerebrum into the left and right hemispheres, each of which controls (for the most part) the activities of the body's opposite side. The crossing of the nerve impulse from one side to the other takes place in the spinal cord, just below the medulla oblongata.

The tentorium cerebelli, a fibrous sheet similar to the falx cerebri, within the occipital region, is at a 90-degree angle to the falx cerebri and separates the cerebrum from the cerebellum. The brainstem perforates the tentorium through an opening called the tentorium incisura.

The oculomotor nerve (CN-III), which controls pupil size, travels along the edge of the tentorium. It is can be compressed when intracranial pressure rises or when the cerebrum is pushed inferiorly (herniated) from edema, a growing mass, or hemorrhage. This compression causes pupillary disturbances that manifest most commonly on the same side as the lesion. If the pressure is great enough, it may affect both sides and both pupils may dilate and become unreactive.

The left cerebral hemisphere is identified as the dominant hemisphere in most of the population with the exception of a few left-handed individuals. It is responsible for mathematical computations (occipital region) and writing (parietal region) and is the center for language interpretation (occipital region) and speech (frontal region). The right, nondominant cerebral hemisphere processes nonverbal imagery (occipital region).

The **cerebellum** is located directly under the tentorium. It lies posterior and inferior to the cerebrum. The cerebellum "fine tunes" motor control and allows the body to move smoothly from one position to another. Additionally, it is responsible for balance and maintenance of muscle tone.

The **brainstem** is an important central processing center and is the communication junction among the cerebrum, spinal cord, cranial nerves, and cerebellum. It includes the midbrain, pons, and medulla oblongata. The **midbrain** makes up the upper portion of the brainstem and consists of the hypothalamus, thalamus, and associated structures. The **hypothalamus** controls much of endocrine function, the vomiting reflex, hunger, thirst, kidney function, body temperature, and emotions. The **thalamus** is the switching

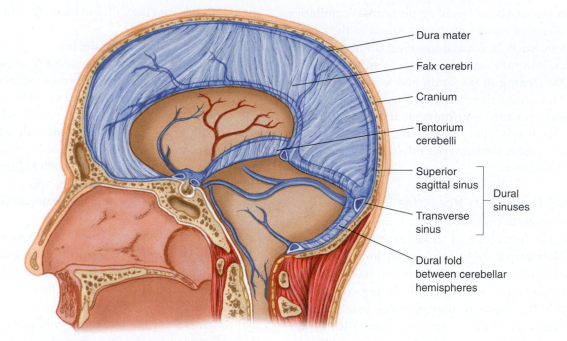

FIGURE 6-4 The partitions extending into the skull, the falx cerebri, and tentorium cerebellum.

center between the pons and the cerebrum and is a critical element in the **ascending reticular activating system**, the system that establishes and maintains consciousness. This region also provides major tracts, or pathways, for optic and olfactory nerves.

The **pons** acts as a communication interchange among various central nervous system components—the cerebellum, the cerebrum, the midbrain, and the spinal cord. It is a bulb-shaped structure directly above the medulla oblongata and appears to be responsible for the sleep component of the reticular activating system.

The last nervous system structure still within the cranial vault is the **medulla oblongata**. It is recognizable as a bulge in the very top of the spinal cord. The medulla contains three important centers—the respiratory center, the cardiac center, and the vasomotor center. The cardiac center regulates the rate and strength of cardiac contractions. The vasomotor center controls the distribution of blood and maintains blood pressure. The respiratory center controls respiratory depth, rate, and rhythm.

To maintain its advanced functioning, the brain has a high metabolic rate. Although the brain accounts for only 2 percent of the body's total weight, it receives about 15 percent of cardiac output and consumes about 20 percent of the body's oxygen supplies. It requires this perfusion whether at rest or engaged in active thought. Furthermore, the blood supply must be constant because the brain has no stored energy sources. It needs constant availability of glucose, thiamine (to help metabolize glucose), and oxygen and relies almost solely on aerobic metabolism. If the blood supply stops, unconsciousness

follows within 10 seconds and brain death will ensue within 4 to 6 minutes.

Central Nervous System (CNS) Circulation

Four major arterial vessels provide blood flow to the brain. The first two are the internal carotid arteries. These vessels divide from the common carotid at the carotid sinus and then enter the cranium through its base. Two posterior vessels, the vertebral arteries, ascend along and through the vertebral column. They then enter through the skull's base where they join and form a single basilar artery that, in turn, joins the circle of Willis.

The internal carotid and basilar arteries interconnect through the circle of Willis at the base of the brain. This structure is an arterial circle that ensures adequate circulation to the brain, even if one of the large feeder vessels is obstructed. Various arteries branch out from the circle of Willis and supply the brain's substance.

Venous drainage occurs initially through bridging veins that drain the cerebral surface. They "bridge" with the dural sinuses (large, thin-walled veins) and ultimately drain into the internal jugular veins and then into the superior vena cava.

Blood–Brain Barrier

The term **blood–brain barrier** refers to the fact that central nervous system capillary walls are thicker, more complete, and not as permeable as those found elsewhere in the body. They do not permit the interstitial flow of proteins and other materials as freely as do normal capillaries. This ensures that many substances found in the circulatory system, such as some hormones, do not affect the cells of the central nervous system. Lymphatic circulation is also lacking in the brain and is replaced by the cerebrospinal fluid flow system. This results in a very special and protected environment for central nervous system cells. If frank blood seeps into the CNS tissue, it acts as an irritant, initiating an inflammatory response, resulting in edema.

Cerebral Perfusion Pressure

Adequate cerebral perfusion is exceptionally critical for proper brain function and depends on many factors. There is normally a slight pressure within the cranium. This intracranial pressure (ICP) is normally less than 10 mmHg and does not significantly impede cerebral blood flow. The pressure that provides cerebral blood flow is termed **cerebral perfusion pressure (CPP)**. It is the **mean arterial pressure (MAP)** minus the ICP. If the mean arterial blood pressure falls below 50 mmHg, normal ICP will reduce CPP to critical levels. Under normal circumstances, when CPP drops, the brain stimulates the circulatory system to increase cardiac output and peripheral vascular resistance, and thereby, increases the blood pressure in order to maintain CPP. This increasing blood pressure to maintain CPP and cerebral perfusion is termed **autoregulation**.

THE MONROE-KELLIE DOCTRINE Intracranial pressure is the pressure within the cranial vault that is exerted on brain tissue, cerebrospinal fluid, and the circulating blood volume within the cranial vault. The ICP is dynamic—constantly changing to variations in body physiology. The relationship among these components is explained by the Monroe-Kellie doctrine, which states:

Intracranial Volume (fixed) = Brain Volume (to include any mass or lesion volume) + CSF Volume + Blood Volume

The intracranial volume is fixed because it is defined by the rigid cranial vault. At any given time, the cranium's fixed volume is filled with brain tissue (80 percent), arterial and venous blood circulating through the intracranial vessels and dural sinuses (10 percent), and CSF in the ventricles and subarachnoid spaces (10 percent). Any increase in one of these, or a developing lesion, is met by a corresponding decrease in another, or the ICP will begin to rise. Fluids, such as CSF and blood (especially venous blood), can be pushed out of the cranium with very slight rises in intracranial pressure. However, this compensatory mechanism is very limited. If cerebral edema continues or there is an extrinsic factor (hemorrhage, hematoma, brain tumor, or other lesion), the expanding mass displaces blood and CSF to their limits and then causes ICP to rise, compressing the brain, and reducing CPP and blood flow to and through the brain.

Should a traumatic brain injury cause the ICP to increase significantly, the increased ICP impedes normal blood flow and limits central nervous system tissue perfusion. As rising ICP reduces cerebral blood flow, autoregulation subsequently raises the systemic blood pressure to ensure that there is enough CPP to provide adequate cerebral perfusion. However, an increased blood pressure causes intracranial pressure to rise still higher and CPP to again fall. As this cycle of increasing intracranial pressure and increasing blood pressure continues, brain injury and death are close at hand.

In general, the brain's structural components are fixed in position. However, if an expanding mass within the cranium—such as cerebral edema or hemorrhage—exerts pressure to surrounding structures, they may become displaced. In some cases, the increasing pressure pushes cranial contents from the lesion site through the tentorium incisura and toward the foramen magnum, as it is the largest opening in the cranium. Movement of brain tissue through such an opening is called *herniation* and leads to progressive and predictable signs and symptoms. However, in most cases, the expanding lesion merely pushes brain tissue away from itself and toward the opposite side of the cranium. Though potentially just as detrimental as herniation, this more common scenario produces less-characteristic signs and symptoms.

Cranial Nerves

The cranial nerves are nerve roots originating within the cranium and along the brainstem. They comprise 12 distinct pathways that account for some of the more important senses, innervate the facial area, and control significant body functions (see Table 6-1 and Figure 6-5).

Ascending Reticular Activating System

The ascending reticular activating system is a tract of neurons within the upper brainstem, pons, and midbrain that is responsible for the sleep–wake cycle. It is a complex control system that monitors the amount of stimulation the body is receiving. It also plays a role in regulating important bodily functions such as respiration, heart rate, and peripheral vascular resistance. Injury to the midbrain may result in unconsciousness or coma, whereas injury to the pons may result in a protracted waking state.

Anatomy and Physiology of the Face

The face is a part of the head. However, there are several specialized concerns related to facial trauma. These include airway complications, injuries to the sensory organs, and similar issues.

Table 6-1 Cranial Nerves

Nerve	Nerve Name	Nerve Function
CN-I	Olfactory	Responsible for the sense of smell and actually branches from the cerebrum.
CN-II	Optic	Responsible for image transmission from the retina to the brain.
CN-III	Oculomotor	Controls four of the six oculomotor muscles and is responsible for most eyeball motion, iris constriction, and the movement of the upper eyelid. As a result of its pathway within the skull, the third cranial nerve may be compressed, causing pupillary dilation and limiting eye movement.
CN-IV	Trochlear	In conjunction with the oculomotor and abducens nerves, this nerve results in conjugate gaze (the eyes looking in the same direction and moving together).
CN-V	Trigeminal	Innervates and receives sensation from the facial region and the gums, teeth, and palate, and controls the muscles of chewing.
CN-VI	Abducens	Responsible for moving the eyeball downward.
CN-VII	Facial	Controls the muscles responsible for facial expression and receives sensation from the anterior tongue.
CN-VIII	Acoustic	Innervates the cochlea and vestibule of the ear and is responsible for hearing as well as positional sense, motion sensation, and balance.
CN-IX	Glossopharyngeal	Innervates the posterior tongue and pharynx and is important in swallowing; also monitors the baro- and chemoreceptors within the major blood vessels.
CN-X	Vagus	Major nerve of the parasympathetic nervous system that monitors and controls the heart, respiration, and much of the abdominal viscera.
CN-XI	Spinal Accessory	Controls the major muscles of the neck, as well as some of the muscles associated with swallowing, and the vocal cords.
CN-XII	Hypoglossal	Exercises voluntary muscular control over the tongue.

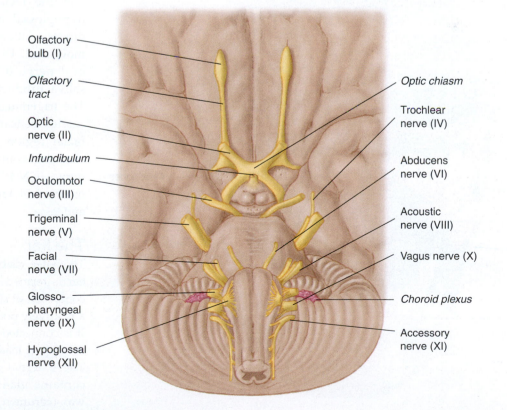

FIGURE 6-5 The cranial nerves as they exit the base of the brain.

The Face, Nasal Cavity, and Oral Cavity

Facial bones make up the anterior and inferior structures of the head and include the **zygoma**, **maxilla**, **mandible**, and nasal bones (Figure 6-6).

The facial region, like most other areas of the body, is covered with skin that serves to protect the tissue underneath from trauma and against adverse environmental effects. In the facial region, the skin is very flexible and relatively thin. It also has a very good vascular supply and hemorrhages readily when injured. Underneath the skin is a minimal layer of subcutaneous tissue. Beneath that are numerous small muscles that control facial expression and the movements of the mouth, eyes, and eyelids.

The external carotid artery and its branches—the facial, temporal, and maxillary arteries—provide circulation to the facial region. The facial artery crosses the mandible and travels up and along the nasal bone. The maxillary artery runs under the mandible and zygoma and provides circulation to the cheek area. The temporal artery runs anterior to the ear just posterior to the zygoma. Each major artery has an associated vein.

The most important of the cranial nerves traversing this area are the trigeminal (CN-V) and the facial (CN-VII) nerves. The trigeminal nerve provides sensation for the face and some motor control over eye movement, as well as enabling the chewing process. The facial nerve provides motor control to facial muscles and contributes to the sensation of taste.

The nasal cavity is formed by the juncture of the ethmoid, nasal, and maxillary bones. It is a channel running posteriorly with a bony septum dividing it into left and right chambers and plates protruding medially from the lateral sides. These plates, called turbinates, form the support for the vascular mucous membranes in the nasal cavity that serve to warm, humidify, and collect particulate matter from the incoming air. The lower nasal cavity is bordered by the bony hard palate and, posteriorly, by the more flexible cartilaginous soft palate. The soft palate moves upward to close the posterior nasal cavity opening during swallowing. The nasal bone lies anterior and inferior to the eyes and provides a base for the nasal cartilage. The nasal cartilage defines the shape of the nose and divides the nostrils and their openings, called the **nares**.

The oral cavity is formed by the concave shape of the maxillary bone, the palate, and the upper teeth meeting the lower teeth of the mandible. The floor of the oral cavity consists of muscles and connective tissue that span the mandible and support the tongue. The tongue connects with the hyoid bone, a free-floating U-shaped bone located inferiorly and posteriorly to the mandible.

Prominent cranial nerves serving the oral area include the hypoglossal, the glossopharyngeal, the trigeminal, and the facial nerves. The hypoglossal nerve (CN-XII) directs swallowing and tongue movement. The glossopharyngeal nerve (CN-IX) controls saliva production and taste. The trigeminal nerve (CN-V) carries sensations from the facial region and assists in chewing control. The facial nerve (CN-VII) controls the muscles of facial expression and taste.

The Ear

The outer, visible portion of the ear is termed the **pinna**. It is composed of cartilage and has a relatively poor blood supply. It is connected to the auditory canal that leads the eardrum. The external auditory canal contains glands that secrete wax (cerumen) for protection. The ear's important structures

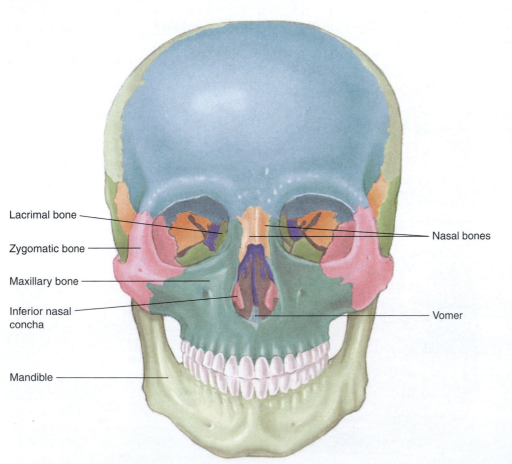

Lacrimal bone

Zygomatic bone

Maxillary bone

Inferior nasal concha

Mandible

Nasal bones

Vomer

FIGURE 6-6 The facial bones.

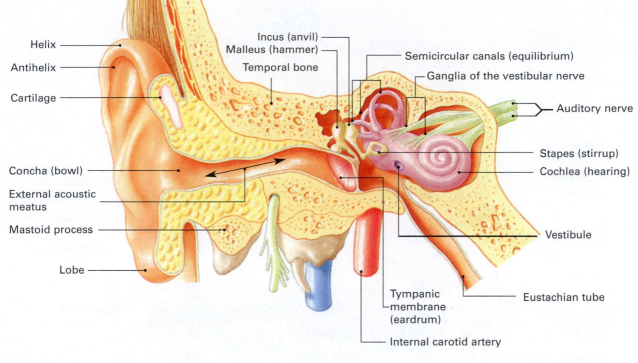

FIGURE 6-7 The anatomy of the ear.

are interior and exceptionally well protected from virtually all types of trauma (Figure 6-7). Only injuries resulting from great pressure differentials (e.g., blast and diving injuries), objects inserted directly into the auditory canal, or basilar skull fractures are likely to damage the ear.

The ear provides the body with two very important functions: hearing and positional sense. The middle and inner ear contain the structures required for hearing. Hearing occurs when sound waves cause the tympanic membrane (eardrum) to vibrate. The eardrum transmits these vibrations through three very small bones (the ossicles) to the cochlea—the organ of hearing. These vibrations stimulate the auditory nerve that transmits impulses to the brain.

The **semicircular canals** are responsible for sensing position and motion. They are three hollow, fluid-filled rings set at different angles. When the head moves, fluid in these rings shifts. Small cells within the semicircular canals, with hairlike projections, sense the motion and position and signal the brain to help maintain balance. This positional sense is present even when the eyes are closed. If injury or illness disturbs this area, it transmits excess signals to the brain. Patients then experience a continuous moving sensation known as *vertigo*.

The Eye

The eyes provide much of the information used to interact with our environment. Although they are placed prominently on the face, the eyes are well protected from trauma by a series of facial bones. The frontal bones project above

the globe of the eye while the nasal bones and cartilage protect medially. The bone of the cheek, or zygoma, completes the physical protection of the eye both laterally and inferiorly. These bones collectively form the eye socket, or **orbit**. The soft tissue of the eyelid and eyelashes give additional protection to the very sensitive and critical ocular surface.

The eye is a spherical globe, filled with liquid (Figure 6-8). Its major compartment (the posterior chamber) contains a crystal-clear gelatinous fluid called **vitreous humor**. Lining the compartment's posterior is a light- and color-sensing tissue known as the **retina**. Images focused on the retina are transmitted to the brain via the optic nerve. The eye's lens separates the posterior and anterior chambers. The lens is responsible for focusing light and images on the retina by the action of small muscles that change its central thickness. A fluid called **aqueous humor**, which is similar to vitreous humor, fills the anterior chamber. The anterior chamber also contains the **iris**, the muscular and colored portion of the eye that regulates the amount of light reaching the retina. Light enters the eye through the dark opening in the center of the iris called the **pupil**.

By examining the eye, you can easily identify several of its components, such as the colored iris and the central black pupil. Bordering the iris is the **sclera**, the white and vascular area that forms the remaining, underlying surface of the exposed eye. The **cornea**, a very thin, clear, and delicate layer, covers both the pupil and iris. Contiguous with the cornea and extending out to the eyelid's interior

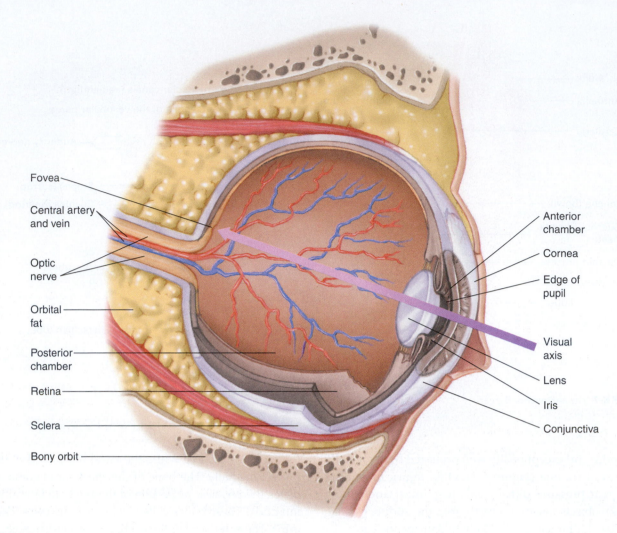

FIGURE 6-8 The anatomy of the eye.

surface is the **conjunctiva**, another delicate, smooth layer that slides over itself and the cornea when the eye closes or blinks.

The eye is bathed in **lacrimal fluid**, which is produced by almond-shaped lacrimal glands located along the brow ridge just lateral and superior to the eyeball. Lacrimal fluid flows through lacrimal ducts and then over the cornea. Because the cornea does not have blood vessels, the fluid provides crucial lubrication, oxygen, and nutrients. If injury or some other mechanism—for example, a contact lens left in an unconscious patient's eye—prevents this fluid from reaching the cornea, the surface of the eye (cornea) may be damaged. The lacrimal fluid is drained from the eye into the lacrimal sac, located along the medial orbit, and empties then into the nose.

The last major functional elements of the eye are the extraocular muscles that move them. These muscles are controlled by three of the cranial nerves. These small muscles are attached to the globe in the region of the conjunctival fold and are hidden within the orbit under the zygomatic arch. The oculomotor (CN-III), trochlear (CN-IV),

and abducens (CN-VI) nerves control these muscles, which, in turn, control the eye's motion. The oculomotor nerve controls pupillary dilation, conjugate movement (movement of the eyes together), and most of the eye's movements through their normal range of motion. The trochlear nerve moves the eye downward and inward, and the abducens nerve is responsible for eye abduction (outward gaze).

Anatomy and Physiology of the Neck

The neck contains numerous essential structures and is vulnerable to trauma. These essential structures are described in this section.

CONTENT REVIEW

➤ Anatomic Components of the Neck
- Larynx
- Trachea
- Esophagus
- Carotid arteries
- Jugular veins
- Cranial nerves
- Lymphatic and thoracic ducts
- Thyroid gland
- Brachial plexus
- Muscles, fascia, soft tissues

Vasculature of the Neck

The major blood vessels in the neck are the carotid arteries and jugular veins. The carotid arteries arise from the brachiocephalic artery on the right and the aorta on the left. They travel upward and medially along the trachea and split into the internal and external carotid arteries at about the level of the upper border of the larynx. The carotid bodies and carotid sinuses are located at this bifurcation. These are responsible for monitoring carbon dioxide and oxygen levels in the blood and the blood pressure, respectively. The jugular veins are paired on each side of the neck. The internal jugular vein runs in a sheath with the carotid artery and vagus nerve, whereas the external jugular vein runs superficially just lateral to the trachea. The jugular veins join the brachiocephalic veins just beneath the clavicles.

Airway Structures

The airway structures in the neck include the larynx superiorly. The larynx is a prominent hollow cylindrical structure made up of the thyroid and cricoid cartilages and resides atop the trachea. The thyroid opening is covered during swallowing by a cartilaginous and soft-tissue flap—the epiglottis. The vocal cords, two folds of connective tissue sitting atop the laryngeal opening, further protect the airway. These cords vibrate with air passage and form sounds. They may also close during swallowing to prevent foreign bodies from entering the lower airway. The cricoid cartilage is a circular ring between the thyroid cartilage and the trachea. The trachea consists of numerous C-shaped cartilages that serve to keep the trachea open. The posterior trachea shares a common border with the anterior esophageal surface. The trachea extends inferiorly to just below the sternum, where it divides into the left and right mainstem bronchi at the carina.

Other Neck Structures

Other structures within the neck include the esophagus, cranial nerves, lymphatic and thoracic ducts, thyroid and parathyroid glands, and brachial plexus. The esophagus is located behind the trachea, with the anterior border continuous with the posterior tracheal border. Some cranial nerves, including the glossopharyngeal (CN-IX) and the vagus (CN-X) nerves, traverse the neck. The vagus nerve is essential for many parasympathetic activities, including speech, swallowing, and cardiac, respiratory, and visceral function. The glossopharyngeal nerve innervates the carotid bodies and carotid sinuses, monitoring blood oxygen levels and blood pressure. The right lymphatic and left thoracic ducts deliver lymph to the venous system at the juncture of the jugular and subclavian veins. The thyroid gland sits over the trachea just below the cricoid cartilage and controls the cellular metabolic rate, as well as systemic

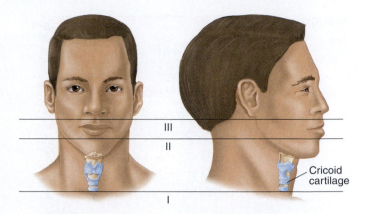

FIGURE 6-9 Zones of the neck.

calcium levels. The brachial plexus is a network of nerves in the lower neck and shoulder responsible for arm, forearm, and hand function. Finally, numerous muscles (including the sternocleidomastoid, platysma, and upper trapezius), fascia, and soft tissues are found in the neck. The thin platysma muscle covers most of the anterior and lateral neck. Penetration of this muscle suggests injury to the important structures beneath it. The neck muscles, like those of the extremities, are contained within fascial compartments. In the presence of soft tissue injury, rapid swelling may increase pressure within a compartment and restrict blood flow.

The neck can be divided into three zones. Zone I is below the cricoid ring; Zone II is above the cricoid ring and below the angle of the jaw; Zone III is above the angle of the jaw (Figure 6-9). Zone I injuries carry the highest mortality, as they involve the great vessels and the trachea. Zone II injuries are more common, because of the limited protection offered by anterior neck structures, and frequently involve the carotid arteries or larynx. Zone III injuries are also of concern because they may involve both cranial nerves and larger vascular structures and are often hidden from view.

Anatomy and Physiology of the Spine

The major components of the spine are the spinal column (and its components) and the spinal cord. These are detailed in the following section.

Vertebral Column

The **vertebral column**, also called the spinal column, consists of 33 bones and provides the main support for the axis of body. Each bone of the vertebral column is called a **vertebra**. By adulthood, nine of the lower vertebrae have fused, forming the **sacrum** and the **coccyx**, respectively (Figure 6-10). This leaves a total of 26 bones (24 separate vertebrae, the sacrum, and the coccyx). The vertebral column

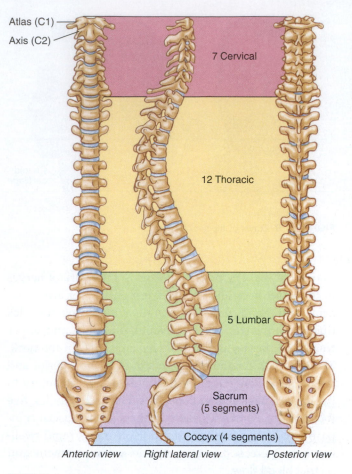

Atlas (C1)
Axis (C2)

7 Cervical

12 Thoracic

5 Lumbar

Sacrum
(5 segments)

Coccyx (4 segments)

Anterior view   Right lateral view   Posterior view

FIGURE 6-10 The anatomic dimensions of the vertebral column (anterior, left lateral, and posterior).

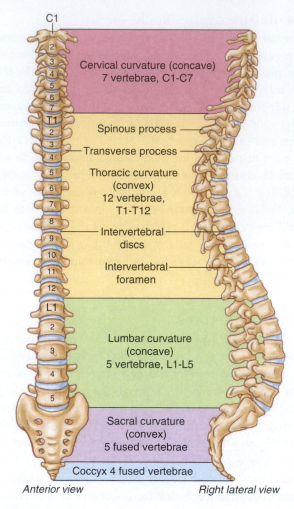

C1

Cervical curvature (concave)
7 vertebrae, C1-C7

Spinous process

Transverse process

Thoracic curvature
(convex)
12 vertebrae,
T1-T12

Intervertebral
discs

Intervertebral
foramen

Lumbar curvature
(concave)
5 vertebrae, L1-L5

Sacral curvature
(convex)
5 fused vertebrae

Coccyx 4 fused vertebrae

Anterior view   Right lateral view

FIGURE 6-11 The vertebral column. Note the four curvatures of the spine in the right lateral view.

extends from the base of the skull to the pelvis. The weight supported by each vertebra progressively increases as you move inferiorly down the spine. Thus, the **cervical vertebrae** are much smaller in width than the **thoracic vertebrae** and the **lumbar vertebrae**.

An **intervertebral disk** separates each pair of vertebrae, except the first and second cervical vertebrae and the fused vertebrae of the sacrum and coccyx. The intervertebral disks account for 25 percent of the total spinal column height and serve to absorb energy and cushion the vertebrae. The intervertebral disk contains an inner sphere called the nucleus pulposus, which is surrounded by an outer collar called the annulus fibrosus. The nucleus pulposus is gelatinous and absorbs compressive stress, whereas the purpose of the annulus fibrosus is primarily to contain the nucleus pulposus.

The vertebral column, when examined from an anterior or posterior perspective, is relatively straight. However, when examined laterally, curvatures are noted. These curvatures are normal and are referred to as the cervical concavity, the thoracic convexity, lumbar concavity, and the sacral convexity (Figure 6-11). The body's weight is eventually transmitted through the spine, then the pelvis, to the lower extremities.

Each vertebra is different, yet they share common features. Anteriorly, the vertebra consists of a vertebral body (or body). Posteriorly, each vertebra has a vertebral arch. Together, the vertebral body and the vertebral arch form the **spinal canal**, also called the **vertebral foramen**, which contains and protects the spinal cord. The vertebral arch is formed by two pedicles and two laminae. The pedicles protrude superiorly and contain the superior articular processes and facets that help to form the joint between one vertebra and the vertebra immediately above it. The laminae are lower and consist of the spinous process, the transverse processes, and the inferior articular facets. The inferior articular facets form the joint between the vertebra and the vertebra immediately below it (Figure 6-12).

The vertebral column is held in place by various ligaments. The major supporting ligaments are the anterior longitudinal ligament and the posterior longitudinal ligament (Figure 6-13). The anterior longitudinal ligament runs vertically along the anterior surfaces the vertebrae from the sacrum to the first cervical vertebra and onto the occipital bone of the skull. This ligament helps to prevent

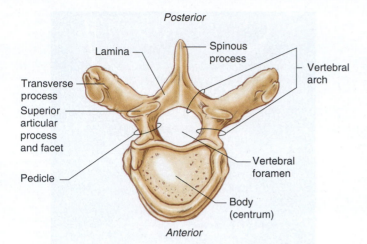

FIGURE 6-12 Structure of a typical vertebra (superior view).

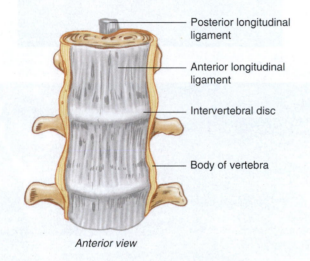

FIGURE 6-13 Anterior view of the spinal column showing anterior and posterior longitudinal ligaments.

hyperextension of the vertebral column. The posterior longitudinal ligament is narrower and weaker than the anterior longitudinal ligament. It runs vertically along the posterior surfaces of the vertebral bodies in the vertebral canal from the sacrum to the second cervical vertebra. The posterior longitudinal ligament helps to prevent hyperflexion of the vertebral column.

Other ligaments help to support the vertebral column. These are primarily located posteriorly and connect the vertebrae together. The strongest of these is the ligamentum flavum. The ligamentum flavum helps to maintain the normal curvatures of the spine and helps to straighten the spine after flexing. The interspinous ligament is a thin ligament that connects the spinous processes of two adjoining vertebrae together. The supraspinous ligament runs posteriorly along the spinous processes

from the seventh cervical vertebra to the sacrum. A similar ligament, the nuchal ligament, protects and supports the neck. It runs from the seventh cervical vertebra to the occipital bone of the skull (Figure 6-14). In addition to the ligaments, the back, chest and pelvic muscles also provide support for the vertebral column.

The physical shape of each vertebra, the intervertebral joint surfaces, and the ligaments holding the intervertebral joints together permit significant spinal column motion, especially in the cervical region. This type of joint structure also provides anatomic barriers to motion beyond the normal range of motion and protects the spinal cord from injury.

Vertebral Column Divisions

The vertebral column can be divided into five specific anatomic regions: the cervical spine, thoracic spine, lumbar spine, sacrum, and coccyx. The individual vertebrae of the column are identified by the first letter of their region and are numbered from superior to inferior. For example, the most inferior of the seven cervical vertebrae is identified as C-7.

CERVICAL SPINE   The cervical spine consists of seven cervical vertebrae located between the base of the skull and the shoulders. The cervical spine is the sole skeletal support for the head, which weighs about 16 to 22 pounds (7 to 10 kilograms). The cervical vertebrae are wider laterally than they are in an anteroposterior width. With the exception of C-7, the spinous process is short and bifid (split). The spinal canal is triangular in shape. Each transverse process contains a hole, called the transverse foramen, that contains the vertebral blood vessels (Figures 6-15 and 6-16).

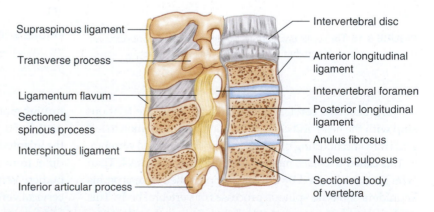

FIGURE 6-14 Ligaments and intervertebral discs of the spine. Lateral view of the spinal column (anterior to the right). The lower vertebrae have been cut sagittally to reveal the spinal canal and some of the ligaments.

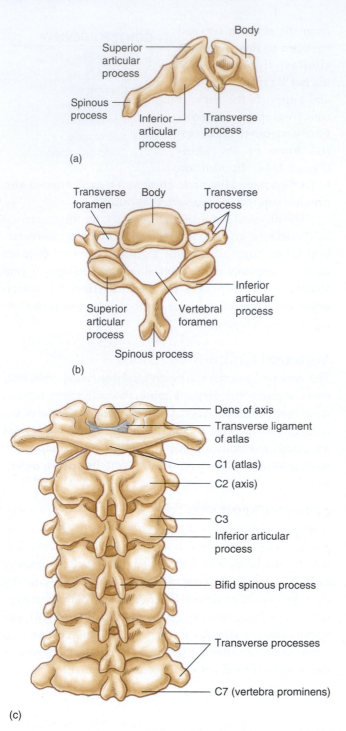

FIGURE 6-15 The cervical vertebrae: (a) right lateral view of vertebra; (b) superior view of vertebra; (c) cervical spine articulations.

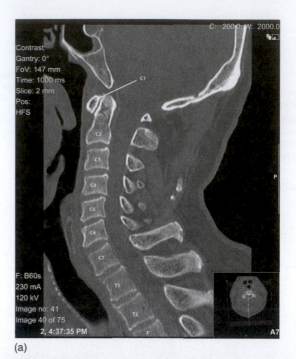

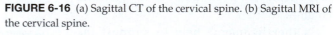

FIGURE 6-16 (a) Sagittal CT of the cervical spine. (b) Sagittal MRI of the cervical spine.

(Photos: Dr. Bryan E. Bledsoe)

The first two cervical vertebrae have a unique relationship with the head and each other that permits rotation to left and right and nodding of the head. The first cervical vertebra, C-1, is called the *atlas*, named after the mythical Greek Titan who was condemned by Zeus to support the heavens on his shoulders. It has no spinous processes or vertebral body. This ring-shaped bone supports the head. This is the atlantooccipital joint. It is securely affixed to the occipital bone and permits nodding but does not accommodate any twisting or

turning motion (Figure 6-17). The highest percentage (approximately 50 percent) of neck flexion and extension occurs at the atlantooccipital joint. The atlas and the next vertebra, C-2, differ from most vertebrae in not having discernible vertebral bodies. Vertebra C-2, called the *axis*, is the strongest of the cervical vertebrae and has a small bony tooth, called the *odontoid process* or *dens*, that projects upward (Figure 6-18). This projection provides a pivotal point around which the atlas and head can rotate from side to side (Figure 6-19).

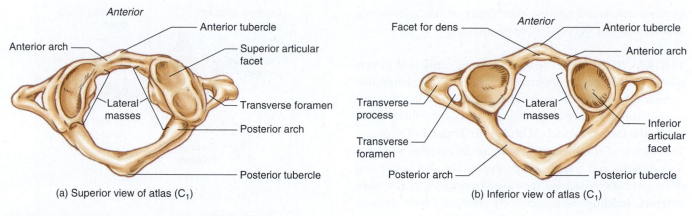

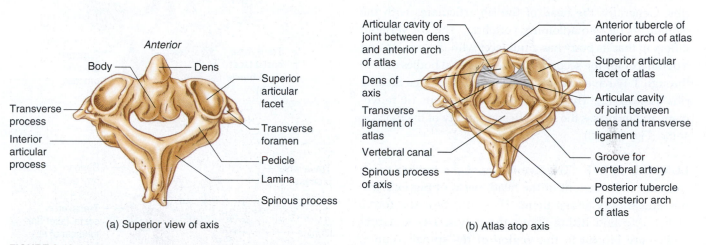

FIGURE 6-18 (a) The axis (superior view); (b) the atlas seated on the axis.

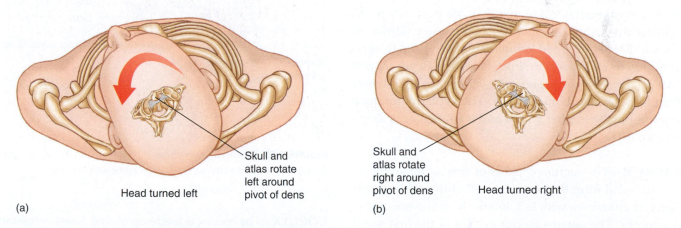

FIGURE 6-19 Relationship between the atlas and the axis. The dens of the axis provides a pivotal point around which the atlas and head can rotate (a) left and (b) right.

The remaining cervical vertebrae permit some rotation, as well as flexion, extension, and lateral bending. The range of motion provided by the cervical spine is greater than that allowed by any other portion of the spinal column, despite the fact that the portion of the spinal cord traveling through this region is critical to virtually all body functions. The last cervical vertebra (C-7) is quite

noticeable, as its spinous process, called the vertebral prominens, is quite pronounced and can be felt as the first bony prominence along the spine and just above the shoulders. The spinal canal diameter in the cervical region is normally 17 mm. The cord becomes compromised when the diameter is reduced to less than 13 mm as occurs in trauma such as when the spinal foramina of two vertebrae become displaced against each other or when bleeding and swelling of the cord increase its size.

THORACIC SPINE The thoracic spine consists of 12 vertebrae. The thoracic vertebrae contain a readily identifiable vertebral body that is heart-shaped. Because the thoracic spine supports more of the human body than the cervical spine, the thoracic vertebral bodies are larger and stronger. The vertebral foramen in this region is circular in shape. The spinous and transverse processes are also larger and more prominent because they are associated with the musculature, holding the upper body erect, and with thoracic cage movement during respiration.

On each side of the thoracic vertebral bodies are specialized facets, called *demifacets*, that articulate with the ribs. Generally, the head of the rib articulates with the demifacets on two adjoining vertebrae. The T-1 vertebra differs in that its body has a full facet with the first rib and a demifacet for the second rib. The vertebral bodies of T-10 through T-12 have only a single facet for the three floating ribs (ribs 10–12). This system of fixation limits rib movement and increases the strength and rigidity of the thoracic spine (Figure 6-20).

LUMBAR SPINE The five bones of the lumbar spine each carry the weight of the head, neck, upper extremities and thorax above them. They also bear the forces of bending and lifting above the pelvis. The vertebral bodies are largest in this region of the spinal column, and the intervertebral disks are also the thickest and bear the greatest stress. In addition, the anterior parts of the vertebral bodies are higher than the posterior parts, causing the normal lumbar spine curvature (lordosis). The lumbar pedicles and laminae are shorter and thicker. The spinous processes are short, flat, and hatchet-shaped and project straight posteriorly. Thus, they are stouter than those in the thoracic spine. The vertebral foramen is largest in the lumbar region and is triangular in shape (Figure 6-21).

SACRUM The sacrum consists of five sacral vertebrae that fuse and form the posterior wall of the pelvis. Superiorly, it articulates with L-5. Inferiorly, it is connected to the coccyx. The anterosuperior margin of the first sacral vertebral remnant projects into the pelvic cavity and is called the *sacral promontory*. The body's center of gravity is approximately 1 centimeter posterior to this landmark. The sacrum, in conjunction with the bones of the pelvis, protects the urinary and reproductive organs. It also serves as the points of attachment between the spinal column and the lower extremities. The articulation with the pelvis is called the *sacroiliac joint* and is very strong. The sacroiliac joint is normally fused and does not allow movement (Figure 6-22).

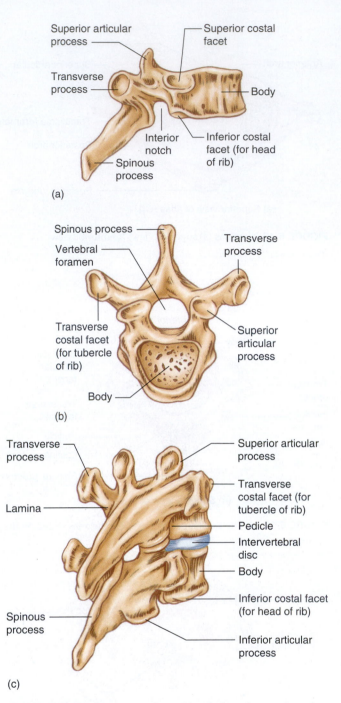

FIGURE 6-20 The thoracic vertebrae: (a) right lateral view of vertebra; (b) superior view of vertebra; (c) thoracic spine articulations.

COCCYX The coccyx is made up of four fused vertebrae that represent the evolutionary remnants of a tail. It is small and triangular in shape and comprises the short skeletal end of the vertebral column. The coccyx serves no major function. It is, however, occasionally fractured during a fall or with childbirth.

The Spinal Cord

The **spinal cord** is the principal central nervous system (CNS) pathway responsible for transmitting sensory input from the body to the brain and for conducting motor and

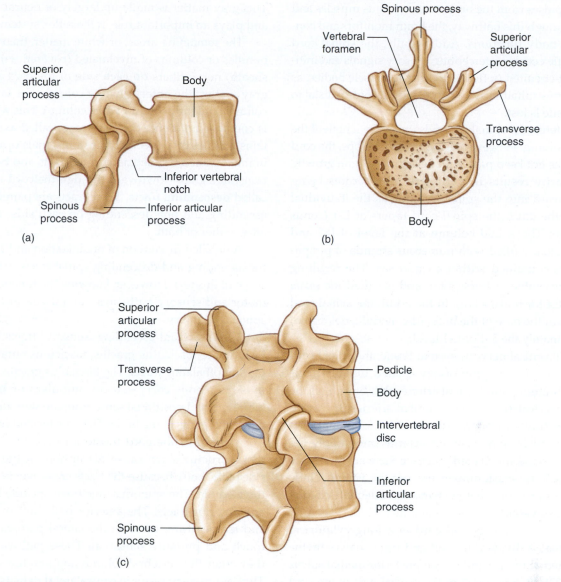

FIGURE 6-21 The lumbar vertebrae: (a) right lateral view of vertebra; (b) superior view of vertebra; (c) lumbar spine articulations.

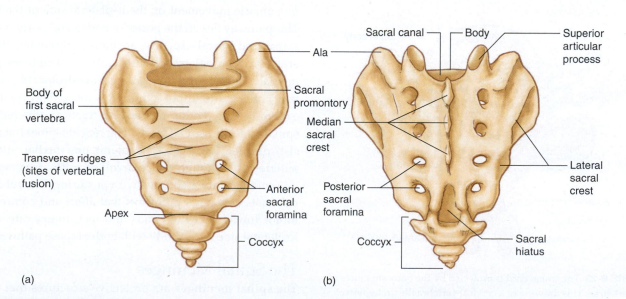

FIGURE 6-22 The sacrum and coccyx: (a) anterior view; (b) posterior view.

control impulses from the brain to the various muscles and organs. Through this pathway, the brain monitors and controls most body functions. Additionally, the spinal cord acts as a reflex center intercepting sensory signals and initiating short-circuited (reflex) signaling to muscle bodies, as needed. If this spinal cord is compromised, control distal to the injury site is lost.

In the fetus, the spinal cord fills the entire length of the vertebral column. However, as the fetus develops, the cord growth does not keep pace with vertebral column growth. This disparity results in peripheral nerve roots being pulled upward into the spinal foramen as the individual grows. In the adult the spinal cord tapers at L-1 (conus medullaris). The spinal column at the level of L-2 and below is actually filled with numerous strands of peripheral nerves contained within a dural sac. The resulting structure resembles a horse's tail and is called the *cauda equina* (Latin for horse's tail). In the adult, the spinal cord extends from the base of the brain (the medulla oblongata) to approximately the L-1 or L-2 level.

Like all central nervous system tissue, the spinal cord requires a constant supply of oxygenated blood. This is supplied through paired spinal arteries that branch off the vertebral, cervical, thoracic, and lumbar arteries. These spinal arteries travel through intervertebral foramina, then split into anterior and posterior arteries and supply the cord itself. On the spinal cord's surface there are numerous interconnections (anastomoses) between the arteries. These anastomoses provide a better chance for adequate circulation in case of vascular blockage or injury.

Anatomically, the spinal cord is a long cylindrical structure that is divided into left and rights halves by the anterior medial fissure and by the posterior medial sulcus (Figure 6-23). In cross section, the central part of the cord has a butterfly or "H" shape and appears gray in color.

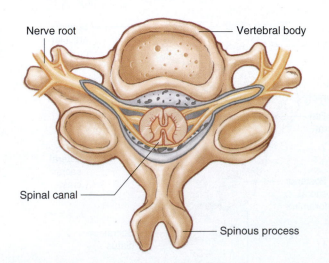

FIGURE 6-23 The spinal cord is protected by the bony structures of the vertebrae. This drawing of a cervical vertebra illustrates nerve roots and protective structures.

Nerve root — Vertebral body
Spinal canal —
Spinous process

This gray matter is made up largely of neural cell bodies and plays an important role in the reflex system.

The remaining areas, or white matter, then form three bundles or columns of myelinated (covered with a protein sheath) nerve fibers on each side of the cord around the gray matter: the anterior white column, the lateral white column, and the posterior white column. This white matter is composed of nerve cell pathways, called **axons**. It contains bundles of axons that transmit signals upward to the brain in what are called **ascending tracts** and bundles that transmit signals downward through the cord in what are called **descending tracts**. These tracts are paired, with one ascending and one descending on each side. Injury may affect either or both.

A detailed discussion of organization and functions of the ascending and descending spinal tracts is beyond the scope of this text. However, knowing the functions of some motor and sensory pathways can aid you in recognizing spinal cord injury.

The important ascending (sensory) tracts or fasciculi include the fasciculus gracilis, fasciculus cutaneous, and the spinothalamic tracts. The fasciculus gracilis and fasciculus cutaneous carry sensory impulses of light touch, vibration, and positional sense from the skin, muscles, tendons, and joints to the brain. They are located on the posterior portion of the cord (posterior columns). Injuries to these structures can cause disruption on the **ipsilateral** side of the body because the tracts cross over at the level of the medulla. The spinothalamic tracts include both lateral and anterior tracts. The anterior pathway conducts pain and temperature, whereas the lateral pathway conducts touch and pressure sensation. These pathways cross as they enter the vertebral column and join the spinal cord. Thus, injury may result in **contralateral** deficits.

The important descending (motor) spinal nerve tract is the corticospinal tract. It is responsible for voluntary and fine muscle movement on the ipsilateral side of the body. This pathway lies on the posterior and lateral portion of the spinal cord. Sacral structures are more peripheral in the lateral corticospinal tracts with cervical structures more medial. This is why central cord syndrome (discussed later) affects the upper extremities more than the lower extremities. Two other descending tracts are the reticulospinal and rubrospinal tracts. The reticulospinal tract consists of three subtracts—one lateral, one medial, and one anterior. It is thought to be involved with sweating and muscular activity associated with posturing. The rubrospinal tracts are lateral pathways that affect and control fine motor function of the hands and feet. Injury affects the ipsilateral side of the body with both of these pathways.

The Spinal Meninges

The **spinal meninges** are protective structures that cover the spine and are contiguous with the meninges that cover and protect the brain. They consist of the dura mater, the arachnoid membrane, and the pia mater. The meninges cover the entire spinal cord and the peripheral nerve roots as they leave the spinal column. However, the spinal meninges are not as strongly secured to the interior spinal column as the meninges of the brain are to the cranium. The dura mater is firmly attached to the base of the skull and to a collagen fiber called the coccygeal ligament at the top of the sacrum. These attachments and the dura mater's attachments associated with each pair of peripheral nerve roots help position the cord centrally within the spinal canal yet permit the column to move around the cord (Figure 6-24).

As in the brain, cerebrospinal fluid bathes the spinal cord by filling the subarachnoid space. The fluid provides a medium for nutrient and waste product exchange and absorbs the shocks of sudden movements. Cerebrospinal fluid is produced in the ventricles of the brain and then circulates through the ventricles and through the arachnoid space of the spinal meninges. The fluid is absorbed by specialized cells (the arachnoid villi) in the lower portion of the lumbar meninges—a region called the spinal cistern.

The distance between the spinal cord and the interior of the vertebral foramen varies in the different spinal regions. The region with the closest tolerance between the

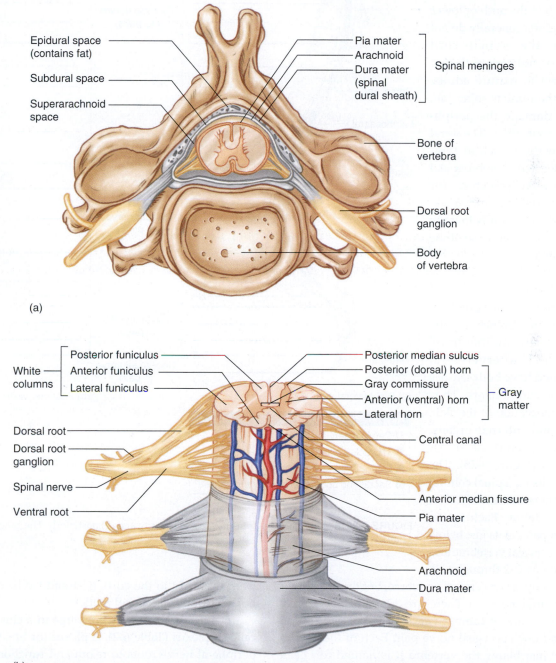

FIGURE 6-24 Anatomy of the spinal cord: (a) cross section through the spinal cord in the cervical region; (b) three-dimensional anterior view of the spinal cord and the meningeal coverings.

cord and the interior surfaces of the spinal foramen is the thoracic spine, where spinal column movement is most limited. Although this region is only rarely injured, even a slight intrusion into the vertebral foramen is likely to cause spinal cord injury. The greatest space between the cord and vertebral canal interior is found in upper lumbar and upper cervical (C-1 and C-2) regions.

Injuries to the mid- or lower lumbar regions generally do not endanger the spinal cord because the cord ends at the L-1 or L-2 level in mature adults. Injury to the lumbar spine can, however, damage the peripheral nerve roots there. The dural sac within the vertebral foramen is filled with cerebrospinal fluid. Lumbar puncture for diagnostic testing and anesthetic administration below the L-2 level is safest because of the cauda equina.

Spinal Nerves

Spinal nerves are the peripheral nerve roots that branch in pairs from the spinal cord. They travel through the intervertebral foramina and have both sensory and motor components. They provide innervation of the skin, muscles, and internal organs. There are 31 pairs of spinal nerve roots (Figure 6-25). The first pair exits the spinal column between the skull and the first cervical vertebra. Each of the next seven pairs exits just below one of the cervical vertebrae and is identified as C-2 through C-8.

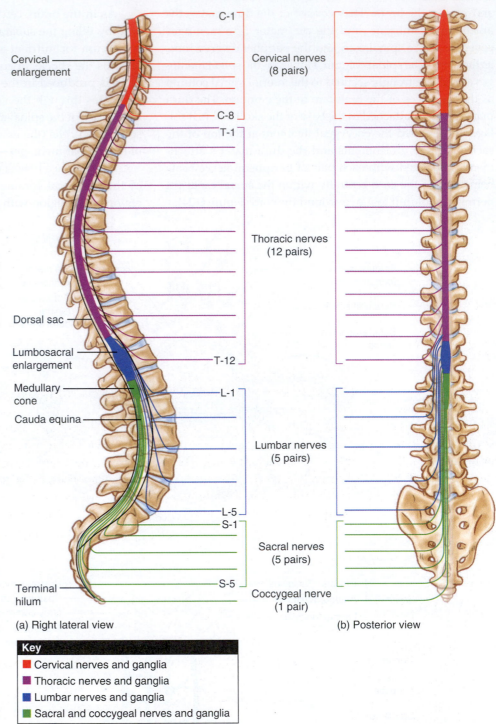

(a) Right lateral view

(b) Posterior view

Key
- ■ Cervical nerves and ganglia
- ■ Thoracic nerves and ganglia
- ■ Lumbar nerves and ganglia
- ■ Sacral and coccygeal nerves and ganglia

FIGURE 6-25 Illustration of the spinal nerves (a) laterally and (b) posteriorly. The ganglia are detailed as well.

(There are only seven cervical vertebrae, but there are eight cervical spinal nerves.) There are 12 pairs of thoracic nerves, five pairs of lumbar nerves, five pairs of sacral nerves, and one coccygeal nerve pair. Each of these pairs originates just below the vertebra it is named for. Each spinal nerve pair has two dorsal and two ventral roots. The ventral roots carry motor impulses from the cord to the body, and the dorsal roots carry sensory impulses from the body to the cord. (C-1 and Co [coccygeal]-1 do not have dorsal [sensory] roots.)

The nerve roots often converge in a cluster of nerves called a plexus (Table 6-2). A plexus (or braiding) permits peripheral nerve roots to rejoin and function as a group. The cervical plexus is made up of the first five cervical nerve roots. It innervates the neck and produces the phrenic nerve. The phrenic nerve (consisting of peripheral

Table 6-2 Spinal Nerve Plexuses

Plexus	Origin	Nerve	Control	Result of Injury
Cervical	C-1 to C-5	Phrenic	Diaphragm	Respiratory paralysis
Brachial	C-5 to C-8, T-1	Axillary	Deltoid/skin of shoulder	Deltoid muscle paralysis
		Radial	Triceps/forearm	Wrist drop
		Median	Flexor muscles, forearm, arm	Decreased usage
		Musculocutaneous	Flexor muscles of arm	Decreased usage
		Ulnar	Wrist/hand	Claw hand; inability to spread fingers
Lumbar	T-12 to L-4	Femoral	Lower abdomen, gluteus, thighs	Inability to extend leg, flex hip
		Obturator	Abductor muscles, medial thigh	Decreased usage
Sacral	L-4 to S-3	Sciatic	Lower extremity	Decreased usage

nerve roots C-3 through C-5) is responsible for control of the diaphragm. The brachial plexus joins the nerves controlling the upper extremity (C-5 through T-1). The lumbar and sacral plexuses control the innervation of the lower extremity.

The sensory components of the spinal nerves innervate specific and discrete surface areas. These areas are called **dermatomes** and are distributed from the occiput of the head to the heel of the foot and buttocks (Figure 6-26). Key locations to recognize for assessments include the collar region (C-3), the little finger (C-7), the nipple line (T-4), the umbilicus (T-10), and the small toe (S-1).

Motor components of the spinal nerve roots also innervate discrete tissues and muscles of the body in regions called **myotomes**. However, as the body grows and matures, some muscles merge and their control is not as specific as it is with the dermatomes. Key myotomes for neurologic evaluation include arm extension (C-5), elbow extension (C-7), small finger abduction (T-1), knee extension (L-3), and ankle flexion (S-1). Evaluation of areas controlled by both dermatomes and myotomes can help to identify the spinal cord region associated with an injury.

The spinal cord also performs some primary processing functions. It aids in speeding body responses and helping the brain maintain balance and muscle tone. These responses, called reflexes, occur as special neurons in the cord, called *interneurons*, intercept sensory signals (Figure 6-27). For example, if you touch a hot stove, the severe pain sends an intense signal to the brain. This

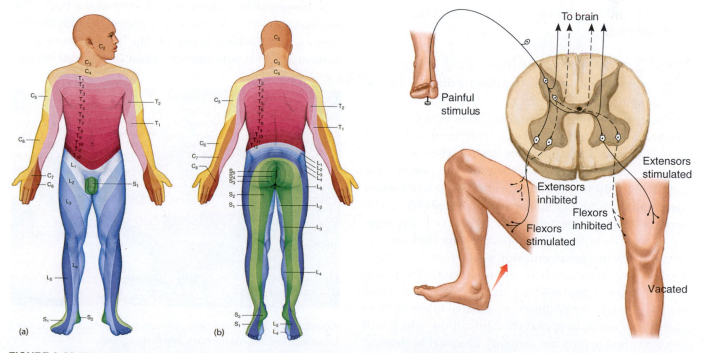

FIGURE 6-26 The dermatomes: (a) anterior view; (b) posterior view.

FIGURE 6-27 The reflex arc.

strong signal simultaneously triggers an interneuron in the spinal cord to direct a signal to the flexor muscles, telling them to contract. The limb withdraws without waiting for the signal to be sent to the brain, be processed there, and then trigger a command that is sent back to the limb. The speed of this reflex action reduces the seriousness of injury. Other reflexes help stabilize the body if it stands in one position for a length of time. As the stretch receptors report that the body is moving, interneurons signal muscles to counteract the movement to help maintain position. This again reduces body reaction time and allows the body to stand or maintain a steady position.

The spinal nerves can be further subdivided according to the division of the autonomic nervous system they serve and to their spinal origin. The parasympathetic nervous system, which controls rest and regenerative functions, consists of peripheral nerve roots branching from the sacral region and cranial nerves (predominantly the vagus nerve). Parasympathetic stimulation slows the heart and increases digestive system activity; this stimulation also plays a role in sexual stimulation. The sympathetic nervous system branches from nerves originating in the thoracic and lumbar regions. It adjusts body metabolic rate to waking activity and provides "fight-or-flight" functions when the body comes under threat or extreme stress. This system decreases digestive activity through vasoconstriction, constricts venous blood vessels, and increases the body's metabolic rate through release of the adrenal hormones norepinephrine and epinephrine. In shock, the sympathetic nervous system causes systemic vasoconstriction to reduce venous blood volume and increases peripheral vascular resistance. It also increases heart rate to increase cardiac output in response to dropping preload and blood pressure.

Blood Supply to the Spinal Cord

Blood to the spinal cord is supplied primarily by the anterior spinal artery and the two posterior spinal arteries. The anterior spinal artery arises from branches of the vertebral arteries and supplies the anterior two-thirds of the spinal cord. Each posterior artery arises primarily from a branch of the vertebral arteries and perfuses the posterior one-third of the spinal cord. The anterior spinal artery and the posterior spinal arteries supply blood primarily to the superior part of the spinal cord. The anterior two-thirds of the lower aspects of the cord are also perfused by the great anterior segmental medullary arteries (medullary artery of Adamkiewicz). The posterior one-third is perfused by the posterior segmental medullary artery. An occlusion or damage to any of these arteries can result in spinal cord infarction, which will give signs and symptoms virtually identical to those of spinal cord injury.

Head, Neck, and Spinal Pathophysiology

Head, neck, and spinal injuries can be difficult to assess in the prehospital setting, yet commonly threaten life or result in lifelong disability. A clear appreciation of the injury mechanisms affecting these regions and of the specific pathological processes related to head, facial, neck, and spinal column injury can help to anticipate, assess, and manage these injuries.

General Mechanisms of Injury to the Head, Neck, and Spine

As with other forms of trauma, injuries to the head, neck, and spine are divided by mechanisms of injury into blunt (closed) and penetrating (open).

Blunt Injury

The head, neck, and spine are fairly well protected from most forms of blunt trauma. At times, however, the forces associated with blunt trauma can exceed this protection and result in serious injury. The most serious of these injuries affects the central nervous system—the brain and spinal cord—but may also affect other structures in these regions. For example, traumatic brain injury frequently results from motor vehicle collisions, accounting for more than half of vehicle crash mortality. Sports-related injuries, falling objects, explosions, falls, and acts of violence, like assault with a club, are less common, but are still significant mechanisms associated with these injuries (Figure 6-28).

The head is frequently injured in blunt trauma because it is anatomically prominent at the top of the body. The trauma victim may flex the neck to protect the face, but this then exposes the head to impact. The head is the frequent point of impact in auto collisions when an occupant impacts

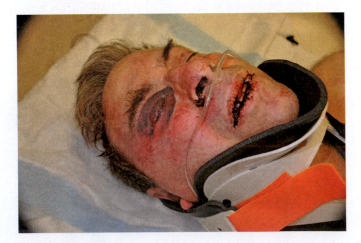

FIGURE 6-28 Blunt injury to the face can produce hemorrhage, soft tissue injuries, internal fractures, and brain injuries.

(© Edward T. Dickinson, MD)

the windshield or steering wheel, or in diving mechanisms or in falls. Blunt trauma can be more localized when caused by weapons such as clubs, sticks, pipes, or other objects wielded by an assailant. Because of the structure of the scalp, a glancing blunt blow can tear the edges of the scalp, resulting in an open wound with a flap of tissue. Head injury is especially prevalent in very young patients. The size of the head relative to the rest of the body, the flexibility of the neck, and the inability of very young patients to protect them contribute to the increased incidence and severity of blunt head trauma in pediatric patients.

The face is frequently injured. Significant facial injury occurs less frequently than head injury in auto impacts because the head's frontal or parietal regions are more likely than the face to impact the windshield. The same holds true for falls, as the arms, chest, or head absorb energy as the conscious victim tries to protect the facial area and head from injury. Intentional violence is less likely to spare the facial region. The face is often the target of blows from a fist or other weapons, such as sticks or clubs. The middle and inner ears and the eyes are very well protected against most blunt trauma, although ear injury may be caused by the pressure changes associated with diving or explosions. The eyes may occasionally be injured by impacts from smaller blunt objects such as a racquetball, baseball, or tennis ball.

The neck is anatomically well protected from most blunt trauma because the head, face, and chest protrude more anteriorly. Laterally, the neck is protected, as the shoulders protrude a significant distance from the neck. The neck is, however, a point of impact in certain situations. For example, during an auto crash the neck may strike the steering wheel or be injured by a shoulder strap that is worn without a lap belt. During a rear impact vehicle collision, the neck may be injured by extremes of extension or flexion. The region may also be impacted by objects during fights or injured during an attempted suicide by hanging.

The spine is vulnerable to numerous types of injury. Injurious forces may tear tendons, muscles, and ligaments, causing pain and possibly destabilizing the vertebral column. Those forces may cause displacement of the vertebrae from their normal position, resulting in a subluxation (partial or incomplete dislocation) or dislocation. The injury process may fracture the spinous or transverse processes, the pedicles, the laminae, or the vertebral body itself. Trauma, especially axial loading, may damage the intervertebral disks and the connective and bony tissues of the vertebral column. They may or may not be associated with injury to the spinal cord itself.

Penetrating Injury

Penetrating injuries to the head, face, neck, and spinal column are not as common as those resulting from blunt trauma. However, they can be more severe and life threatening. In addition, a penetrating injury to the head suggests that the meninges have been opened, producing a route for introduction of serious infections.

Penetrating injuries to the head, face, neck, and spine are usually due to shootings or stabbings. Gunshot wounds are the most common and are especially injurious because bullets release a tremendous amount of energy as they slow during collision with skeletal and central nervous tissues. Similarly, explosions propel projectiles, either intrinsic to the explosive device or from debris produced by the blast, that may penetrate and damage this region. Knife wounds to the head and face tend to be superficial because of the region's extensive skeletal components. The anterior and lateral neck, however, is not as well protected. Neck wounds may compromise the airway, esophagus, and major blood vessels, quickly threatening the patient's life.

Pathophysiology of Brain Injury

Traumatic brain injury (TBI) is defined by the National Head Injury Foundation as "a traumatic insult to the brain capable of producing physical, intellectual, emotional, social, and vocational changes." It is classified as a direct or indirect injury to the tissue of the cerebrum, cerebellum, or brainstem.

Direct Injury

Direct (or primary) injury is caused by a variety of mechanisms. Rapid acceleration (or deceleration) or penetrating injury can cause mechanical injury to the neurons and supporting cells and impair function. These injuries can also disrupt blood vessels, both restricting blood flow through the injured area and causing central nervous tissue irritation as blood flows into the affected areas. Remember that the brain is specially protected from contact with some of the blood's content by the blood–brain barrier. Injury can disrupt this barrier. Finally, serious jarring may damage capillary walls, adversely affecting their permeability, and cause a fluid shift to the interstitial space, or tissue edema. Most frequently, a combination of these processes is associated with direct brain injury.

Two specific types of direct brain injury are coup and contrecoup injury (Figure 6-29). **Coup injuries** are

> **CONTENT REVIEW**
>
> ➤ Types of Direct Brain Injury
>
> **Focal**
> - Cerebral contusion
> - Intracranial hemorrhage
> - Epidural hematoma
> - Subdural hematoma
> - Intracerebral hemorrhage
>
> **Diffuse**
> - Concussion (mild to moderate diffuse axonal injury)
> - Moderate diffuse axonal injury
> - Severe diffuse axonal injury (formerly, brainstem injury)

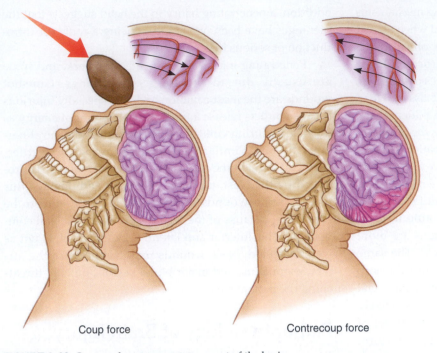

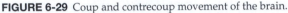

FIGURE 6-29 Coup and contrecoup movement of the brain.

injuries that occur directly at the point of impact as the brain moves toward and collides with the interior of the skull. These are most common in the frontal region because its interior surface is rough and irregular. In contrast, the occipital areas are smooth and coup injuries occur less frequently here. Coup injury may also occur as the brain slides along the rough contours at the base of the skull.

Contrecoup injuries cause injury away from the primary impact point as the brain, floating in cerebrospinal fluid inside the cranium, "sloshes" toward the impact, then away from it, again impacting the interior of the skull. For example, a blow to the forehead might cause injury to the occipital region (visual center) and produce visual disturbances ("seeing stars"). Contrecoup injury in the frontal region is most common (from an impact to the occipital region) because the frontal bones have an irregular inner surface.

Direct brain injuries can be further assigned to one of two specific categories—focal or diffuse.

FOCAL INJURIES   Focal injuries occur at a specific location in the brain and include contusions and intracranial hemorrhages.

Cerebral Contusion   A cerebral contusion is caused by blunt trauma to brain tissue that produces capillary bleeding into the brain's substance. Contusion is relatively common with blunt head injuries and often produces confusion and other types of neurologic deficit—which are usually transient. This injury may result from a coup or contrecoup mechanism and may occur at one or several sites in the brain. The localized injury manifests with

dysfunction related to the injury site. For example, a patient who suffers a frontal lobe contusion after trauma to the forehead may experience personality changes. (Remember, the frontal lobe is the most commonly injured lobe.) A cerebral contusion may be small and isolated or may be large and/or widespread. The more brain tissue involved, the greater the extent of injury and the signs, symptoms, and neurologic deficit.

Intracranial Hemorrhage   Bleeding can occur at several locations within the brain, each presenting with a different pathological process. These injuries—proceeding from the most superficial to the deepest—are epidural, subdural, and intracerebral hemorrhages. In contrast to patients with concussions and contusions, expect the intracranial hemorrhage patient to deteriorate during your assessment and care because of associated indirect injury, such as progressing hemorrhage and increasing intracranial pressure.

Bleeding between the dura mater and the skull's interior surface is called an **epidural hematoma** (Figure 6-30). It usually involves arterial vessels—often the middle meningeal artery in the temporal region. Because the bleeding is from a relatively high-pressure vessel, intracranial pressure builds rapidly, compressing the brain. As pressure builds, the patient often becomes unresponsive. The hemorrhage-induced increase in intracranial pressure reduces cerebral perfusion pressure and oxygenated

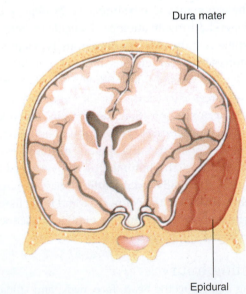

FIGURE 6-30 Epidural hematoma.

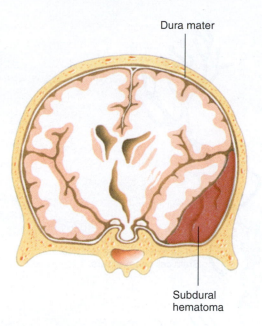

Dura mater

Subdural
hematoma

FIGURE 6-31 Subdural hematoma.

circulation to the nerve cells (indirect injury). Bleeding may be so significant that it displaces the brain away from the injury site. Although the progression is both rapid and life threatening, immediate surgery can sometimes reverse it.

Bleeding within the meninges, specifically beneath the dura mater and within the subarachnoid space, is called **subdural hematoma** (Figure 6-31). This type of hemorrhage occurs very slowly and may have a subtle presentation because blood loss is usually due to small venous vessel rupture—often one of the small bridging vessels between the cerebral cortex and dural sinuses. The vessel most commonly involved is the superior sagittal sinus. Because subdural hemorrhage occurs above the pia mater, it does not cause the cerebral irritation associated with intracerebral hemorrhage. Free blood in the cerebrospinal fluid may clog structures responsible for the fluid's reabsorption, which can result in an increasing cerebral spinal fluid volume and an increasing ICP. The patient sometimes does not show overt signs and symptoms of this injury until hours, or even days, after injury. Because of this delay, subdural hemorrhage can at times be difficult to detect in the prehospital setting.

Suspect subdural hematoma in a "non-trauma" patient who demonstrates neurologic signs and symptoms (e.g., changes in level of consciousness or headache). Obtaining a careful history may uncover a recent mechanism of injury, such as a fall or head trauma, that could cause this presentation. Such injuries are occasionally encountered in elderly patients or with chronic alcoholics. Because both the aging process and chronic alcoholism reduce brain size, head injury may cause greater and less controlled brain motion within the cranium. This increases the likelihood of injury and a subdural hematoma.

Intracerebral hemorrhage results from a ruptured blood vessel (most frequently an artery) that releases blood into the substance of the brain. Although blood loss is generally minimal, it can be particularly damaging. Tissue edema results because free blood, outside a blood vessel, irritates nervous tissues. Intracerebral hemorrhage often presents much like a stroke, with signs and symptoms occurring very quickly. The particular presentation relates to the brain area involved. Normally, signs and symptoms will progressively worsen with time.

Two other localized conditions in the brain that can result in increasing intracranial pressure are cerebral edema and hydrocephalus. Injury to the brain tissue initiates the inflammation response. The inflammation process permits fluid and proteins to pass through cerebral capillary walls. These proteins exert an osmotic pressure and draw water into and expand the interstitial space (cerebral edema). As the inflamed area swells, it exerts pressure on surrounding tissue.

Hydrocephalus may occur with hemorrhage into the subarachnoid space. Blood cells then clog the arachnoid villa, the small structures that permit fluids in the cerebral spinal fluid to reenter the bloodstream. This causes an accumulation of cerebrospinal fluid and an increase in ICP.

DIFFUSE INJURIES Diffuse injuries involve a more generalized mechanism of injury than do focal injuries. They include mild (concussions), moderate, and severe axonal disruptions. During head injury, a stretching, shearing, or tearing force may be applied to nerve fibers and cause damage to axons—the long nerve cell communication pathways. This injury is frequently distributed throughout the brain and thus is called **diffuse axonal injury** (DAI). Diffuse axonal injuries are common among severe acceleration/deceleration mechanisms such as motor collisions and auto/pedestrian collisions. DAI may also result from severe compression, then decompression, as an explosion's overpressure passes through the victim (Figure 6-32). DAIs can range from the mild (a concussion) to the severe and life threatening.

Concussion A **concussion** is a mild to moderate form of DAI and is the most common result of blunt head injury. It represents nerve dysfunction without substantial anatomic damage (e.g., a normal head CT scan). Concussion may cause a transient episode of neuronal dysfunction (confusion, disorientation, and event amnesia) that rapidly returns to normal neurologic activity. Prehospital concussion management consists of frequent neurologic assessments with attention to the airway and respiratory effort, and looking for subtle changes in the level of consciousness. Most patients survive with no neurologic impairment.

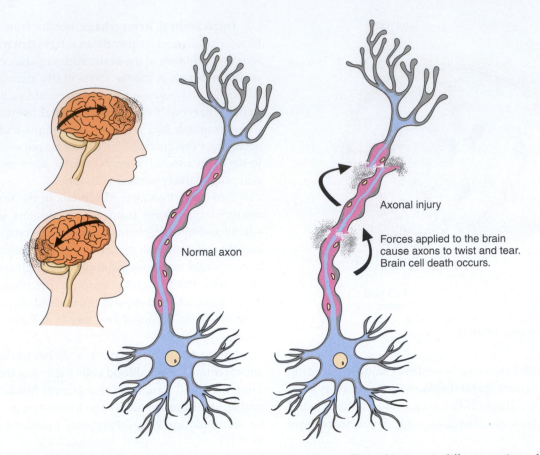

Normal axon

Axonal injury

Forces applied to the brain cause axons to twist and tear. Brain cell death occurs.

FIGURE 6-32 A diffuse axonal injury (DAI) is a type of brain injury caused by shearing forces that occur in different portions of the brain as a result of compression, acceleration, and/or deceleration.

A concussion, contusion, intracerebral hemorrhage, subdural hematoma, and epidural hematoma may occur alone or in combination with one another. For example, an injury may cause a concussion and an epidural hematoma concurrently. The concussion results in immediate unconsciousness that usually resolves after only a few minutes. The patient becomes conscious and alert but then later exhibits a deteriorating level of consciousness as the epidural hematoma expands and increases intracranial pressure. This interim period of consciousness, called a *lucid interval*, is a classic (if rarely seen) sign of epidural hematoma. There is a danger of increasing injury if the impact occurs again before the victim has an opportunity to completely recover from a mild DAI.

Moderate Diffuse Axonal Injury Moderate DAI is caused by shearing, stretching, or tearing of the nerve fibers, but is also associated with minute brain bruising. This injury is often referred to as the "classic concussion." If the cerebral cortex or reticular activating system of the brainstem is involved, the patient may become unconscious. This type of injury is more severe than a mild concussion. It occurs in 20 percent of all severe head injuries and comprises 45 percent of all DAI cases. Moderate DAI can be associated with basilar skull fracture. Although most patients survive this injury, some degree of residual neurologic impairment is common.

Short- and long-term signs and symptoms associated with moderate DAI include immediate unconsciousness followed by persistent confusion, inability to concentrate, disorientation, and retrograde and anterograde amnesia. The victim may also complain of headache, focal neurologic deficits, light sensitivity (photophobia), and disturbances in smell and other senses. Anxiety may be present and the patient may experience significant mood swings.

Severe Diffuse Axonal Injury Severe DAI (previously known as brainstem injury) is a significant mechanical disruption of multiple axons in both cerebral hemispheres with extension into the brainstem. Approximately 16 percent of all severe head injuries and 36 percent of all cases of DAI are classified as severe. Many patients do not survive this type of injury. Of those who do, many will have some degree of permanent neurologic impairment. The patient experiencing severe DAI will usually remain unconscious for a prolonged period of time. The patient may display signs of increased ICP (Cushing's response).

Indirect Injury

Indirect (or secondary) injuries are the result of factors that occur because of, although after, the initial (or primary) injury. These pathophysiological processes are progressive and cause the patient deterioration often associated with serious head injuries. Indirect injuries may be as or more damaging than the initial injury because of the skull's unique design and the delicate nature of central nervous system tissue.

Two distinct pathophysiologic processes cause indirect injuries. The first process is a diminishing circulation to brain tissue (intracranial perfusion) caued by an increasing intracranial pressure—possibly exacerbated by hypoxia, hypercarbia, and systemic hypotension. The second process is progressive pressure against, or physical displacement of, brain tissue secondary to an expanding mass (often blood) within the cranial vault. As these mechanisms continue and increase nervous tissue injury, they cause many of the progressive signs and symptoms often associated with head injury.

Intracranial Perfusion

The brain is the body's most perfusion-sensitive organ. Any injury that affects perfusion has a rapid and devastating effect on the brain and its control of body systems. Cerebral, cerebellar, and brainstem perfusion may be disrupted both by increasing intracranial pressure and by low systemic blood pressure (hypotension).

As mentioned earlier, the cranial volume is fixed and does not vary. The cerebrum, cerebellum, and brainstem account for 80 percent (1,200 mL) of this volume. Venous, capillary, and arterial blood accounts for most of the remaining space, or about 12 percent (150 mL) of intracranial volume. Cerebrospinal fluid accounts for roughly the remaining 8 percent (90 mL). Any increase in the size of one internal component must be matched by a similar reduction in another component (Monroe-Kellie doctrine). If it is not, the intracranial pressure rises.

Venous blood vessels are the first intracranial space to be compressed as a mass expands within the cranium. If the mass continues its expansion, the next intracranial volume affected is the cerebrospinal fluid. It is pushed out of the cranium and into the spinal cord. These two mechanisms respond very quickly to ICP changes and maintain an ICP very close to normal. However, once these mechanisms reach their compensatory limits, intracranial pressure rises quickly and begins to restrict arterial blood flow. Any reduction in cerebral blood flow triggers a rise in the systemic blood pressure as the body tries to ensure adequate cerebral perfusion (autoregulation). As the systolic blood pressure rises, so does ICP. This increase in ICP further increases the resistance to cerebral blood flow, reducing cerebral circulation and producing more cerebral hypoxia and hypercarbia. These factors result in an additional rise in systolic blood pressure, and then ICP—leading to a worsening, eventually deadly, cycle (Figure 6-33). If the mass, fluid accumulation (edema), or hemorrhage continues to expand, the ICP becomes so high that cerebral circulation all but stops.

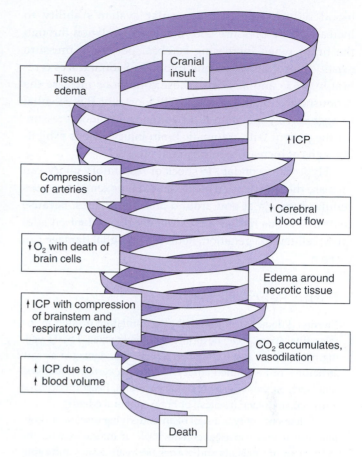

FIGURE 6-33 Pathway of deterioration following central nervous system insult.

Another factor affecting ICP and circulation through the brain is the carbon dioxide level in the cerebrospinal fluid. As carbon dioxide levels rise, cerebral arteries vasodilate to provide increased blood flow and reduce hypercarbia. In the presence of an already high ICP, this process can quickly make matters worse. The brain's response to hypercarbia and increasing ICP causes the classic hyperventilation and hypertension associated with head injury. Hypocarbia can also have dire consequences. Hypocarbia triggers cerebral arterial vasoconstriction. When combined with reduced CPP, arterial vasoconstriction further reduces cerebral circulation. In extreme cases, the resulting vasoconstriction can significantly slow circulation through the brain. Maintaining near-normocapnia is critical to optimizing CPP. This is the reason why capnography is such a valuable tool in guiding ventilation for head injury patients.

Two systemic problems frequently associated with trauma, and sometimes related to brain injury, are hypotension and hypoventilation. These problems seriously compound any existing head injury through a tertiary injury mechanism.

Hypotension is especially damaging for the patient with traumatic brain injury. Any physiologic compensation to maintain blood pressure in the patient who is losing blood reduces the cardiovascular system's ability to increase blood pressure and maintain circulation through the brain when increasing cerebral perfusion pressure exists. The resulting cerebral hypoperfusion induces cerebral hypoxia and acidosis. These conditions increase the seriousness of brain injury and TBI mortality. It is essential to aggressively maintain fluid volume and blood pressure for the patient with traumatic brain injury who is exhibiting signs of increasing intracranial pressure.

Hypoxia, secondary to shock or respiratory injury, can increase the severity of a head injury. Hypoxemia increases cellular hypoxia at and around any injury sites. Because central nervous tissues are extremely dependent on adequate cellular oxygenation, neuronal and glial damage can worsen.

Patho Pearls

Edema. Edema (swelling) is the accumulation of fluid in the interstitial space. It can be localized or generalized. Local swelling may appear at the site of an injury (e.g., damaged airway structures or a sprained ankle) or within a certain organ system, such as the lungs (pulmonary edema), heart (pericardial effusion), abdomen (ascites), or brain (cerebral edema).

Edema not only is a sign of an underlying disease or problem, but it also causes problems itself. It interferes with the movement of nutrients and wastes between tissues and capillaries. It may diminish capillary blood flow, depriving tissues of oxygen. In turn, this may slow the healing of wounds, promote infection, and facilitate formation of pressure sores. Edema affecting organs such as the brain, lung, heart, or larynx may be life threatening. Body water that is retained in the interstitial spaces is body water not available for metabolic processes in the cells. Therefore, even if the total body water is normal, edema can cause a relative condition of dehydration. Damage to the airway, where development of edema is life threatening, requires that the patient be intubated before the swelling develops to the point of airway obstruction.

Edema that occurs with injury to the brain is especially dangerous. Because the brain is confined within the bony skull, there is no room for expansion, so edema places pressure on the brain tissues, especially the brainstem. As the edema progresses, it causes herniation, in which brain tissues are pushed out through the foramen magnum, the opening through which the spinal cord connects to the brain.

Pressure and Structural Displacement

As hemorrhage or edema increases in a part of the brain, the expansion pushes uninjured tissue away from the injury site. Even in the absence of increased ICP, such expansion puts pressure on adjacent brain tissue—often the brainstem. As the mass continues to increase in size, it may physically compress brainstem components. With further expansion, it may push (herniate) the brain tissue against and around the falx cerebri and the tentorium cerebelli. Because these are basically immobile structures within the skull, displacement results in a process called *herniation*. With herniation, a portion of a brain structure is pushed into and through an opening, thus physically injuring brain tissue and compromising its blood supply. If displacement affects the upper brainstem by pushing it through the tentorium incisura (uncal herniation), it may cause vomiting, altered mental status, and pupillary dilation. If the displacement affects the medulla oblongata by pushing it into the foramen magnum (cerebellar herniation), it may cause disturbances in breathing, blood pressure, and heart rate.

Injury Progression and Development of Signs and Symptoms

Direct injury, increasing intracranial pressure, and compression and displacement of brain tissue can cause alterations in mental status and consciousness. These injuries also produce specific signs and symptoms related to the central nervous system structure(s) affected. The actual brain injury process can be mapped as pressure increases and the injury moves from the cortical surface and down to the brainstem.

As a portion of the cerebral cortex is injured, the specific functions it controls are affected. For example, if the frontal lobe is injured, the patient may present with alterations in personality. If the occipital region is affected, visual disturbances may be seen. A large region of cortical disruption may cause confusion and affect the patient's mental status. The patient may forget the circumstances of the event itself (**event amnesia**), those leading up to (before) the incident (**retrograde amnesia**), or those following (after) the incident (**anterograde amnesia**). The patient may also become disoriented (to time, place, person, and one's own person), confused, or combative. Focal deficits, such as hemiplegia or hemiparesis (one-sided weakness), or seizures may also result. When intracranial injury extends to components of the ascending reticular activating system in the brainstem, the patient may have an altered level of consciousness manifest as lethargy, somnolence, or coma.

If compression results from an expanding mass along the central region of the cerebrum, increased pressure is first seen in the midbrain, then the pons,

CONTENT REVIEW

➤ Signs and Symptoms of Brain Injury
- Altered level of consciousness
- Alterations in personality
- Amnesia
  - Retrograde
  - Anterograde
- Chusing's triad
  - Increasing blood pressure
  - Slowing pulse rate
  - Irregular respirations
- Vomiting (often without nausea)
- Body temperature changes
- Changes in reactivity of pupils
- Decorticate posturing

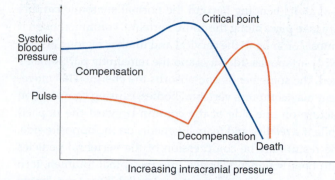

FIGURE 6-34 Cushing's reflex: how systolic blood pressure and pulse rate respond to increasing intracranial pressure.

and finally in the medulla oblongata. The signs and symptoms of this progressive pressure and structural displacement are somewhat predictable and are known as the *central syndrome.*

In the central syndrome, upper brainstem compression produces an increase in blood pressure to maintain cerebral perfusion pressure (called **Cushing's reflex**) and a reflex decrease in heart rate in response to vagus nerve (parasympathetic) stimulation of the SA node and AV junction (Figure 6-34). The patient may also exhibit a characteristic cyclical breathing pattern called **Cheyne-Stokes respirations**. This consists of increasing, then decreasing, respiratory volumes, followed by a period of apnea. The combination of an increasing blood pressure, slowing pulse, and irregular respirations is a classical sign of brainstem pressure or injury called **Cushing's triad**. If the brain injury involves the hypothalamus, the patient may experience vomiting (frequently without nausea) and body temperature changes. The pupils remain small and reactive. Decorticate posturing (body extension with arm flexion) in response to painful stimuli may occur as the neural pathways through the upper brainstem are disrupted (herniation).

As the middle brainstem becomes involved, the pulse pressure widens and the heart rate becomes bradycardic. Respirations now may be deep and rapid (central neurologic hyperventilation). Increasing intracranial pressure may also induce pupil sluggishness or nonreactivity (bilaterally, because the injury involves compression from above) as the oculomotor nerve (CN-III) is compressed. The patient may develop extension (decerebrate) posturing. Few patients ever regain normal function once they have reached this ICP level.

Finally, as the pressure reaches the lower brainstem, the pupils become fully dilated and unreactive. Respirations become ataxic (erratic with no characteristic rhythm) or may even cease altogether. The pulse rate is often very irregular, with great swings in rate. ECG conduction disturbances become apparent, including QRS complex, S–T segment, and T-wave changes. As control over blood pressure is disrupted, the patient becomes hypotensive. The patient

will no longer respond to painful stimuli and the skeletal muscles will become flaccid. Patients rarely survive once the ICP rises to this level.

If the mass causing the compression is located more laterally than in the central syndrome just described, the signs and symptoms occur in a less predictable sequence. The pupillary responses—sluggishness, nonreactivity, and dilation—are usually ipsilateral (on the same side) to the expanding mass.

Pediatric Head Trauma

Head trauma in the pediatric patient has a very different pathophysiologic process than that seen in the older patient. The skull is not fully formed at birth and is still rather cartilaginous. It distorts more easily with trauma and transmits injury forces more directly to the central nervous tissues. However, incomplete skull formation, with its "soft spots" (the anterior and posterior fontanelles), allows some intracranial expansion. Fontanelles are likely to bulge outward with increasing intracranial pressure. Generally speaking, this softer skeletal structure increases the direct injury associated with head trauma in the very young pediatric patient but slows the progression of increasing intracranial pressure and secondary injury.

As noted earlier, blood and cerebrospinal fluid represent about 20 percent of the total adult cranium's volume (about 240 mL). As a rule, blood loss into the cranial vault cannot account for a significant component of hypovolemia in the adult. However, the pediatric patient has a proportionally larger head, an ability to accommodate increased fluids because of the fontanelles, and a much smaller total body fluid volume and reserves. In the pediatric patient, therefore, intracranial hemorrhage may significantly contribute to hypovolemia.

Pathophysiology of Spinal Injury

Spinal injuries can involve the spinal column, spinal cord, peripheral nerve roots, ligaments, muscles, or any combination of these. Spinal injuries can vary significantly from relatively minor compression fractures without spinal cord involvement to significant vertebral fractures with transection of the spinal cord and resultant paralysis. It is important to note that spinal column injury does not necessarily mean that the cord is injured. Conversely, it is possible to have a cord injury without a spinal column fracture or displacement. However, a spinal column injury reduces the stability of the column and further movement may endanger or further endanger the cord.

Mechanisms of Spinal Injury

Numerous mechanisms of injury have been associated with spinal injuries. These include extremes of normal anatomic range of motion, such as hyperflexion and hyperextension, as well as rotation and lateral bending. In addition, compression (axial loading) or traction (distraction) along the axis of the spine can cause serious spinal injury. As with injuries to the head, face, and neck, spinal column injury may occur as a direct result of either blunt or penetrating trauma.

EXTREMES OF RANGE OF MOTION Hyperextension or hyperflexion injuries bend the spine forcibly beyond its normal range of motion. These injuries occur most commonly in the cervical or lumbar regions. A classic example of a hyperextension injury mechanism is a rear-impact auto collision (e.g., whiplash). The patient's head remains stationary while the upper torso rapidly moves forward as the auto impact accelerates the seat forward. The head moves backward and subsequently hyperextends the unsupported neck. The hyperextension places compressive forces on the posterior vertebral structures (spinous processes, laminae, and pedicles). In addition, it stretches the anterior longitudinal ligament. Hyperextension injuries may cause disk disruption, compression of the interspinous ligaments, and fracture of the posterior vertebral elements. If the forces are great enough, ligaments may tear or the vertebra may fracture, resulting in instability and bone displacement. The bone fragments may also penetrate the spinal canal and injure the spinal cord.

In frontal impact crashes, the shoulder strap may restrain the patient's body while the head continues forward. The neck, in turn, restrains the head and flexes the spine with the movement. The process is frequently forceful enough to hyperflex the spine and causes a patient to literally "kiss the chest" (sometimes demonstrated by the patient's lipstick print on her shirt front). Hyperflexion may lead to anterior vertebral body wedge fractures, posterior longitudinal and interspinous ligament stretching or rupture, compression injury to the cord, pedicle fracture, and disruption of the intervertebral disks with dislocation of the vertebrae.

Excessive rotation beyond normal anatomic barriers may occur in the cervical and lumbar spine. Anatomically, the head is attached to the vertebral column at the foramen magnum, located well posterior of the neck's midline and the head's center of mass. With lateral impact, the head often turns toward the impacting force as the body moves to the side and out from under it. The cervical spine attachment restrains the motion and turns the head violently. Rotation injury normally affects the upper aspects of the cervical spine, but may also be transmitted to the lumbar spine as, for example, when a tackled football player's thorax twists while his feet are firmly planted. The result is a rotational injury that may include stretching or tearing of the ligaments, rotational subluxation or dislocation, and vertebral fracture. Rotational injury can also occur in a motor vehicle collision in which multiple impacts and force vectors are involved.

Lateral bending beyond the normal anatomic barriers may take place along the entire vertebral column, though it is most common in the cervical and lumbar regions. As one body part moves sideways and the remaining part remains fixed, the spine bends and absorbs the energy. This movement may compress vertebral bodies, causing compression fracture on one side of the column (toward the impact) while it stretches and tears ligaments on the opposite side. The result may be compression of the vertebral pedicles with bone fragments driven into the spinal foramen, torn ligaments, and possibly vertebral instability. An example of this mechanism is a lateral impact auto collision, in which the forces of the collision move the thorax to the side and out from under the head, placing severe lateral stress on the cervical spine. Because of the spine's structure, forces necessary to cause injury from lateral bending are generally less than those needed to cause flexion/extension injury.

AXIAL STRESS Axial stress occurs when either compression or distraction forces are applied to the spine. Compression stress, most commonly called *axial loading*, may occur when a person lifts a weight too great for the strength of the lumbar spine. The weight of the upper torso, head, and neck, in addition to the weight of the object being lifted, pushes against the pelvis, legs, and feet. The lumbar spine is compressed and a vertebra can fracture. Similar compression injuries can also occur when a person falls from a height and lands on the heels. The resulting force is transmitted up the lower extremities to the pelvis, the sacrum, and the lumbar spine. Axial loading injuries are also common in helicopter crashes, where the crash energy is transmitted to the lumbar spine. (Figure 6-35). Another frequent mechanism of axial loading injury is the shallow water dive. In this case, the diver hits the bottom of the pool, lake, or river with the head while the weight of the lower body and the energy of the dive continues to drive

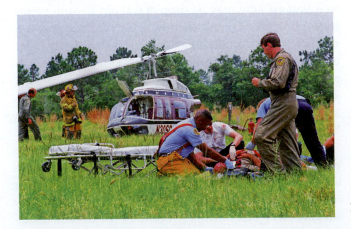

FIGURE 6-35 Axial compression injuries are common in falls from a height and in helicopter crashes.

(© Craig Jackson/In the Dark Photography)

the thorax into the head, crushing the cervical spine. This mechanism also occurs in auto crashes when an occupant is propelled into the windshield by the collision forces. In this case, the impact is likely to compress, fracture, and crush the vertebrae and possibly herniate (rupture) disks. This will often release the gelatinous centers into the vertebral foramina—sometimes compressing the spinal cord. The most common sites of axial loading injuries are between T-12 and L-2 (for lifting injuries and heel-first falls) and the cervical region (for head impacts).

Distraction is the opposite of axial loading. A force, such as gravity applied during a hanging or at the end of a bungee jump, stretches the spinal column and can disrupt ligaments. The process may also stretch and damage the spinal cord without causing physical damage to the spinal column. The upper cervical spine is most commonly affected by this mechanism of injury.

Often, the actual spinal injury process involves complicated combinations of the various injury mechanisms discussed. Hanging may suspend the victim from the side of the head, causing injury from distraction and severe lateral bending directed at the C-1/C-2 region (causing a "hangman's fracture"). The lateral impact auto crash may produce both lateral bending and rotational injuries affecting the cervical spine. The shallow water dive may result in both axial loading and hyperflexion of the neck as the body pushes against and bends the neck. (Note that the cervical spine is posterior to the midline of both the head and chest. In-line impacts frequently cause the head and neck to flex as the body pushes forward.)

Be aware of the distinctions among connective tissue, skeletal, and spinal cord injuries. Connective tissue and skeletal injuries do not necessarily result in spinal cord injuries—although they can. They do represent potential instability of the spinal column and the danger that any subsequent motion may have on the spinal cord and spinal cord injury. Spinal cord injury can also occur without noticeable injury to the ligaments, disks, and vertebrae of the spinal column—particularly in children. This is why a patient who shows signs or symptoms of spine injury, or has experienced a mechanism that suggests the possibility of spine injury, should receive immediate spinal immobilization as soon as possible. Maintain immobilization during all of your assessment, care, and transport.

OTHER MECHANISMS OF SPINAL COLUMN INJURY

As already noted, spinal column injuries can also result from both direct blunt and penetrating trauma. A direct blow to the spine may injure the spinal column, spinal cord, and/or associated structures. Penetrating injuries, caused by objects such as knives, ice picks, or bullets, may also injure the spine. The penetrating object can damage vertebral ligaments, fracture vertebral bodies, force bone fragments directly into the spinal cord, or directly damage

the cord. However, unlike blunt trauma, penetrating injury infrequently causes ligamentous instability of the vertebral column.

As a result of trauma, the tissues adjacent to the spinal cord may swell or otherwise encroach on the vertebral foramen. Because of the close tolerances between the interior surfaces of the vertebral foramen and the cord, this swelling may place pressure on the cord, either causing a direct compression injury or interrupting blood flow through the compressed tissues. Such an injury may also involve the spinal nerve roots close to the injury.

Electrocution, on rare occasions, can cause spinal injury. The extreme and uncontrolled muscle contractions associated with this mechanism of injury can tear tendons and ligaments and fracture vertebrae, resulting in column instability and possible spinal cord injury.

A direct injury to the spinal or vertebral blood vessels, or any swelling from soft tissue or skeletal injuries, can interfere with circulation to portions of the spinal cord. This will likely cause tissue ischemia and compromise of spinal cord function.

The coccygeal region of the spinal column can also be injured. Although it does not contain the spinal cord or many peripheral nerve roots, injury to the region can be painful. Such injuries are usually related to direct blunt trauma, such as a fall onto the upper buttocks region. The coccyx is often fractured during childbirth.

Blunt and penetrating injury mechanisms have different injuries, depending on the structures they involve. The following sections discuss the pathological processes of injuries as they affect the head, face, neck, and spinal column.

Pathophysiology of Spinal Cord Injury

Central nervous system injury—in addition to injury to the brain itself—can involve the spinal cord, which is the principal communications pathway to and from the brain. Any injury along the length of the spinal cord can disrupt these communications and leave the distal organs and muscles without central nervous system control. Spinal cord injury also prevents sensory nerves from communicating with the brain, thereby preventing the brain from accurately perceiving the environment.

Damage to the spinal cord generally occurs in two phases. The initial damage is a direct result of a mechanical event that injures the cord or causes hemorrhage and edema within the substance of the cord itself. Secondary injury is additional or continued tissue destruction that results when hemorrhage and edema compress the cord and reduce circulation to the substance of the cord. Secondary injury can occur within hours of the injury. Remember, the spinal cord is highly dependent on a constant supply of oxygenated blood. Both the primary injury and the secondary injury can compromise spinal cord blood flow.

Spinal Cord Injuries

Spinal cord injuries include concussion, contusion, compression, laceration, hemorrhage, and transection.

CONCUSSION Concussion of the cord, like a concussion of the brain (mild DAI), can cause a temporary and transient disruption of cord function. It does not result in structural damage to the spinal cord itself and, unless there are associated injuries, cord concussion generally resolves over time without any deficits.

CONTUSION A spinal cord contusion is simply a bruising of the spinal cord. It is associated with some tissue damage, vascular leakage, inflammation, and edema. When blood crosses the blood–brain barrier, more significant edema may occur. In general, however, this injury is likely to repair itself with limited residual deficits, if any. The resolution of a cord contusion usually takes longer to resolve than a cord concussion.

COMPRESSION Spinal cord compression may occur secondary to the displacement of a vertebral body, through herniation of an intervertebral disk, displacement of a vertebral bone fragment (Figure 6-36), or swelling of adjacent tissues. The pressure caused by these mechanisms can cause restricted perfusion, ischemic damage, and possibly physical damage to the cord.

LACERATION Cord laceration can occur as bony fragments or other sharp objects are driven into the vertebral foramen or spinal cord and the affected tissues are lacerated or stretched to the point of tearing. Laceration is likely to cause hemorrhage into the cord, swelling from the injury, and disruption of some portions of the cord and their associated communication pathways. In very minor lacerations, some recovery may be expected. Significant or severe lacerations, however, usually result in permanent neurologic deficits.

HEMORRHAGE Spinal cord hemorrhage is often associated with a contusion, laceration, or stretching injury. It can cause injury by disrupting blood flow, causing increased pressure from accumulating blood and irritation caused by blood passing through the blood–brain barrier. Injury to some of the arteries supplying the cord may affect circulation distant from the injury, resulting in an ischemic injury above the level of physical injury.

TRANSECTION Cord **transection** is an injury that partially or completely severs the spinal cord. In a complete transection, the cord is totally cut and the potential to send and receive nerve impulses below the injury site is lost. With a spinal cord transection in the thoracic spine, the signs and symptoms can include incontinence and **paraplegia**. A transection in the cervical spine region can cause **quadriplegia**, incontinence, and partial or complete respiratory paralysis.

Spinal Cord Syndromes

The signs and symptoms seen following a spinal cord injury are directly related to the level of the spinal cord affected and the degree of damage that results from the injury (Figure 6-37). Spinal cord injuries can be classified in various ways, depending on the type of injury and residual deficits. They are often classified as complete or incomplete, depending on the degree of spinal cord interruption. The loss of spinal reflexes after injury to the spinal cord that affects muscles innervated by the cord segments below the site of the injury is called *spinal shock*.

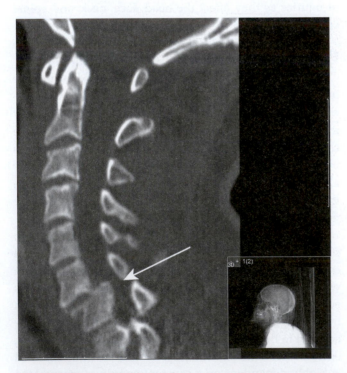

FIGURE 6-36 A displaced bone fragment (as indicated by the arrow) can compress the spinal cord.

(© Dr. Bryan E. Bledsoe)

Effects of Spinal injury

Level of Injury	Effect*
C1 to C5	Paralysis of muscles used for breathing and of all arm and leg muscles, usually fatal
C5 to C6	Legs paralyzed, slight ability to flex arms
C6 to C7	Paralysis of legs and part of wrists and hands; shoulder movement and elbow bending relatively preserved
C8 to T1	Legs and trunk paralyzed; eyelids droop; loss of sweating to the forehead (Horner's syndrome); arms relatively normal, hands paralyzed
T2 to T4	Legs and trunk paralyzed; loss of feeling below the nipples
T5 to T8	Legs and lower trunk paralyzed; loss of feeling below the rib cage
T9 to T11	Legs paralyzed, loss of feeling below the umbilicus
T12 to L1	Paralysis and loss of feeling below the groin
L2 to L5	Different patterns of leg weakness and numbness
S1 to S2	Different patterns of leg weakness and numbness
S3 to S5	Loss of bladder and bowel control; numbness in the perineum

*Loss of bladder and bowel control can occur with severe injury anywhere along the spinal column.

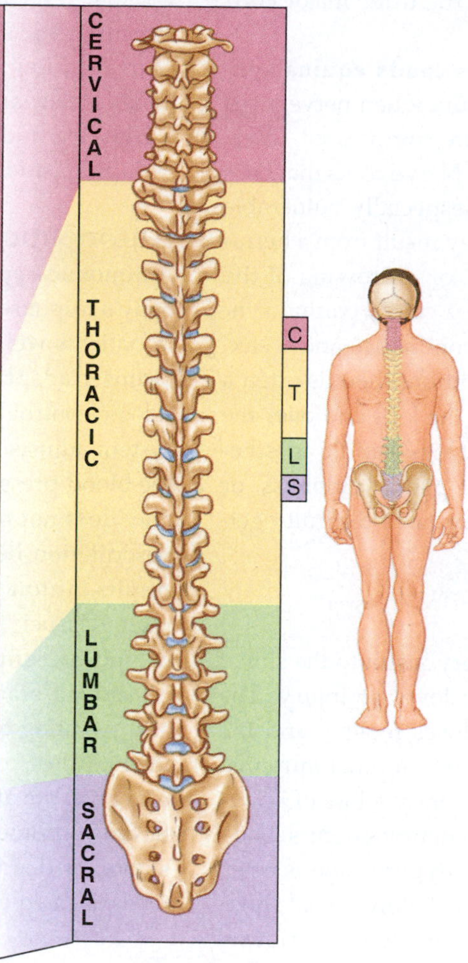

FIGURE 6-37 The effects of a spinal cord injury by spinal level.

Complete cord transection results from a total severing of the spinal cord. The signs and symptoms are related to the level of the cord injured. The signs and symptoms of a complete transection occur in phases.

During the acute phase of a high cervical spine injury, expect to see respiratory insufficiency, quadriplegia, absent upper and lower extremity reflexes (areflexia), lack of sensation below the affected level (anesthesia), and loss of rectal and bladder sphincter tone. Hypothermia is common because the sympathetic nervous system can no longer control the arterioles distributing blood to the skin's surface. These arterioles dilate and increase heat loss to the environment. Injuries to the lower cervical spine will often spare the respiratory muscles. High thoracic lesions may cause lower extremity paralysis (paraplegia) or weakness (paraparesis) instead of the quadriplegia or quadriparesis associated with cervical lesions. With lower thoracic and lumbar lesions, urinary and bowel retention are common and hypotension is rare.

The next phase is the subacute phase. During this phase (usually within 3 to 4 weeks), muscle flaccidity is replaced by the return of intrinsic activity of spinal neurons, and spasticity (muscle spasms and/or stiffness resulting in awkward movement) develops. The signs and symptoms of spinal shock may persist. Autonomic hyperreflexia (discussed in a following section) is also common in the subacute phase.

Anterior cord syndrome results from bony fragments or pressure compressing arteries that perfuse the anterior spinal cord. Anterior cord syndrome is usually caused by a flexion–extension injury that results in damage to the vertebral artery. Thus, the cord is damaged by vascular disruption and subsequent ischemia and infarction. The potential for recovery is poor. The injury generally involves loss of motor function and of sensation to pain, light touch, and temperature below the injury site. The patient is likely to retain motion, positional, and vibration sensation. Anterior cord syndrome is the second most common type of spinal injury.

Central cord syndrome usually results from hyperextension of the cervical spine, as might occur with a forward fall and facial impact. It is often associated with a preexisting degenerative disease, such as arthritis, that has narrowed the vertebral canal. This syndrome causes motor weakness that is more likely to affect the upper rather than the lower extremities, as well as possibly causing bladder incontinence. This syndrome usually occurs in patients older than 50 years of age.

Brown-Séquard syndrome is usually caused by a penetrating injury that affects one side of the cord (hemitransection). The damage to one side results in sensory and motor loss to the ipsilateral side of the body. Pain and temperature perception are lost on the contralateral side of the body. This occurs because of the crossing over of certain nerve fibers as they enter the spinal cord. This injury is rare and is usually associated with some recovery, except in cases of direct penetrating trauma. Brown-Séquard syndrome has the best prognosis of the three major cord syndromes.

Another form of spinal injury is **cauda equina syndrome**. Cauda equina syndrome occurs when nerve roots at the lower end of the spinal cord are compressed, interrupting sensation and motor control. Nerve roots that control bladder and bowel function are especially vulnerable to injury. Cauda equina syndrome may result from a herniated disk, tumor, infection, fracture, or narrowing of the spinal canal. Signs and symptoms of cauda equina syndrome include bowel or bladder incontinence and weakness in the lower extremities. In addition, there is often a loss of or altered sensation between the legs and over the buttocks, the inner thighs and back of legs (saddle anesthesia), and the feet/heels. Because of pain, numbness, or weakness, the patient may stumble or have difficulty getting up from a chair.

Spinal Shock

Spinal shock results from a temporary insult to the spinal cord affecting the body below the level of injury. The affected area becomes flaccid and loses feeling, and the patient is unable to move the extremities or other musculature (flaccid paralysis). There is frequently a loss of bowel and bladder control, and priapism sometimes occurs. Body temperature control is affected, and hypotension is often present as a result of peripheral vasodilation. Spinal shock is often a transient problem if the cord is not seriously damaged.

Neurogenic Shock

Neurogenic shock occurs when injury to the spinal cord or brain or hemorrhage disrupts the brain's ability to control the body—particularly autonomic functions. The interruption of signals limits vasoconstriction, most noticeably in the skin below the level of injury. Lack of sympathetic tone causes the arteries and veins to dilate, expanding the vascular space, resulting in a relative hypovolemia. With the reduced cardiac preload, the heart fails to fill adequately. With inadequate ventricular filling, contraction does not stretch the ventricular walls thus reducing the strength of ventricular contraction (Frank-Starling reflex). Cardiac output is reduced. The process is further compounded as the autonomic nervous system loses sympathetic control over the adrenal medulla and can no longer control the release of epinephrine and norepinephrine. These hormones are responsible for increasing the heart rate against direct parasympathetic stimulation. Their absence restricts the increase in heart rate that normally follows reduced cardiac preload and falling blood pressure. The result of all these factors is a patient in relative hypovolemia without

the compensatory mechanisms to correct it. The patient is unable to maintain blood pressure becaused of a reduced cardiac output, as the body is unable to increase peripheral vascular resistance through vasoconstriction. The patient in neurogenic shock is thus likely to present with a slow heart rate, low blood pressure, and shock-like symptoms (cool, moist, and pale skin) above the cord injury, and warm, dry, and flushed skin below the injury, as well as with priapism in the male.

Autonomic Hyperreflexia Syndrome

Autonomic hyperreflexia syndrome is associated with the body's response to the effects of neurogenic shock. It occurs in patients well after the initial spinal injury as the body begins to adapt to the problems associated with loss of neurologic control below the injury. After a time, the vascular system adjusts to the lack of sympathetic stimulation and the blood pressure returns to normal. However, the body now does not respond to increases in blood pressure with vasodilation below the cord injury, so only bradycardia results. Autonomic hyperreflexia syndrome is most commonly associated with injuries at or above T-5. The syndrome presents with sudden hypertension, as high as 300 mmHg, bradycardia, pounding headache, blurred vision, and sweating and flushing of the skin above the point of injury. Nasal congestion, nausea, and bladder and rectum distention are also frequently present in autonomic hyperreflexia syndrome. The patient is at risk of developing seizures, stroke, or death. Autonomic hyperreflexia syndrome is a medical emergency and must be treated immediately.

Transient Syndromes

There are a few transient (temporary) syndromes associated with spinal cord injury—particularly with injury to the cervical region. These most often result from sporting events. The most common of these is the stinger. A stinger is a sports-related injury to nerves in or near the neck or shoulder. It is sometimes called a burner or nerve pinch injury. However, the the term *stinger* is most descriptive of the symptoms that an athlete experiences, including painful electrical sensations radiating through the neck or one of the arms. Although the stinger is technically a spine injury, it is not a spinal cord injury. The stinger occurs most commonly in contact sports. It is not as catastrophic as a spinal cord injury and does not result in paralysis in the arms or legs.

A more serious condition is *transient quadriplegia*. Transient quadriplegia results from a more serious, but temporary, injury to the cervical spinal cord. Nervous dysfunction can occur in one or both arms, one or both legs, all four extremities, or an arm and leg on the same side of the body. Patients can have numbness or pain, with or without weakness, or complete paralysis. The typical episode of transient quadriplegia usually lasts less than 15 minutes. However, in certain situations it can take up to 48 hours to resolve.

Typically, there is complete return of motor function and sensation and full, pain-free range of motion of the spine. When this dramatic condition occurs, the patient should be treated with all the precautions for a cervical spine injury, including immobilization of the head and neck and transport to an emergency facility. Once a person has experienced an episode of transient quadriplegia, there is a 40 percent chance of a second episode. However, as long as there is no evidence of abnormal motion between the vertebrae or spinal cord compression, athletes are allowed to return to sporting activities without increased risk of permanent nerve injury.

Other Causes of Neurologic Dysfunction

Not all injuries that cause neurologic dysfunction along a dermatome or myotome are related to spinal cord injuries. An injury may occur anywhere along a nerve's path. For example, the C-7 nerve roots travel from just below the seventh cervical vertebra through the shoulder, arm, and forearm before innervating the little finger. The nerve may be damaged by a vertebral fracture or disk protrusion. It can also be damaged distal to the spinal cord through a shoulder, arm, or forearm fracture, soft tissue injury and swelling, penetrating trauma, or compartment syndrome anywhere along the nerve's course.

Any of the injuries previously described may interrupt sensory signals to the brain from the little finger region and motor signals to the region from the brain (to initiate movement and maintain muscle tone). The most obvious difference between nerve root injury and spinal cord injury is the size of the region affected. Remember, however, that an injury that is affecting only a single dermatome may have created a vertebral column instability that threatens the entire cord.

There are also several nontraumatic processes that affect the spinal cord. Refer to the chapter "Neurology" for further information.

Pediatric Spinal Injuries

Pediatric patients are also at risk for spinal injuries, although they occur less frequently than in other age groups. Overall, the incidence of pediatric spine trauma is 10 percent or less of total spine injuries.

There are numerous anatomic differences between the pediatric and the adult spine. These differences account for different injury patterns seen in the various pediatric age groups. The infant's spine has tremendous mobility and elasticity that is due to underdevelopment of the neck muscles as well as incompletely calcified, wedge-shaped vertebrae and shallow, horizontally oriented facet joints. In addition, the relatively large size of the child's head with respect to the torso increases the likelihood of cervical spine injuries, especially between the skull and the first cervical vertebra (atlanto-occipital joint).

Between the ages of 2 and 10, tremendous changes occur in the spinal column. Muscles and ligaments strengthen, bones grow and attain a mature shape and size, and areas of cartilage and soft bone are replaced with normal, calcified bone. In addition, the head becomes smaller in proportion to the torso. These changes shift the focus of injury from the upper cervical spine (skull to C-1–C-2) to the lower cervical spine (C-5–C-6). It appears that age-related maturation in the upper pediatric cervical spine is usually completed by approximately age 10 and maturation of the lower cervical spine occurs by approximately age 14.

The elasticity of the pediatric spine provides more protection against spinal cord trauma than in older patients. This mobility and elasticity help to explain the relatively low incidence of spinal column injuries and the proportionately high incidence of spinal cord injuries without radiographic abnormalities (discussed in the next paragraph). In essence, the young spinal column will stretch, but not break. However, this places the spinal cord at increased risk for distraction injuries.

Children are at risk for the same sort of injuries as adults. However, because the spinal column is more flexible and the ligaments stretch more easily, it is possible for a child to sustain a spinal cord injury despite having normal spinal X-rays. This phenomenon, referred to as spinal cord injury without radiographic abnormality (SCIWORA), is defined as the presence of a spinal injury despite normal radiographic studies (plain X-rays, flexion–extension X-rays, and CT and MRI scans). A young child's vertebral column can withstand elongation without evidence of vertebral column injury even though the spinal cord is injured. The mismatch of elasticity between the vertebral column and spinal cord is the major factor contributing to the high incidence of SCIWORA injuries in young children.

Specific Injuries to the Head, Neck, and Spine
Scalp Injury

The most superficial head injuries involve the scalp (Figure 6-38). A scalp injury may also be the only overt indication of deeper, more serious injury beneath. The scalp overlies the firm skull and is very vascular. The blood vessels lack the ability to constrict as effectively as those found elsewhere in the body. Thus, scalp wounds tend to bleed heavily and persistently. It is said that head injuries do not often result in shock. This, however, assumes that the hemorrhage is easy to control. In fact, any serious blood loss from scalp wounds can contribute to shock and, if left uncontrolled, may cause hypovolemia and shock. Scalp wounds further provide a route for infection because emissary veins drain from the dural sinuses through the skull

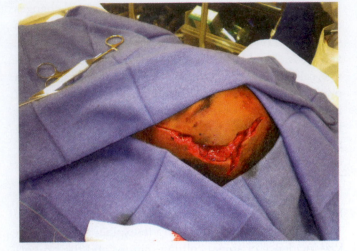

FIGURE 6-38 Scalp wounds can bleed heavily.

(© Dr. Bryan Bledsoe)

and into the superficial venous circulation. Because of rich circulation to the area, scalp wounds tend to heal quickly.

Scalp wounds may confound patient assessment (Figure 6-39). Usually, blunt trauma creates a contusion that, because of the firm skull underneath, expands outwardly in a very rapid and noticeable way. However, blunt trauma may also tear underlying fascia and areolar tissue, causing it to separate. This can leave an elevated border surrounding a depression, mimicking the contour of a depressed skull fracture. However, the scalp's blood vessels may bleed under the skin and into a depressed skull fracture, fill any depression, and conceal the injury. It is therefore important to assess and record the nature of a head wound early in the assessment.

A common and special type of scalp wound is the avulsion. Areolar tissue is only loosely attached to the skull, and glancing blows can create a shearing force against the scalp's border. Such blows frequently tear a flap of scalp loose and fold it back against the uninjured scalp, exposing a portion of the cranium. The mechanism of injury may also seriously contaminate the wound and may cause moderate hemorrhage unless the avulsed tissue folds back sharply, compressing the blood vessels.

Cranial Injury

Because of its spherical shape and skeletal design, the skull does not fracture unless there is significant trauma. Such fractures may present as linear, depressed, comminuted, or basilar in nature (Figure 6-40). Linear fractures are small cracks in the

Scalp/Head Injury Presentations

Scalp
Fascial
Skull

Hematoma The blow disrupts blood vessels, resulting in accumulating blood and a hematoma.

Depression The blow may tear fascial layers under the scalp and result in a depression, with or without a depressed skull fracture.

Normal Scalp Contour Blood may fill the space vacated by the torn fascia layers, or ...

Depressed Fracture Blood may fill the area vacated by a depressed skull fracture.

FIGURE 6-39 A scalp/head injury can present as a raised hematoma, a depression, or disguised by a normal scalp contour.

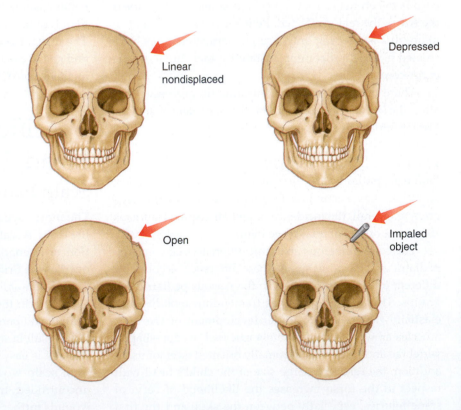

Linear nondisplaced

Depressed

Open

Impaled object

FIGURE 6-40 Various types of skull fractures.

cranium and represent about 80 percent of all skull fractures. The temporal bone is one of the thinnest and most frequently fractured cranial bones. If there are no associated intracranial or vascular injuries, a linear fracture poses very little danger to the patient. In contrast, a depressed fracture represents an inward skull displacement and results in a greater likelihood of intracranial injury. Comminuted fractures involve multiple skull fragments that may penetrate the meninges and cause physical harm to the structures beneath. Remember, severe traumatic brain injury can occur without skull fracture.

A common type of skull fracture involves the base of the skull. This area is permeated with foramina (openings) for the spinal cord, cranial nerves, and various blood vessels. The basilar skull also has hollow or open structures such as the sinuses, orbits of the eye, nasal cavities, external auditory canals, and middle and inner ears. These spaces weaken the skull and leave the basilar area prone to fracture.

Signs of basilar skull fracture vary with the injury's location (Figure 6-41). If a fracture involves the auditory canal and lower lateral areas of the skull, hemorrhage may appear at the mastoid region (just posterior and slightly

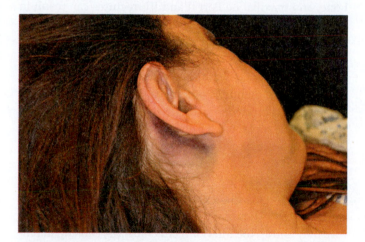

FIGURE 6-41A Retroauricular ecchymosis (Battle's sign).

(© Edward T. Dickinson, MD)

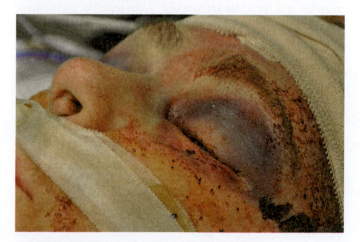

FIGURE 6-41B Periorbital ecchymosis (raccoon eyes).

(© Edward T. Dickinson, MD)

inferior to the ear). This causes a characteristic black and blue discoloration called **retroauricular ecchymosis** or Battle's sign. Another classic basilar skull fracture sign is **bilateral periorbital ecchymosis**, sometimes referred to as "raccoon eyes." This is a dramatic discoloration around both eyes associated with orbital fractures and hemorrhage into the surrounding tissue. Both retroauricular ecchymosis and bilateral periorbital ecchymosis require time to develop. Neither is likely to visible during the period after an injury when the patient is under paramedic care.

Basilar skull fractures can tear the dura mater, causing an opening between the brain and the body's surface. Such a wound may permit cerebrospinal fluid to leak out through the nasal cavity or the external auditory canal and thus provide a possible route for infection to enter the meninges. This wound type may also provide an escape for cerebrospinal fluid in the presence of increasing intracranial pressure. Escaping cerebrospinal fluid may mitigate an increased ICP and somewhat limit damage to the brain. (Cerebrospinal fluid is an important medium, but the body can regenerate it very rapidly.) Although it is not a reliable sign of basilar skull fracture, blood mixed with cerebrospinal fluid and flowing from the nose, mouth, or ears may produce the target or "halo" sign (a dark red circle surrounded by a lighter yellowish ring) when dropped on a pillow or towel.[3,4] Normal blood produces a narrow ring of yellowish coloration around the red circle produced by the less mobile erythrocytes. If cerebrospinal fluid is mixed with the blood, this outer yellowish ring is much larger. Be aware, however, that other fluids, such as lacrimal or nasal fluids or saliva, may cause a similar response. Hence, the halo sign is most reliable when associated with fluid leaking from the ear.

Bullet wounds can cause specific types of cranial fracture. The entrance wound often produces a small, comminuted fracture that often forces bone fragments into the brain. If the bullet's kinetic energy is sufficient to allow the bullet to exit from the skull and cause a second fracture, this exit wound site is usually blown outward and is often more severe in appearance than the entrance wound.

In many cases, the energy of a projectile passing through the skull causes a cavitational wave of pressure that is contained by the rigid cranial vault. This can result is significant damage to the brain, and, if the transmitted kinetic energy is strong enough, the skull may fracture and "explode" outward.

Another wound type occurs when a bullet enters the skull at an angle and is deflected along the skull's interior until its energy is completely exhausted. This process often results in devastating damage to the brain and is rarely survivable.

A special type of head injury is an impaled object. As is the case with objects impaled in most other regions of the body, any further movement of the object motion may cause additional hemorrhage and injury. An impaled object in the head is a serious situation. Brain tissue is much more delicate than other body tissues, does not immobilize the object as well, and is easily injured by object motion. As with objects impaled elsewhere, impaled object removal from the head may cause further injury and increase the rate of blood loss and of subsequent blood accumulation.

Remember that a skull fracture is a skeletal injury that will heal with time. It does not always injure the brain. Rather, it is the possibility of injury beneath the fracture that is of greatest concern. The forces necessary to fracture the skull are significant and likely to cause serious injury within.

Facial Injury

Facial injuries can be serious, not only because of the cosmetic appearance, but also because of the vasculature and airway. In addition, facial injuries can also affect the organs of sight, smell, taste, and hearing. Remember that serious facial injuries suggest associated brain and spinal injuries.

Facial Soft Tissue Injury

Facial soft tissue injury is common and can sometimes threaten both the patient's airway and physical appearance. Because of the ample arterial and venous supply, injuries in the region may bleed heavily, possibly contributing to hypovolemia. Facial injuries are often the result of violence (e.g., bullet or knife wounds). Superficial injuries and hemorrhage rarely affect the airway. With deep lacerations, however, blood may accumulate and threaten the airway or be swallowed, causing vomiting. Serious injuries of the soft tissues and bones supporting the pharynx may reduce the patient's ability to control his airway, increasing the likelihood of foreign body or fluid aspiration with resultant airway compromise. Aspiration and hypoxia are more likely to be due to blood and vomitus rather than physical obstruction.

Remember, inspiration creates a negative pressure in the chest. This negative pressure may cause collapse of damaged structures along the airway that are normally held open by bony or cartilaginous formations. Soft tissue swelling may also rapidly restrict the airway or close it completely. Swelling and deformity from trauma may distort the facial features so landmarks become hard to recognize, thus making airway management even more difficult. In serious facial soft tissue injury, always consider the likelihood of associated injury, especially basilar skull fracture and spinal column injury.

Facial Dislocations and Fractures

Trauma may cause open or closed facial fractures with significant associated pain, swelling, deformity, crepitus,

and hemorrhage. Common injuries include mandibular, maxillary, nasal, and orbital fractures and dislocations.

Mandibular dislocation occurs as the condylar process is displaced from the temporomandibular joint. This dislocation may result in the malocclusion and misalignment of teeth, deformity of the facial region at or around the joint, immobility of the jaw, and pain.

Mandibular fractures are painful and present with deformity along the jaw's surface, and may result in the loosening of teeth. An open mandibular fracture may produce bloodstained saliva. Mandibular fracture may represent a serious life threat if the patient is placed supine. Always look for a second fracture site when you encounter a patient with a mandibular fracture.

Maxillary fractures are classified according to **Le Fort criteria** (Figure 6-42). A slight instability involving the maxilla alone usually has no associated displacement and is classified as a Le Fort I fracture. A Le Fort II fracture involves fractures of both the maxilla and nasal bones and results in instability of the maxilla and nasal region. Le Fort III fractures characteristically involve the entire facial region below the brow ridge, including the zygoma, nasal bone, and maxilla. Le Fort II and III fractures can result in cerebrospinal fluid leakage and may endanger the patency of the nasal and oral aspects of the airway.

Dental injury is commonly associated with serious blunt facial trauma. Teeth may chip, break, loosen, or dislodge from the mandible or maxilla. They may become foreign objects aspirated into the airway. Note that a dislodged tooth may be replanted if fully intact and handled properly during prehospital care.

Orbital (blowout) fractures most commonly involve the inferior shelf of the orbit. This fracture is most common as pressure on the globe fractures the weakest region—the inferior shelf extending into the maxillary sinus. The fracture may entrap the inferior rectus muscles, causing inability of the eye to look upward (when compared to the other eye). Zygomatic arch fractures may also entrap other facial muscles and limit jaw movement. With maxillary fractures, the patient often experiences significant swelling and pain in the maxillary sinus region. Although these injuries are not life threatening, they warrant evaluation by emergency department staff.

Most injuries to the face are limited to soft tissue injuries. The face is very vascular and is supported by skeletal structures underneath. Swelling tends to be rapid and pronounced, deforming the region very quickly. The area is also prone to rapid and significant hemorrhage.

CONTENT REVIEW

➤ Le Fort Facial Fractures
- I—slight instability to maxilla; no displacement
- II—fracture of both maxilla and nasal bones
- III—fracture involving entire face below brow ridge (zygoma, nasal bone, maxilla)

Le Fort I   **Le Fort II**   **Le Fort III**

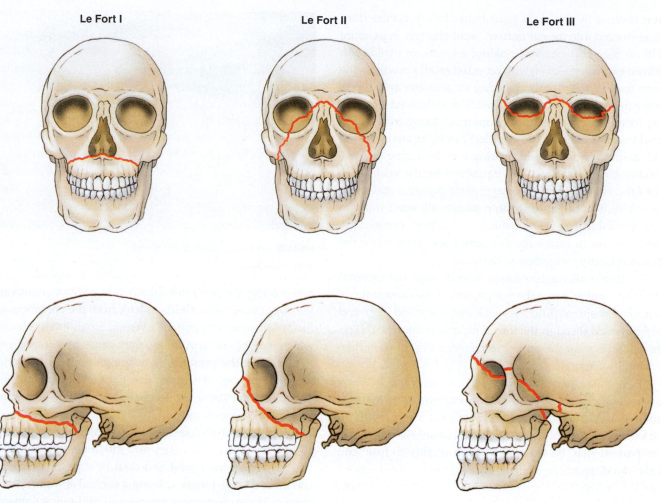

FIGURE 6-42 Le Fort facial fracture classification.

A special type of facial injury is that associated with a suicide attempt using a rifle or shotgun. Typically, the victim places the gun barrel under the chin, but in an effort to pull the trigger, stretches and tilts the head back. The gunshot blast is then directed under the chin and at the facial region, but may be deflected from entering the cranial vault. The result is a very disrupted face with much of the tissues damaged or destroyed. The patient may still be conscious and there is often heavy bleeding that makes it difficult to locate and manage the airway. With such a patient, the airway is in serious danger of obstruction and attempts to secure it can be very challenging.

Nasal Injury

Nasal injuries are painful and often create a deformed appearance, but are not life threatening. Dislocation or fracture of the cartilage and nasal bone may interfere with nasal air passage, and the swelling and associated hemorrhage can be a threat to the airway. However, the conscious and alert patient is usually able to control the airway without problem.

Epistaxis (nosebleed) is a common nasal problem associated with facial trauma. Bleeding can be spontaneous as well as traumatic, and can be further classified as either anterior or posterior. Anterior hemorrhage comes from the nasal septum and is usually due to bleeding from a network of vessels called *Kiesselbach's plexus*. Such hemorrhage bleeds slowly and is usually self-limited. Posterior hemorrhage may be severe and cause blood to drain down the back of the patient's throat. In epistaxis secondary to severe head trauma with likely basilar skull fracture, the nasal cavity's posterior wall integrity may be compromised. Attempts at nasal airway, nasogastric tube, or nasotracheal tube insertion may cause the tube to enter the cranial vault and injure the brain.

Ear Injury

The external ear, or *pinna*, which is exposed to the environment, is often injured. It has a minimal blood supply and often does not bleed heavily when lacerated. In glancing blows, the pinna may be partially or completely avulsed. In a folding type of injury, the cartilage may separate. Because of the poor blood supply, external ear injuries do not heal as well as other facial wounds.

The internal portions of the ear—the external auditory canal and the middle and inner ear—are well protected from trauma by the skull's structure. Injury occurs from objects forced into the ear or from rapid changes in pressure as in diving accidents, water skiing impacts, or explosions. With an explosion—even with repeated small arms fire—the pinna focuses the rapidly changing air pressure and directs it into the external auditory canal. This enhanced pressure may irritate or rupture the tympanum. If strong enough, the small bones of hearing (the ossicles) can be injured, causing a temporary or permanent hearing loss. In diving injuries, the changing pressure is not equalized by the eustachian tube (also called the pharyngotympanic passage) and eventually builds until the eardrum ruptures, allowing water to enter the middle ear. The patient may experience vertigo, which can be an extremely dangerous sensation when the patient is nearly weightless underwater.

Basilar skull fractures may also disrupt the external auditory canal and tear the tympanum. If the dura mater is torn, cerebrospinal fluid may leak into the middle ear and seep outward through the torn tympanum (otorrhea) (Figure 6-43). As with the other mechanisms described earlier, hearing loss may result.

Tympanic injuries are not life threatening and, in many cases, repair themselves—even a rupture that tears as much as half the tympanum. However, a victim with an acute hearing loss can be quite apprehensive and anxious. The patient may be frustrated when unable to hear and understand questions or instructions.

Eye Injury

Although the orbits are effective in protecting the eye, penetrating and some blunt trauma may cause serious injury. The eye structures are specialized, and like most specialized tissues, do not regenerate rapidly. If significant penetrating injury occurs, especially if accompanied by loss of the eye's fluids—aqueous or vitreous humor—the patient's sight is threatened, possibly with permanent loss. A penetrating object is likely to disturb the integrity of the anterior

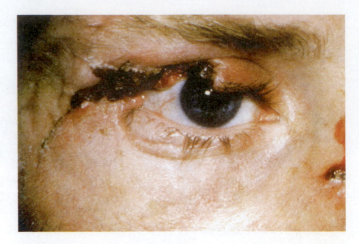

FIGURE 6-44 Laceration of the eyelid.

(© Dr. Bryan Bledsoe)

and possibly the posterior chamber. In addition, removal of the object may allow fluids to leak from the chambers and further threaten the patient's vision. Small foreign bodies, which may be difficult to see, may cause penetrating injuries. Suspect the presence of a foreign body if the patient reports a history of sudden eye pain and a foreign body sensation after using a power saw or grinder—especially when working with metal.

Similarly, small foreign particles that land on the eye's surface can also cause injury and inflammation. The object may embed in the eyelid and then be dragged across the cornea as the eye blinks, causing a corneal abrasions or laceration. These often cause intense and continuing pain even after the object is removed from the eye. These injuries are usually superficial, but they can be deep (Figure 6-44).

Blunt trauma to the eye may result in several types of injuries. Hemorrhage may occur in the anterior chamber and pool, displaying a collection of blood in front of the iris and pupil. This condition, called **hyphema**, is a potential threat to the patient's vision. It requires evaluation by an ophthalmologist and may result in hospital admission.

A less serious, but equally dramatic, eye injury is a subconjunctival hemorrhage. This may occur after a strong sneeze, vomiting episode, or direct eye trauma, such as orbital contusion. It occurs when a small blood vessel in the subconjunctival tissue ruptures, leaving a portion of the eye's surface blood red (Figure 6-45). Subconjunctival hemorrhage often clears without intervention and rarely causes any residual scars or impairment.

Blunt trauma may fracture the orbit and produce an injury called *eye avulsion*. In such a case, the eye is not really avulsed but appears to protrude from the wound as the orbital structure is crushed and depressed. If the eye, nerves, and vasculature remain intact, sight in the eye can often be salvaged. Blunt trauma from such mechanisms as a racquetball or baseball may compress the orbital contents, fracturing the inferior orbital wall, entrapping the inferior rectus muscles, and displacing orbital contents (fat) and

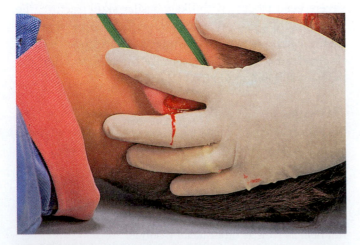

FIGURE 6-43 Blood or fluid draining from the patient's ear suggests basilar skull fracture.

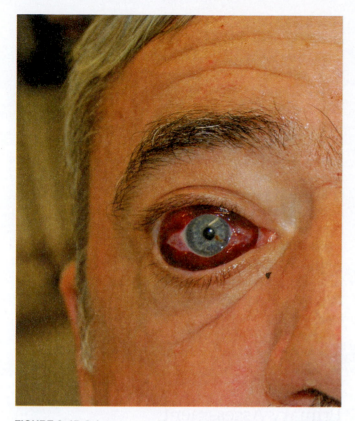

FIGURE 6-45 Subconjunctival hemorrhage.
(© Edward T. Dickinson, MD)

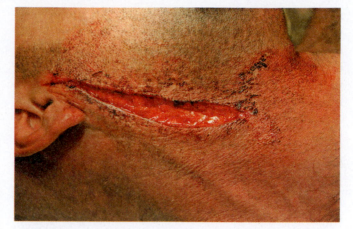

FIGURE 6-46 Laceration to the neck.
(© Edward T. Dickinson, MD)

blood into the maxillary sinus. These injuries may present with a depressed eye, called *enophthalmos*.

Trauma can also cause **retinal detachment**, in which the retina separates from the eye's posterior wall. The patient typically complains of a dark curtain obstructing part of the field of view. This is a true sight-threatening emergency.

Soft tissue lacerations can occur around the eye and involve the eyelid. If not properly identified and repaired, such an injury may disrupt lacrimal duct function and interrupt corneal lubrication and oxygenation. Another soft tissue problem may occur if a contact lens is left in the eye of an unconscious patient. The contact lens will then obstruct the normal lacrimal fluid flow across the eye. This circulation loss may dry out the eye's surface and cause hypoxic injury. The result is usually severe eye pain and possible corneal damage.

Neck Injury

The neck is protected from impact by the more anterior head and chest and by skeletal and muscular structures. The neck's major skeletal component is the cervical vertebral column, which is supported by interconnecting ligaments. The neck muscles provide additional protection to the vital structures in the neck. They include the muscles that support and move the head, as well as the shoulder muscles that help move the upper extremities. The skeletal structures and muscles of the neck protect the airway, carotid and jugular blood vessels, and the esophagus well from all but anterior blunt trauma and deep penetrating trauma. Penetrating trauma may result in serious injuries to the airway, spine, blood vessels, and other structures in the region.

Trauma to Blood Vessels of the Neck

Blunt trauma to a blood vessel can cause a serious and rapidly expanding hematoma. This hematoma may be trapped within the fascia of the region and restrict the jugular veins. Laceration of the external jugular vein, or deep laceration involving the internal jugular vein or the carotid arteries, usually results in severe hemorrhage as a result of the large vessel size (Figure 6-46). Laceration of these structures and subsequent hemorrhage can rapidly lead to hypovolemia and shock. Arterial injury may cause subsequent brain hypoxia and infarct, mimicking signs and symptoms of a stroke. An open neck wound involving the internal jugular vein may allow formation of an air embolism as the venous pressure drops below atmospheric pressure with deep respirations.

Airway Trauma

Trauma may also injure the larynx and trachea. Severe blunt or penetrating trauma may separate the larynx from the trachea, fracture or crush either of these two structures, or open the trachea to the environment. These injuries may result in serious hemorrhage that threatens the airway, also causing vocal cord contusion or swelling, irritation and injury to the epiglottis (epiglottitis), destruction of the integrity of the airway, disruption of normal airway landmarks, and restrictive soft tissue swelling.

Other Neck Trauma

The neck may also demonstrate subcutaneous emphysema from tension pneumothorax (air pushed into the skin from intrathoracic pressure that migrates to the neck) or from tracheal injury in the neck. Penetrating trauma may also involve the esophagus, perforating it and permitting gastric contents or undigested material to enter the fascia. Because the fascia communicates with the mediastinum, this foreign material can physically harm mediastinal structures or provide the medium for infection (mediastinitis), which may cause devastating results. Deep penetrating trauma may injure the vagus nerve, causing tachycardia and gastrointestinal disturbances. More anterior and superficial injuries may damage the thyroid and parathyroid glands.

Spinal Column Injury

Several areas of the spinal column are especially subject to injury. The cervical region accounts for over half of all spinal injuries, with the atlas/axis (C-1/C-2) joint being the site of the majority of fatal spine injuries. This is due to the very delicate nature of these two vertebrae, the mobility of the joint, and the weight of the head they support. C-7 is also injured frequently because it is located at the transition between the flexible cervical spine and the more rigid thoracic spine.

Similar injuries can occur at the transition point between the thoracic and lumbar vertebrae (T-12/L-1). The lumbosacral area (L-5/S-1) likewise can be injured because the pelvis effectively stabilizes the sacral spine. Spinal injuries not associated with the cervical spine are about equally divided between the thoracolumbar and lumbosacral regions.

Remember that the spinal cord ends at the L-1/L-2 region. Below this point, the spinal nerve roots extend until they exit the spinal column (cauda equina). These spinal nerve roots are more mobile than the cord and less likely to be injured within the spinal foramen during spinal column injury.

Assessment of the Patient with a Head, Neck, or Spine Injury

Assessment of the patient with a potential central nervous system (brain and spinal cord) injury should progress through the normal patient assessment steps: scene size-up, primary assessment, secondary assessment (rapid or focused trauma assessment), and periodic reassessments. The mechanisms and physical signs of injury associated with these injuries are the greatest reasons to suspect central nervous system injury. If they are found, suspect and treat for traumatic brain and spinal cord injury as well. Patient assessment and care as presented in this chapter are for patients who do not otherwise have overt signs and symptoms of physical injury to the region, yet may have a CNS injury that presents with a more subtle and specific presentation.

Scene Size-up

Analyze the mechanism of injury to identify the probability of injury to the head, neck, and back. Try to mentally visualize movements of the brain and spine during any collision process. Typical MOIs that might cause brain and spinal cord injury are auto collisions, falls, sports injuries, explosions, assaults, and penetrating trauma. These mechanisms are likely to cause soft tissue wounds and other evidence of the injury. However, consider the possibility of severe flexion, extension, lateral bending, rotation, axial loading, or distraction injuries. Often. traumatic brain injury—and, sometimes, spinal cord injury—can occur without obvious external evidence. If a likely mechanism is found or suspected, anticipate these and prepare to assess and treat as required. However, be alert for brain and spinal cord injuries. Remember, the soft tissue injuries to the head and neck and skeletal injuries to the skull and vertebral column will usually heal uneventfully. It is the central nervous system injury that is the most significant threat to the patient's life and quality of life. Even if the incident does not appear to involve a significant mechanism of injury, look for and ensure that there are no signs or symptoms of spinal cord or brain injury during the early assessment.

Primary Assessment

If the scene survey identifies any reason to suspect spinal injury, apply spinal stabilization as determined by your local protocols. These may range from placement of a cervical collar to full backboard application. These precautions can be discontinued later if the patient meets the criteria established by a spinal clearance protocol. Full spinal precautions are generally ineffective and can cause some patient discomfort and extend scene time. Generally, a patient sustaining any serious injury should receive spinal stabilization as determined by local protocols. However, recognize that a progressing traumatic brain injury requires care only available at a neurosurgical center.

Begin to form an initial patient impression with the primary assessment. Carefully determine the patient's level of consciousness and orientation (person, place, and time). Any deviation from rapid and clear answers to any questions should raise suspicions for possible brain injury. Even though determining the patient's mental status may add a few seconds to the primary assessment, detecting trends can be critical to rapid identification of a traumatic brain injury. Question the patient about the event and identify any retrograde, event, or anterograde amnesia. Make sure any questions and answers from the patient are appropriate to the circumstances. Suspect brain injury if you can identify any reduced mental acuity in your patient.

Note the patient's facial skin color, respiratory effort, and level of responsiveness throughout the primary assessment, as these factors can aid in recognition of brain injury.

Table 6-3 Simplified Motor Score (SMS)

SMS Score	Definition	Sample Patient Response(s)
SMS 2	Obeys commands	Responds appropriately to a request to move an extremity or blink
SMS 1	Localizes pain	Makes a purposeful movement toward a painful stimulus, such as reaching across the midline and above a clavicle when supraorbital pressure is applied
SMS 0	Withdraws from pain or worse	Merely moves hand or other body part when the flesh between thumb and first finger is squeezed, or—worse—maintains a decorticate or decerebrate posture or has no response to any stimulus.

Throughout the primary assessment continue to develop an impression of the patient's injury and refine this impression with any and all information gathered during any subsequent questioning and assessment.

Simplified Motor Score

If the MOI or initial impression suggests a traumatic brain injury, consider performing a **Simplified Motor Score (SMS)** evaluation. This simplified system is used to predict possible brain injury and appears to have similar clinical validity when compared to the Glasgow Coma Scale (discussed later under "Secondary Assessment"), yet the SMS is simple and rapid enough to include during the early primary assessment.

The SMS (Table 6-3) considers three elements of the motor component of GCS:

- Obeys commands = 2
- Localizes pain = 1
- Withdraws to pain or worse = 0

A patient is given an SMS score of 2 if he can respond to a request to move an extremity or other body part, like blinking his eyes. The patient receives an SMS score of 1 if he makes a purposeful movement toward a painful stimulus. For example, his hand crosses the midline and moves above a clavicle when supraorbital pressure is applied. The patient receives an SMS score of 0 if he simply withdraws his hand or moves another part of the body when the soft tissues between the thumb and first finger are firmly squeezed, or—worse—if he maintains a decorticate or decerebrate posture, or if he makes no response to any stimulus.

A score of less than 2 (i.e., 1 or 0) suggests transport to a neurology or trauma center. A score of 0 suggests the need for endotracheal intubation.

Airway

Airway maintenance in the brain injury patient is critical.[5] A reduced level of consciousness may leave the patient unable to protect his airway. If the patient does not withdraw to painful stimuli, it may be necessary to protect the airway with an extraglottic airway or endotracheal tube while using spinal precautions.[5] If the patient does withdraw to painful stimuli and is not fully conscious and alert, monitor the airway carefully, with large-bore suction ready in case of vomiting. If not contraindicated by injuries, consider placing the patient in either the recovery position or with the head and shoulders elevated 15 degrees. Both positions reduce the risk of aspiration. Always be prepared to protect the airway if the patient's level of consciousness diminishes to a point at which the protective airway reflexes are lost. As suspected brain injury patients are also likely to have spinal injury, maintain spinal precautions and neutral spinal positioning during any airway procedure.

Breathing

Closely monitor the patient's breathing to ensure that he is moving an adequate volume of air. Determine the respiratory rate, depth, and rhythm.

If the patient is breathing fewer than 10 times per minute, moving significantly less than 500 mL of air with each breath, or has a minute volume of less than 4 liters, consider ventilating the patient. Remember that head injury is likely to produce irregular breathing patterns and that hypoxia and hypercarbia both contribute to morbidity and mortality with traumatic brain injury. Ventilations for any head injury patient should be guided by capnography.[6] For the head injury patient without signs of herniation, adjust ventilation rates to maintain a capnography reading of between 35 and 40 mmHg (adults at about 10 breaths per minute, children at about 20 breaths per minute, and infants at about 25 breaths per minute). For patients with suspected herniation (increasing blood pressure, slowing pulse rate, and erratic respirations), capnography readings should range between 30 and 35 mmHg, using ventilation rates about 10 breaths per minute faster than for patients without herniation.[6,7] Remember, too little or too much CO_2 can have dire effects on the head injury patient.[8] Carefully guide ventilations with capnography. For a patient who is breathing adequately, use pulse oximetry to monitor oxygenation. If saturation is below 96 percent, apply supplemental oxygen to maintain a saturation of at least 96 percent. It is essential to keep oxygen saturation above 95 percent with a traumatic brain injury patient.[9]

Circulation

Carefully evaluate the patient's pulse. If the rate is below 60 beats per minute and strong (and the patient is not a well-conditioned athlete), suspect brain injury. If the rate is normal (between 60 and 100 beats per minute) and there are injuries or hemorrhage that would suggest hypovolemia and shock, control any significant hemorrhage noted during the primary assessment, as hypovolemia can be especially devastating when associated with brain injury.

Recognition of Herniation

It is important to try to recognize the signs of brain herniation early. It is a significant threat to the patient's life and requires prompt intervention. The patient experiencing brain herniation is likely to have an increasing systolic blood pressure (noted by a very strong, bounding pulse), slow and decreasing pulse rate, and respirations that become dramatically irregular (Cushing's triad). The patient will most certainly have a decreasing level of consciousness (Glasgow Coma Scale score ≤8 or SMS score <2 and dropping), singular or bilaterally dilated and fixed pupils, and posturing (decerebrate or decorticate) or no movement at all with noxious stimuli. These patients require immediate ventilation, guided by capnography, to a carbon dioxide level of 30 to 40 mmHg. They also require immediate transport to a neurology or trauma center.

At the conclusion of the primary assessment, categorize the possible brain injury patient as unstable and provide rapid transport to the nearest appropriate trauma center. The suspected traumatic brain-injured patient should receive a rapid trauma assessment and a careful evaluation of vital signs and Glasgow Coma Scale.

Patient Priority

At the end of the primary assessment, you must identify the patient's category for care and transport. One such system is CUPS. It is an acronym for four patient categories. A critical (C) patient is one who has a problem with airway, breathing, and/or circulation and does not ever make it out of the primary assessment process, as he requires immediate transport. Unstable (U) and potentially unstable (P) patients receive the rapid trauma assessment, whereas stable (S) patients may receive the focused trauma assessment. With most head, face, and neck injury patients, try to perform a rapid trauma assessment because of the increased likelihood of airway, vascular, special sense organ, or central nervous system injuries. If there is no significant mechanism of injury and injuries appear minor and superficial, perform a focused trauma exam directed at the specific location(s) of injury.

Secondary Assessment/Rapid Trauma Assessment

Complete the rapid trauma assessment for patients with suspected central nervous system injury, along with the special neurologic assessment elements described here. Remember, the patient with suspected head, neck, and spinal column injury is likely to have a brain and/or spinal cord injury as well. In contrast, patients with brain and/or spinal cord injuries are likely to have head, neck, and spinal column injuries.

Eye Exam

In general, eye reactivity reflects the brain's oxygenation status. Watch for bright and sparkling eyes and briskly reactive pupils. Shine a bright light into the eyes—or in bright sunlight, shade them—and watch for sluggishness, non-reactivity, and constriction (or dilation). Ensure that reactivity is bilateral. Note that both eyes should respond to changes in light intensity affecting only one eye (**consensual reactivity**). Both eyes should track together and, at rest, directly forward. Usually, an affected pupil is on the same side (ipsilateral) as a head injury. If the head is turned during assessment or care, watch eye movement. Normally, the eyes will move more slowly as the head is turned. If the eyes move with the head, it is suggestive of head injury and is called the doll's eyes (oculocephalic) response. If spine injury cannot be ruled out, do not try to elicit this response.

Pay close attention to the eyes when evaluating a patient with possible head trauma. The eyes can provide indications of problems with cranial nerves CN-II, III, IV, and VI and with perfusion associated with cerebral blood flow. The eyes also give quick, highly visible signs of the patient's demeanor—anxiety, fear, anger, and so forth.

Pupil size and reactivity also give clues to underlying conditions. Depressant drugs or cerebral hypoxia will reduce pupillary responsiveness, whereas extreme hypoxia causes them to dilate and remain fixed. An expanding cranial lesion can place progressive pressure on the oculomotor nerve (CN-III), causing the ipsilateral (same side) pupil to become sluggish and subsequently dilated and fixed. This occurs because the outer oculomotor nerve contains parasympathetic fibers. As increasing pressure interferes with these nerve fibers, the pupil dilates and is unable to constrict. If one pupil is fixed yet shows some response to consensual stimulation (light variations in the other eye), the problem most likely lies with the oculomotor nerve.

Full-Body Physical Exam

During the full-body exam, carefully observe and palpate each body region. With spinal cord injury, there may be a transverse line across the body beneath which the skin is flush and warm and above which the skin is cool and clammy. This is the result of the loss of nervous control below the level of injury. It also suggests that the body is unable to regulate blood flow movement below the injury and suggests blood pooling there, even in the presence of shock. Above the level of injury, peripheral vascular constriction, compensating for hypovolemia, limits blood flow to the skin. This patient has a limited ability to compensate for shock and is in danger of early decompensation.

During the full-body physical assessment, look for any line of demarcation between normal sensation and paresthesia or anesthesia and any differences in muscle tone. Begin the exam with the feet, and work up the body toward the head. Try not to alarm the patient, because if he recognizes that he cannot sense touch, his anxiety and fear may increase. Use a sharp object not likely to cause injury, and move upward. A splintered tongue blade or wooden applicator stick works nicely and has the advantage of being disposable. Note the level where the patient first identifies sensation or pain and relate it to the dermatomes. Mark the level at which sensation is first noticed with a felt-tipped pen and compare with subsequent exams.

In addition, evaluate the myotomes to determine the level of muscular control. Suspect muscle flaccidity if a body area has muscle masses with a more relaxed tone than the rest of the body. These neurologic signs provide a good indication of the level of spinal cord injury. Examine both sides of the body because there may be differences from side to side both in sensation and in levels of voluntary and involuntary (muscle tone) motor activity.

Continue the exam, inspecting each distal extremity and evaluating both motor and sensory function. If there is any extremity injury, perform what spinal assessment is possible while working around the injuries and ensuring that no further harm occurs.

For each upper extremity, test finger abduction/adduction (T-1) by having the patient spread the fingers of each hand while you squeeze the second, third, and fourth fingers together. There should be bilaterally equal and moderate resistance. Test finger or hand extension (C-7) by having the patient hold the fingers and/or wrists fully extended. Place pressure against the back of the fingers while holding the forearm in place. Again, there should be bilaterally equal and moderate resistance. Finally, have the patient squeeze your first two fingers in his hand and ensure that the grip is firm and bilaterally equal.

To assess for limb sensation, first ask about any abnormal feelings in the limb—inability to move (paralysis), weakness (paraparesis), numbness (anesthesia), tingling (paresthesia), or pain. Have the patient close both eyes and check his ability to distinguish between sensations of pain and light touch. To check pain perception (the spinothalamic tract), use a pointed object not likely to cause injury and yet induce slight point pain. To check for light touch (involving several tracts), use a cotton swab or a gentle touch with the pad of a finger. Responses to both pain and touch stimulation should be bilateral and equal.

Also test motor and sensory function for the lower extremities. Place your hand against the ball of the patient's foot and have him push firmly against it (plantar flexion, S-1 and S-2). Then place your hand on top of the toes and have the patient pull the toes and foot upward (dorsiflexion, L-5).

Table 6-4 Cervical Spine Exam Reminder

Nerve Root	Muscle Group/Function
C-5	Deltoid
C-6	Wrist extension
C-7	Wrist flexion
C-8	Finger Flexors
T-1	Interossei (flaring of fingers)

To evaluate pain sensation, use the same techniques you used in testing the upper extremities. Lower limb strength and sensations should be present and bilaterally equal.

Check for Babinski's sign by stroking the lateral aspect of the bottom of the foot and watch for toe and great toe movement. Fanning of the toes and dorsiflexion (lifting) of the great toe is a positive sign and suggests injury along the pyramidal (descending spinal) tracts.

If discrete areas of neurologic deficit exist, correlate these to an injury along the nerve pathway or suspect injury to the spinal nerve root as it emerges from the spinal column. A nerve root injury suggests a vertebral column injury and a need for spinal immobilization. Also consider that the source of a deficit may be peripheral nerve damage related to soft-tissue or skeletal damage along its pathway to the affected area. Again, try to identify the associated dermatome and myotome and, thus, the likely location of the lesion along the spinal column, spinal root, or peripheral nerve (Table 6-4 and Table 6-5).

Always check the blood glucose level in patients with suspected head injury. Research has found that hypoglycemia increases the morbidity and mortality rate in these patients. It may be prudent to perform a quick blood glucose check to ensure the glucose level is above 60 mg/dL. If not, administer small amounts of IV glucose ($D_{50}W$ or $D_{10}W$) to maintain a glucose level between 60 and 100. Avoid hyperglycemia, as it is associated with poor outcomes in head injured patients.

Vital Signs

Monitor the patient's vital signs very carefully and look for any evidence of increasing intracranial pressure. Carefully

Table 6-5 Lumbar Spine Exam Reminder

Nerve Root	Muscle Group/Function
L-2/L-3	Quadriceps muscles
L-4	Ankle dorsiflexion/inversion
L-5	Great toe extension
S-1	Foot plantar flexion and eversion

note the pulse rate and strength. A strong and especially slow pulse suggests increasing ICP. Monitor the blood pressure carefully and pay close attention to the pulse pressure. A wide pulse pressure (a high systolic blood pressure and a normal diastolic pressure) is a sign of increasing intracranial pressure and cardiovascular compensation to ensure adequate cerebral perfusion pressure. Record the pulse rate and blood pressure readings and recognize that a slowing pulse rate and an increasing systolic blood pressure represent an ominous trend. Apply the ECG monitor and look for arrhythmias. On the other hand, hypotension in the traumatic brain injury patient can be especially dangerous. An increasing systolic blood pressure is a reflex to ensure that cerebral blood flow in the presence of increased intracerebral pressure is adequate. If the cardiovascular system cannot respond with this reflex because it is already compensating for blood loss and hypovolemia, cerebral perfusion may drop to critical levels, resulting in increased morbidity and mortality. In a suspected traumatic brain injury patient, it is essential to maintain a systolic blood pressure of at least 90 mmHg with aggressive fluid resuscitation.

Finally, note the respiratory pattern. An increased respiratory rate and volume or erratic respiration—Cheyne-Stokes, central neurologic hyperventilation, or ataxic respirations—suggest brainstem injury. Be alert for Cushing's triad—a combination of a slowing pulse rate, increasing systolic blood pressure, and irregular respirations.

Body temperature is also an important consideration when evaluating the potential spinal injury patient. Spinal injury patients are subject to fluctuations in body temperature related to ambient temperature changes. This is because these patients lose the ability to control the skin's heat conservation/dissipation function below the level of the spinal cord lesion. Although this does not result in an obvious sign, the patient is still highly susceptible to body temperature fluctuations. Cover the patient with blankets in all but the warmest environments, watch for any patient complaint of being cold, and monitor the patient's temperature carefully.

At the rapid trauma assessment's conclusion, determine the need for rapid transport. A history of head trauma coupled with any history of unconsciousness, a degradation in the level of orientation or consciousness, or any vital sign suggestive of traumatic brain injury requires rapid transport to the closest appropriate facility. If such signs and symptoms of brain injury exist, begin rapid transport and contact medical direction for approval to transport to the nearest trauma center.

Glasgow Coma Scale

As already noted, with a mechanism of injury that has caused or is likely to cause head, neck, or spinal column injury, a central nervous system injury must be considered. A commonly used tool for scoring neurologic deficits is the **Glasgow Coma Scale (GCS)** score. However, although it has been a mainstay in neurologic assessment for decades, the GCS has been more recently considered not to be the predictor of patient outcome it was once thought to be. Consult local system protocols and medical direction to identify how this evaluation tool is used in your system. (Some systems are beginning to use the Simplified Motor Score [SMS], described earlier, along with or instead of the GCS.) See further notes about use of the GCS in the paragraph at the end of this section.

If your system uses the GCS, it is important to determine the patient's initial GCS score and repeat the evaluation frequently. This will aid in detection of any patient deterioration and the possibility of progressing brain injury.

The GCS is a standardized evaluation method used to measure a patient's level of consciousness. It is often used to determine the patient's criticality, the need for intubation, and how quickly transport is required. The scale assesses the best eye opening, verbal, and motor response and awards points for the various responses, with a total score that will range between 3 and 15 points (see the adult GCS in Table 6-6 and the pediatric GCS in Table 6-7). A patient with a score of 13 or 14 is considered to have a mild

Table 6-6 Glasgow Coma Scale

Eye Opening	
Spontaneous	4
To verbal command	3
To pain	2
No response	1
Verbal Response	
Oriented and converses	5
Disoriented and converses	4
Inappropriate words	3
Incomprehensible sounds	2
No response	1
Motor Response	
Obeys verbal commands	6
Localizes pain	5
Withdraws from pain (flexion)	4
Abnormal flexion in response to pain (decorticate rigidity)	3
Extension in response to pain (decerebrate rigidity)	2
No response	1

Table 6-7 Pediatric Glasgow Coma Scale

		>1 Year	<1 Year	
Eye Opening	4	Spontaneous	Spontaneous	
	3	To verbal command	To shout	
	2	To pain	To pain	
	1	No response	No response	
		>1 Year	**<1 Year**	
Best Motor Response	6	Obeys		
	5	Localizes pain	Localizes pain	
	4	Flexion–withdrawal	Flexion–withdrawal	
	3	Flexion–abnormal (decorticate rigidity)	Flexion–abnormal (decorticate rigidity)	
	2	Extension (decerebrate rigidity)	Extension (decerebrate rigidity)	
	1	No response	No response	
		>5 Years	**2–5 Years**	**0–23 Months**
Best Verbal Response	5	Oriented and converses	Appropriate words and phrases	Smiles, coos, cries appropriately
	4	Disoriented and converses	Inappropriate words	Cries
	3	Inappropriate words	Cries and/or screams	Inappropriate crying and/or screaming
	2	Incomprehensible sounds	Grunts	Grunts
	1	No response	No response	No response

head injury. A score of 9 to 12 indicates moderate injury, whereas a score of ≤8 represents severe head injury. Most patients with a GCS of ≤8 are in a coma and are likely to need endotracheal intubation.

GCS points are awarded as follows:

- For eye-opening response (E), award 1 point for no response, 2 points for eye opening in response to pain, 3 points for eye opening in response to verbal command, and 4 points for spontaneous eye opening.

- For verbal response (V), award 1 point for no sound or response; 2 points for incomprehensible, garbled sounds; 3 points for inappropriate words and speech that make no sense; 4 points for confused or disoriented speech; and 5 points for clear and oriented speech.

- For motor response (M), award 1 point for no movement or response, 2 points for decerebrate posturing, 3 points for decorticate posturing, 4 points for withdrawal of a body part from pain, 5 points for purposeful movement (of the hand) to localize pain, and 6 points for following simple verbal commands.

The lowest total GCS value is 3, which represents a completely unresponsive patient. The maximum GCS value is 15, which represents the conscious, but not necessarily fully oriented, patient.

Record the best response for each of the GCS criteria (for example, as E_3, V_4, M_5), and note any differences, either from side to side or in the upper versus lower extremities. Record any asymmetry in your GCS findings, and monitor for any trends. Determine the GCS score every 5 minutes (with reassessments) in the patient with any GCS less than 15.

The pediatric patient is a special challenge to GCS assessment. To arrive at an accurate value, modify your evaluation of the child's best verbal response as appropriate for the developmental age.

Again, as noted at the beginning of this section, there has recently been research noting that the GCS is an imperfect means of assessing level of consciousness. First, there is wide variability in the ability of providers of all types (physician, nursing, prehospital) to accurately and reproducibly measure the GCS in patients.[10] Secondly, the GCS does not detect subtle but important changes in the level of consciousness—for example, the otherwise lucid patient who is fully oriented to person and place, but not time. Finally, and perhaps most important for prehospital trauma care, the GCS is an imperfect measure of when airway protection and intubation are indicated. Other factors, including objective assessment of airway patency (e.g., presence of airway reflexes such as cough, handling of secretions, and evidence of obstructed airflow), may be more important. Continue to use the GCS in your assessment and treatment decisions based on local system standards.[11]

Other Signs of Nervous System Injury

A sign sometimes associated with spinal injury in the male is priapism. This prolonged, possibly painful, nonsexual erection of the male genitalia is due to unopposed parasympathetic stimulation. Disruption of the sympathetic (thoracolumbar) pathways following a cervical spine injury inhibits sympathetic tone, allowing parasympathetic tone to predominate. This produces priapism. Often, though, pain sensation here is lost because of disruption of the sensory pathways.

Infrequently, a patient with midcervical spine injury presents in the "hold-up" position. In this case the patient's arms rise to a position above the shoulders and head. This occurs because injury paralyzes adductor and extensor muscles, while the patient maintains control over the abductors and flexors. Without adductor and extensor opposition, normal muscle tone impulses or any attempt by the patient to move the limb cause it to move toward the flexed position. When treating such a patient, simply secure the patient's wrists to his belt to hold the limbs down for transport.

If the patient (who is not elderly or very young) is able to reliably report information about the injury and does not show any signs or symptoms of spinal injury, or the mechanism of injury does not suggest spinal injury, ask the patient to gently move his neck. If the patient experiences any pain or discomfort with neck motion or shows any neurologic deficit, employ spinal precautions and consider transport to a trauma center for further evaluation. Also continue to monitor the extremities for signs of neurologic impairment. If any are found, immediately employ spinal precautions.

Traumatic brain injury may cause seizures. Seizures are serious complications because they may compromise the airway and respirations, increase intracranial pressure, and exacerbate any existing brain injury. If a seizure is observed, or the patient or bystanders describe one, determine as much about the episode to be prepared to describe the seizure in detail, including its origin and progression, to the attending physician. Protect any patient with seizures from further injury and be especially cognizant of the airway. Consider the administration of diazepam or lorazepam if needed.

Patient Questioning

While carrying out the rapid trauma assessment, question the responsive patient regarding headache and increased light sensitivity (photophobia), which are common symptoms of brain injury. Also question the patient regarding memory of the events preceding and following the injury to identify any retrograde and anterograde amnesia. Note any repetitive questioning by the patient to identify what happened (inability to establish short-term memory) and any unusual behavior or confusion.

In addition to evaluating signs and symptoms (the S in SAMPLE history), question the patient regarding the elements of the AMPLE history (allergies, medications, pertinent past history, last oral intake, events leading to the injury), with special focus on any information regarding pre-incident nervous system injury or illness. Alcohol or drug intoxication will make assessment more difficult and mask signs of central nervous system injury.[11] Also be especially cognizant of any recent history of anticoagulant therapy, such as aspirin, warfarin (Coumadin), dabigatran (Pradaxa), rivaroxaban (Xarelto), or enoxaparin (Lovenox). These medications are anticoagulants and may make the patient more prone to bleeding associated with any brain or spine injury.

Reassessment

Perform reassessments every 5 minutes for patients with potentially serious injuries. Be especially alert for a slowing pulse, increasing systolic blood pressure (an increasing pulse pressure), and development of deeper, more rapid, or erratic respirations (Cushing's triad). Carefully monitor the patient for changes in consciousness and orientation as well. Perform serial GCS or SMS evaluations and note any changes or trends. Finally, watch the eyes for signs of cerebral hypoxia—they become dull and lackluster—or of increasing intracranial pressure—one pupil becomes sluggish, nonreactive, then dilated. Also look for any changes in the dermatomes and myotomes affected by the injury. Note any changes in any element of patient presentation and track any trends to identify whether the patient's condition is deteriorating, improving, or remaining the same (Figure 6-47).

Monitor pulse oximetry, capnography, and blood pressure readings to ensure that the patient does not become hypoxic and/or hypovolemic. Both these conditions are associated with increased mortality and morbidity in traumatic brain injury. If there are any signs of deterioration, provide rapid transport. Monitor capnography readings to ensure that the carbon dioxide level remains between 35 and 40 mmHg. Monitor the pulse oximetry to ensure that oxygen saturation remains above 96 percent and administer supplemental oxygen as needed.

several studies have shown that commonly used extrication techniques actually cause more spinal movement than simply asking the patient to exit the vehicle on his own (with assistance as needed). As a result, many EMS systems have significantly altered their approach to potential spinal injuries. Circumstances on scene—either concerns about scene safety or the need for rapid transport to a trauma center—preclude spending the time required for standard spinal immobilization as previously practiced. In such cases, use a rapid extrication procedure.[12,13]

With whatever personnel are available, stabilize the patient's spine, shoulders, pelvis, and legs with the patient's nose, navel, and toes kept in line. Ensure that providers are coordinated and understand what movement is to take place. One provider, usually at the patient's head, should direct the move, counting a cadence to permit the crew to work together. Ensure that personnel involved in the extrication move the patient while maintaining patient alignment of the nose, navel, and toes. Then, on the leader's count, move the patient from a seated or other position to a waiting spine board or stretcher.

Remember the objectives of spinal movement and stabilization: Keep the spine in the neutral, in-line position by keeping the patient's eyes facing directly forward and keeping the shoulders and pelvis in a plane perpendicular to that of the gaze. Be sure to prevent any flexion/extension, rotation, or lateral bending.

Although the rapid extrication technique does not provide maximum protection for the spine, it does permit rapid movement of the patient with a spinal injury when other considerations demand it. Rapid extrication from the confined space of a wrecked automobile is difficult at best. Plan the move carefully and execute rapid extrication by carefully explaining the process and individual responsibilities to your team members.

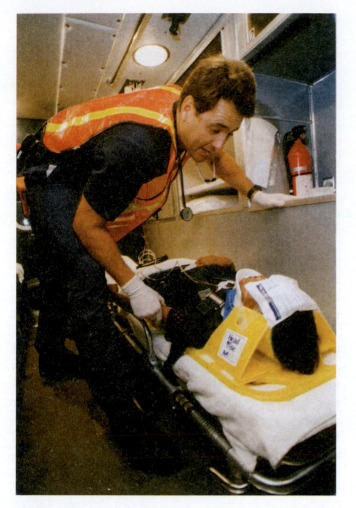

FIGURE 6-47 Repeat the ongoing assessment every 5 minutes with seriously injured patients.

(© Craig Jackson/In the Dark Photography)

Management of Head, Neck, and Spinal Injuries

This section details an overview of the prehospital management of head, neck, and spinal injuries. It is important to remember that these injuries often occur with other injuries to other body structures (e.g., spleen, liver). The primary prehospital treatment of patients with head, neck and spinal injuries includes extrication, assessment, spinal stabilization (if indicated), and transport. Some of these patients may require medications for pain, to facilitate airway management, and for the management and prevention of seizures.

Rapid Extrication in Motor Vehicle Collisions

Applying spinal immobilization can be a time-consuming process. Furthermore, research has demonstrated that it is relatively ineffective and, in some cases, harmful. In addition,

Patho Pearls

Historically, spinal immobilization practices were based on rational conjecture. The actual origin of this concept has remained elusive, although some articles in the 1960s suggested the practice. In 1985, the U.S. Department of Transportation published a curriculum for EMT education that strongly recommended full spinal immobilization for patients who had even the slightest potential for spinal injury. This was the primary impetus for the detailed spinal immobilization practices that have prevailed in EMS. More recently, scientific studies of common prehospital immobilization practices have found these to be ineffective and, in some cases, harmful.[14] Because of this, many EMS systems and EMS organizations have markedly changed their approach to patients with potential spinal injuries. The scientific evidence has shown the following[15-19]:

1. *It is virtually impossible to immobilize the spine.* The spine consists of numerous joints that allow movement in

numerous planes of motion. Even with the best immobilization techniques, there is still significant movement of the spine. Even the highest quality cervical collars still allow a fair amount of motion.

2. *Spinal mobilization may be harmful.* Certainly, being immobilized on a backboard for any period of time can cause pain. Ultimately, pain leads to tenderness, which can lead to additional evaluation, including imaging (X-rays, CT). In addition, several studies have shown that immobilization, as previously practiced, can actually impair respiratory function and cause pressure sores.

3. *Spinal immobilization practices and rigid cervical dollars can impair airway management.* The application of a simple rigid collar can reduce mouth opening by up to 25 percent in certain individuals. Attempting to place an endotracheal tube in a patient firmly secured to a backboard is difficult and, in some cases, impossible.

4. *Rigid cervical collars appear to increase intracranial pressure.* Properly fitted and placed cervical collars can impair venous drainage of the head through the jugular veins. (They do not affect arterial blood flow to the head through the carotid and vertebral arteries, as these structures are deeper and more protected than the veins.) By restricting venous blood flow out of the head and not restricting arterial inflow, these rigid collars can cause an increase in intracranial pressure. In patients with coexisting head injuries, placement of a rigid cervical collar can actually make the patient's condition worse.

5. *Rigid cervical collars can actually make high cervical spine injuries worse.* Studies have shown that application of a rigid cervical collar can actually cause a distraction type injury in patients with high cervical spine injuries (C-1–C-2). The amount of distraction (separation between the vertebrae) varies but can potentially worsen these already devastating injuries.

6. *The process of applying cervical collars and spinal immobilization can cause more movement than allowing patients to self-extricate.* Several studies have shown that common extrication techniques used in prehospital care actually cause more spinal movement than simply asking the patient to exit the vehicle (with assistance, if needed).[20,21]

7. *Lawsuits will follow the lack of spinal immobilization.* This has been a common mantra. However, there is no significant evidence that medical liability is increased or decreased with current spinal mobilization practices. Furthermore, with the evolving scientific evidence showing that current spinal mobilization practices may be harmful, the pendulum may swing the other way, with accusations that full spinal mobilization actually worsens an injury.

Various strategies have been developed in an attempt to limit spinal immobilization. At this point, a definitive answer is still elusive. Generally, the use of long spine boards has no significant role in prehospital care other than for emergent extrication and patient movement. In these instances, scoop-type stretchers and vacuum mattresses may be a better alternative. Because of problems with rigid cervical collars, some systems have elected to go back to the older soft cervical collars as used in the early days of modern EMS.[22] These do more to remind the patient not to move his head and neck than to provide any significant level of immobilization. Some systems have elected to use rigid cervical collars only. EMS providers must always follow local protocols in regard to treatment of spinal injuries.

Spinal Precautions

Neutral, in-line positioning is very important in spinal injury patient care because it maintains the best spinal column positioning and the greatest clearance between the cord and the spinal foramen interior. This positioning permits the best circulation and thus lessens the impact of local injury and edema. As patient assessment progresses, gently and smoothly move any body segment that is out of alignment toward alignment when examined. If the patient feels any increase in pain or if there is a significant resistance to movement, immobilize the head and neck or other portion of the body in the position achieved. Do not continue movement, as doing so may compromise the spinal cord. Maintain the patient's head and body position using manual immobilization until mechanical immobilization can be applied.

Spinal Clearance Protocols

The decision to continue spinal precautions is predicated on an evaluation of the injury mechanism and of patient findings suggestive of injury. Recent research has demonstrated that prehospital personnel, using a standardized and validated protocol, can reliably identify patients who are likely to have spinal injury, and those who are not. Various **spinal clearance protocols** have been developed and proven reliable, one of the first being the Maine protocol (Figure 6-48). Many of these spinal clearance protocols are based on a protocol used in emergency departments to determine whether cervical spine imaging is required. The protocol was produced through a research project, termed the National Emergency X-Radiography Utilization Study (NEXUS), and has been used by emergency physicians to determine which patients need spinal imaging and which do not. It seemed intuitive that if a patient did not meet criteria for emergency department spinal imaging, prehospital spinal immobilization is probably unwarranted. The NEXUS criteria are essentially the same criteria used in the Maine protocol (Figure 6-49). There are several derivations of these protocols, but all have common features. The Canadian C-Spine Rule is commonly used and has been found somewhat superior to the

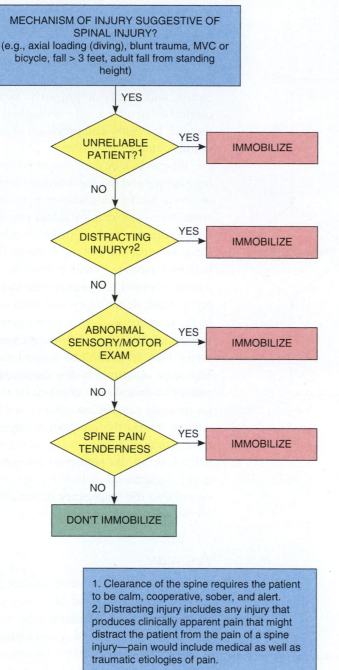

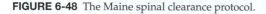

FIGURE 6-48 The Maine spinal clearance protocol.

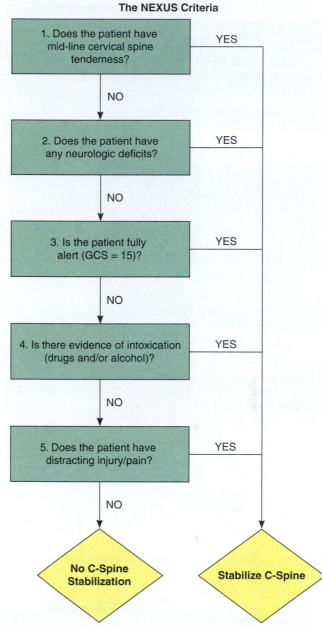

FIGURE 6-49 The NEXUS criteria for assessing for spinal injury. Patients who meet these criteria have a high likelihood (99.8% negative predictive value) of not having a spinal injury.

NEXUS criteria in several studies (Figure 6-50). It evaluates for mechanisms of injury associated with spinal injury. It does not use distracting injury/pain as a criteria. Both the NEXUS criteria and the Canadian C-Spine Rule are highly effective in detecting patients with spinal injuries. Spinal precautions may be discontinued if the following three criteria are met:

- The patient is alert and fully oriented, is not intoxicated or under the influence of drugs (including alcohol), has a Glasgow Coma Scale score of 15, and is not significantly affected by the "fight-or-flight" response.

- The patient is free of significant distracting injuries, such as a significant fracture or joint injury, or symptoms such as abdominal pain or dyspnea.

- The patient is free of any signs or symptoms of spinal injury.

An additional criterion to consider regarding discontinuance of spinal precautions is the patient's age. Those at both ends of the age spectrum—the very young and the very old—may be unreliable reporters of spinal symptoms. The elderly are not good reporters of spinal symptoms because preexisting disease and medical problems, as well

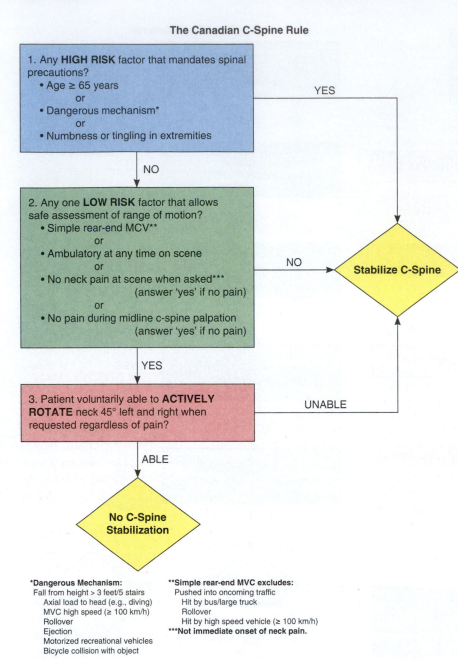

The Canadian C-Spine Rule

1. Any **HIGH RISK** factor that mandates spinal precautions?
   • Age ≥ 65 years
      or
   • Dangerous mechanism*
      or
   • Numbness or tingling in extremities

YES → Stabilize C-Spine

NO ↓

2. Any one **LOW RISK** factor that allows safe assessment of range of motion?
   • Simple rear-end MCV**
      or
   • Ambulatory at any time on scene
      or
   • No neck pain at scene when asked***
      (answer 'yes' if no pain)
      or
   • No pain during midline c-spine palpation
      (answer 'yes' if no pain)

NO → Stabilize C-Spine

YES ↓

3. Patient voluntarily able to **ACTIVELY ROTATE** neck 45° left and right when requested regardless of pain?

UNABLE → Stabilize C-Spine

ABLE ↓

No C-Spine Stabilization

***Dangerous Mechanism:**
   Fall from height > 3 feet/5 stairs
   Axial load to head (e.g., diving)
   MVC high speed (≥ 100 km/h)
   Rollover
   Ejection
   Motorized recreational vehicles
   Bicycle collision with object

****Simple rear-end MVC excludes:**
   Pushed into oncoming traffic
   Hit by bus/large truck
   Rollover
   Hit by high speed vehicle (≥ 100 km/h)
*****Not immediate onset of neck pain.**

FIGURE 6-50 The Canadian C-Spine Rules is another guideline for determining the need for assessing for spinal injury. It considers the mechanism of injury but does not consider distracting injuries/pain.

as reduced sensitivity to pain, affect their ability to recognize and report pain. The elderly are also more likely to sustain spinal column injury from limited mechanisms of injury, and the distance between the spinal cord and the spinal column interior may be limited because of aging and degenerative disease. Very young patients may simply cry as a result of pain or may be too young to accurately articulate spinal symptoms. Again, consult local protocols to determine whether, and under what circumstances, spinal precautions for either the elderly or the very young can be discontinued.

If there is any doubt about the patient's potential for spinal injury or the patient's ability to accurately report any symptoms of such an injury, use spinal precautions as dictated by local protocols.

If spinal precautions are to be continued, maintain manual spinal stabilization and apply a properly sized cervical collar after a full examination of the neck for injury and provision of any needed emergent care there.

Whenever a trauma patient is wearing a helmet and has sustained moderate or severe head injury, suspect a cervical spine injury and employ spinal precautions as directed by local protocols. Consider whether or not to remove the helmet based on local protocols. A patient's helmet use reduces the likelihood of soft tissue injury and skull and facial fracture and also significantly reduces the incidence of traumatic brain injury. However, don't be lulled into a false sense of security by the absence of a patient's outward signs of injury. Be alert for the early signs of brain injury and be sure to inform the emergency department staff that the patient was wearing a helmet. Bring the helmet to the emergency department with the patient or describe to the emergency department physician any damage it sustained.

Airway

As with other patient conditions, assurance and maintenance of the airway is a primary concern for patients who have sustained head neck and spinal injuries. Studies have shown that the presence of hypoxia and hypercapnia in the prehospital setting worsens outcomes and survival of patients with these injuries. However, studies have also shown that prehospital intubation may actually worsen neurologic outcomes and survival of patients with traumatic brain injuries. Thus, it is essential that the paramedic pay particular attention to the airway and ventilation. For patients with a Glasgow Coma Scale score of 8 or less, an airway device may be indicated (Figure 6-51). Although it is been standard practice to use endotracheal intubation, there appears to be a role for expanding use of extraglottic airways for these patients. The use of sedation and neuromuscular blockers may facilitate intubation of head-injured patients. Regardless, mechanical ventilation and airway maintenance remain the cornerstones of care for patients with neurologic injuries.

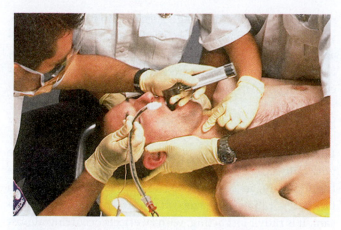

FIGURE 6-51 Oral intubation is difficult in the patient with facial trauma because landmarks may be distorted, blood may flow into the airway, and the head must remain in the neutral position.

Rapid Sequence Induction/Intubation

Head injury patients are often unable to care for their airway and are likely to vomit. If they are unresponsive, an extraglottic airway or endotracheal intubation is indicated. However, if they are unable to protect their airway but are not completely unresponsive, they may require intubation using a rapid sequence intubation (RSI) procedure. RSI may also be required for patients with airway concerns whose teeth are clenched (trismus) and for patients with serious oral trauma and the risk of swelling and progressive airway obstruction. The role of RSI in the prehospital management of a head injury patient remains controversial. Some studies have shown that prehospital RSI improves outcomes when compared to routine airway management. Other studies seem to question its use, especially when not performed often by a provider and when capnography is not closely monitored for hyperventilation. RSI may be best suited for services that encounter more frequent head trauma or ones that have a limited number of paramedics who perform the procedure, to ensure that the provider remains competent in the skill. Above all, the decision to use prehospital RSI rests with the system medical director, and local protocols should be followed.

Breathing

Maintaining near-normal ventilation is essential for patients with severe traumatic brain injury. This may require simply monitoring the patient's ventilatory status. In some cases, it may require mechanical ventilation. If mechanical ventilation is required, it is essential to avoid hypercapnia. In addition, it is also important to avoid hypoxia, as well as hyperoxia. Because of this, all patients with the neurologic injury should be monitored with pulse oximetry and waveform capnography. These parameters will help to guide ventilation. Remember, the

minute ventilation is a function of the respiratory rate and the tidal volume. The respiratory rate is easy to measure in the prehospital setting. However, unless the patient is on a mechanical ventilator, you can only estimate the tidal volume.

Ventilation should be monitored during treatment and transport. If the patient begins to show signs of herniation, consider hyperventilation if local protocols allow it. Hyperventilation should be used only if there are signs and symptoms of herniation.

Circulation

It is now standard practice in prehospital trauma care to use permissive hypotension for trauma patients. The purpose of this is to restore blood flow to affected organs, yet not return the blood pressure to a normal level. An increased blood pressure actually worsens bleeding. However, a blood pressure that is too low will not adequately perfuse critical organs.

In the case of traumatic brain injury, this practice must be modified to ensure adequate perfusion of the brain. As discussed in this chapter, perfusion of the brain is related to the mean arterial pressure and the prevailing intracranial pressure (ICP). The amount of blood necessary to adequately perfuse the brain is the cerebral perfusion pressure (CPP). As the ICP increases, as seen in trauma, it takes an increase in mean arterial pressure to adequately perfuse the brain. Thus, the practice of permissive hypotension must be modified to account for this. In patients with traumatic brain injury it is important to increase the blood pressure to a point at which cerebral perfusion pressure is maintained. This is certainly hard to determine in the field. However, serial examination of vital signs, Glasgow Coma Scale findings, and other parameters will help with this. Once the patient is in the trauma center, an ICP monitor will be placed so that the ICP can be accurately measured. This will allow hospital personnel to determine the patient's response to treatment and other therapies.

Blood Pressure Maintenance

Adequate circulation for the brain and spinal cord injury patient is essential to arrive at a good outcome. The brain is very dependent on receiving a continuous supply of oxygenated blood. Hypovolemia and any associated hypotension reduce oxygen transport to the brain. This condition also reduces both circulation through the brain and the blood's ability to remove the products of metabolism. Because brain tissue is especially sensitive to oxygen deprivation, any further circulatory loss might prove devastating to head injury patients who have already suffered some damage to brain tissue. The problems of hypovolemia and hypotension are compounded if there is any increase in intracranial pressure. Such an increase further restricts cerebral blood flow, and the body's autoregulatory mechanisms cannot compensate in a preexisting state of hypotension.

Care for the patient in whom you suspect increased intracranial pressure with fluid resuscitation, even though the patient's other injuries might not suggest that step. For example, the patient with penetrating chest trauma might not receive aggressive fluid resuscitation until the systolic blood pressure drops to below 80 mmHg. If that patient also has a serious head injury with increasing intracranial pressure, waiting for the blood pressure to drop to that level would be life threatening. Therefore, provide rapid fluid (electrolyte) administration and other shock care measures to maintain a systolic blood pressure of 90 mmHg.

Provide fluid resuscitation for any patient with significant head injury in whom you suspect brain injury and who shows signs of shock compensation—rapid, thready pulse, slowed capillary refill, lowered level of consciousness, anxiety, or restlessness. Insert a large-bore catheter and administer normal saline at a wide-open rate through nonrestrictive trauma IV tubing. In rapid succession, administer serial boluses of 500 mL of an isotonic solution, titrated to blood pressure, to maintain a systolic blood pressure of 90 mmHg. In the child (6–12 years), young child (2–5 years), and infant (0–1 year), maintain a systolic blood pressure of at least 80, 75, or 65 mmHg, respectively and use proportionally sized fluid boluses. Periods of hypotension, as well as hypoxia, are associated with a poor outcome from serious traumatic brain injury.

In serious brain injury, the blood pressure may rise. This elevation in blood pressure is a reflex response to increasing intracranial pressure and represents an attempt by the body to maintain perfusion of the brain. In the patient with probable brain injury, do not treat hypertension beyond elevating the head 30 degrees.

Medications

The role of prehospital medications in the treatment of the patient with a head, neck or spinal injury is limited. However, some medications are common. These include oxygen and, to a limited degree, topical anesthetic sprays. Other medications that may be useful for patients with central nervous system injury include osmotic diuretics (e.g., mannitol),

neuromuscular blockers (e.g., succinylcholine, atracurium, vecuronium), sedatives (e.g., diazepam, lorazepam, midazolam, etomidate, ketamine), analgesics (e.g., morphine, fentanyl, ketamine), and others. These medications are discussed in detail in the chapter "Emergency Pharmacology."

Sedatives

DIAZEPAM Diazepam (Valium) is a benzodiazepine with both antianxiety and muscle relaxant qualities. In prehospital care, it is often used to premedicate patients to facilitate intubation. Diazepam is also a potent anticonvulsant. It is rather fast acting, with IV effects occurring almost immediately and reaching peak effectiveness in 15 minutes. Its duration is from 15 to 60 minutes.

The effects of diazepam (and lorazepam and midazolam) may be reversed by the administration of flumazenil.

LORAZEPAM Lorazepam (Ativan) is one of the most potent of the benzodiazepines and yet has a shorter sedative half-life than diazepam. Paradoxically, its antiseizure effects last longer; it is otherwise much like diazepam.

Analgesics with Sedative Properties

MORPHINE Morphine (Duramorph, Astramorph) is an opium alkaloid used to relieve pain (narcotic analgesic), to sedate, and to reduce anxiety. It may mask the signs and symptoms of head injury and mildly increase intracranial pressure. It also reduces cardiac preload by increasing venous capacitance and thus may decrease blood pressure in the hypovolemic patient. Its major side effects are hypotension, respiratory depression, and possible nausea and vomiting.

FENTANYL Fentanyl is an opiate narcotic, chemically unrelated to morphine, that provides immediate and effective pain control. Fentanyl's onset of action is more rapid than morphine's and it is considerably more potent, thus requiring lower doses. Fentanyl does not cause hypotension to the same degree as morphine, which makes it an ideal agent for trauma.

Naloxone (Narcan) is a narcotic antagonist that can quickly reverse the effects of narcotics and should be available anytime you use morphine sulfate or fentanyl. Naloxone is a shorter-acting drug than morphine, so repeat doses may be necessary.

KETAMINE Ketamine is an analgesic and sedative with a very predictable dose-related response. It does not cause hypotension, as some other agents do. However, it may induce hypertension and tachycardia. Use it with care in head injury patients, especially if they have any hypertension. Ketamine has several beneficial effects, and its use in emergency medicine and EMS is increasing.

Other Medications

MANNITOL   Mannitol is an osmotic diuretic that draws water from the interstitial space and into the cardiovascular system. The kidneys then eliminate the water, along with sodium. In head injury, this draws fluid from the cerebrum and may reduce cerebral edema and ICP. It is sometimes indicated in severe head injury with the signs of herniation. However, use mannitol with caution in patients with reduced kidney function, as it may induce hypertension, and do not use it in patients who already have hypotension (a systolic blood pressure below 90 mmHg), as it will further reduce blood pressure.

DEXTROSE   In general, significant hypoglycemia is especially detrimental to the patient with head injury. Current practice calls for identifying the blood glucose level on all unresponsive head injury patients, especially those with a possible history of chronic alcoholism or diabetes. If significant hypoglycemia is found, administer 25 mg of glucose and 100 mg of thiamine. It may be prudent to use small doses of dextrose in the head injury patient to prevent hyperglycemia. Consult your protocols and medical direction for guidance regarding dextrose administration to the head injury patient.

Medications and Spinal Cord Injury

In the past, corticosteroids have been used to combat the inflammation frequently associated with spinal cord injury. Research and other information now suggest that this treatment is not as effective as once thought, and high-dose steroid treatment is not without significant side effects. Therefore, the routine use of steroids for the treatment of spinal injury is no longer recommended.

Consult with your medical director and protocols for any system-specific recommendations regarding the treatment of spinal injury and the use of medications.

Medications and Neurogenic Shock

The loss of sympathetic control leads to both a relaxation of the blood vessels (vasodilation) below the level of the lesion and the inability of the body to increase the heart rate. This expanded vascular system leads to a relative hypovolemia and lower blood pressure. The problem is further compounded as the heart, without sympathetic stimulation and in the presence of this relative hypovolemia, displays a normal or bradycardic heart rate.

Frequently, the hypovolemia is treated with a fluid challenge, followed by careful use of a vasopressor such as dopamine, norepinephrine, or phenylephrine. The slow heart rate is treated with atropine to reduce any parasympathetic stimulation.

The initial treatment for hypovolemia from suspected neurogenic shock is by fluid challenge (Figure 6-52).

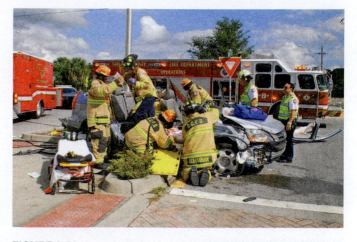

FIGURE 6-52 Aggressive fluid resuscitation may be necessary for the patient in neurogenic shock.
(© Ed Effron)

Establish an IV with a 1,000-mL bag of normal saline, a nonrestrictive administration set, and a large-bore IV catheter. Administer 250 to 500 mL of solution quickly, monitor the blood pressure and heart rate, and auscultate the lungs for signs of developing pulmonary edema (crackles). If the patient responds with an increasing blood pressure, a slowing heart rate, and signs of improved perfusion, consider a second bolus, or monitor the patient and administer a second bolus if the patient's signs and symptoms begin to deteriorate. If the patient does not improve with one or two fluid challenges, consider vasopressor therapy, as allowed by your protocols.

Medications and the Combative or Seizing Patient

Frequently, the patient who has sustained potentially serious spinal cord or traumatic brain injury is intoxicated or is otherwise very uncooperative or combative. In some of these cases, sedatives may be indicated to reduce anxiety and because the patient actively resists spinal precautions and further motion endangers the spine. Such patient motion may compromise efforts to immobilize the spine and may increase the potential for further damage. Consider using a benzodiazepine (e.g., diazepam, midazolam) to calm the patient. Sedatives should be administered as permitted by your system's protocols and under the close and direct supervision of an on-line medical direction physician.

Transport Considerations

There are special considerations to observe when transporting the patient with serious head injury to the hospital. Some suggest that the use of red lights, siren, rough ride (high speed), and other patient stimulation may agitate the patient, increase intracranial pressure, and induce seizures. Although there is little evidence to support this claim, it is probably prudent to reduce speed and use red lights and siren sparingly.

Be cautious in considering head injury patients as candidates for air medical service transport. Even though the time saved by helicopter transport may be very important, the head injury patient is prone to seizures, especially with physical stimulation (noise and vibration) associated with this mode of transport. Seizures aboard any type of aircraft are very dangerous. If you elect to transport by air, ensure that the patient is firmly secured to a long spine board (including feet and hands) and that his airway is protected by endotracheal intubation.

Emotional Support

Identify someone to remain with the patient with the specific role of providing calming reassurance during care and transport. Remember, head injury patients may have trouble remembering events preceding and immediately following the incident, as well as having difficulty laying down short-term memory. Providing the patient with information helps to reduce the patient's anxiety.

Head injury patients may be very confused, distressed, abusive, or even combative. Do not take this behavior personally. Maintain a professional demeanor and provide emotional support during assessment, care, and transport.

Summary

The head, neck, and spinal column contain very special and important structures—key elements of the central nervous system, the airway, the alimentary canal, and major organs of sensation. Serious trauma to these regions may endanger these structures and demands special assessment and care. During the scene size-up, identify possible mechanisms of injury and the injuries they suggest. If the MOI suggests spine injury, provide spinal precautions unless you have a reliable reporter (fully conscious and alert, without any intoxication or distracting injury, not elderly or very young) and without any spinal cord injury signs. Establish a general patient impression and determine his level of consciousness and orientation early. Ensure that the airway is clear and protected from aspiration and physical obstruction. Administer supplemental oxygen, if needed, and ventilate, as necessary, being careful not to under- or overventilate the patient. Guide ventilation by capnography. Provide rapid transport for the patient with possible intracranial hemorrhage or serious lesion.

Once the airway, breathing, and circulation have been addressed, address skeletal fractures, minor bleeding, and open wounds. Provide complete immobilization for the potential spine injury patient and move the patient carefully. Provide emotional support and information during patient care.

You Make the Call

You are called to a scene where a young woman, in an attempt to end her life, has deeply lacerated her anterior and lateral neck. The wound is deep and produces severe flowing hemorrhage with bubbling on expiration. She also has blood gurgling and spattering from her mouth with expiration.

1. What structures are most likely injured?

2. What care would you employ?

3. What are serious life threats associated with this injury?

See Suggested Responses at the back of this book.

Review Questions

1. Retroauricular ecchymosis over the mastoid bone is also called _____
   a. Battle's sign.
   b. raccoon eye.
   c. Goblet's sign.
   d. periorbital ecchymosis.

2. Periorbital and retroauricular ecchymosis indicate that what type of injury has occurred?
   a. Tension pneumothorax
   b. Basilar skull fracture
   c. Abdominal injury
   d. Impending shock

3. An eye injury involving hemorrhage into the anterior chamber pools is known as _____
   a. ecchymosis.
   c. erythema.
   b. blepharospasm.
   d. hyphema.

4. Your patient has been involved in serious trauma and has received an open wound to the neck, exposing and damaging blood vessels. Your concern should be directed toward the danger of exsanguination and _____
   a. pulmonary edema.
   b. tension pneumothorax.
   c. air embolism.
   d. subcutaneous emphysema.

5. What type of eye injury from a traumatic mechanism may cause the patient to complain of a dark curtain obstructing part of his field of view?
   a. Ocular hyphema
   b. Acute retinal artery occlusion
   c. Retinal detachment
   d. Corneal abrasion

6. A classic sign of increasing intracranial pressure, which includes a slowing pulse, increasing systolic blood pressure, and irregular respirations, is referred to as _____
   a. Cheyne-Stokes respirations.
   b. Cushing's triad.
   c. Kernig's sign.
   d. Babinski's sign.

7. The connective tissue sheet covering the superior aspect of the cranium is called the galea _____
   a. pericranium.
   b. periosteum.
   c. aponeurotica.
   d. subaponeurotica.

8. The most common sites of axial loading injuries from heel-first falls are located between _____
   a. T-12 and L-2.
   c. C-5 and T-4.
   b. C-1 and C-7.
   d. L-3 and L-5.

9. When the patient has injuries to the head and face, what life threat should you constantly be assessing and reassessing for?
   e. Respiratory arrest
   a. Airway occlusion
   b. Stroke
   c. Irreversible shock

10. All of the following are primary functions of the intervertebral disks except _____
    a. limiting bone wear.
    b. absorbing shock.
    c. accommodating motion of adjacent vertebrae.
    d. elevating the diaphragm during inspiratory efforts.

11. The major weight-bearing component of a vertebra is the _____
    a. pedicle.
    b. laminae.
    c. vertebral body.
    d. spinal canal.

12. Which of the following statements regarding cervical collar use is true for trauma patients?
    a. It serves as an adjunct to full cervical immobilization.
    b. It serves to accentuate axial loading and prevent any flexion/extension.
    c. It serves to immobilize the cervical, thoracic, and lumbar spine.
    d. It serves to prevent axial loading when used before manual stabilization.

13. Which of the following structures of a vertebra articulates with the ribs?
    a. Spinous process
    b. Vertebral pedicle
    c. Intervertebral disk
    d. Demifacets

14. Generally, if a patient presents with a Glasgow Coma Scale score of less than _____, the patient will likely need advanced airway management.
    a. 8
    c. 12
    b. 10
    d. 14

15. The inability to remember events that occurred after a traumatic event is known as _____
    a. anterograde amnesia.
    b. retrograde amnesia.
    c. transient amnesia.
    d. morbid amnesia.

16. During a trauma assessment, you notice that a patient has no sensation below the lower border of the rib cage. This would suggest spinal pathology between which vertebral areas?
    a. C-1 and C-3
    b. C-3 and T-4
    c. T-4 and T-10
    d. T-10 and S-1

17. Which of the following vital signs would most likely indicate a potential spinal cord injury?
    a. Hypotension, bradycardia, and shallow respirations
    b. Hypertension, bradycardia, and shallow respirations
    c. Hypotension, tachycardia, and deep respirations
    d. Hypertension, tachycardia, and deep respirations

18. The three layers of the meninges are the pia mater, the dura mater, and the _____
    a. tentorium.
    b. falx cerebri.
    c. zygomatica.
    d. arachnoid.

19. Which of the following drugs may cause fasciculations and raise ICP?
    a. Succinylcholine
    b. Solu-Medrol
    c. Mannitol
    d. Rocuronium

20. The largest portion of the brain, which controls consciousness and higher mental functions, is the _____
    a. brainstem.
    b. cerebellum.
    c. cerebrum.
    d. hypothalamus.

21. For the head injury patient without signs of herniation, you should adjust ventilation rates to maintain an end-tidal CO_2 reading of between _____
    a. 20 and 25.
    b. 25 and 30.
    c. 30 and 35.
    d. 35 and 40.

22. Rate, depth, and rhythm of respirations are controlled by the _____
    a. pons.
    b. cerebellum.
    c. aponeurotica center.
    d. brainstem.

23. For which of the following patients would the anticholinergic agent atropine be best suited?
    a. A patient in early spinal shock
    b. A patient with an injury to the upper spinal cord
    c. A patient with an injury to the lower spinal cord
    d. A patient with autonomic hyperreflexia syndrome

24. The primary management objective in a patient with a suspected spinal cord injury, as evidenced by vertebral instability, pain, and loss of appropriate motor and sensory function, is to _____
    a. administer medications to prevent further paralysis.
    b. apply a cervical collar independent of spinal stabilization.
    c. initiate mechanical stabilization followed by manual immobilization.
    d. maintain the patient in a neutral, in-line position as well as possible.

25. Priapism is defined as _____
    a. a sustained erection of the penis.
    b. clear discharge from the nose.
    c. an occasional variant of angina.
    d. respiratory paralysis.

26. The most accurate definition of dermatomes is _____
    a. spinal nerves that innervate specific and discrete areas of the body surface.
    b. spinal nerves that innervate specific organs and organ systems.
    c. spinal nerves that pinpoint the exact location of the injury site.
    d. spinal nerves that innervate discrete tissues and muscles in the body.

27. All of the following are signs or symptoms of spinal shock except _____
    a. priapism.
    b. hypertension.
    c. loss of bladder control.
    d. flaccid paralysis.

28. Which of the following best defines spinal shock?
    a. An insult to the cord that affects the body above the level of the injury
    b. An insult to the cord that affects the body through extravasation of blood volume
    c. An insult to the cord that affects the body above and below the level of the injury
    d. An insult to the cord that affects the body below the level of the injury

29. The central nervous system is made up of the _____
    a. brain and cervical spine.
    b. brain and spinal cord.
    c. spinal cord only.
    d. brain and meninges.

30. A patient presents with abnormal motor findings after falling out of a tree. You note that he can walk but is unable to use his arms. This motor finding is most characteristic of what injury?
    a. Posterior cord syndrme
    b. Lateral cord syndrome
    c. Central cord syndrome
    d. Anterior cord syndrome

See Answers to Review Questions at the end of this book.

References

1. Trafton, P. G. "Spinal Cord Injuries." *Surg Clin North Am* 62(1) (Feb 1982): 61–72.]

2. Rasouli, M. R., et al. "Preventing Motor Vehicle Crashes Related Spine Injuries in Children." *World J Pediatr* 7(4) (Nov 2011): 311–317.

3. Dula, D. J. "The Ring Sign: Is It a Reliable Indicator for Cerebral Spinal Fluid?" *Ann Emerg Med* 22(4)(Apr 1993): 718–720.

4. Ray, A. M. "Halo Sign Is Neither Sensitive nor Specific for Cerebrospinal Fluid Leak." *Ann Emerg Med* 53(2) (Feb 2009): 288.

5. Davis, D. P., et al. "The Relationship between Out-of-Hospital Airway Management and Outcome among Trauma Patients with a Glasgow Coma Scale Score of 8 or Less." *Prehosp Emerg Care* 15(2) (Apr–Jun 2011): 184–192.

6. Dumont, T. M., et al. "Inappropriate Prehospital Ventilation in Severe Traumatic Brain Injury Increases In-Hospital Mortality." *J Neurotrauma* 27(7)(Jul 2010): 1233–1241.

7. Caulfield, E. V., et al. "Prehospital Hypocapnia and Poor Outcome after Severe Traumatic Brain Injury." *J Trauma* 66(6) (Jun 2009): 1577–1582.

8. Warner, K. J., J. Cuschieri, M. K. Copass, G. J. Jurkovich, and E. M. Bulger. "The Impact of Prehospital Ventilation on Outcome after Severe Traumatic Brain Injury." *J Trauma* 62(6) (Jun 2007): 1330–1336.

9. Davis, D. P., J. V. Dunford, M. Ochs, K. Park, and D. B. Hoyt. "The Use of Quantitative End-Tidal Capnography to Avoid Inadvertent Severe Hyperventilation in Patients with Head Injury after Paramedic Rapid Sequence Intubation." *J Trauma* 56(4) (Apr 2004): 808–814.

10. Bledsoe, BE, Casey M, Feldman J, Johnson L, Diel S, Forred W, Gorman C. Glasgow Coma Scale Scoring is often inaccurate. *Prehosp Disaster Med* 2015;30:1-8.

11. Shahin, H., S. P. Gopinath, and C. S. Robertson. "Influence of Alcohol on Early Glasgow Coma Scale in Head-Injured Patients." *J Trauma* 69(5) (Nov 2010): 1176–1181.

12. Benger, J. and J. Blackham. "Why Do We Put Cervical Collars on Conscious Trauma Patients?" *Scand J Trauma Resusc Emerg Med* 17(2012): 44.

13. Farrington, J. D. "Extrication of Victims—Surgical Principles." *J Trauma* 8 (1968): 493–512.

14. Hauswald, M. "A Re-Conceptualisation of Acute Spinal Care. *Emerg Med J* 30 (9)(2013):720-723.

15. Ay, D., C. Aktas, S. Yesilyurt, S. Sarikaya, et al. "Respiratory Effects of Spinal Immobilization Devices on Pulmonary Function in Healthy Volunteer Individuals." *Turkish J Trauma Emerg Surg* 17 (2011): 103–107.

16. Goutcher, C. M. and V. Lochhead. "Reduction in Mouth Opening with Semi-Rigid Cervical Collars." *Br J Anaesth* 95 (2005): 344–348.

17. Davies, G., C. Deakin, and A. Wilson. "The Effect of a Rigid Collar on Intracranial Pressure." *Injury* 27 (1996): 647–649.

18. Stone, M. B., C. M. Tubridy, and R. Curran. "The Effect of Rigid Cervical Collars on Internal Jugular Vein Dimensions." *Acad Emerg Med* 17 (2010): 100–102.

19. Ben-Galim, P., N. Dreiangel, K. L. Mattox, C. A. Reitman, et al. "Extrication Collars Can Result in Abnormal Separation Between Vertebrae in the Presence of a Dissociative Injury." *J Trauma* 69 (2010):447-450.

20. Perry, S. D., B. McLellan, W. E. McIlroy, B. E. Maki, et al. "The Efficacy of Head Immobilization Techniques during Simulated Vehicle Motion." *Spine (Phila Pa 1976)* 24 (1999): 1839–1844.

21. Engsberg, J. R., J. W. Standeven, T. L. Shurtleff, J. L. Eggars, et al. "Cervical Spine Motion during Extrication." *J Emerg Med* 44 (2013): 122–127.

22. Miller, C. P., J. E. Bible, K. A. Jegede, P. G. Whang, and J. N. Grauer. "Soft and Rigid Collars Provide Similar Restriction in Cervical Range of Motion during Fifteen Activities of Daily Living." *Spine (Phila Pa 1976)* 35 (2010): 1271–1278.

Further Reading

American College of Surgeons, Committee on Trauma. *Advanced Trauma Life Support Course: Student Manual.* 9th ed. Chicago: American College of Surgeons, 2012.

Bledsoe, B. E., and D. Clayden. *Prehospital Emergency Pharmacology.* 7th ed. Upper Saddle River, NJ: Pearson/Prentice Hall, 2011.

Bledsoe, B. E., B. J. Colbert, and J. E. Ankney. *Essentials of A & P for Emergency Care.* Upper Saddle River, NJ: Pearson/Prentice Hall, 2010.

Ivatury, R. R. and G. C. Cayten, eds. *Textbook of Penetrating Trauma.* Media, PA: Williams & Wilkins, 1996.

Martini, F. *Fundamentals of Anatomy and Physiology.* 10th ed. San Francisco: Pearson, 2014.

Marx, J., R. Hockberger, and R. Walls. *Emergency Medicine: Concepts and Clinical Practice.* 8th ed. St. Louis: Mosby, 2013.

National Association of EMTs. *Prehospital Trauma Life Support.* 8th ed. Burlington: Jones & Bartlett Learning, 2014.

Tintinelli, J. E., ed. *Emergency Medicine: A Comprehensive Study Guide.* 7th ed. New York: McGraw-Hill, 2012.

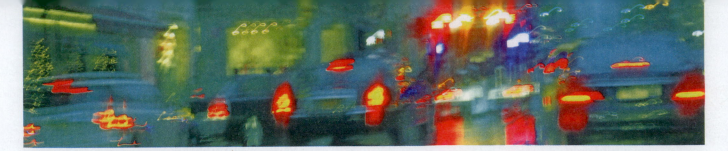

Chapter 7
Chest Trauma

Bryan E. Bledsoe, DO, FACEP, FAAEM, EMT-P

Robert S. Porter, MA, EMT-P

STANDARD
Trauma (Chest Trauma)

COMPETENCY
Integrates assessment findings with principles of epidemiology and pathophysiology to formulate a field impression to implement a comprehensive treatment/disposition plan for an acutely injured patient.

∨ Learning Objectives

Terminal Performance Objective: After reading this chapter, you should be able to assess and manage patients with thoracic trauma.

Enabling Objectives: To accomplish the terminal performance objective, you should be able to:

1. Define key terms introduced in this chapter.

2. Discuss the epidemiology of chest trauma.

3. Describe the anatomy and physiology of the thorax and the structures within it.

4. Identify how blunt and penetrating mechanisms can result in thoracic trauma.

5. List and describe common pulmonary and chest wall injuries seen in the prehospital environment.

6. List and describe common cardiac and vascular injuries that can occur secondary to thoracic trauma.

7. Identify the phases and the steps of assessment for patients that have suffered chest wall trauma and present with various injuries.

8. Given a variety of scenarios, discuss the management of patients with thoracic injuries.

KEY TERMS

Case Study

Medic 101 responds to a shooting call at a Southside tavern. A man was reportedly shot during a robbery attempt. Victoria and Christian are the responding paramedics. On arrival, they quickly size up the scene and determine it to be safe. Police are on scene, have an assailant in custody, and have controlled the gathering crowd.

At the patient's side, paramedics find a supine male, just inside the tavern door. The tavern owner reports that the man had tried to take cash from the register when the owner shot him with a .38 caliber handgun at close range. Primary assessment reveals a confused, yet weakly combative, patient with pale, ashen skin. He says his name is Conrad and his age is 34. Conrad's speech is not broken by his respirations and he appears conscious, alert, and oriented. His trachea is midline, jugular veins are flat, and he is breathing with only slight distress. Victoria notes minimal bleeding without air leak from four wounds found just below the left clavicle along the midclavicular line, just left of the upper sternum, just right of the lower sternum, and close to the right nipple (and fifth intercostal space) along the midclavicular line. Conrad is slightly tachypneic with symmetrical chest rise and slightly diminished breath sounds on the right. During assessment, his level of consciousness begins to diminish. Radial pulses are not palpable, but weak, thready carotid pulses are present. No exit wounds are noted when Conrad is lifted quickly from the floor to the stretcher. The carotid pulse suggests a systolic blood pressure between 60 and 80 mmHg. Pulse oximetry reads erratically between 88 and 92 percent.

Conrad is immediately placed on 100 percent oxygen and his color improves somewhat. He is rapidly loaded into the ambulance, where bilateral antecubital large-bore IV lines are initiated and run wide open.

Christian administers a 500 mL bolus en route to Southside Hospital. After the bolus, Victoria rechecks the vital signs and notes that the pulse remains rapid and weak and blood pressure is 72 by palpation. Conrad now only mumbles to verbal stimuli. Christian alerts medical direction and asks to have a trauma team standing by.

As Victoria addresses potential life threats identified during the primary assessment, she quickly reassesses the chest and notes more labored respirations and that chest rise is no longer symmetrical. The right chest is somewhat hyperexpanded, exhibiting decreased breath sounds in comparison to the left. Conrad appears more ashen, with carotid pulses now absent. His trachea appears somewhat deviated to the left with increasing jugular venous distention. Christian, suspecting tension pneumothorax, asks Victoria to decompress the right chest. Victoria inserts a 3-inch-long 14-gauge IV catheter into the right second intercostal space along the midclavicular line and notes a significant outrush of air. She now observes improvement in Conrad's color and chest rise with less labored breathing. A subsequent reassessment finds that weak, thready carotid pulses have returned as the ambulance arrives at the hospital.

The emergency physician and trauma team take over Conrad's care, initiate a transfusion of packed red blood cells, intubate him, and place bilateral chest tubes for hemopneumothoraces. A trauma X-ray series reveals one bullet in the area of the left scapula, another right of the thoracic spine, one in the right upper abdominal quadrant, and one in the midline upper abdomen. Bedside FAST ultrasound examination reveals blood in the abdomen. Conrad is rapidly transferred to an operating room and an abdominal exploration is performed, revealing a liver laceration and partial abdominal aorta laceration. These injuries are repaired, and Conrad survives.

Introduction to Chest Trauma

The thoracic cavity (chest) contains many vital structures including the heart, great vessels, esophagus, **tracheobronchial tree**, and lungs. Trauma to any one of these structures could be life threatening. It has been estimated that 45 to 50 percent of unrestrained drivers sustain blunt chest trauma. Twenty-five percent of all motor vehicle deaths are due to thoracic trauma (about 8,000 per year in the United States). The majority of these deaths are secondary to injuries to the heart and great vessels. The distribution of organ injury in blunt thoracic trauma is detailed in Table 7-1. In addition to life threats from intrathoracic injuries, abdominal injuries are also common in patients with chest injury and can cause significant **comorbidity.**

An increase in penetrating trauma associated with violent crime has also been observed in urban areas (Figure 7-1). The distribution of organ injury in penetrating thoracic trauma is detailed in Table 7-2. Cheap "Saturday night special" weapons (usually single-fire handguns)

Table 7-1 Distribution of Organ Injury in Blunt Thoracic Trauma

Organ/Structure	Percentage
Chest wall	70
Lung	21
Heart	7
Diaphragm	7
Esophagus	7
Aorta	4.8
Tracheobronchial	0.8

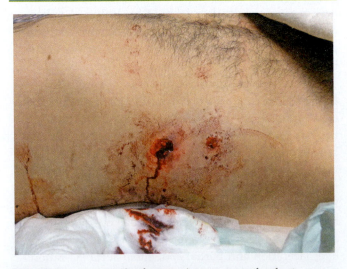

FIGURE 7-1 An example of penetrating trauma to the chest.

(© Dr. Bryan E. Bledsoe)

Table 7-2 Distribution of Organ Injury in Penetrating Thoracic Trauma

Thoracic Cavity	Percentage
Chest wall	100
Lung	65–90
Heart	49
Diaphragm	30
Abdominal Cavity	**Percentage**
Liver	20
Stomach	8
Small intestine	7
Colon	6
Kidney	5

have been replaced by semiautomatic handguns and high-velocity semiautomatic rifles with large magazine capacities. This has increased the incidence of patients receiving multiple chest wounds—often with high-energy weapons. With multiple wounds, there is an increased likelihood of striking vital structures resulting in a higher mortality rate. Numerous advances in penetrating thoracic trauma treatment have been made during recent military conflicts and mortality from penetrating thoracic wounds has decreased from 8 to 40 percent during World War II to 3 to 18 percent today.

In this chapter, chest trauma (both penetrating and blunt injuries) will be discussed. These mechanisms of injury are not just simple injury categories but have real clinical significance for prehospital care. Certain injuries are almost exclusively associated with one type of chest trauma but are unlikely with the other. For example, pericardial tamponade is almost exclusively associated with penetrating thoracic trauma, whereas cardiac rupture is almost exclusively caused by blunt trauma. Considering the mechanism of injury, understanding injury pathophysiology, and awareness of the patient's signs and symptoms, will help to predict, identify, and treat potentially life-threatening chest trauma.

Thoracic Anatomy and Physiology

The thoracic cavity moves air in and out of the respiratory tree for oxygen and carbon dioxide exchange to support metabolism. This chest consists of the thoracic skeleton, diaphragm, and associated musculature. It is also the location of the heart, major blood vessels, trachea, bronchi, lungs, and other important structures essential for body function. Finally, thoracic dynamics (ventilation) are controlled by a series of brain centers and lung and blood vessel sensors.

Thoracic Skeleton

The thoracic skeleton forms the thoracic cage and is defined by 12 pairs of ribs that articulate posteriorly with the thoracic spine and then extend in an anterior and inferior direction (Figure 7-2). The upper seven rib pairs join the sternum at their costochondral joints. The 8th through 10th ribs have indirect cartilage connections at their anterior ends where they join the 7th rib at the inferior sternal margin. The 11th and 12th ribs are often termed *floating ribs* and have no anterior attachment. The sternum completes the anterior bony thorax structure and is made up of three sections: the manubrium, the sternal body, and the xiphoid process. The manubrium is the sternum's superior portion and is the medial endpoint of the clavicle and first rib. The sternal angle (also known as the angle of Louis) is the junction of the manubrium and sternal body and is palpable through the skin as an elevated ridge or prominence. This ridge has clinical significance, as it is the attachment site of the second rib and topographical landmark to help identify the second intercostal space. Knowing this location is important, because it helps you locate where to perform needle chest decompression in case of a tension pneumothorax. The xiphoid process, the most inferior portion of the sternum, meets the sternal body just below the costal cartilages of the lower ribs (**xiphisternal joint**).

The thorax is divided into imaginary vertical lines used to describe positions lateral to the sternum. These lines include the midclavicular line, anterior axillary line, midaxillary line, posterior axillary line, and medial scapular line. When combined with a rib level, these lines serve as accurate landmarks for describing wounds, for locating underlying structures, and for identifying locations to perform procedures. The space just inferior to each rib is called an *intercostal space* and is given the number of the rib above it. For example, the anterior axillary line extends from the anterior margin of the axilla (armpit) inferiorly along the thoracic wall. Its intersection with the fifth intercostal space is generally used as the site to place a thoracostomy tube in patients with pneumo- or hemothorax. This location is not frequently used for prehospital needle decompression, because it is often obscured by a patient's arms or may interfere with immobilization devices, strapping, and blankets.

The thoracic outlet is the superior thorax opening. It is narrow in comparison to the overall thoracic diameter and outlet and is defined by the curvature of the first rib, with its posterior attachment to the first thoracic vertebra and ending anteriorly, at the manubrium. The thoracic outlet is formed posteriorly by the 12th vertebra, laterally by curvature of the 12th rib, and extends anteriorly and superiorly along the costal margin to the xiphisternal joint.

Diaphragm

The diaphragm is a domelike, muscular sheet that separates the abdominal cavity from the thoracic cavity. It is affixed to the rib cage's lower border; its central and superior margin may extend to the fourth intercostal space anteriorly and sixth intercostal space posteriorly during maximal expiration. This superior positioning may allow penetrating wounds to the mid- and lower thorax to penetrate the diaphragm and enter the abdominal cavity. The aorta, esophagus, and inferior vena cava exit the thoracic cavity through separate openings in this structure. The diaphragm is the major respiratory muscle. When contracted, it displaces the thoracic cavity floor downward during inspiration and relaxes and moves upward with expiration.

Associated Musculature

The chest wall structure also includes the shoulder musculature, clavicles, scapula, and humerus. These provide additional protection to vital structures within the upper thorax. The clavicles articulate laterally with the acromion process of the scapula. The scapula covers the posterior and lateral aspects of the first six ribs and articulates with the humerus to complete the shoulder girdle. The chest wall muscles found between ribs, called *intercostal muscles*, along with the diaphragm and sternocleidomastoid muscles, are major muscles of respiration. The sternocleidomastoid muscles raise the upper rib and sternum and, with the sternum, raise the anterior attachments of the next nine ribs. The intercostal muscles contract to further elevate the ribs and increase the thorax's anterior–posterior dimension. Simultaneously, the diaphragm contracts and flattens

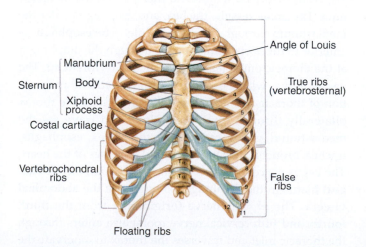

FIGURE 7-2 Skeletal components of the thorax.

to further increase thoracic cavity volume. As thoracic volume increases, intrathoracic pressure falls to less than atmospheric pressure. Air then enters the respiratory tree and fills the lungs and alveoli. This continues until the pressure is equalized.

As the naturally elastic musculature relaxes and recoils, the diaphragm again pushes upward into the thoracic cavity, the ribs and sternum move inferiorly, and the ribs move closer together in an inferior and posterior direction. This decreases the thoracic volume and increases the intrathoracic pressure. When pressure within the thorax exceeds that of the surrounding atmosphere, air exits the respiratory system. Therefore, exhalation in a resting state is largely passive, aided by elastic lung recoil. Gravity helps facilitate exhalation with downward displacement of the ribs and abdominal contents in either the upright or the supine position. This changing of volume to move air in and out is called the *bellows effect*.

Changing intrathoracic volume and pressure also assists in moving blood into the systemic circulation and back to the heart. Increasing intrathoracic pressure during exhalation pushes blood away from the heart and thorax, while decreasing intrathoracic pressure during inspiration draws venous blood toward the thorax and heart. The changing intrathoracic pressure also affects blood pressure and pulse strength. Normally, systolic blood pressure and pulse strength fall slightly during inspiration and rise again during expiration.

Although the diaphragm is the primary respiratory muscle, the intercostal muscles are also important to increase respiratory depth and volume. As oxygen consumption and carbon dioxide production increase during exercise or stress from trauma or infection, the respiratory system increases the respiratory rate, depth, and work. To accommodate this increased need for greater respiratory exchange, more accessory respiratory muscles are recruited. These include the sternocleidomastoid and scalene muscles of the neck for inspiration and the anterior abdominal muscles to aid in forceful exhalation. The rhomboid muscles lift, abduct, and rotate the scapulae to help lift the upper chest with inspiration. The cough reflex, a special respiratory reflex that is important to keeping the airways clear and alveoli expanded, depends on the addition of the latissimus dorsi muscles located along the posterior and lateral thoracic wall and the erector spinae muscles along the spine to allow for forceful thoracic contraction.

Trachea, Bronchi, and Lungs

The tracheobronchial tree and lungs are within the chest. The tracheobronchial tree is a series of progressively narrowing and dividing airways, beginning with the trachea and ending at the alveoli. The trachea enters through the thoracic inlet and divides into right and left mainstem bronchi at the carina, located in the upper central thorax. Right and left mainstem bronchi extend for about 3 centimeters and enter each respective lung at the **pulmonary hilum**. The pulmonary hilum is also where pulmonary arteries enter and pulmonary veins exit and is the lung's sole fixation point in the thoracic cage. Bronchi then further divide into bronchioles, which ultimately terminate in alveoli—the basic unit of lung structure and function.

Each lung occupies one side of the thoracic cavity and is divided into lobes. The right lung has three lobes: upper, middle, and lower. The left lung has two lobes: upper and lower. The left upper lobe contains the cardiac notch against which the heart rests. The lower section of the left upper lobe (the lingula) projects around the lateral border of the heart and corresponds to the right lung's middle lobe.

The lungs are covered with a thin, smooth membrane called the *visceral pleura*. It folds over on itself at the pulmonary hilum and then lines the thoracic cavity's interior, where it is called the *parietal pleura*. The potential space that is formed between these dual layers of pleura contains a small amount of serous (pleural) fluid. This fluid lubricates the pleural layers and permits the lungs to move effortlessly against the interior thoracic wall during inspiration and expiration. The dual layer of pleura and pleural fluid also creates a seal between the lungs and the thoracic cage that causes lungs to expand and contract with changing thoracic cavity volume. If air is allowed to enter this potential space freely, the lung collapses, producing a pneumothorax.

Mediastinum

The mediastinum is the central space within the thoracic cavity bounded laterally by the lungs, inferiorly by the diaphragm, and superiorly by the thoracic inlet (Figure 7-3). The heart is located within and fills most of the mediastinum. The **great vessels**, trachea, and esophagus enter the mediastinum through the thoracic inlet. The esophagus is anterior to the aorta before it exits through the diaphragm at the thoracic outlet (esophageal hiatus or foramen). The vagus nerve, which provides parasympathetic innervation of thoracic and abdominal viscera, enters the thorax bilaterally through the thoracic inlet and traverses the mediastinum, giving branches to the larynx, esophagus, trachea, bronchi, and supraventricular tissues of the heart. The vagus nerve then exits the thorax through the esophageal hiatus in the diaphragm to innervate the abdominal viscera. The phrenic nerve (originating from the third, fourth, and fifth cervical nerve roots) also enters through the thoracic inlet and traverses the thorax to innervate the diaphragm.

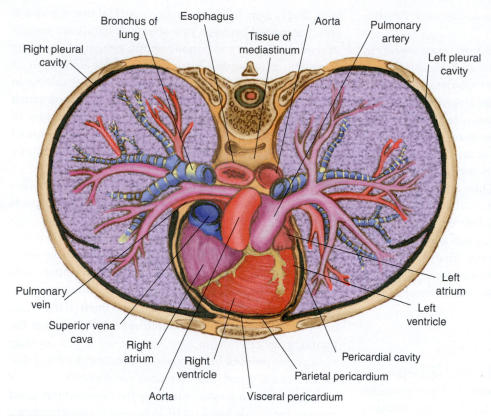

Bronchus of lung · Esophagus · Tissue of mediastinum · Aorta · Pulmonary artery · Right pleural cavity · Left pleural cavity · Pulmonary vein · Superior vena cava · Right atrium · Right ventricle · Aorta · Visceral pericardium · Parietal pericardium · Pericardial cavity · Left ventricle · Left atrium

FIGURE 7-3 Structures of the mediastinum and thorax.

The thoracic duct (part of the lymphatic system) also traverses the thorax from the thoracic outlet, where it enters through the aortic opening in the diaphragm. It typically crosses the midline from the right side of the aorta in the posterior mediastinum at the level of the fifth thoracic vertebra and then ascends above the level of the left clavicle before arching back downward to empty into the left internal jugular vein. The thoracic duct carries most of the body's lymphatic drainage (all but the right side of the head, neck, thorax, and right upper extremity).

Heart

The heart is located in the mediastinum and receives its blood supply via coronary arteries that rise from the aorta just above the aortic semilunar valve leaflets. The coronary arteries fill primarily during diastole. Any changes in afterload (peripheral vascular resistance) play a direct role in determining coronary perfusion pressure. Tachycardia can also limit coronary artery blood flow because excessive heart rates decrease ventricular filling time (diastole) and coronary artery filling time. Endocardial (within the heart muscle) vessels are also compressed by **myocardium** contraction, further limiting coronary blood flow. Atherosclerosis of these vessels accentuates any limitation in coronary blood flow. Epicardial blood flow is not affected by cardiac muscle contraction because epicardial vessels lie on the heart's surface and are not compressed with

myocardial contraction. Cardiac muscle tissue in the interior of the heart is, therefore, more susceptible to ischemia.

A membranous lining, the **pericardium**, surrounds the heart and space containing it and is similar to pleura of the lungs. The portion of this lining that covers the heart's outer surface is the **epicardium**, or visceral pericardium. It then extends to the root of the great vessels before folding back on itself. This folding back forms the parietal pericardium, which is the pericardial sac's outer lining that surrounds the heart. These two layers make up serous pericardium and, like pleura, also form a potential space, the pericardial space. This space usually contains a small amount (up to 35 to 50 mL) of straw-colored fluid. Pericardial fluid functions as a lubricant between the visceral and parietal layers and permits the heart to move easily against the lungs during contractions. It also may provide some protection against local infection from adjacent structures such as the lungs or pleural space. External to the serous pericardium is a tough fibrous sac called the fibrous pericardium that, unlike the serous pericardium, resists distention. The fibrous pericardium originates at the base of the great vessels and surrounds the heart and serous pericardium before fusing with the central tendon of the diaphragm. This pericardial structure fixes the heart in the mediastinum and prevents kinking of great vessels. If the pericardial space rapidly fills with blood, the fibrous pericardium resists passive heart filling during diastole and thereby reduces cardiac output (pericardial tamponade).

Great Vessels

The great vessels are the large arteries and veins that enter and exit the heart and are found in the mediastinum. These are the aorta, superior and inferior vena cava, pulmonary arteries, and pulmonary veins. Injury to these large vascular structures can lead to rapid exsanguination and death if the condition is not quickly recognized and repaired. The aorta, which is fixed at three points within the thorax, is not only susceptible to penetrating injury but also to blunt injury by rapid deceleration or shear forces. It is fixed at the annulus, where it leaves the heart; at the **ligamentum arteriosum** near the bifurcation of the pulmonary artery;

and at the aortic hiatus, where it passes through the diaphragm and enters the abdomen.

Other major vessels that branch from great vessels in the upper chest include the subclavian arteries and veins, the jugular veins, the common carotid arteries, and the brachiocephalic artery (which is the first large branch off the aortic arch dividing into right common carotid and right subclavian arteries). The internal mammary arteries are inferior branches of the subclavian arteries and run along the anterior surface of the pleura, posterior to the costochondral (rib–cartilage) junction. They are often used in coronary bypass grafting. The intercostal arteries are thoracic aorta branches (except for the first two, which arise from branches of the subclavian) that run along lower rib margins along with intercostal nerves. Finally, the bronchial arteries (one right and two left) are usually branches of the thoracic aorta that nourish the nonrespiratory (parenchymal) lung tissues.

Esophagus

The esophagus is a smooth muscular tube that enters the thorax through the thoracic inlet with, and just posterior to, the trachea. It continues for the length of the mediastinum and exits through the esophageal hiatus of the diaphragm. It is contiguous with the posterior tracheal wall and transports food and drink from the oropharynx to the stomach. It moves food and liquid toward the stomach through peristalsis. During vomiting, peristalsis reverses and propels emesis up the esophagus and out through the mouth.

Pathophysiology of Thoracic Trauma

Thoracic trauma, as with other forms of trauma, is classified into two major categories by mechanism: blunt and penetrating. It is important to consider these injury mechanisms and their effects on thoracic organs.

Blunt Trauma

Blunt thoracic trauma is injury resulting from kinetic energy forces transmitted through tissues. These injuries may be further subdivided into other classifications. Blast injuries result from an explosive chemical reaction that creates a pressure wave traveling outward from the explosion's epicenter. This pressure wave causes tissue disruption by dramatic compression and then decompression as the wave passes and may be particularly damaging to hollow, air-filled structures. Crush injuries occur when the body is compressed between an object and a hard surface. This can lead to direct injury or disruption of the chest wall, diaphragm, heart, or tracheobronchial tree. If a victim remains pinned between two objects, a significant restriction in ventilation and venous return, known as traumatic asphyxia, may occur. Crush injuries may also result in impaired organ and soft tissues perfusion, resulting in organ ischemia and cellular acidosis. Prolonged crush injury may also result in **rhabdomyolysis** and release of degraded muscle fiber contents into circulation. Some of these contents—myoglobin, in particular—can be highly toxic to the kidneys.

Deceleration injuries occur when the body is in motion and impacts a fixed object, such as when the chest impacts against the steering column in a front-end collision (Figure 7-4). This impact causes a direct blunt chest wall injury while the internal thoracic organs continue in forward motion. The organs and other structures then impact with the internal thoracic cavity surface and may be compressed as more posterior structures collide with them. If the organ or structure has points of fixation, as with the aorta at the ligamentum arteriosum, the force of the organ moving against this point of fixation (shear force) can lead to a disruption of the vessel. These sudden deceleration and shear forces can cause injury or rupture of the myocardium, great vessels, lungs, trachea, and bronchi. Rapid chest compression, especially against a closed glottis, may also cause alveolar and tracheobronchial rupture and pneumothorax, a phenomenon referred to as "paper bag syndrome."

Age and a patient's general health status may alter the effects of the forces causing blunt trauma. The cartilaginous nature of the pediatric chest often spares infants and children from rib fractures, but more easily transmits trauma energy to vital organs below. This can result in a less significant chest wall injury, yet an increased chance of serious internal injury. Geriatric patients respond very differently to blunt chest trauma. They suffer more frequent rib fractures than younger adults because of skeletal calcification and brittleness. Although the greater incidence

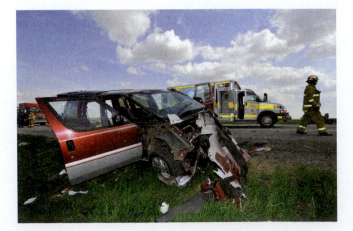

FIGURE 7-4 Frontal impact auto crashes frequently result in blunt chest trauma.

(© Kevin Link/Science Source)

of rib fracture may somewhat protect the underlying organs, preexisting disease and progressive reduction of respiratory and cardiac reserves result in a greater morbidity and mortality from serious chest trauma.

Penetrating Trauma

Penetrating thoracic trauma results when an object enters the chest, causing either direct or secondary injury from transmitted forces. Penetrating chest trauma can be subdivided into three categories: low-energy, high-energy, and shotgun wounds.

Low-energy wounds are those caused by arrows, knives, smaller handguns, and other relatively slow-moving objects (Figure 7-5). They cause injury by direct contact or very limited temporary cavity creation. Injury that occurs from this wound type is related to the direct path that missiles or objects take.

High-energy wounds are caused by military and hunting rifles, and some high-powered handguns at close range, that fire projectiles at very high velocity. Their velocity gives the projectile very high kinetic energy. As a projectile passes through tissue, it creates a shock wave, tissue movement (including compression and stretching), and a large temporary cavity, a phenomenon known as cavitation. These wounds cause extensive tissue damage perpendicular to the projectile's track. The effect is accentuated by bullet construction that "mushrooms" on striking tissue, thereby increasing its profile (presenting surface) and causing greater cavitation. Tumbling—a bullet rotating along its long axis—also accentuates cavitation but greatly decreases projectile penetration.

Shotgun wounds are classified according to the distance between the victim and the shotgun. A smaller gauge (larger barrel size) of shotgun and a larger size of shot also increase the weapon's effective range, penetrating power, and potential to cause tissue damage. Type I injuries are those for which the target is more than 7 meters from the gun barrel at discharge. Pellets usually penetrate the skin and subcutaneous tissue but rarely penetrate deep fascia to cause body cavity penetration. An exception to this rule is larger shot sizes, typically known as "buckshot." A 2¾-inch 12-gauge shotgun round may contain up to nine 00 buckshot pellets, each of which is ballistically equivalent to a .32 caliber pistol round. Type II injuries occur at a distance of 3 to 7 meters and often permit the pellets to penetrate deep fascia with internal organ injury possible. Type III injuries occur at a distance of less than 3 meters and usually involve massive tissue destruction and life-threatening injury.

The severity of penetrating thoracic trauma is often related to the structures involved. Lung tissue is very resilient when impacted by high-energy projectiles. The "spongy" nature of the air-filled alveoli absorbs the cavitation wave energy and reduces the temporary cavity size and injury associated with compression and stretching. The great vessels and heart (if it is distended with blood) react much differently. Fluid transmits kinetic energy readily and may cause cardiac or vessel rupture. On the other hand, simple penetration may occur with slower-moving projectiles or if the heart is struck while in diastole. Although a projectile tends to move in a straight line, it is easily deflected by contact with bony structures within the chest. Contact with bones also fragments the projectile (as well as the skeletal structure it strikes), increasing the energy exchange rate and injury seriousness. Penetrating trauma frequently leads to pneumothorax, which may be bilateral, depending on the missile or knife track. Table 7-3 lists common injuries associated with penetrating thoracic trauma. Intraabdominal and

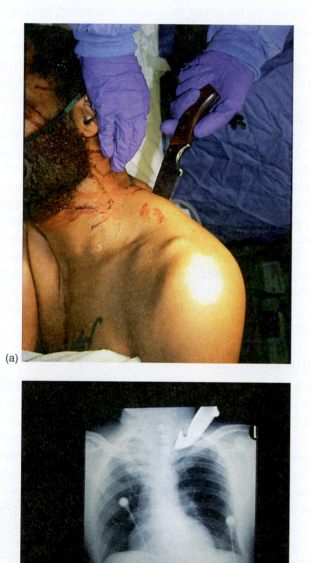

(a)

(b)

FIGURE 7-5 (a) Penetrating (stab) wound to the chest. (b) X-ray shows deep penetration.

(Both: © Edward T. Dickinson, MD)

Table 7-3 Injuries Associated with Penetrating Thoracic Trauma

Closed pneumothorax
Open pneumothorax (including sucking chest wound)
Tension pneumothorax
Pneumomediastinum
Hemothorax
Hemopneumothorax
Laceration of vascular structures, including the great vessels
Tracheobronchial tree lacerations
Esophageal lacerations
Penetrating cardiac injuries
Pericardial tamponade
Spinal cord injuries
Diaphragmatic penetration/laceration/rupture
Intraabdominal penetration with associated organ injury

diaphragmatic injuries often occur in conjunction with penetrating chest trauma. (Figure 7-6).

Chest Wall Injuries

Chest wall injuries are by far the most common injuries encountered in blunt chest trauma. As previously discussed, an intact and moving chest wall is necessary to develop pressures essential for air movement into and out of the lungs (the bellows effect). Chest wall injury may disrupt this motion and result in respiratory insufficiency. Closed chest wall injuries include contusions, rib fractures, sternal fractures/dislocations, and flail chest. Open chest wall injuries are almost entirely the result of penetrating trauma and are often associated with injury of deeper

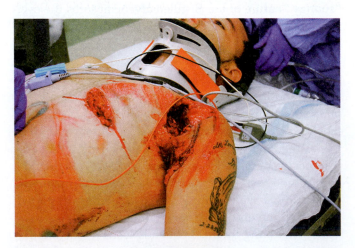

FIGURE 7-6 Penetrating wounds to the chest often will involve the abdomen or abdominal organs.

(© Edward T. Dickinson, MD)

structures, in addition to disruption of the changing intrathoracic pressure necessary for respiration.

Chest Wall Contusion

A chest wall contusion is the most common result of blunt thoracic injury. Injury damages the soft tissue covering the thoracic cage and causes pain with respiratory effort. Like contusions elsewhere, a chest wall contusion may present initially with erythema, then ecchymosis. Discoloration may outline the object that caused the injury; the affected ribs, as soft tissue is trapped between the ribs and the source; and/or a combination of both. The most common symptom of chest wall contusion is pain. Typically, the pain is worse with deep breathing and may reduce chest expansion. The contusion site is often tender and associated with chest wall movement because of the pain. You may auscultate diminished breath sounds because of the hypoventilation resulting from limited chest expansion. Hypoventilation may not be apparent in a young, otherwise healthy individual and may not pose a significant life threat because of the individual's significant pulmonary reserves. Older patients, however, often have preexisting medical problems and little pulmonary reserve, and do not tolerate this injury as well. Some patients may become hypoxemic. Pediatric patients have very flexible ribs that resist fracture and easily transmit trauma forces. The result may be chest wall contusion and internal injury without rib fracture.

Rib Fractures

Rib fractures are found in more than 50 percent of serious blunt chest trauma. Rib fractures are likely to occur at the impact point or along the object's border as it contacts the chest (Figure 7-7). Fractures may also occur at a location remote from the injury site. The thoracic cage is a hollow structure with some flex to it. As compressional blunt trauma force deforms the thorax, ribs flex and may fracture at their weakest point, the posterior angle (along the posterior axillary line).

Ribs 4 through 8 are most commonly fractured because they are least protected by other structures and are firmly fixed at both ends (to the spine and sternum). It takes great force to fracture ribs 1 through 3 because the shoulder, scapula, and heavy musculature of the upper chest protect them. Their fracture is sometimes associated with severe intrathoracic injuries (tracheobronchial tree injury, aortic

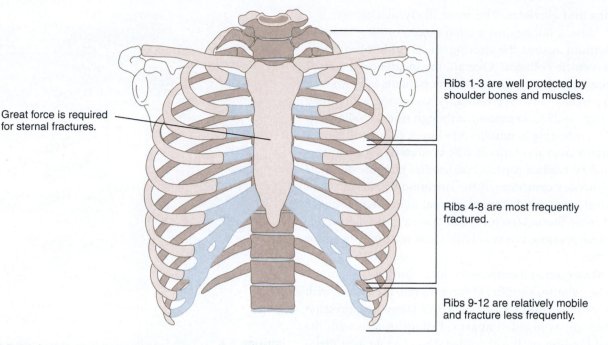

Great force is required for sternal fractures.

Ribs 1-3 are well protected by shoulder bones and muscles.

Ribs 4-8 are most frequently fractured.

Ribs 9-12 are relatively mobile and fracture less frequently.

FIGURE 7-7 Rib fractures.

rupture, and other vascular injuries), especially if multiple ribs are involved. Ribs 9 through 12 are less firmly attached to the sternum, relatively mobile, and thus less likely to fracture. However, they more easily transmit trauma energy to internal organs and may permit more intraabdominal injury without fracture. Fractures of ribs 9 through 12 are frequently associated with serious trauma and splenic or hepatic injury.

The incidence and significance of rib fracture vary with age. Pediatric patients have very cartilaginous ribs that bend easily. Their ribs resist fracture and transmit forces to the thoracic and abdominal structures underneath. Pediatric patients thus have a decreased incidence of rib fractures, but have a higher incidence of pulmonary contusions. Geriatric patients, however, have ribs that are calcified, less flexible, and more easily fractured and are more likely to have comorbidities like COPD, which reduces respiratory reserves and compounds the effects of rib injury. If multiple rib fractures are noted in a young adult, they are probably associated with significant trauma and may lead to significant pain, splinting, hypoventilation, and inadequate cough. They may also be associated with significant internal injuries. The mortality associated with rib fractures increases with the number of fractures, extremes of age (the very young or very old), and associated chronic respiratory or cardiac problems, especially in elderly trauma victims.

Rib fractures are likely to be associated with an overlying chest wall contusion and present with similar signs and symptoms. The fracture site may also demonstrate a grating sensation (crepitus) as bone ends move against each other, either during chest wall movement or during direct palpation (although this is uncommon). Pain associated with rib fracture is often greater than that with chest wall contusion and will more greatly limit respiratory excursion. Pain with deep inspiration in patients with rib fractures may also inhibit the sigh reflex, the body's physiologic response to **atelectasis**. Pediatric patients may grunt during exhalation if atelectasis is present. Grunting, or partial expiration against a closed glottis, increases positive end-expiratory pressure (PEEP) and helps limit atelectasis. This reduced chest wall excursion may cause hypoxia, hypoventilation, and muscle spasms at the fracture site.

Hypoventilation can result in a progressive alveolar collapse (atelectasis). This collapse reduces lung surface available for gas exchange and can contribute to hypoxia. These atelectatic segments also may become filled with blood or tissue fluid from the injury and set the stage for secondary infection, such as pneumonia. Although pneumonia does not develop in the emergency setting, it causes significant mortality in blunt chest injury patients. Serious internal injuries may also result as jagged rib ends may lacerate structures beneath them. Intercostal artery laceration may result in hemothorax, whereas intercostal nerve damage may result in a focal neurologic deficit (numbness or weakness) of the affected intercostal muscle and associated skin and soft tissue structures. Lower rib fracture and displacement may injure the liver (right) or spleen (left).

Sternal Fracture and Dislocation
Sternal fractures and dislocations are usually associated with blunt anterior chest trauma. Sternal fractures result only from severe impact, as this chest region is well supported by

the ribs and clavicles. The most likely mechanism is a direct blow, a fall against a fixed object, or blunt force of the sternum against the steering wheel or dashboard in a motor vehicle collision. Overall, the incidence of sternal fracture in serious thoracic trauma patients is between 5 and 8 percent. However, mortality associated with it may be as high as 25 to 45 percent, although recent studies suggest that mortality is significantly lower. Almost all sternal fracture-related mortality is due to underlying blunt cardiac injury, cardiac rupture, pericardial tamponade, and/or pulmonary contusion. If the surrounding ribs or costochondral joints are disrupted, sternal injury may result in a flail chest. Sternal fractures can cause a noticeable deformity and possible crepitus with chest wall movement or palpation.

Dislocation at the sternoclavicular joint is uncommon and also requires significant force. It, too, may occur with blunt anterior chest trauma or with a lateral compression mechanism, as in side impact collisions or falls with the patient landing on the shoulder. The clavicle may dislocate from the sternum in one of two ways, anteriorly or posteriorly. Anterior dislocation creates a noticeable deformity anterior to the manubrium. Posterior dislocation displaces the clavicle head behind the sternum, leaving a void just lateral to the manubrium. (Any deformity is more difficult to identify, although the shoulder may noticeably displace anteriorly and medially.) Posterior clavicular dislocation may compress or lacerate underlying great vessels or compress or injure the trachea and esophagus. Tracheal compression may result in stridor and voice change.

Flail Chest

A **flail chest** is a chest segment that becomes free to move independently with respiratory pressure changes. The condition occurs when three or more adjacent ribs fracture in two or more places (Figure 7-8). It is one of the most serious chest wall injuries because it is often associated with severe underlying pulmonary injury (contusion) and it reduces respiratory volume while increasing respiratory effort. This underlying injury adds to morbidity and mortality in serious thoracic trauma (between 20 and 40 percent), as do age, head injury, shock, and other associated injuries. The most common injury mechanisms causing flail chest are blunt traumas from falls, motor vehicle crashes, industrial injuries, and assaults.

The flail segment is no longer an intact, controlled part of the chest wall. Increasing intrathoracic pressure associated with expiration moves the flail segment outward while the rest of the chest moves inward (paradoxical movement). This moves air from uninjured alveoli to alveoli under the flail segment. This movement, in turn, reduces the tidal volume, increases respiratory effort associated with ventilation, and can move the mediastinum

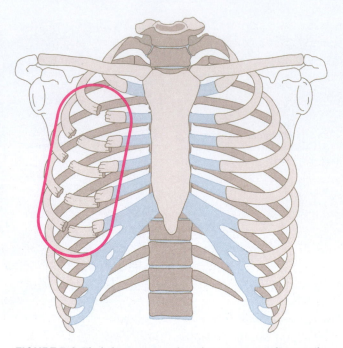

FIGURE 7-8 Flail chest occurs when three or more adjacent ribs fracture in two or more places.

toward the injury. During inspiration, intrathoracic pressure falls as respiratory muscles move the chest wall outward and the diaphragm drops caudally (toward the tail). Reduced intrathoracic pressure draws the flail segment inward as the adjacent chest wall moves outward. Lung tissue beneath the flail segment moves inward with the inward-moving segment, reducing the air volume moving into the thorax and displacing the mediastinum away from the injury. In summary, the injury produces a chest wall segment that moves in opposition to the chest's normal respiratory effort, reduces air volume moved through the airway, and displaces the mediastinum toward and then away from the injury site with each breath (Figure 7-9). In flail chest, the patient takes more energy to move less air, and respiratory volume is further reduced as rib fracture pain produces chest wall splinting.

It takes tremendous energy to cause a flail chest (three or more ribs fractured in two or more places). As a result, it

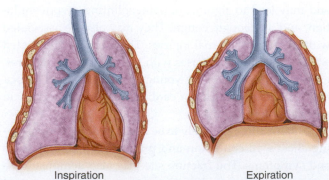

| Inspiration | Expiration |

FIGURE 7-9 Paradoxical movement of the chest wall seen in flail chest.

is often associated with serious internal injuries. In addition, flail segment movement, which is opposite to the rest of the chest wall, can be damaging to surrounding tissue. With each breath, fracture sites move against one another, causing further muscle damage, soft-tissue damage, and pain. Small flail segments may go undetected as associated intercostal muscle spasm naturally splints the segment. With time, however, these muscles suffer further injury and fatigue and the flail segment's paradoxical movement becomes more and more apparent.

Positive-pressure ventilation of a flail chest patient can reverse the pressures that cause paradoxical chest wall movement, restore tidal volume, and reduce the pain of chest wall movement. It accomplishes this by pushing the chest wall and flail segment together and outward with positive pressure. Passive expiration then causes both the flail segment and the remaining chest to move inward together. However, with underlying injury, positive-pressure ventilation may cause a pneumothorax. It must also be noted that positive pressure ventilation may limit blood return through the vena cava (by increasing intrathoracic pressure). Blood flow in the vena cava is normally enhanced by the negative intrathoracic pressure that occurs during normal inspiration. Careful monitoring for changes in hemodynamic status is necessary.

Pulmonary Injuries

Pulmonary injuries are injuries to lung tissue and/or the tissues that support the lung and allow it to contact the interior of the thoracic cavity. Pulmonary injuries include simple pneumothorax, open pneumothorax, tension pneumothorax, hemothorax, and pulmonary contusion.

Simple Pneumothorax

A simple **pneumothorax** (also known as closed pneumothorax) occurs when lung tissue is injured and air leaks into the pleural space (Figure 7-10). Simple pneumothorax can result from penetrating or blunt trauma. However, air does not enter through the wound, but through airway injuries the trauma caused. In simple pneumothorax, the intrathoracic pressure does not exceed normal expiratory pressures and there is no mediastinal shift. As more and more air accumulates in the pleural space, the lung eventually collapses. With lung collapse (pneumothorax), there is associated alveolar collapse (atelectasis) and blood shunted past the collapsed alveoli without undergoing respiratory gas exchange. As more and more alveoli collapse, this condition, called ventilation/perfusion mismatch, becomes more pronounced and begins to cause hypoxemia and hypercarbia (acidosis). This could become life endangering, especially if there are other associated injuries or shock.

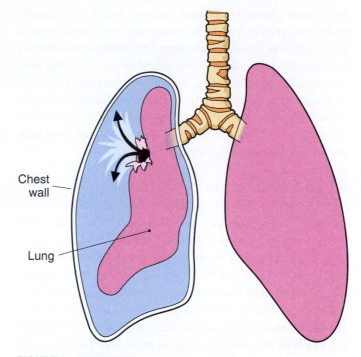

FIGURE 7-10 Simple (closed) pneumothorax.

As mentioned earlier, simple pneumothorax can occur with penetrating and blunt mechanisms. Blunt trauma may cause a pneumothorax when a rib fracture directly punctures the lung. Another mechanism may cause alveolar rupture from a sudden increase in intrathoracic pressure as the chest impacts the steering column with fully expanded lungs and a closed glottis (much like a paper bag filled with air and compressed suddenly between two hands). The incidence of pneumothorax in serious thoracic trauma is reported to be between 10 and 30 percent; its morbidity is related to the degree of atelectasis and ventilation/perfusion mismatch present. Penetrating chest trauma is frequently associated with simple pneumothorax or with an injury that allows air to enter the pleural space through an external wound (open pneumothorax).

A simple pneumothorax reduces respiratory efficiency and may lead to hypoxia. Hypoxia and increases in CO_2 blood levels trigger the medulla to increase respiratory rate (tachypnea) and volume. If the pneumothorax is small, there may be no apparent signs or symptoms. A larger pneumothorax may cause mild dyspnea, however, and complete lung collapse may result in severe dyspnea and hypoxia. The signs, symptoms, and significance of simple pneumothorax increase with any preexisting disease. A pneumothorax may produce local chest pain with respiration as pleurae become irritated (respirophasic pain). This injury may cause the chest to hyperinflate and breath sounds to diminish on the affected side (usually in the extremes of the upper and lower lung first). A small pneumothorax involving less than 15 percent of the affected lung may be difficult to detect clinically and requires only supportive measures. Often, a small pneumothorax will seal itself and air in the pleural cavity will be reabsorbed. A larger pneumothorax is often clinically apparent and requires more aggressive therapy, such as supplemental oxygen chest tube placement (in the emergency department).

Open Pneumothorax

An open pneumothorax is more common in military injuries when a high-velocity bullet creates a significant chest wall wound (usually an exit wound). Recently, the use of high-velocity assault weapons has become more common in civilian settings and thus the frequency of these injuries is on the increase. Another cause of open pneumothorax is a shotgun blast at close range, with an associated large chest wall wound. This chest wall disruption leads to free air passage between the atmosphere and pleural space (Figure 7-11). Air is drawn into the wound as the chest moves outward and the diaphragm moves downward during inspiration. Intrathoracic pressure falls and air enters through the wound and into the chest cavity. This air replaces lung tissue, allows lung collapse, and results in a large functional dead space. Inspiratory effort of the contralateral chest pulls the mediastinum toward it and away from the injury. This prevents the uninjured lung from inflating fully. On exhalation, the contracting chest wall and rising diaphragm increase intrathoracic pressure, forcing force air outward through the wound. This air movement is often called a "sucking chest wound."

For air movement to occur through a chest wall opening, the opening must be at least two-thirds the diameter of the trachea. Remember, trachea size is about that of the patient's little finger. This must be the unimpeded size of the chest opening—not the wound size. The chest wall's thickness and resiliency often allow tissues to close around a wound to air movement, thereby limiting air movement (unless the wound is quite large). Such wounds rarely occur with handgun rounds, but may be possible with high-velocity rifle rounds. With these, the defect may allow free air movement and create an open pneumothorax.

An open pneumothorax can be recognized by the large open chest wound and the characteristic air movement (or sound) produced. Air passage through the wound and the wound's associated hemorrhage may produce frothy blood around the opening—another characteristic of an open pneumothorax. The patient is likely to experience increased dyspnea, and possibly hypovolemia, from associated hemorrhage. The patient's condition is further compromised because the reduced intrathoracic pressures developed during inspiration do not assist venous return, as occurs with an intact chest and normal respiratory effort.

Tension Pneumothorax

A **tension pneumothorax** is an open or simple pneumothorax that generates and maintains a pressure greater than atmospheric pressure within the thorax. It may be caused by trauma or possibly by positive-pressure ventilation of a patient with chest trauma or a congenital defect affecting the respiratory tree. A tension pneumothorax may also occur as an open pneumothorax is sealed or when a piece of tissue acts as a one-way valve, allowing air to enter the pleural space but not exit and thus causing a pressure buildup.

Tension pneumothorax occurs because the mechanism of injury (either an external wound or an internal injury) forms a one-way valve. Air flows into the pleural space through the defect during inspiration because the pressure within the intrathoracic pressure is less than atmospheric pressure. With expiration, increasing intrathoracic and pleural pressure closes the defect and does not permit air to escape. With each breath, air volume and pressure within the pleural space increases. Increasing intrapleural pressure will often collapse the lung on the ipsilateral side, which causes intercostal and suprasternal bulging and places pressure on the mediastinum. As pressure continues to build, it displaces the mediastinum, compressing the uninjured lung and crimping the vena cava as

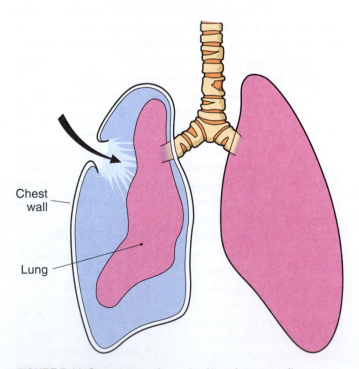

Chest wall

Lung

FIGURE 7-11 Open pneumothorax (sucking chest wound).

CONTENT REVIEW

➤ Signs and Symptoms of Open Pneumothorax
- Penetrating chest trauma
- Sucking chest wound
- Frothy blood at wound site
- Dyspnea
- Hypovolemia

it enters the thorax through the diaphragm and/or where it attaches to the heart. This reduces venous return (which, in turn, reduces cardiac output), resulting in an increase in venous pressure that causes jugular venous distention (JVD) and a narrow pulse pressure. Tracheal shift occurs when the mediastinum is pushed away from the side of the chest with increasing pressure. Tracheal shift is a very late and rare finding and is more commonly seen in young trauma victims, as the younger mediastinum is more mobile than an adult's. Atelectasis occurs in the ipsilateral side from the initial lung collapse and on the contralateral (uninjured or opposite) side from mediastinal shift and compression of the uninjured lung. These mechanisms lead to a ventilation/perfusion mismatch, further hypoxemia, and systemic hypoxia.

A tension pneumothorax begins with simple or open pneumothorax (Figure 7-12). As the pleural space pressure begins to rise, dyspnea, ventilation/perfusion mismatch, and hypoxemia develop. The ipsilateral chest becomes hyperinflated and hyperresonant to percussion and respiratory sounds become very faint, then absent. Increasing intrathoracic pressure may cause the intercostal tissues to bulge outward. The contralateral chest becomes somewhat dull to percussion, with progressively fainter respiratory sounds as the tension pneumothorax worsens.

Severe hypoxia will cause cyanosis, diaphoresis, and altered mental status, while increased intrathoracic pressure reduces venous return and may cause JVD and hypotension. If the condition is not quickly recognized and promptly treated, it may lead to death. Often the most obvious clinical finding is a pneumothorax and associated hemodynamic compromise.

Tension pneumothorax is a serious, progressive, and immediate threat to life. It is corrected by relieving the intrapleural pressure by inserting a needle through the chest wall to convert a tension pneumothorax to an open pneumothorax. As long as the catheter remains open, it will relieve any building pressure, ensure venous return, and help to maintain adequate ventilation.

CONTENT REVIEW

➤ Signs and Symptoms of Tension Pneumothorax
- Chest trauma
- Severe dyspnea
- Ventilation/perfusion mismatch
- Hypoxemia
- Hyperinflation of affected side of chest
- Hyperresonance of affected side of chest
- Diminished, then absent breath sounds
- Cyanosis
- Diaphoresis
- Altered mental status
- Jugular venous distention
- Hypotension
- Hypovolemia

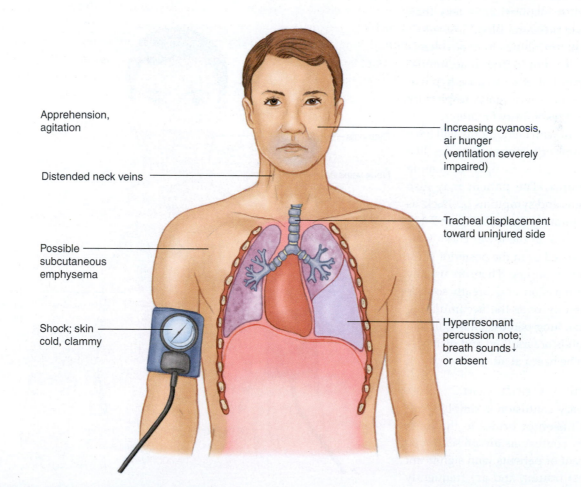

Apprehension, agitation

Distended neck veins

Possible subcutaneous emphysema

Shock; skin cold, clammy

Increasing cyanosis, air hunger (ventilation severely impaired)

Tracheal displacement toward uninjured side

Hyperresonant percussion note; breath sounds↓ or absent

FIGURE 7-12 Physical findings of tension pneumothorax.

Hemothorax

A **hemothorax** is simply an accumulation of blood in the pleural space from internal hemorrhage. It can be very minor and not detectable in the field or, when associated with serious or great vessel injury, may result in rapid patient deterioration. Serious hemorrhage may displace a complete lung and accumulate more than 1,500 mL of blood rapidly in the chest. The mortality rate is often over 75 percent, with almost two-thirds of those dying at the scene. Hemothorax is primarily a blood loss problem, as each hemithorax may hold up to 3,000 mL of blood (or half the total blood volume). However, blood lost into the thorax also reduces the tidal volume and respiratory efficiency in a patient who has already suffered trauma and is likely to develop shock.

Hemothorax is often associated with rib fractures and seen with either blunt or penetrating mechanisms. It often accompanies pneumothorax (a **hemopneumothorax**) and occurs 25 percent of the time with penetrating trauma. Hemorrhage into the pleural space may occur from a lung laceration (most common) or laceration to the intercostal arteries, pulmonary arteries or veins, great vessels, or the internal mammary artery. Intercostal arteries can bleed at a rate of 50 mL/min. Bleeding into the chest is more rapid than would occur elsewhere because pressure within the chest during inspiration is less than atmospheric pressure. Blood lost into a hemothorax contributes to hypovolemia and displaces lung tissue. If accumulation is significant, it may cause hypovolemia and shock, hypoxemia, respiratory distress, and respiratory failure.

A patient with hemothorax will have either a blunt or penetrating injury like those associated with open or simple pneumothorax. The patient may also display signs and symptoms of shock, as well as respiratory distress (Figure 7-13). Blood will pool in the lower chest if the patient is seated or in the posterior chest if the patient is supine. There are usually normal percussion and breath sounds except directly over the accumulating fluid. There, lung percussion is dull and breath sounds are muffled and distant—if they can be heard at all.

Pulmonary Contusion

A pulmonary contusion is simply a soft tissue contusion or bruise to the lung. Pulmonary contusions are present in 30 to 75 percent of patients with significant blunt chest trauma and are frequently associated with rib fractures. Pulmonary contusions range in severity from very limited, minor, and unrecognizable injuries to those that are extensive and possibly life threatening. They result in a mortality rate of between 14 and 20 percent for serious chest trauma patients.

Two specific injury mechanisms can cause energy transfer to the pulmonary tissue and result in pulmonary contusions. They are deceleration or the pressure wave associated with either passage of a high-velocity bullet or explosion. Deceleration injury is by far the most common etiology and occurs as the moving body strikes a fixed object. A common example of this mechanism is chest impact with the steering wheel during an auto collision or contact with the ground if ejected from a moving vehicle. As the chest wall hits the object and stops, the lungs continue forward, compressing and stretching the alveolar tissues (or shearing them). This causes alveolar/capillary membrane disruption, leading to microscopic hemorrhage and edema.

CONTENT REVIEW

➤ Signs and Symptoms of Hemothorax
- Blunt or penetrating chest trauma
- Signs and symptoms of shock
- Dyspnea
- Dull percussive sounds over site of collecting blood

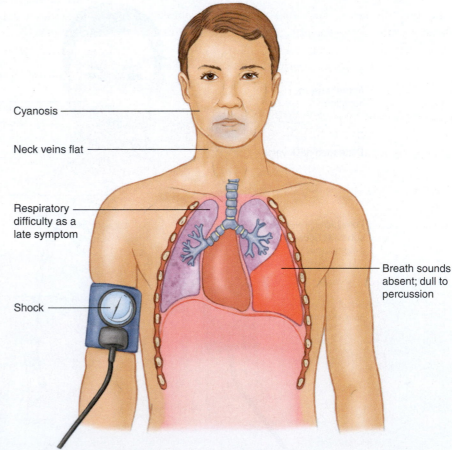

Cyanosis

Neck veins flat

Respiratory difficulty as a late symptom

Shock

Breath sounds absent; dull to percussion

FIGURE 7-13 Physical findings of massive hemothorax.

The second mechanism, an explosion or bullet's pressure wave passage, can compress and stretch lung tissue. Because of the nature of lung tissue (air-filled sacs surrounded by delicate and vascular membranes), pressure passage is partially reflected at the gas/fluid (alveolar/capillary) interface. This leaves small, flame-shaped disruption areas throughout the membrane leading to microhemorrhage and edema (called the *Spalding effect*). Pulmonary contusions are generally not associated with low-speed chest penetration and lung tissue and structure laceration.

The microhemorrhage seen with pulmonary contusion may be extensive and result in up to 1,000 to 1,500 mL of blood loss (although this is uncommon). This hemorrhage also may cause tissue irritation, initiate the inflammation process, and cause fluid to migrate into the interstitial space. Fluid accumulation in the alveolar/capillary membrane (pulmonary edema) adversely affects the rate at which the respiratory gases can diffuse across it. Fluid accumulation also stiffens the membrane, making the lung less compliant and increasing the work of breathing. Edema development also increases the pressures necessary to move blood through pulmonary capillary beds. This increases the pulmonary vascular system pressure (pulmonary hypertension) and the workload of the right heart. In combination, these effects lead to atelectasis, hypovolemia, ventilation/perfusion mismatch, hypoxemia, hypotension, and, possibly, respiratory failure and shock. Although isolated pulmonary contusions can occur, they are frequently associated with other injuries.

A patient with pulmonary contusion will report a mechanism of injury and evidence of blunt or penetrating chest injury. Although associated injuries may display immediate signs and symptoms (as in rib fracture pain), the signs and symptoms of a pulmonary contusion take time to develop. A patient will likely complain of increasing dyspnea, have increasing respiratory effort, and show progressing hypoxia, as evidenced by gradually falling oxygen saturation levels. Careful chest auscultation may reveal increasing crackles and fainter breath sounds. Serious pulmonary contusion may cause **hemoptysis** and possibly signs and symptoms of shock.

Cardiovascular Injuries

Cardiovascular injuries are associated with the mortality rate in chest trauma victims. These include blunt cardiac injury, pericardial tamponade, myocardial aneurysm or rupture, aortic aneurysm or rupture, and other vascular injuries.

Blunt Cardiac Injury

Blunt cardiac injury carries a high mortality rate and occurs most commonly with severe blunt anterior chest trauma. When the chest strikes an object or an object strikes the chest, the heart, which is relatively mobile within the chest, strikes the anterior chest wall and then is compressed between the sternum and thoracic spine as the thorax flexes with impact. The resulting contusion will most likely affect the right atrium and ventricle (the portions of the heart that are the most anterior in the chest) (Figure 7-14).

A cardiac contusion is similar to any other muscle contusion. The injury disrupts muscle cells and microcirculation, resulting in muscle fiber tearing and damage, hemorrhage, and edema. Injury may reduce the cardiac contractile strength and reduce cardiac output. Because of cardiac muscle automaticity and conductivity, contusion may also disturb the cardiac conductive system. If injury is significant, it may lead to hematoma, pericardial tamponade, and necrosis and may result in cardiac irritability, ectopic (abnormal origin) beats, and conduction system defects, such as bundle branch blocks and arrhythmias. If the injury is very extensive, it may lead to tissue necrosis (death), decreased ventricular compliance, congestive heart failure, cardiogenic shock, myocardial aneurysm, and acute or delayed myocardial rupture. In contrast to a myocardial infarction from coronary artery disease, cellular damage from blunt cardiac injury heals with less scarring and there is limited injury progression in the absence of associated coronary artery disease.

A patient experiencing blunt cardiac injury usually will have experienced significant blunt chest trauma—most likely affecting the anterior chest. The patient will likely complain of chest or retrosternal pain, very much

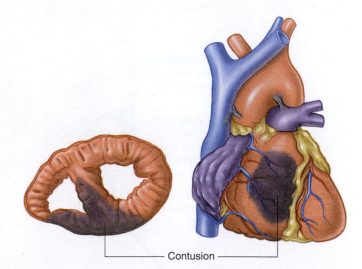

— Contusion —

FIGURE 7-14 Blunt cardiac injury most frequently affects the right atrium and ventricle as they collide with the sternum.

CONTENT REVIEW

➤ Signs and Symptoms of Pulmonary Contusion
- Blunt or penetrating chest trauma
- Increasing dyspnea
- Hypoxia
- Increasing crackles
- Diminishing breath sounds
- Hemoptysis
- Signs and symptoms of shock

like that of myocardial infarction, and may have associated chest injuries such as anterior rib or sternal fractures. Cardiac monitoring usually reveals a sinus tachycardia (though it may be caused by the fight-or-flight response, pain, hypovolemia, or hypoxia from associated chest injury). Other arrhythmias associated with blunt cardiac injuries are atrial flutter or fibrillation, premature atrial or ventricular contractions, tachyarrhythmias, bradyarrhythmias, bundle branch patterns, T wave inversions, and ST segment elevations. A pericardial friction rub and murmur may be auscultated over the **precordium** but is more likely to occur weeks after injury and is associated with development of inflammatory pericardial effusion.

COMMOTIO CORDIS **Commotio cordis** is a rare event in which ventricular fibrillation is induced by a direct chest blow. Often the impact is seemingly modest, such as being struck in the chest by a baseball. Although commotio cordis is rare, it is the second leading cause of sudden death in young athletes. Historical data have shown that approximately 95 percent of cases occurred in males and 87 percent in whites. The average age of occurrence is 14 years, with a range of 3 months to 52 years. Approximately 15 percent of victims are successfully resuscitated. Survival rates are low because the condition is initially unrecognized or misdiagnosed during the time when CPR or defibrillation should be provided. Treatment for commotio cordis is the same as for ventricular fibrillation and should include CPR and immediate defibrillation.

Pericardial Tamponade

Pericardial tamponade is a restriction to cardiac filling caused by blood (or other fluid) filling the pericardial sac. It occurs in less than 2 percent of all serious chest trauma patients and is almost always related to penetrating injury. Low-velocity wounds, such as stabbings and low-energy weapons, are the most frequent mechanism and carry a high overall mortality. High-velocity gunshot wounds to the heart result in significant tissue destruction and almost certain death.

Pericardial tamponade begins with a tear in a superficial coronary artery or following penetration of the myocardium by an object. Blood leaks into the pericardial space and accumulates (Figure 7-15). The fibrous pericardium

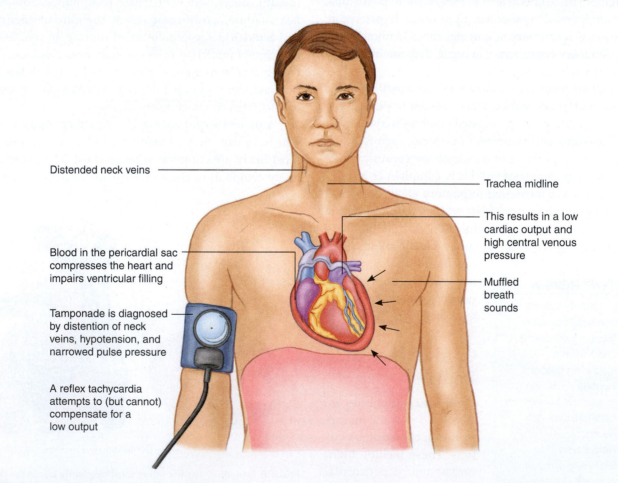

Distended neck veins

Trachea midline

This results in a low
cardiac output and
high central venous
pressure

Blood in the pericardial sac
compresses the heart and
impairs ventricular filling

Muffled
breath
sounds

Tamponade is diagnosed
by distention of neck
veins, hypotension, and
narrowed pulse pressure

A reflex tachycardia
attempts to (but cannot)
compensate for a
low output

FIGURE 7-15 Physical findings of cardiac tamponade.

does not stretch and the accumulating blood exerts pressure on the heart. Even limited pressure limits cardiac filling. This first affects the right ventricle, where filling pressure is the lowest. As pericardial tamponade develops, the increasing pressure slows venous return to the heart, increases central venous pressure, and causes JVD. Reduced right ventricular output limits outflow to pulmonary arteries and then venous return to the left heart. Cardiac tamponade results in a decreasing cardiac output and systemic hypotension. Pressure exerted by blood in the pericardium also restricts blood flow through coronary arteries and to the myocardium. This may result in myocardial ischemia and infarct. It takes about 150 to 300 mL of blood to exert a pressure necessary to induce frank tamponade, whereas removing as little as 20 mL may provide significant relief. The progression of pericardial tamponade depends on the rate of blood flow into the pericardial sac. It may occur very rapidly (as occurs with a stab wound) and result in death before emergency medical services arrival, or may gradually progress over hours (usually from a medical condition or recent cardiothoracic surgery).

The patient with pericardial tamponade will likely have a penetrating injury to the anterior or posterior chest, although blunt trauma can also cause this problem. Although projectile and knife blade trajectories are difficult to predict, always consider the possibility of pericardial tamponade with any thoracic or upper abdominal penetrating wound—especially if it is over the precordium (central lower chest) (Figure 7-16).

Pericardial tamponade diminishes the pulse strength, decreases the pulse pressure, and distends the jugular veins. The patient will likely be agitated, tachycardic, diaphoretic, and ashen in appearance. Cyanosis may be noted in the head, neck, and upper extremities. Heart tones may be muffled or distant sounding. Beck's triad (JVD, distant heart tones, and hypotension) is indicative of pericardial tamponade but may not be recognized early after the injury. Another sign of pericardial tamponade is Kussmaul's sign—a decrease or absence of JVD during inspiration. As a patient inspires, reduced intrathoracic pressure increases venous return and decreases the pressure from the accumulating pericardial fluid. This translates to a better venous return and cardiac output during inspiration, and the effect can be seen in the jugular veins.

Other findings suggesting pericardial tamponade can include pulsus

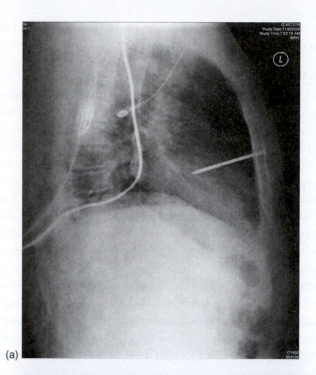

(a)

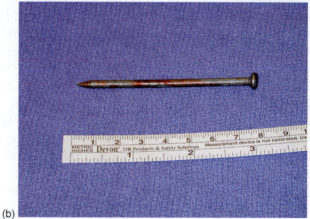

(b)

FIGURE 7-16 Penetrating trauma to the heart (nail) (a) as seen on lateral chest X-ray and (b) following surgical removal.
(Both: © Edward T. Dickinson, MD)

CONTENT REVIEW

➤ Signs and Symptoms of Pericardial Tamponade
- Dyspnea and possible cyanosis
- Jugular venous distention
- Weak, thready pulse
- Decreasing blood pressure
- Shock
- Narrowing pulse pressure

paradoxus and electrical alternans. **Pulsus paradoxus** is an abnormally large decrease in a systolic blood pressure during inspiration. With pulsus paradoxus the drop in systolic pressure can exceed 10 mmHg as the patient inspires during the normal respiratory cycle. (Normally, systolic blood pressure drops just slightly with each inspiration.) Pulsus paradoxus results from an increase in cardiac output as the intrapericardial pressure increases with tamponade. This ultimately causes reduced intrathoracic inspiration pressure. As the systolic pressure varies with pulsus paradoxus, there may be an alternation between strong and weak pulse called **pulsus alternans**. **Electrical alternans**, which is only rarely seen in acute pericardial tamponade, is noted on a cardiac rhythm strip as P, QRS, and T amplitude decreases with every other cardiac cycle. In profound pericardial tamponade, the heart displays a rhythm without producing a pulse (pulseless electrical activity [PEA]).

Myocardial Aneurysm or Rupture

Myocardial **aneurysm** or rupture occurs almost exclusively in extreme blunt thoracic trauma, such as automobile collisions. It also has been reported in cases when blunt forces are not extreme—for example, as a result of CPR. The condition can affect any of the heart's chambers, the interatrial septum, or the interventricular septum, or can involve the valves and their supporting structures. Multiple heart chambers or structures are involved 30 percent of the time. Myocardial aneurysm and delayed myocardial rupture also occur secondary to necrosis from a myocardial infarction, repaired penetrating injury or surgery, or blunt cardiac injury. Necrosis usually develops around two weeks after injury as inflammatory cells replace the weakening or dead myocardial tissue with scar tissue that can lead to ventricular wall aneurysm and/or subsequent rupture. Myocardial rupture can also occur with high-velocity projectile injuries.

A patient who experiences myocardial rupture will likely have suffered serious blunt or penetrating trauma to the chest and may have rib or sternal fractures. Specific symptoms may depend on the actual pathology. The victim may have signs and symptoms of pericardial tamponade if the rupture is contained within the pericardial sac. If the process affects only ruptured valves, the patient may present with right or left heart failure. If there is a myocardial aneurysm, rupture may be delayed. However, when it happens, the patient will suddenly develop absent vital signs or signs and symptoms of pericardial tamponade. Death usually follows.

Traumatic Dissection or Rupture of the Aorta

Aortic dissection and rupture are extremely life-threatening injuries resulting from either blunt or penetrating trauma. Aortic injury is most commonly caused by blunt trauma and carries an overall mortality of 85 to 95 percent. It is responsible for 15 percent of all thoracic trauma deaths. Dissection and rupture are usually associated with high-speed automobile crashes (most commonly, with lateral impact) and in some cases with falls from heights. Unlike myocardial rupture, a significant number, possibly as high as 20 percent, of these victims will survive the initial insult and aneurysm. Some 30 percent of these initial survivors will die within 6 hours if not treated, increasing to about 50 percent at 24 hours, and slightly less than 70 percent by the first week's end. It is often the patient subset that survives the initial impact and is alive when EMS arrives that is the most likely to benefit from recognition of the potential injury and then by rapidly extricating, packaging, and transporting the patient to a trauma center.

Table 7-4 Incidence and Anatomic Location of Traumatic Aortic Rupture

Aortic annulus	9 percent
Aortic isthmus	85 percent
Diaphragm	3 percent
Other	3 percent

The aorta is a large, high-pressure vessel that provides outflow from the left ventricle for distribution to the systemic circulation. It is fixed at three points as it passes through the thoracic cavity and, because of this, experiences shear forces secondary to severe chest deceleration. The fixation points are where the aorta joins the heart (aortic annulus), where it is joined with the ligamentum arteriosum (aortic isthmus), and where it exits the chest (through the diaphragm) (Table 7-4). Traumatic aortic dissection occurs infrequently to the ascending aorta and most commonly to the descending aorta. With severe deceleration, shear forces separate the arterial layers, specifically the interior surface (tunica intima) from the muscle layer (the tunica media). This allows blood to enter and, because it is under great pressure, begins to dissect the aortic lining, forming a false lumen. It is likely to rupture if it is not surgically repaired.

A patient with an aortic rupture will be severely hypotensive and may rapidly lose all vital signs and die unless moved into surgery immediately. Aortic dissection progresses more slowly, although a dissection may rupture at any moment. The patient will probably have a history of a high fall or severe auto collision and deceleration. A lateral impact is an especially high risk factor for aortic dissection or rupture. The patient may complain of severe tearing chest pain that may radiate to the back. The patient may have a pulse deficit between the left and right upper extremities and/or reduced pulse strength in the lower extremities. The blood pressure may be high (hypertension) because of the stretching of sympathetic nerve fibers present in the aorta near the ligamentum arteriosum, or the pressure may be low because of leakage and hypovolemia. Auscultation may reveal a harsh systolic murmur caused by turbulence as blood exits the heart and passes the disrupted blood vessel wall.

Other Vascular Injuries

Pulmonary arteries and venae cavae are other thoracic vascular structures that can sustain injury during chest trauma. Injury to these vessels and resulting hemorrhage may cause a significant hemothorax, possibly leading to hypotension and respiratory insufficiency. Blood may also flow into the mediastinum and compress the great vessels, esophagus, and heart. Penetrating trauma is a primary cause of injury to the pulmonary arteries and venae cavae.

A patient with pulmonary artery or vena cava injury will likely have a penetrating chest or neck wound with a likelihood of central chest involvement. These injuries present with signs and symptoms of hypovolemia and shock and result in hemothorax or hemomediastinum and signs and symptoms associated with those injuries.

Other Thoracic Injuries

Other thoracic injuries worthy of mention include diaphragmatic rupture, esophageal rupture, tracheobronchial disruption, and traumatic asphyxia.

Traumatic Rupture or Perforation of the Diaphragm

Traumatic rupture or perforation of the diaphragm can occur in both high-energy blunt and penetrating thoracoabdominal trauma. The incidence is estimated as being between 1 and 6 percent of all victims of multiple trauma. It is more common in patients who have sustained penetrating trauma to the lower chest. These injuries have an incidence of abdominal organ and tissue involvement as great as 30 to 40 percent. Remember that during expiration the diaphragm may move superiorly to the fourth intercostal space (nipple level) anteriorly and sixth intercostal space posteriorly. Any penetrating injuries at these levels or below may penetrate the diaphragm. Diaphragmatic perforation and herniation occur most frequently on the left side, as the liver tends to protect the right diaphragm. The liver is also unlikely to herniate through a torn diaphragm unless the defect is large.

If traumatic diaphragmatic rupture occurs, the abdominal organs may herniate through the defect into the thoracic cavity. This herniation may cause bowel strangulation or necrosis, ipsilateral lung restriction, and mediastinal displacement. Mediastinal displacement occurs when the displaced abdominal contents place pressure on the lung and mediastinal structures, moving them toward the contralateral side in a mechanism similar to that seen in tension pneumothorax.

Diaphragmatic rupture presents with signs and symptoms similar to those of tension pneumothorax, including dyspnea, hypoxia, hypotension, and JVD. The patient will have blunt abdominal or penetrating trauma to the lower chest or upper abdomen. The abdomen may appear hollow (scaphoid) and bowel sounds may be noted in one side of the thorax (most commonly, the left). The patient may be hypotensive and hypoxic if the herniation is extensive. The patient may complain of upper abdominal pain, although this symptom is often overshadowed by other injuries. If the diaphragmatic tear is small, there may be no herniation. Even with serious tearing, herniation may not occur or it may be delayed by months to years. Without serious herniation, it may be difficult to recognize a diaphragmatic rupture.

Traumatic Esophageal Rupture

Traumatic esophageal rupture is a rare blunt thoracic trauma complication. Esophageal rupture occurs with only about 0.4 percent of penetrating chest trauma. Because the esophagus is centrally located within the chest, injury to this structure usually coincides with other mediastinal injuries. (Esophageal rupture may also result from medical problems such as violent emesis, carcinoma, anatomic distortion, or gastric reflux.) Esophageal rupture carries a 30 percent or greater percent mortality rate, even if quickly recognized. The mortality rate is much greater if this injury is not diagnosed and treated promptly. The mortality from esophageal rupture is related to material from the esophagus entering the mediastinum. This results in serious infection or chemical irritation and serious mediastinal structure damage. Air may also enter the mediastinum through an esophageal rupture, especially during positive-pressure ventilation.

Trauma patients with esophageal rupture will likely have deep penetrating trauma to the central chest and may complain of difficult or painful swallowing, respirophasic chest pain, and pain radiating to the midback. Patients may also display subcutaneous emphysema around the lower neck.

Tracheobronchial Injury (Disruption)

Tracheobronchial injury is a relatively infrequent finding in thoracic trauma, with an incidence of less than 3 percent in patients with significant chest trauma. It may occur from either blunt or penetrating injury mechanisms and carries a high mortality rate (similar to that for esophageal rupture). In contrast to patients with esophageal rupture, who usually die days after injury, 50 percent of tracheobronchial injury patients die within an hour or so of injury. Disruption can occur anywhere in the tracheobronchial tree, but is most likely to occur within 2.5 cm of the carina.

A patient with a tracheal or mainstem bronchial disruption is generally in respiratory distress with cyanosis, hemoptysis, and, in some cases, massive subcutaneous emphysema. The patient may also experience a pneumothorax and/or a tension pneumothorax. Intermittent positive-pressure ventilation can force air into the pleura or mediastinum, making the condition worse.

Traumatic Asphyxia

Traumatic asphyxia occurs when a severe compressive force is applied to the chest. It can lead to a reverse blood flow from the right heart into the superior vena cava and into venous vessels of the upper extremities. (Traumatic asphyxia is not as much a respiratory problem as it is a vascular problem.) Traumatic asphyxia causes engorgement of the veins and capillaries of the head and neck with desaturated venous blood, turning the skin in this region a deep red, purple, or blue. Blood backflow damages

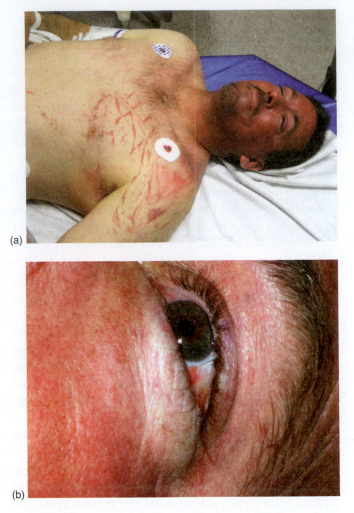

(a)

(b)

FIGURE 7-17 (a) Traumatic asphyxia. (b) Subconjunctival hemorrhage associated with traumatic asphyxia.

(Both: © Dr. Bryan E. Bledsoe)

microcirculation in the head and neck, producing petechiae (small hemorrhages under the skin—Figure 7-17a) and subconjunctival hemorrhages (to the whites of the eyes—Figure 7-17b), and stagnating blood above the compression point.

Backflow may damage cerebral circulation, resulting in numerous small strokes in the older patient whose venous vessels are not very elastic. If flow restriction continues, toxins and acids accumulate in the blood. These toxins may have a devastating effect when they return to the central circulation with the release of pressure. If thoracic compression continues, it restricts venous return and may prevent or seriously restrict the victim's respirations. This results in hypotension, hypoxemia, and shock. Death may follow rapidly. Patient extrication may result in rapid hemorrhage at the injury with pressure release. Compression release may likewise result in rapid patient deterioration and death from internal hemorrhage.

Patients with traumatic asphyxia suffer severe chest compression that is likely to continue until extrication. Compression-induced blood flow restriction and backflow

are dramatic and can cause the classic head and neck discoloration. The victim's face appears swollen (plethora), eyes bulge, and there are numerous subconjunctival hemorrhages. The patient may have severe dyspnea related to the compression and injuries associated with severe chest impact. Once pressure is released, the patient may show signs of hypovolemia, hypotension, and shock as well as signs related to any coexisting respiratory problems.

Patho Pearls

Detecting the Effects of Thoracic Trauma. The thoracic cavity contains three general regions: the pericardial region, the pulmonary region, and the mediastinum. The pericardial region contains the heart and the origin of the great vessels. The pulmonary region contains the lungs, the airways, and the pulmonary vasculature. The mediastinum contains the esophagus, the vagus nerve, the thoracic duct, and other essential structures. Despite these, the thoracic cavity primarily involves respiratory and cardiac functions. Thus, with any thoracic injury, you would expect to see first a variation in respiratory function, cardiac function, or both. With a pneumothorax, you initially will see a subtle increase in respiratory rate and then, as the process progresses, increased respiratory effort and, finally, signs and symptoms of poor oxygenation. If this is allowed to progress untreated, cardiovascular impairment will follow. Cardiovascular impairment can result from incomplete ventricular filling caused by increased intrathoracic pressure or from blood loss within the lung parenchyma.

Similarly, a penetrating injury to the heart can lead to cardiovascular collapse. With low-energy wounds, such as knife stab wounds, the pericardial sac may fill with blood, thus preventing adequate ventricular filling (pericardial tamponade). This will be manifest as an initial increase in heart rate, narrowing of the pulse pressure (resulting from restricted ventricular filling), and distended neck veins. As cardiac efficiency declines, the pulmonary vasculature can become congested, resulting in poor oxygenation. High-energy wounds, such as gunshot wounds, that penetrate the heart are usually mortal wounds—even in the best of EMS systems and trauma centers.

Any time you have a patient with a suspected thoracic injury, first look at the respiratory and circulatory systems for signs of impairment. These findings can help guide you to the nature of your patient's injury.

Assessment of the Chest Injury Patient

Proper assessment of the chest injury patient is critical to anticipating and detecting injury and providing correct interventions. Chest injury patient assessment follows the standard prehospital assessment process, but special considerations regarding chest injury occur during the scene size-up, primary assessment, and especially during the rapid trauma assessment. Reassessment is also critical for injury progression during serious chest trauma.

Scene Size-Up

Chest injury care, like that for any other serious trauma, requires Standard Precautions with gloves as a minimum. Consider a face shield if you will be attending to the airway and a gown for splash protection with serious penetrating thoracic trauma. Ensure a safe scene, including protection from any assailant, if violence is suspected.

Examine the mechanism of injury carefully and determine if the central chest (heart, great vessels, trachea, and esophagus) might be in the path of any penetrating trauma. In gunshot injuries, determine the weapon type, caliber, distance between the gun barrel and victim, and the probable projectile pathway. Determine the direction of blunt trauma impact, as it may also have a bearing on which organs have sustained injury. Anterior impact may rupture lung tissue and contuse the lung and heart. Lateral impact or landing on one's feet from a great height may tear the aorta as the heart displaces laterally and stresses the aorta's ligamentous attachments.

Primary Assessment

During primary assessment, determine a patient's mental status, potential for spine injury, and the airway, breathing, and circulation status. Intervene as necessary to correct life-threatening conditions. It is during primary assessment that first signs and symptoms of serious chest trauma should be identified. Be watchful for any dyspnea and/or any asymmetrical, paradoxical, exaggerated, or limited chest movement. Look for chest hyperinflation or an abdomen that appears hollow. Notice abnormal skin color indicative of hypoxia, such as cyanosis or an ashen discoloration. Look for distended jugular veins, intercostal or suprasternal retractions, and use of accessory muscles of respiration. Also look for any changing neck and facial features caused by subcutaneous emphysema.

Ensure that ventilation is adequate and administer supplemental oxygen as needed to maintain an aequate SpO_2. Provide positive-pressure ventilations with care, if needed. Remember that a thoracic injury may weaken the lung tissues and makes the patient prone to pneumothorax or tension pneumothorax. Positive-pressure ventilations may cause these problems as a side effect of therapy Be suspicious of internal hemorrhage and plan to initiate at least one large-bore intravenous catheter and line or nonrestrictive saline lock in anticipation of hypovolemia, hypotension, and shock. With anterior blunt or penetrating trauma that may involve the heart, attach the ECG electrodes and monitor for arrhythmias. Attach a pulse oximeter and monitor oxygen saturation to evaluate respiratory effectiveness. Waveform capnography may also be useful in detecting early or minute changes in ventilation and perfusion. If there is any mechanism suggesting serious chest trauma or any physical signs of either hypoventilation or hypovolemia compensation, perform rapid trauma assessment with a special focus on the chest and prepare for rapid patient transport to the trauma center.[2]

Secondary/Rapid Trauma Assessment

During rapid trauma assessment, examine the patient's chest in detail, carefully observing, questioning about, palpating, and auscultating the region.

Observe

Observe the chest for impact evidence. Look for erythema that has developed as a result of the injury, especially as it outlines ribs or forms a pattern reflecting contours of the object the chest hit. Look carefully for penetrating trauma and try to determine the entry angle and penetration depth. Also look for exit wounds. A lateral chest injury is likely to involve the lungs, whereas a penetrating injury through the central chest is likely to involve the heart, great vessels, trachea, or esophagus. Injury to the mediastinal structures is also likely to cause serious hemorrhage, hypovolemia, and shock. Look for intercostal and suprasternal retractions, as well as external jugular venous distention. Remember, JVD is normally present in supine normotensive patients and may be exaggerated or may continue if the patient is moved to a seated position if venous pressure is elevated. The jugular veins are usually flat in hypovolemic chest trauma patients.

Watch chest movement carefully during respiration. The chest should rise and the abdomen fall smoothly with inspiration and return to their positions during expiration. Any limited motion, either bilaterally or unilaterally, suggests a problem. Watch for paradoxical motion of a flail chest. That movement will be limited initially because of muscle spasm during early care, but continued respiration may further damage surrounding soft tissues and result in intercostal muscle fatigue. This may lead to progressive and more obvious paradoxical motion and greater respiratory impairment. Look for any hyperinflation of one side of the chest and any deformity that may exist from a rib fracture, sternal fracture or dislocation, or subcutaneous emphysema. Assess the volume of air movement with each breath and ensure that the minute volume is greater than 6 liters. If not, consider gentle supportive ventilation with the bag-valve mask. Assess pulse oximetry and, should saturation begin to drop, consider more aggressive airway and respiratory support, as well as supplemental oxygen administration, as determined by the SpO_2. Examine any open wounds for air movement that may be indicative of an open pneumothorax. Observe the general color of the patient. If a patient's skin is dusky, ashen, or cyanotic, suspect respiratory compromise. Suspect traumatic asphyxia if a patient's head and neck are swollen and red, dark red, or blue.

Question

Question a patient about any pain, pain on motion, pain with breathing effort (respirophasic pain), or dyspnea. Note if the pain is crushing, tearing, or described otherwise by the patient. Have the patient describe the exact location of the pain, its severity, and any radiation of the pain. Question the patient regarding other sensations and carefully monitor the patient's consciousness and orientation levels. Obtain a complete patient history, if possible, and identify any serious preexisting conditions, especially those affecting respiration, such as COPD or asthma.

Palpate

Palpate the thorax carefully and completely, feeling for any injury signs. (Figure 7-18). Feel for any swelling, deformity, crepitus, or crackling. Compress the thorax between your hands with pressure directed inward. Then apply downward pressure on the midsternum. Such pressure will flex the ribs and should elicit pain from any fracture site along the thorax. (Apply pressure only if you have found no signs or symptoms of chest injury. If you suspect rib or sternal fracture, provide appropriate care but do not aggravate the injury.) Rest your hands on the lower thorax and let the chest lift your hands with inspiration and let them fall with expiration. (Figure 7-19). The motion should be smooth and equal. If not, determine the nature of any asymmetry. If appropriate, have the patient take a deep breath and ask him about any discomfort or pain.

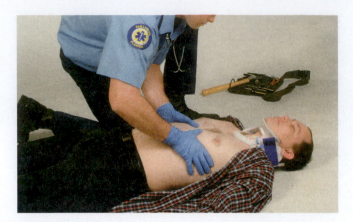

FIGURE 7-19 Place your hands on the lower thorax and let them rise and fall with respiration.

Auscultate

Auscultate all lung fields, both anteriorly and posteriorly (Figure 7-20). Listen for both inspiratory and expiratory air movement and note any crackles, indicating edema from pulmonary contusion or congestive heart failure, and/or any diminished breath sounds, suggesting hypoventilation. Compare one side to the other and one field to another. Listen carefully for distant or muffled heart sounds or decreased breath sounds.

Percuss

Percuss the chest and note the responses. (Figure 7-21). Determine whether the area percussed is normal, hyperresonant, or dull. A dull response suggests blood or other fluid collection, whereas hyperresonance suggests air under pressure, as in tension pneumothorax.

The findings from the rapid trauma assessment may suggest an injury or multiple injuries. Identify the likely cause of any signs and symptoms found and suspect and anticipate the worst. There may be evidence of chest wall injury and some signs of internal injuries if they exist. As

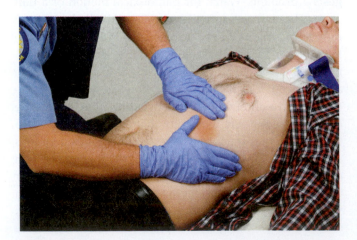

FIGURE 7-18 Carefully palpate the thorax of a patient with a suspected injury to the region.

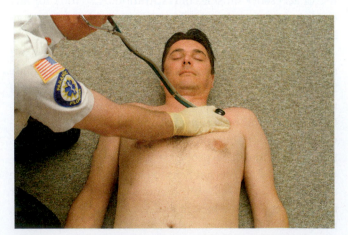

FIGURE 7-20 Auscultate all lung lobes, both anteriorly and posteriorly.

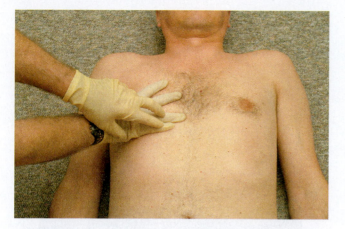

FIGURE 7-21 Percuss all lung lobes, listening for a dull response or hyperresonance.

mentioned earlier, blunt and penetrating trauma typically cause different types of injuries.

Blunt Trauma Assessment

In blunt trauma, there may be a slight chest wall discoloration indicative of a contusion or contusions. Contusions may also cause pain—generally in a specific area or region—and somewhat limit respiration. As the energy of impact increases, there may be fractures of ribs 4 through 8 and a greater possibility of underlying injury. If the upper ribs or ribs 9 through 12 are fractured, suspect a serious underlying injury. Sternal fractures also require great energy and are associated with a higher incidence of internal injury. Rib fractures generate point-specific pain (at the fracture site) and crepitus on deep breathing or palpation of the patient's chest during rapid trauma assessment. That pain may further limit chest excursion during respiration. As energy causing trauma increases, more ribs may be fractured, causing a flail chest. Remember that the paradoxical motion seen with a flail chest is initially limited by muscular splinting and becomes more noticeable and causes more respiratory distress as the time following the injury increases.

In blunt chest injury, anticipate and assess for additional signs suggesting internal injury. Specific signs of lung injury include increasing dyspnea, signs of hypoxemia, accessory muscle use, and intercostal and suprasternal retractions. Auscultation may help differentiate between pulmonary contusion and pneumothorax. Pulmonary contusions may manifest as progressively increasing crackles, whereas a pneumothorax presents with diminishing breath sounds on the ipsilateral side. Further, with pneumothorax, the affected side may be hyperinflated and resonant to percussion. If pneumothorax progresses to tension pneumothorax, there will likely be progressing dyspnea and hypoxia, hemodynamic compromise, accessory muscle use, distended jugular veins, tracheal shift toward the contralateral side (a late finding), and ipsilateral chest hyperresonance on percussion. Subcutaneous emphysema

may develop, especially if a lung defect was caused by, or is associated with, rib fractures. Hemothorax is noticeable because of blood loss from the injury. Suspect this if hypovolemia is associated with blunt chest trauma. Hemothorax, when sizable, may cause dyspnea and a lung field that is dull to percussion.

Blunt mediastinal injury can affect the heart, great vessels, and trachea. Heart injury may present with chest pain similar to a myocardial infarction and, if serious enough, with heart failure or cardiogenic shock signs. An ECG may reveal tachycardia, bradycardia, or PVCs, and, in cases of severe myocardial contusion, may demonstrate ST-segment elevation. Cardiac rupture usually causes sudden death, whereas pericardial tamponade is unlikely in blunt chest trauma. Injury to great vessels (dissection) is most frequently associated with lateral impacts or feet-first falls (from a height) and may produce a tearing chest pain and pulse deficits in the extremities. If the dissection ruptures, rapidly progressing hypovolemia, hypotension, shock, and death follow. Tracheobronchial injury may cause a rapidly developing pneumomediastinum or pneumothorax and possible subcutaneous emphysema, hemoptysis, dyspnea, and hypoxia. Positive-pressure ventilations may worsen the signs and symptoms of this. Traumatic asphyxia presents with jugular vein distention, head and neck discoloration, severe dyspnea, and possible hypovolemia and shock signs.

Penetrating Trauma Assessment

Penetrating injury results in different signs and symptoms depending on the injury. Inspect a chest wound for frothy blood or air exchange sounds with respirations (open pneumothorax). Remember that a wound needs to be rather large (high-velocity bullet exit wound or close-range shotgun blast) for this injury to occur. A penetrating wound, however, commonly causes a simple pneumothorax with its associated signs and symptoms. A hyperinflated chest, distended jugular veins, tracheal shift away from the injury, distant or absent breath sounds, hyperresonance to percussion, and severe dyspnea and hypotension all suggest a tension pneumothorax. Tension pneumothorax may push air outward through a penetrating wound or cause subcutaneous emphysema around the wound.[3] Some degree of hemothorax is likely to be associated with penetrating chest trauma and, if extensive, may present with diminished or absent breath sounds and a chest region that is dull to percussion. Hemothorax also causes, or significantly contributes to, hypovolemia and shock.

Penetrating heart trauma is likely to cause pericardial tamponade and present with jugular vein distention, distant heart sounds, and hypotension (Beck's triad). Pulsus paradoxus may be present, and jugular filling may occur with inspiration (Kussmaul's sign). Both pulsus paradoxus and jugular filling are indicative of pericardial tamponade. Additionally, with pericardial tamponade, heart sounds

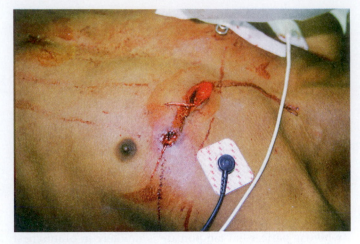

FIGURE 7-22 Gunshot wound to the chest.
(© Edward T. Dickinson, MD)

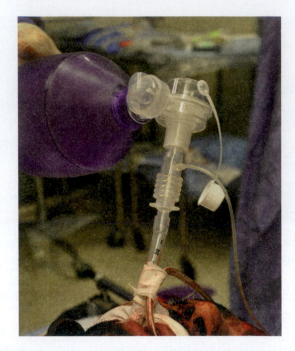

FIGURE 7-24 With pulse oximetry and capnography, you can continuously monitor the patient's oxygenation and ventilation status.
(© Edward T. Dickinson, MD)

are often distant or muffled, the pulses are weak, and the patient experiences increasing hypotension and shock (Figure 7-22). Penetrating heart trauma may also cause myocardial rupture and immediate death (Figure 7-23). These patients have vital signs that fall precipitously as vascular volume is lost into the mediastinum.

Reassessment

Reassessments simply repeat the elements of the primary assessment and vital signs and reexamine injuries discovered during earlier assessment. Reassessment takes on great importance for the chest trauma patient. With any serious chest impact or any penetrating chest injury, observe respiratory depth, rate, and symmetry. Auscultate

both lung fields for equality and crackles and monitor distal pulses, oxygen saturation, ventilation status, skin color, and blood pressure for progressing hypovolemia signs (Figure 7-24). If any signs change between reassessments, search out a cause and care for any additional injuries. Be especially suspicious of a developing tension pneumothorax, pericardial tamponade, extensive and evolving pulmonary contusion, and hypovolemia associated with hemothorax. If any of these is suspected, institute the appropriate management steps.

Management of the Chest Injury Patient

General patient management for significant chest injury focuses on ensuring adequate oxygenation and respiratory volume and rate. Administer supplemental oxygen, if needed, based on the SpO_2. Ensure that the airway is patent and consider endotracheal intubation if there is any significant deterioration in mental status. Consider intubation early in care, as patients with thoracic trauma are likely to get worse over time. Rapid sequence intubation may be needed for the combative patient. Endotracheal intubation also makes ventilation easier for the patient with flail chest or pulmonary contusion.

Carefully evaluate the minute volume (breaths per minute times volume); if it is less than 6,000 mL, consider assisting. Ventilate the conscious patient with severe dyspnea at a rate of 10 to 12 breaths per minute, trying to

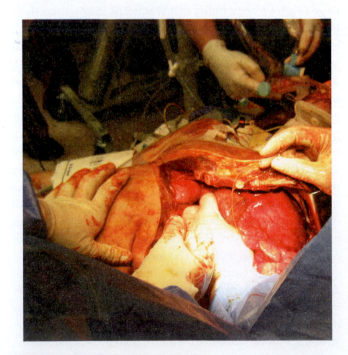

FIGURE 7-23 Stab wound to the chest.
(© Michael Casey, MD)

match the patient's respiratory rate. Closely monitor pulse oximetry, mental status, and skin color. Also monitor capnography to ensure physiologic CO_2 levels. Bag-valve mask ventilation may also be beneficial for patients with serious rib fractures and flail chest. Positive pressure displaces the chest wall outward, potentially reducing fracture site movement and moving the flail segment with the chest. It may also be beneficial to the patient who is exhausted from an increased work of breathing associated with a pulmonary contusion. In this case, positive-pressure ventilations (PPV) may help move fluids back into the vascular system, thereby relieving edema. Remember, however, that positive-pressure ventilations change respiratory dynamics from a less-than-atmospheric to a greater-than-atmospheric process and may exacerbate respiratory problems such as tracheobronchial injury, pneumothorax, and tension pneumothorax. Positive pressure ventilation may also impair venous return to the heart.

Anticipate heart and great vessel compromise with thoracic injury and be ready to support the patient's cardiovascular system. Initiate at least one large-bore IV site if the patient has a serious chest trauma mechanism and place two lines if there are any hypovolemia or compensation signs. Be prepared to administer fluids quickly (in 250- to 500-mL boluses) if the patient's systolic blood pressure drops below 80 mmHg.

IV fluid infusion for the chest trauma patient must be titrated carefully. Excessive fluid administration may increase the blood loss rate and dilute clotting factors, thus prolonging and possibly increasing any hemorrhage. Additional fluid also may worsen the edema associated with pulmonary contusion, increasing the rate and extent of the injury. Whenever you administer fluids to the chest trauma patient, do so incrementally, periodically auscultating all lung fields carefully, and slow or stop fluid resuscitation if you hear crackles or dyspnea increases. The technique of hypotensive resuscitation also demands careful titration of fluid boluses to keep the systolic BP at or below 80 mmHg.

Care is specific for thoracic injuries, including rib fractures, sternoclavicular dislocation, flail chest, open pneumothorax, tension pneumothorax, hemothorax, blunt cardiac injury, pericardial tamponade, aortic dissection, tracheobronchial injury, and traumatic asphyxia.

Rib Fractures

Rib fractures, either isolated or associated with other respiratory injuries, may produce pain that significantly limits respiratory effort and leads to hypoventilation. In these patients, you may consider administering analgesics to afford greater patient comfort and improve chest excursion. Ensure that the patient is hemodynamically stable, there is no associated abdominal or head injury, and the

patient is fully conscious and oriented. Consider administration of morphine sulfate, fentanyl, or meperidine as described in the chapter "Orthopedic Trauma." Note that nitrous oxide use is contraindicated in chest trauma, as nitrous oxide may migrate into a pneumothorax or tension pneumothorax, making them worse.

Sternoclavicular Dislocation

Supportive therapy is usually all that is required for an isolated sternoclavicular dislocation. However, hemodynamic instability may indicate associated injuries requiring rapid transport to a trauma center with aggressive resuscitation measures instituted en route. If you suspect posterior sternoclavicular dislocation and note the patient to be in significant respiratory distress that is not effectively treated with initial airway maneuvers and supplemental oxygen (as determined by the SpO_2), transport immediately. It may help to place the patient in the supine position with a sandbag between the shoulder blades. This helps to pull the shoulders back and move the clavicular head laterally and away from the trachea. Do not perform this procedure on multiple-trauma patients because of the risk of spine injury. An alternative field-expedient method of reducing impingement is to place the patient supine and grasp the clavicle near the sternum. Pull it upward and laterally, directly perpendicular to the sternum. This distracts the clavicle forward, alleviating its airway impingement.

Flail Chest

Place the flail chest injury patient on the injured side if spinal stabilization is not required. If spinal injury is suspected, secure a large and bulky dressing with bandaging against the flail segment to stabilize it. Use supplemental oxygen monitored by pulse oximetry and monitor the ECG. If there is significant dyspnea, evidence of underlying pulmonary injury, or signs and symptoms of respiratory compromise, these measures will not suffice. Consider endotracheal intubation and positive pressure ventilations with high-concentration oxygen. Positive-pressure ventilations can internally splint the flail segment, expand atelectatic lung areas, and also treat any underlying pulmonary contusion. Monitor waveform capnography, if possible. Use of sandbags to support a flail segment is not indicated because they may diminish chest movement, adding to hypoventilation, atelectasis, and subsequent hypoxemia. Rapid transport to the trauma center is indicated, as this injury and associated complications and injuries can be life threatening.

Open Pneumothorax

Provide supplemental oxygen for the patient with an open pneumothorax. Monitor the oxygen saturation and

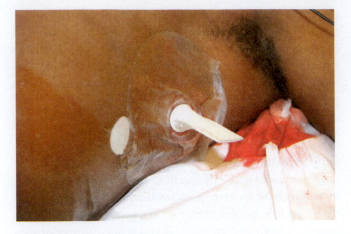

FIGURE 7-25 An Asherman chest seal in place on a patient.

(© *Edward T. Dickinson, MD*)

respiratory effort. If there is a penetrating injury, cover it with a sterile occlusive dressing (sterile plastic wrap) taped on three sides or with a commercially available one-way valve dressing such as the Asherman Chest Seal (Figure 7-25). This process converts an open pneumothorax into a closed pneumothorax, prevents further air aspiration, and relieves any building pressure (tension pneumothorax) through the valvelike dressing.

If dyspnea diminishes somewhat but still continues, provide positive-pressure ventilations and intubate as needed. Carefully monitor the patient when you use intermittent positive-pressure ventilation because it may lead to a tension pneumothorax. If, after a dressing has been applied, the patient has progressive difficulty breathing, appears to be hypoventilating and hypoxemic, has decreasing breath sounds on the injured side, and has increasing jugular vein distention, remove the occlusive dressing. If you hear air rush out and the patient's respirations improve, reseal the wound, monitor breathing carefully, and again remove the dressing if any dyspnea redevelops. If removing a dressing does not relieve increasing signs and symptoms, suspect and treat for tension pneumothorax using needle decompression.

Tension Pneumothorax

Confirm a possible tension pneumothorax by auscultating the lung fields for diminished breath sounds, percussing for hyperresonance, and observing for severe dyspnea, chest hyperinflation, and jugular vein distention.[4] Successful treatment depends on rapid recognition and then pleural decompression. As you prepare to decompress the affected (ipsilateral) side, apply supplemental oxygen if the airway is intact and the patient is able to demonstrate adequate ventilatory effort. Pleural decompression should be employed only if the patient demonstrates significant dyspnea and distinct signs and symptoms of tension pneumothorax.

If necessary, provide ventilations with a bag-valve mask and supplemental oxygen and intubate if the patient is unable to maintain an airway or continues to show hypoxemia while on high-concentration oxygen. Perform needle thoracentesis by inserting a long (e.g., 3-inch) 14-gauge intravascular catheter into the second intercostal space, midclavicular line on the side of the thorax with decreased breath sounds and hyperinflation (Figure 7-26).[5,6] In the supine patient, this location is most appropriate for pleural decompression, as any air in the thorax will move to the anterior regions of the thorax. This location is easy to identify by finding the angle of Louis and palpating the intercostal space just lateral to it. Then, advance the catheter in a straight posterior trajectory (in the supine patient, this is straight toward the floor) through the chest wall. Ensure that the needle enters the thoracic cavity by passing the needle just over the rib. The intercostal artery, vein, and nerve pass just under each rib and may be injured if the needle's track is too high. As the pleural space is entered, there will be a pop and there may be a rush of air. Advance the catheter into the chest and then withdraw the needle.[7,8]

If the patient remains symptomatic, place a second or third catheter in the third or fourth intercostal space, midaxillary line to ensure proper decompression. Secure the catheter in place with tape, being careful not to block the port or kink the catheter. Leaving the catheter open to air converts tension pneumothorax into a simple pneumothorax and stabilizes the patient. Monitor the patient's respirations and breath sounds for a recurring tension pneumothorax. If signs and symptoms again appear, decompress the chest again. Frequently, the initial catheter clogs or kinks and requires replacement.

Rapidly transport the patient to the trauma center for definitive treatment (usually a chest tube). Avoid infusing IV crystalloid boluses if the patient is hemodynamically stable. An underlying pulmonary contusion may lead to edema and can be made worse with overaggressive fluid therapy. If the patient remains significantly hypotensive (SBP < 80 mmHg) after chest decompression and respirations are ineffective, consider the possibility of internal hemorrhage and a need for fluid resuscitation. If respirations do not dramatically improve, assess for a contralateral tension pneumothorax or pericardial tamponade as the cause.

Hemothorax

Treat the suspected hemothorax with oxygen administration and ventilatory support, as needed. Initiate two large-bore intravenous catheters, readied to infuse fluid in 250 to 500 mL boluses. Be conservative in fluid administration. Maintain a systolic blood pressure of 80 mmHg but do not attempt to return it to preinjury levels. Carefully listen to

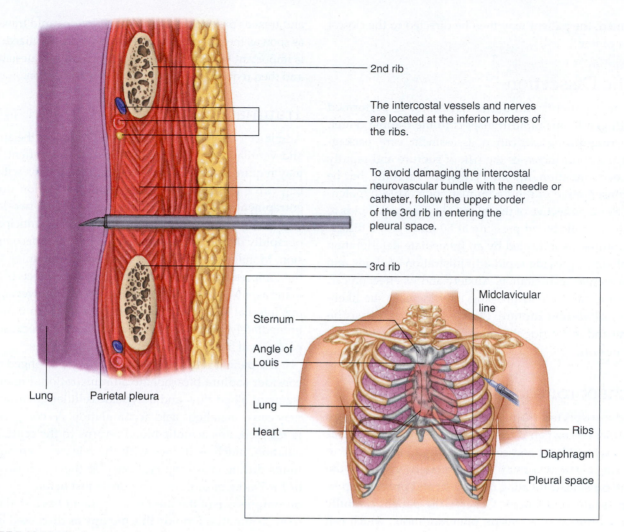

FIGURE 7-26 Needle decompression of a tension pneumothorax.

breath sounds during any infusion because increasing vascular volume may increase edema and pulmonary contusion size and density. It may also increase the pressure, rate, and volume of internal hemorrhage. If pulmonary contusion is extensive and the patient cannot be adequately oxygenated by high-concentration oxygen, positive-pressure ventilations are indicated and may limit further edema that contributes to the injury. Positive end-expiratory pressure (PEEP) and, more likely, continuous positive airway pressure (CPAP) may also benefit a patient experiencing hemothorax. Increased intrathoracic pressure may serve to expand collapsed alveoli, slow hemorrhage, push edema fluid back into the circulatory system, and increase the oxygen partial pressure.

Blunt Cardiac Injury

Suspect blunt cardiac injury in serious frontal impact collisions and administer supplemental oxygen if the patient is hypoxic by SpO₂. Monitor the ECG and watch for arrhythmias and conduction defects. Establish an IV line if antiarrhythmics (such as amiodarone) are needed, and monitor

the patient for great vessel injury. Use pharmacological care measures recommended for advanced cardiac life support (see the chapter "Cardiology"). Rapidly transport the patient to the trauma center for further evaluation and continued monitoring.

Pericardial Tamponade

Maintain a high index of suspicion for pericardial tamponade in the patient with central thoracic penetrating trauma. Appropriate prehospital care includes oxygen (if needed) and IV fluid administration to maximize oxygenation and venous return. Definitive care is to remove some of the accumulating pericardial fluid through pericardiocentesis. This action is rarely permitted in the field. Thus, the patient needs to be transported as rapidly as possible to the emergency department. Note that a relatively simple procedure can relieve this problem and can be adequately administered by an emergency physician. If a physician-staffed emergency department is significantly closer to you than a trauma center, it may be the best choice for a patient with isolated pericardial tamponade. After pericardiocentesis is performed, the patient may then be directed to the closest trauma center.

Aortic Dissection

Care for a patient with aortic dissection is performed through gentle but rapid transport to the trauma center. Any jarring during extrication, assessment, care, packaging, or transport increases the risk of rupture and rapidly fatal exsanguination. Initiate IV therapy en route, but be very conservative in fluid administration. Mild hypotension may be protective of the injury site. Titrate IV fluids to keep the systolic blood pressure at 80 mmHg. If a dissection ruptures, as indicated by an immediate deterioration in vital signs, provide rapid administration of fluids and cardiovascular resuscitation. Anxiety and its effect on cardiac output and blood pressure may increase the likelihood of dissection rupture. Place a special emphasis on calming and reassuring the patient during very gentle care and transport.

Tracheobronchial Injury

Treat the suspected tracheobronchial injury patient with supplemental oxygen if the patient is hypoxic, and clear the airway of blood and secretions. If you are unable to maintain a patent airway or adequately ventilate the patient, consider intubating the patient and providing positive-pressure ventilations. Observe the patient carefully for development of a tension pneumothorax, which can occur as a complication of positive-pressure ventilations,

and treat as previously prescribed. Provide rapid transport as soon as the patient can be extricated and stabilized. This is important because these patients can rapidly destabilize and then require emergency surgical intervention.

Traumatic Asphyxia

Administer supplemental oxygen and support the airway and ventilations of the traumatic asphyxia patient. This may require using positive-pressure ventilations with the bag-valve mask to ensure adequate ventilation during entrapment and possibly thereafter. Establish two large-bore IV lines for rapid crystalloid infusion in anticipation of rapidly developing hypovolemia with chest decompression. Monitor the ECG for evidence of arrhythmias. Once the compressing force is removed, the direct effects of traumatic asphyxia may spontaneously resolve. However, serious internal hemorrhage may begin. Prepare to transport immediately after release from entrapment because the patient will likely have severe coexisting injuries.

If a patient remains entrapped for a prolonged time, consider sodium bicarbonate administration. Prolonged stagnant blood flow and a hypoxic cellular environment may cause metabolic acid accumulation. As compression is released, this acidotic blood returns to the central circulation, much as it does with the release of entrapped limbs during crush injury. Consider the administration of 1 mEq/kg of sodium bicarbonate just before or during decompression of the chest if entrapment has lasted more than 20 minutes. Employ this therapy as discussed in the chapter "Soft Tissue Trauma."

Summary

Thoracic trauma by either blunt or penetrating mechanisms has a great potential for posing a threat to a patient's life. In fact, 25 percent of all traumatic deaths are secondary to thoracic injuries. In assessing these patients, the mechanism of injury, when considered along with the clinical findings, may help in differentiating among the many possible injuries. Assessment, in turn, helps guide the needed interventions and determines the priority for rapid extrication and transport. Aggressive airway management, oxygenation, ventilation, and fluid resuscitation, when indicated, can make the difference between patient survival and death. Specific interventions, such as pleural decompression or flail segment stabilization, can also affect mortality and morbidity from chest trauma. Understanding the pathophysiology of chest trauma and employing proper assessment and care measures will ensure the best possible outcome for the patient.

You Make the Call

The Medic 101 team responds to the interstate, where they have been called to a crash scene. An older pickup truck has struck a bridge abutment, apparently after the driver fell asleep while driving home from the night shift. The scene survey reveals that the State Patrol has deployed appropriate warning flares and controlled traffic to allow safe access to the scene. The paramedics approach the truck and find a 20-year-old male patient unconscious behind the wheel. The paramedics note that no seat belt had been worn and no air bag had deployed. The steering wheel is displaced somewhat upward and bent inward against the dash. The windshield is starred.

The primary assessment reveals an unconscious male patient with central cyanosis, poor air exchange, and no peripheral (radial) pulses palpable. With in-line stabilization, the patient is rapidly extricated to a long board, the airway is opened by a jaw thrust (with cervical precautions), and an oral airway is then placed with respiratory assistance provided via BVM with supplemental oxygen. Little improvement is noted in the patient's color, air exchange, level of consciousness, and peripheral pulses. The trachea appears midline, but jugular vein distention is present. As the patient's clothes are cut away, subcutaneous emphysema is palpable along the left anterior and lateral chest wall. There is a pronounced inward movement of a section of anterior chest wall with the patient's inspiratory efforts.

1. Considering the mechanism of injury and what is known about the patient, what thoracic pathophysiology may explain the patient's presentation?

2. As the treating paramedic, what is your next step in stabilizing this patient?

3. What further emergency treatment is likely indicated by the absence of breath sounds on the left side and a relatively normal abdominal exam?

See Suggested Responses at the back of this book.

Review Questions

1. The union between the xiphoid process and the body of the sternum is called the _____
   a. manubrium.
   b. thoracic duct.
   c. costal margin.
   d. xiphisternal joint.

2. During a football game, a 17-year-old male is tackled and knocked to the ground; he reports hearing a "bone crack." The team manager summons the paramedics. By the time you arrive, the patient states that he is "feeling funny" and having difficulty breathing, with pain on each breath. Assessment reveals unequal breath sounds, a rapid, weak pulse and a low BP. The patient's appearance suggests that he may be developing shock. You suspect a fractured rib and possibly _____
   a. traumatic asphyxia.
   b. pericardial tamponade.
   c. tension pneumothorax.
   d. traumatic aortic rupture.

3. Secondary to a severe chest wall contusion, which of the following symptoms is most commonly seen?
   a. Pain
   b. Hypoventilation
   c. Nausea
   d. Use of accessory muscles

4. You have elected to apply an occlusive dressing to your patient who has sustained a stab wound to the chest. How should you secure the dressing?
   a. On two sides
   b. On four sides
   c. On three sides
   d. Loosely over the wound

5. Your patient has received significant deceleration trauma to his chest. He presents with absent radial and brachial pulses in the left upper extremity and severe hypotension. He reported that he felt a tearing sensation in his chest before quickly losing consciousness. He most likely has experienced a _____
   a. severe rib fracture.
   b. pericardial tamponade.
   c. pulmonary contusion.
   d. traumatic aortic dissection.

6. What impact pattern during a motor vehicle collision is most likely going to result in a patient sustaining a traumatic aortic dissection or aortic rupture?
   a. Lateral
   b. Frontal
   c. Rollover
   d. Rotational

7. The mechanism of injury most likely to cause traumatic asphyxia is _____
   a. blunt trauma, low impact.
   b. penetrating trauma, low velocity.
   c. penetrating trauma, high velocity.
   d. blunt trauma, compressive force.

8. You and your partner are called to the scene of a motor vehicle collision. When you arrive, you note that a car has struck a parked vehicle. Your 30-year-old female patient complains of difficulty breathing and you note that breath sounds are diminished unilaterally. The patient states that, at the last minute, she anticipated the impending crash and held her breath. You suspect "paper-bag syndrome." What type of injury would this mechanism cause?
   a. Pneumothorax
   b. Flail chest
   c. Splenic rupture
   d. Diaphragm rupture

9. The most appropriate prehospital management for a patient with a flail segment and no other suspected underlying injury is the application or placement of _____
   a. chest tube insertion.
   b. positive-pressure ventilation.
   c. needle decompression.
   d. a sandbag on the injured side.

10. What is the critical intervention for a patient with chest wall trauma, labored breathing, unequal chest wall motion, absent unilateral breath sounds, and hyperresonance?
    a. Initiate a large-bore IV.
    b. Apply oxygen.
    c. Decompress the appropriate portion of the thorax.
    d. Provide full spinal immobilization.

See Answers to Review Questions at the end of this book.

References

1. De Lorenzo, R. A. "Oxygen Therapy and COPD: Prehospital Dilemma Explored." *Journal of Emergency Medical Services (JEMS)* 19(7) (1994): 38–50.

2. Kidler, E., et al. "The Effect of Prehospital Time Related Variables in the Mortality following Severe Thoracic Trauma." *Injury* (May 2011).

3. Leigh-Smith, S. and G. Davies. "Tension Pneumothorax: Eyes May Be More Diagnostic than Ears." *Emerg Med J* 20 (2003): 495–496.

4. Leigh-Smith, S. and T. Harris. "Tension Pneumothorax—Time for a Re-Think?" *Emerg Med J* 22 (2005): 8–16.

5. Stevens, R. L., et al. "Needle Thoracostomy for Tension Pneumothorax: Failure Predicted by Chest Tomography." *Prehosp Emerg Care* 13(1) (Jan–Mar 2009): 14–17.

6. Ball, C. G., et al. "Thoracic Needle Decompression for Tension Pneumothorax: Clinical Correlation with Catheter Length." *Can J Surg* 53(3) (Jun 2010): 184–188.

7. Eckstein, M. and D. Suyehara. "Needle Thoracostomy in the Prehospital Setting." *Prehosp Emerg Care* 2(2) (Apr–Jun 1988): 132–135.

8. Holcomb, J. B., J. G. McManus, S. T. Kerr, and A. E. Pusateri. "Needle versus Tube Thoracostomy in a Swine Model of Tension Pneumothorax." *Prehosp Emerg Care* 13(1) (Jan–Mar 2009): 18–27.

Further Reading

American College of Surgeons, Committee on Trauma. *Advanced Trauma Life Support Course: Student Manual*. 9th ed. Chicago: American College of Surgeons, 2012.

Bickley, L. *Bates' Guide to Physical Examination and History Taking*. 11th ed. Philadelphia: Wolters-Kluwer, 2012.

Bledsoe, B. E., and D. Clayden. *Prehospital Emergency Pharmacology*. 7th ed. Upper Saddle River, NJ: Pearson/Prentice Hall, 2012.

Bledsoe, B. E., B. J. Colbert, and J. E. Ankney. *Essentials of A & P for Emergency Care*. Upper Saddle River, NJ: Pearson/Prentice Hall, 2010.

Campbell, John E. *International Trauma Life Support for Prehospital Care Providers*. 8th ed. Upper Saddle River, NJ: Pearson/Prentice Hall, 2016.

Clemente, C. D. *Anatomy: A Regional Atlas of the Human Body*. 5th ed. Baltimore: Lippincott, Williams & Wilkins, 2006.

Hall-Craggs, E. C. B. *Anatomy as a Basis for Clinical Medicine*. 3rd ed. Baltimore: Lippincott, Williams & Wilkins, 1995.

Martini, Frederic. *Fundamentals of Anatomy and Physiology*. 10th ed. San Francisco: Pearson, 2014.

Marx, J., R. Hockberger, and R. Walls. *Emergency Medicine: Concepts and Clinical Practice*. 8th ed. St. Louis: Mosby, 2013.

National Association of EMTs. *Prehospital Trauma Life Support*. 8th ed. Burlington: Jones & Bartlett Learning, 2014.

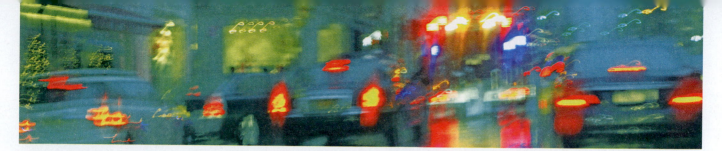

Chapter 8
Abdominal and Pelvic Trauma

Bryan E. Bledsoe, DO, FACEP, FAAEM, EMT-P

Robert S. Porter, MA, EMT-P

STANDARD
Trauma (Abdominal and Genitourinary Trauma)

COMPETENCY
Integrates assessment findings with principles of epidemiology and pathophysiology to formulate a field impression to implement a comprehensive treatment/disposition plan for an acutely injured patient.

Learning Objectives

Terminal Performance Objective: After reading this chapter you should be able to assess and manage patients with abdominal trauma.

Enabling Objectives: To accomplish the terminal performance objective, you should be able to:

1. Define key terms introduced in this chapter.

2. Discuss the epidemiology and trends observed in abdominal and pelvic trauma.

3. Describe the anatomy and physiology of the abdominal cavity and its contents.

4. Identify how blunt and penetrating mechanisms of injury can result in abdominal and pelvic trauma.

5. Discuss the pathophysiology of abdominal trauma as it pertains to hollow, solid, and vascular injury patterns.

6. Identify the stages and discuss the steps necessary for assessment of patients with injuries sustained from trauma to the abdomen and pelvis.

7. Given a variety of scenarios, develop a management plan for patients with abdominal and pelvic injuries.

KEY TERMS

Case Study

Janice and her paramedic partner Doug respond to a "shots fired" call in the early hours of Saturday morning. They arrive at an apartment complex, noting that several police vehicles are on scene. Officers tell the paramedics that the wife is in custody and are directed by an officer to a hallway where a middle-aged male sits propped against a wall. The man holds what appears to be a blood-soaked towel against his abdomen.

Janice introduces herself as a paramedic and begins the patient's primary assessment. The victim, Marty, is a 43-year-old who was shot by his wife during a domestic dispute. He reports "she shot me once with my 9-mm handgun" at close range. Janice coaxes Marty to lift the towel and observes a small entrance wound to the left upper quadrant, above and to the left of the navel. The wound is oozing just a small amount of blood. Inspection of Marty's back and flank reveals no exit wound. Doug assesses vital signs and obtains a blood pressure of 110/86 mmHg, a strong and regular pulse at a rate of 90, and respirations of 22. Marty's ECG traces a sinus rhythm with no abnormalities, and his oxygen saturation is 99 percent. He is alert and oriented to time, place, and person. He describes his abdominal pain as sharp at the entrance wound, although the area surrounding the wound feels "burning" in nature.

Janice does not administer oxygen because of the normal saturation reading. She and Doug prepare to move Marty quickly to the waiting stretcher and then to the ambulance.

As Janice prepares Marty for the ride to the hospital, Doug informs her that the nearest trauma center has just received several seriously injured patients from an auto crash, and Janice and Doug are directed to a more distant Level II trauma center.

En route, Janice initiates an IV line with a large-bore catheter, trauma tubing, and a 1,000-mL bag of normal saline solution, running at a to-keep-open rate. During transport, Janice questions Marty about his symptoms. Janice's reassessment reveals a blood pressure of 112/94 mmHg, a strong pulse at 86, and respirations that are now somewhat shallow at 24. Oxygen saturation remains at 99 percent and the ECG still displays a normal sinus rhythm. Blood is no longer draining from the entrance wound, and further examination does not reveal an exit wound. Janice auscultates the chest and abdomen and, though road sounds limit auscultation clarity, she hears only clear breath sounds in the chest and no bowel sounds.

Janice completes a final set of vital signs as they arrive at the emergency department. Marty's pulse is 88, blood pressure is 112/96 mmHg, and respirations are 22 and somewhat shallow. Janice quickly reports her assessment findings and care to the trauma team. In the emergency department, Marty is crossmatched for blood and prepared for an exploratory laparotomy in the operating room. During Janice's next trip to the trauma center, the staff informs her that Marty's surgery was successful. They found the stomach to be perforated, the spleen to be torn, and more than 400 mL of blood was in the abdomen. Marty did well during surgery, however, and was on his way to a quick recovery.

Introduction to Abdominal and Pelvic Trauma

The abdominal cavity is one of the body's largest cavities and contains many organs essential to life. It is not well protected by the skeletal anatomy, as are most other body cavities. Both blunt and penetrating trauma may damage these vital organs, with large volumes of blood lost in the cavity. However, injuries to the abdomen do not always present as dramatically as they do elsewhere because of the few skeletal structures. Transmitted injury signs—deformity, swelling, and discoloration—take time to develop and are not often seen in the prehospital setting.

These considerations make anticipation of abdominal injuries and careful abdominal assessment critical for patients with abdominal and pelvic trauma.

Over the past decade, the morbidity and mortality for various abdominal injuries has been on the decline as a result of improved surgical and critical care techniques, as well as enhanced diagnostic imaging. Reduced injury-to-surgery times have also contributed to this decline, as EMS systems have recognized the necessity of rapid surgical intervention. Abdominal injury severity and deaths associated with blunt trauma have also decreased thanks to improvements in highway design and vehicle structure and to greater seat belt use and air bag deployment. However, overall morbidity and mortality from penetrating trauma is on the rise as a result of the increasing violence in society, most specifically the growing use and increasing power of guns and other weapons. Penetrating trauma is now approaching trauma associated with auto crashes as the number-one trauma killer. Nowhere is this more apparent than with abdominal injuries.

Most blunt abdominal and pelvic trauma results from vehicle collisions, which cause an estimated 50 to 75 percent of cases. There are three common mechanisms associated with blunt abdominal and pelvic trauma:

- *Deceleration.* Rapid deceleration causes the internal organs to move toward the deceleration point of contact, potentially causing shear injuries and organ rupture.

- *Crushing.* With deceleration, the abdominal organs are crushed against the interior abdominal wall. In crushing injuries, the solid organs (e.g., liver, spleen, kidneys) are particularly vulnerable.

- *Compression.* External compression of the abdominal and pelvic contents can cause organ rupture, particularly of the hollow organs (e.g., intestines, urinary bladder).

Penetrating abdominal and pelvic trauma from gunshot wounds most commonly affects the abdominal and pelvic organs (although the pelvic organs are fairly well protected by the bony pelvis). Table 8-1 details the most commonly affected organs in penetrating abdominal and pelvic trauma.

Prevention of abdominal injuries, as with most other types of trauma, is the best way to reduce morbidity and mortality. As noted, improvements in highway and vehicle design and employing safe practices at home and in the workplace play important roles in reducing both abdominal injury incidence and seriousness.

There remains room for further improvements in safety practices. For example, many people still do not use seat belts. Failure to use the seat belt increases the incidence of

Table 8-1 Organs Most Commonly Affected in Penetrating Abdominal and Pelvic Trauma

Organ	Percentage
Gunshot Wounds	
Small intestine	50
Colon	40
Liver	30
Abdominal vascular structures	25
Stab Wounds	
Liver	40
Small intestine	30
Diaphragm	20
Colon	15

abdominal injury secondary to impact with the steering wheel, dashboard, or other auto interior surfaces or the impact after ejection. (Side-impact air bags have the potential to reduce the incidence of pelvic fracture and internal abdominal injuries frequently associated with this mechanism of injury.)

One area of special concern is proper lap belt application. If the belt rides too high on the abdomen, deceleration may direct forces both to abdominal cavity contents and the lumbar spine. Severe compression may result in serious associated abdominal injury. Proper placement, in which the belt rests on the iliac crests, transmits severe deceleration forces to the pelvis and body's skeletal structure, thus sparing the abdominal contents and the spine from injury. Proper positioning of seat belts is especially important for children. Too low a belt placement may impinge on the femurs and, with severe impact, fracture them near the pelvis.

Abdominal and Pelvic Anatomy and Physiology

The abdominal cavity is bordered by the diaphragm; the pelvis, vertebral column, inferior ribs, and back muscles (psoas and paraspinal muscles); the flank muscles; and the abdominal wall muscles anteriorly (Figure 8-1). The cavity is divided into three spaces: the **peritoneal space**, the **retroperitoneal space**, and the **pelvic space**. The anatomic landmarks include the umbilicus, the xiphoid process, the iliac crests, and the pubic prominence.

The abdomen is divided into four quadrants by vertical and horizontal lines intersecting at the umbilicus and forming the right and left upper and lower

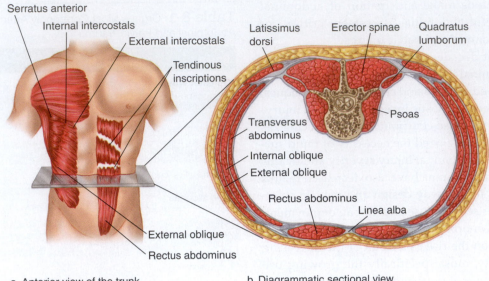

a. Anterior view of the trunk, showing superficial and deep members of the oblique and rectus groups.

b. Diagrammatic sectional view through the abdominal region.

FIGURE 8-1 Muscles protecting the organs of the abdominal cavity.

quadrants. The right upper quadrant contains the gallbladder, right kidney, most of the liver, some small bowel, a portion of the ascending and transverse colon, and a small portion of the pancreas. The left upper quadrant contains the stomach, spleen, left kidney, most of the pancreas, and portions of the liver, small bowel, and transverse and descending colon. The right lower quadrant contains the appendix and portions of the urinary bladder, small bowel, ascending colon, rectum, and the right ovary in females. The left lower quadrant contains the sigmoid colon and portions of the urinary bladder, small bowel, descending colon, rectum, and the left ovary in females.

Digestive Tract

The **digestive tract** is a 25-foot-long hollow muscular tube responsible for digestion and waste products (Figure 8-2). The abdominal components of the digestive tract include the stomach, small bowel (duodenum, jejunum, and ileum), large bowel (or colon), rectum, and anus. These structures fill the anterior and lateral aspects of the abdominal cavity, except for the area occupied by the liver.

Accessory Organs

The liver is the largest organ in the abdomen and is responsible for detoxifying blood, producing bile, manufacturing clotting factors, and storing glycogen and other important agents for body metabolism. The liver also assists in

osmotic fluid regulation and produces proteins used in the clotting process.

The gallbladder is a small hollow organ located behind and beneath the liver. It receives bile and stores it until it is needed during digestion of fatty food. It then contracts and secretes bile through the bile duct and into the duodenum. Bile helps emulsify (break apart and suspend) ingested fats that would otherwise remain as indigestible clumps during the digestive process.

Another accessory digestive organ is the pancreas. It is responsible for production of glucagon and insulin. The pancreas also produces important digestive enzymes. These enzymes pass through the pancreatic duct that joins the bile duct just before entering the duodenum. Like the liver, the pancreas is a solid, though delicate, organ, encapsulated in a serous membrane. It is located in the medial and lower portion of the left upper quadrant and extends into the medial right upper quadrant.

Spleen

The spleen is not an accessory digestive organ, but rather a part of the immune system. It is a very vascular organ about the size of the palm of the hand and is located behind the stomach and lateral to the kidney in the left upper quadrant. The spleen performs important immunologic functions and also stores a large blood volume. Although the spleen is well protected in its location by the rib cage, spine, and flank and back muscles, it can be injured during blunt trauma, especially with impacts affecting the left flank.

The Digestive System

ORGANS OF THE DIGESTIVE SYSTEM

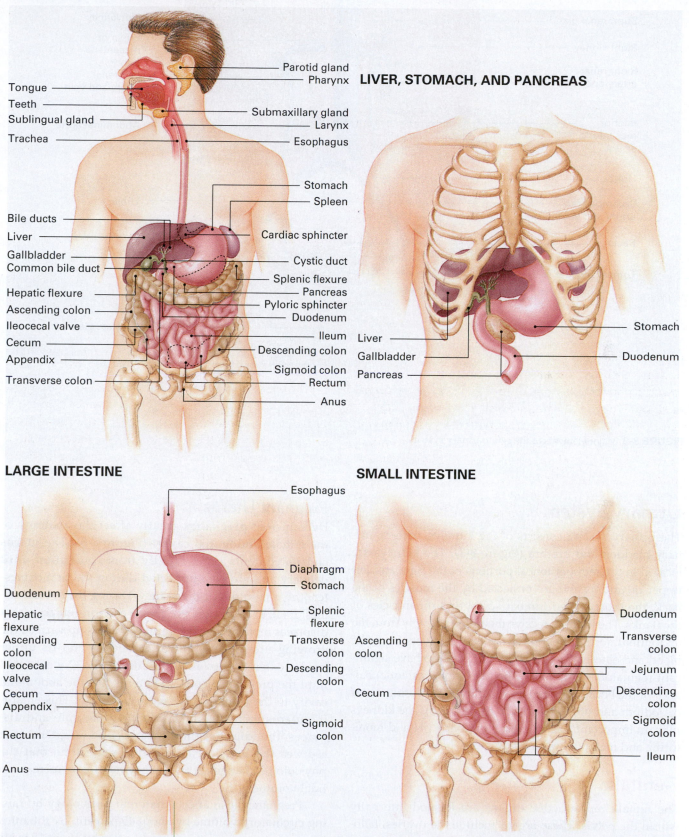

LIVER, STOMACH, AND PANCREAS

Parotid gland
Pharynx
Tongue
Teeth
Sublingual gland
Trachea
Submaxillary gland
Larynx
Esophagus

Stomach
Spleen
Bile ducts
Liver
Cardiac sphincter
Gallbladder
Common bile duct
Cystic duct
Hepatic flexure
Splenic flexure
Pancreas
Ascending colon
Pyloric sphincter
Ileocecal valve
Duodenum
Cecum
Ileum
Appendix
Descending colon
Sigmoid colon
Transverse colon
Rectum
Anus

Liver
Gallbladder
Pancreas
Stomach
Duodenum

LARGE INTESTINE

Esophagus
Duodenum
Diaphragm
Stomach
Hepatic flexure
Ascending colon
Splenic flexure
Ileocecal valve
Transverse colon
Cecum
Descending colon
Appendix
Rectum
Sigmoid colon
Anus

SMALL INTESTINE

Ascending colon
Cecum
Duodenum
Transverse colon
Jejunum
Descending colon
Sigmoid colon
Ileum

FIGURE 8-2 The digestive tract and accessory organs.

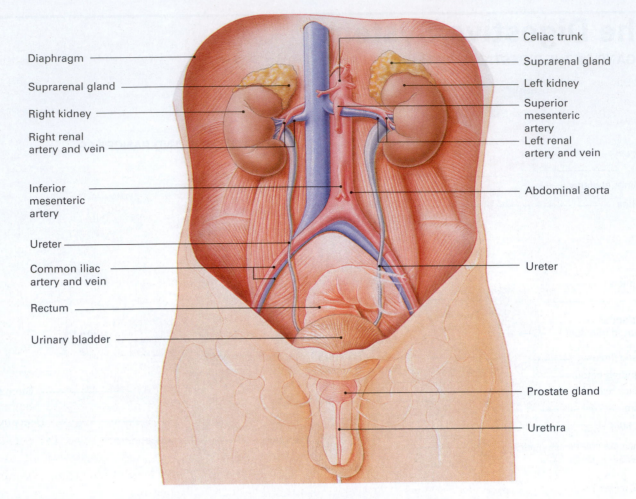

Diaphragm

Suprarenal gland

Right kidney

Right renal
artery and vein

Inferior
mesenteric
artery

Ureter

Common iliac
artery and vein

Rectum

Urinary bladder

Celiac trunk

Suprarenal gland

Left kidney

Superior
mesenteric
artery

Left renal
artery and vein

Abdominal aorta

Ureter

Prostate gland

Urethra

FIGURE 8-3 Major elements of the genitourinary system.

Urinary System

The urinary system consists of the kidneys, ureters, urinary bladder, and urethra (Figure 8-3). The kidneys are located in the retroperitoneal portions of the right and left upper quadrants and are protected by the muscles of the back, the thoracic and lumbar spine, and the muscles of the flanks. The kidneys receive their blood supply from the abdominal aorta. They extract waste products from the blood and eliminate them as urine. They also have significant regulatory control over the salt/water (osmotic) balance of the body, exercised by retaining or releasing water or sodium and other body salts. Additionally, the kidneys play an important role in controlling body pH and monitoring and maintaining blood pressure.

Genitalia

The female reproductive organs are located internally within the pelvis. These organs include the ovaries, fallopian tubes, uterus, and vagina. The male reproductive organs are outside and include the testes, scrotum, and penis (Figure 8-4).

Pregnant Uterus

Dynamics of pregnancy greatly affect the anatomy of the female abdominal cavity (Figure 8-5). The uterus and its contents grow rapidly from conception until delivery and are well protected during the first trimester (three months) of pregnancy. During the second trimester (12 to 24 weeks), progressive uterine enlargement displaces most of the abdominal contents upward as the growing uterus rises out of the pelvis and its upper border extends above the umbilicus. By 32 weeks and until the pregnancy ends, the uterus fills the abdominal cavity to the level of the lower rib margin. This enlarging uterus increases intraabdominal pressure and displaces the diaphragm upward. The displacement reduces the lung capacity at the same time that the physiologic changes of pregnancy require an increase in tidal volume.

Pregnancy also affects maternal physiology by raising circulatory volume by about 45 percent. By the third trimester, pregnancy raises cardiac rate by about 15 beats per minute and cardiac output by up to 40 percent. The increase in vascular volume is accompanied by a less

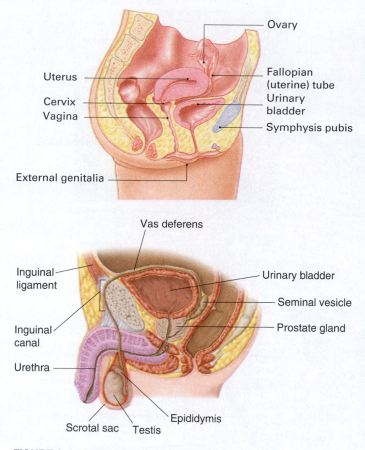

FIGURE 8-4 The female and male reproductive systems.

vena cava, reducing venous return to the heart (cardiac preload) and inducing a temporary hypotension in the supine patient (**supine hypotensive syndrome**) that is easily corrected with repositioning. Finally, the developing fetus means there are now two lives to protect when the mother suffers any trauma, especially trauma involving the abdomen.

Vasculature

The abdominal contents are supplied with blood via the abdominal aorta that is located along the left side of the spinal column. It sends forth many branches to discrete organs and the bowel (Figure 8-6). The abdominal aorta bifurcates at the upper sacral level into two large iliac arteries. These eventually become the femoral arteries as they traverse and then exit the pelvis. The attachment of these arteries to the pelvic structure is quite firm and may result in their tearing if the pelvis is fractured and displaced. The inferior vena cava is located along the right side of the spinal column and drains venous blood from the lower extremities and the abdomen, relatively parallel to the arterial system, returning it to the heart. The abdomen also contains the portal system that collects venous blood and other fluids, as well as nutrients absorbed by the intestines, and transports these to the liver. The liver detoxifies the fluid, stores excess nutrients, adds nutrients when they are deficient, and then sends the blood/nutrient/fluid mixture into the inferior vena cava just below the heart. There, it mixes with venous blood and is circulated through the heart and then to the rest of the body.

significant increase in erythrocytes. The result is a relative anemia that becomes an important consideration with aggressive fluid resuscitation for the mother in shock. In the last trimester of pregnancy, the uterus is significant in both size and weight and may compress the

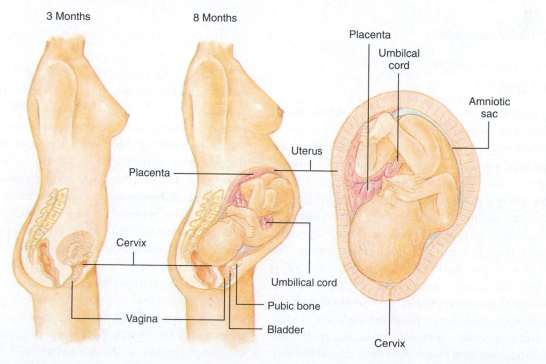

FIGURE 8-5 The pregnant uterus.

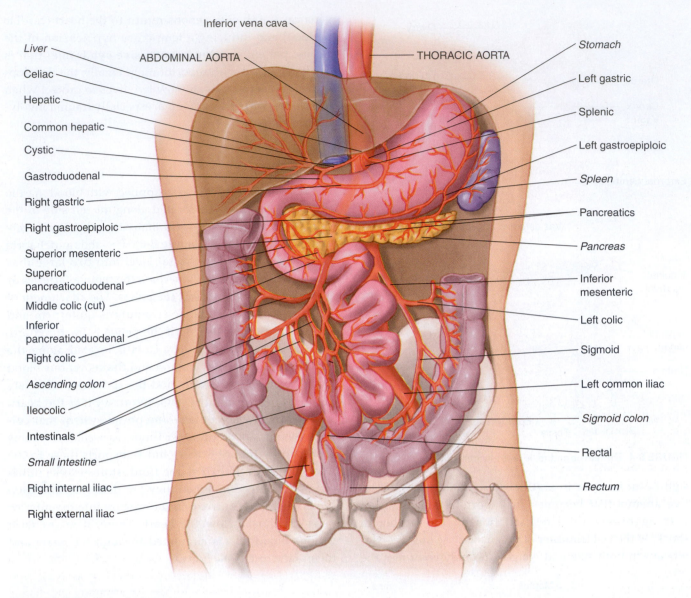

FIGURE 8-6 The abdominal arteries.

Peritoneum

Many abdominal organs are covered by a serous membrane called the **peritoneum** (Figure 8-7). This tissue resembles the lung's pleura and functions in a similar manner. The parietal peritoneum covers most of the interior surface of the anterior and lateral abdominal cavity, whereas the visceral peritoneum covers individual organs. A small amount of fluid is found between the peritoneal layers and permits free bowel movement during digestion. The digestive tract is supported by the **mesentery**. The mesentery is a double peritoneal fold containing blood vessels, lymphatic vessels, nerves, and fatty tissue. It suspends the bowel from the posterior abdominal wall. An additional fold of mesentery, called the *omentum*, covers, insulates, and protects the anterior abdominal cavity. The thickness of the omentum varies with the size and percentage of body fat. It may be several inches thick in an obese

patient or very narrow in a thin and muscular patient. Some abdominal structures are covered by peritoneum, the exception being the retroperitoneal organs, which are the kidneys, spleen, duodenum, pancreas, urinary bladder, the posterior portions of the ascending and descending colon, and the rectum. Most major vascular structures within the abdomen are also retroperitoneal. An organ's relation to the peritoneum becomes important in trauma because peritoneal irritation (peritonitis) caused by free blood in the peritoneal space presents with more apparent signs and symptoms than does hemorrhage or other fluid release into the retroperitoneal space.

The abdominal cavity is a dynamic place. The diaphragm moves up and down, displacing abdominal contents with each breath. With deep expiration, the central diaphragm moves as far upward as the fourth intercostal space anteriorly (the nipple line), and the seventh intercostal

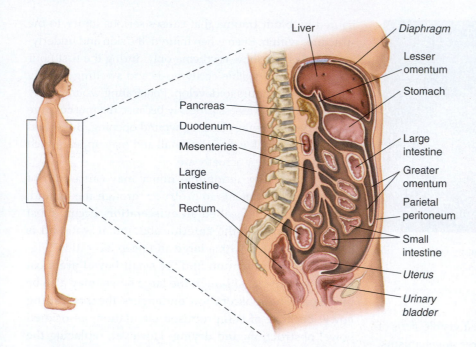

FIGURE 8-7 The peritoneum.

space (the inferior tips of the scapulae) posteriorly. (The diaphragm's edge attaches to the rib cage's border.) During forced and maximal inspiration, the diaphragm moves as much as 3 inches (9 cm) inferiorly. Movement of the diaphragm displaces abdominal contents up and down with each breath. Additionally, the volume of substances within the hollow organs varies—for example, an empty (10 mL) versus a distended (500 mL) bladder or a full (1.5 L) versus an empty stomach. The digestive tract is also suspended from the posterior abdominal cavity and is permitted some movement as it digests food. This dynamic movement becomes an important consideration when anticipating abdominal injury from blunt or penetrating trauma.

Pathophysiology of Abdominal and Pelvic Trauma

Mechanism of Injury

Unlike other major body cavities (skull, spine, and thorax), the abdomen is bound by muscles rather than skeleton. This results in a greater trauma energy transmission to the internal organs and structures. Concurrently, the signs of physical energy transmission signs are limited.

Penetrating Trauma

Penetrating trauma delivers energy directly to tissues that the penetrating object contacts (Figure 8-8) or, as seen with high-velocity projectiles, also transmits energy and injury

some distance from the projectile's path. The bullet injury process causes damage as the projectile contacts and then compresses and stretches the affected tissues. The projectile adds to the damage as it draws debris and contaminants into the wound, potentially causing wound infection or poor healing. Tissue disruption from penetrating trauma may cause uncontrolled hemorrhage, organ damage, spillage of hollow organ contents, and peritonitis. Gunshot wounds to the abdomen, especially those from high-powered weapons and shotguns at close range, transmit a tremendous amount of energy and tend to cause a morbidity and mortality approximately 10 times greater than those associated with the lower velocity of stab wounds.[1] When penetrating trauma causes abdominal injury, it usually affects the liver (40 percent of the time), the small bowel (25 percent of the time), and the large bowel (10 percent of the time). Injuries to the spleen, kidneys, and pancreas follow in decreasing order of incidence.

A special type of penetrating trauma is induced by a shotgun blast. A shotgun often delivers numerous round pellets. The aerodynamics of shot and the rapid expansion of the pellets reduce the energy of impact based on the distance the projectiles travel. Generally, shotgun blasts at short range (under 3 yards) are lethal. Between 3 and 7 yards, projectile penetration is great but often survivable. At distances greater than 7 yards, penetration depth and subsequent injury fall off quickly. These parameters change somewhat with the decreasing gauge size (gun barrel diameter) and the shot size. (See the chapter "Mechanisms of Injury" in this volume.)

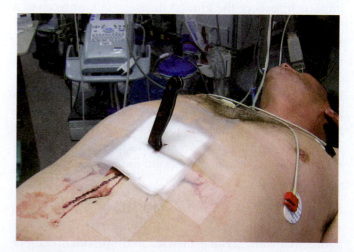

FIGURE 8-8 Stab wound to the upper abdomen.

(© Michael Casey, MD)

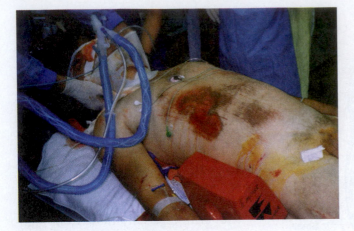

FIGURE 8-9 Blunt trauma to the upper abdomen.

(© Edward T. Dickinson, MD)

Blunt Trauma

Blunt abdominal trauma produces the least visible signs of injury and causes trauma through three mechanisms: deceleration, compression, and shear (Figure 8-9). As the exterior of the abdomen decelerates (or accelerates) during impact, the contents slam into one another in a chain reaction. They are first injured by the force of velocity changes and then by the forces of compression as they are trapped between the impacting object and the more posterior organs. The entire contents of the cavity may be compressed. Shear forces can also cause damage when one part of an organ is free to move while another part is restricted by anatomic attachments. Blunt trauma is responsible for about 40 percent of splenic injury and a little more than 20 percent of hepatic injury. The bowel and kidneys are the next most frequently injured abdominal structures in blunt trauma.

Careful mechanism of injury evaluation is important to assessing injuries within the region. Pay special attention to the potential for seat belt injury or direct injury as the abdomen impacts vehicle structures in a collision, impacts objects or the ground during a fall, or receives a blow during an assault. Remember that the early presentation of a contusion will likely be a simple reddening (erythema) of the affected area and not the more dramatic discoloration of ecchymosis. Thus, it is important to analyze the mechanism of injury, identify a high index of suspicion for intraabdominal injury, and carefully examine the abdomen for signs and symptoms of injury. The abdominal wall, hollow organs, solid organs, vascular structures, mesentery, and peritoneum all respond differently to trauma.

Abdominal Wall Injury

Any injury to the abdominal contents must first involve the abdominal wall. Because the skin and muscular lining of the abdomen are more resistant to injury than many of the internal organs, they are likely to be uninjured or minimally

injured by blunt trauma that causes serious injury to the structures within. Even when injured, the skin and underlying muscle may show erythema only during the first hour or so. The more visible ecchymosis and swelling usually require several hours to develop. Penetrating wounds may also be difficult to assess properly because the musculature and skin tension may close the wound opening. Bullet and knife wounds look especially small and may appear much less lethal than they actually are.

A penetrating abdominal injury may cause part of the abdominal contents to protrude through the wound. This type of injury, called an **evisceration**, occurs most frequently through the anterior abdominal wall and is usually associated with a large and deep laceration (Figure 8-10). The omentum and/or small bowel are most likely to protrude, although the large bowel may also be involved. The evisceration endangers the protruding bowel because of compromised circulation, associated bowel obstruction, and drying. However, replacing the protruding abdominal contents risks introducing bacteria into the peritoneal space. If the bowel is torn, there is an additional danger of its contents leaking into the peritoneal space when it is replaced.

Penetrating trauma to the thorax, buttocks, flanks, and back may also enter the abdomen and cause injury. The abdominal organs extend well into the thorax and move up to the nipple line anteriorly and to the tips of the scapulae posteriorly during deep expiration. Injury to the lower chest may lacerate the diaphragm and injure the stomach, liver, spleen, or gallbladder. Flank, back, and buttock muscles are thick and resist penetrating trauma well. However, deep wounds in these locations can penetrate into the abdominal cavity and cause injury to adjacent organs.

Tears in the diaphragm may also disrupt the abdominal cavity. These tears may occur with penetrating injury to the lower thorax or upper abdomen. Not only may these injuries compromise diaphragmatic function, but they may

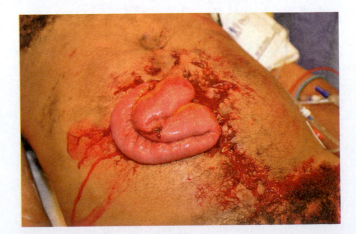

FIGURE 8-10 Abdominal evisceration.

(© Edward T. Dickinson, MD)

also allow the abdominal contents (such as those of the stomach, liver, or a portion of the small bowel) to enter the thoracic cavity. This reduces the available thoracic volume available during respiration and may compromise the blood supply to the herniated organs. Small diaphragmatic tears are unlikely to allow the abdominal contents to enter the thorax and are unlikely to affect respiration. Large tears are likely to do both.

Hollow Organ Injury

Hollow organs such as the stomach, small bowel, large bowel, rectum, urinary bladder, gallbladder, and pregnant uterus may rupture with compression from blunt forces—especially if the organ is full and distended. They may also tear as penetrating objects contact them. The small bowel is the most frequently injured hollow abdominal organ during penetrating trauma because it rests anteriorly and just under the anterior abdominal muscles and omentum. Hollow organ damage can cause hemorrhage and content spillage into the retroperitoneal, peritoneal, or pelvic spaces. The jejunum, ileum, colon, and rectum contain progressively higher bacterial concentrations; rupture and the subsequent leakage of these organs may cause a severe but delayed infection. The other hollow organs are more likely to release contents that cause a chemical irritation of the abdominal lining. Injury to the hollow organs may result in frank blood in the stool (**hematochezia**), blood in emesis (**hematemesis**), and blood in the urine (**hematuria**).

Solid Organ Injury

Solid organs such as the spleen, liver, pancreas, and kidneys are also subject to blunt and penetrating trauma. These organs are especially dense and are prone to contusion, and organ damage may range from minimal bleeding to rupture. If the organ's capsule remains intact, hemorrhage may be limited. However, if the capsule is disrupted by penetrating trauma or torn by the mechanism of blunt trauma, unrestricted hemorrhage may occur.

The spleen is relatively well protected by the lower ribs, back and flank muscles, and spinal column. It may be injured with severe abdominal compression, blunt left flank trauma, or penetrating injury. The spleen can bleed profusely, resulting in shock. Occasionally, blood loss may accumulate against the diaphragm (especially in the supine patient) and result in referred pain to the left shoulder region (Kehr's sign).

The pancreas is in the center of the upper abdomen. It is somewhat less delicate than the spleen and is well protected from blunt trauma by its location deep in the central abdominal cavity. Penetrating trauma may lacerate the pancreas and allow blood and digestive enzymes to enter the abdominal cavity. These pancreatic enzymes may actually begin to digest pancreatic and surrounding tissues, leading to severe injury. Pancreatic injury can result from severe blunt trauma to the upper abdomen because of compression of the pancreas between the trauma force and the vertebral column. This may occur when a patient impacts a steering wheel or the handlebars of a motorcycle during a crash. These patients may complain of upper abdominal pain that may radiate to the back.

The kidneys are equally well protected by their location deep in the retroperitoneal space. They are somewhat more resistant to injury than the pancreas, have a more substantial serous capsule, and are attached by large renal arteries to the aorta. They are most frequently injured with trauma to the back or flanks. Renal injury may cause localized back or flank pain, as well as hematuria.

The liver is the largest single organ within the abdomen and is surrounded by the strong visceral peritoneum. The liver is firmer than both the spleen and pancreas and is somewhat protected by the inferior border of the thorax. With trauma to this region, the liver can be damaged. The liver is restrained from forward motion by the ligamentum teres. During severe deceleration, the liver's weight forces it into the ligament, possibly causing shear injury, laceration, and hemorrhage. Liver injury often presents with tenderness along the right lower thoracic border and, as blood accumulates against the diaphragm, pain in the upper right shoulder. The liver is a very vascular organ and may account for serious internal hemorrhage and the need for massive in-hospital fluid resuscitation.

Vascular Injury

Arteries and veins within the abdomen are prone to injury with serious consequences. The abdominal aorta and its major branches (gastric, superior and inferior mesenteric, splenic, hepatic, renal, gonadal, and iliac) can be injured by direct blunt or penetrating trauma or may be injured as abdominal organs decelerate and pull on their vascular attachments during an auto collision or similar impact. Penetrating trauma does not frequently involve the very large abdominal vessels. However, when the aorta or other major artery is damaged, the resultant internal hemorrhage can be severe. The vena cava and its tributaries, as well as the portal system, can also be injured and may bleed heavily because the limited musculature in the large veins does not close the lumen as well as with arterial vessels. Most vascular injuries (97 percent) are associated with penetrating trauma.

Vascular injury in the peritoneal, retroperitoneal, and pelvic spaces can be serious for several reasons. These spaces expand easily and do not significantly resist continuing hemorrhage, as would occur with a vascular injury within a muscle mass elsewhere in the body. Without this pressure, both the rate and volume of blood loss do not slow initially. These spaces also contain organs that require significant circulation, supplied by rather large arterial and venous vessels. The abdomen's dynamic nature and its anatomic size mean that greater blood volumes can accumulate before swelling becomes noticeable.

Mesentery and Bowel Injury

The mesentery provides the bowel with circulation, innervation, and attachment. Blunt injury occurs as the mesentery stretches or is compressed during impact. This injury occurs most frequently at points of relative immobility such as the duodenal/jejunal juncture (where the small bowel is affixed by the ligament of Treitz) or where the small bowel joins the large bowel at the ileocecal junction. Injuries involving the mesentery may disrupt blood vessels supplying the bowel and eventually cause ischemia, necrosis, and possible rupture. Mesenteric injuries do not usually bleed profusely because the peritoneal layers contain the hemorrhage. Deceleration or compression may tear or rupture the full bowel. With penetrating trauma, the omentum is frequently injured and the bowel may be torn anywhere along its length, although tears to the small bowel (jejunum and ileum) are the most likely because of its central and anterior location. Even though a tear may release bowel contents into the peritoneal space, the signs and symptoms of such release are often delayed. The duodenum is less frequently injured because of its location deep within the abdomen (partially retroperitoneal). Penetrating trauma to the lateral abdomen is likely to injure the large bowel (ascending colon on the right and descending colon on the left).

Peritoneal Injury

The peritoneum is the very delicate and sensitive lining of the anterior abdominal cavity. Inflammation of the peritoneum is called **peritonitis** and can be caused by bacterial and chemical irritation. Bacterial peritonitis is an irritation due to infection and is often caused by bacteria released into the space by a torn bowel or open wound. It typically takes the bacteria between 12 and 24 hours to grow in sufficient numbers to produce inflammation; therefore, the condition is usually not apparent during prehospital care. Chemical peritonitis occurs more rapidly than bacterial peritonitis because of the caustic nature of digestive enzymes and acids (from the stomach or duodenum), blood, and, to a lesser degree, urine. These agents quickly irritate the peritoneum and induce the inflammatory response. Blood induces limited peritoneal inflammation, and serious hemorrhage alone is unlikely to cause this condition.

Peritonitis is a progressive process that presents with characteristic signs and symptoms. It usually begins with a slight tenderness at the injury location. Over time, the area of inflammation expands, as does the area of tenderness. Any abdominal jarring, as occurs with percussion or when you quickly release the pressure of deep palpation, causes a twinge of pain (rebound tenderness). **Rebound tenderness** is a sign of great historical importance, but testing for it is painful and offers no information not gained by ordinary palpation. The practice of eliciting rebound tenderness is considered obsolete and is discouraged in modern care. In response to pain induced by movement of the irritated abdominal tissue, the anterior abdominal muscles contract—even in the unconscious patient. This is called **guarding.** When assessing the abdomen, be aware that trauma-related local muscle injury may result in local or regional abdominal muscle tenderness and spasm that mimics peritonitis. Tenderness or frank pain from the physical injury may coexist with the signs of peritonitis.

Pelvic Injury

A pelvic fracture represents a serious skeletal injury with potentially serious and often life-threatening hemorrhage and potential injury to the pelvic organs. These organs—the ureters, bladder, urethra, female reproductive structure, prostate, rectum, and anus—can all be injured by severe kinetic forces, crushing mechanisms, or displaced bone fragments. Pelvic fracture can also cause serious injury to the pregnant uterus. (Pelvic hemorrhage and fracture are discussed in the chapter "Orthopedic Trauma" in this issue.)

Trauma and sexual assault may also injure the reproductive structures. Direct trauma to the female genitalia or injury caused by objects inserted into the vagina may tear the soft tissues of this region. Because these tissues are both very sensitive and vascular, the injury may bleed heavily and be very painful. The same is true for the male genitalia, which are more prone to injury because of their external location.

Injury During Pregnancy

Trauma is the number-one killer of pregnant women. Penetrating abdominal trauma alone accounts for as much as 36 percent of overall maternal mortality. Gunshot wounds to the abdomen of the pregnant woman also account for fetal mortality rates of between 40 and 70 percent. In blunt trauma, auto collisions are the leading cause of maternal and fetal mortality and morbidity. Proper seat belt placement can significantly reduce injury to the pregnant mother and fetus, whereas improper placement increases the incidence of both uterine rupture and placental separation from the uterine wall. Unrestrained mothers in serious auto collisions are four times more likely to suffer fetal mortality.

Physiologic changes associated with pregnancy protect both the mother and her abdominal organs. With the increasing uterine size, most abdominal organs are displaced higher in the abdominal cavity (Figure 8-11). This generally protects them unless blunt or penetrating trauma to the upper abdomen occurs. If that happens, then the injury may involve numerous organs, with increased morbidity and mortality. Direct penetrating injury to the central and lower abdomen in late pregnancy often spares the mother from serious injury. The resulting injury, however, often damages the uterus and endangers the fetus.

The late-term pregnant woman is at additional risk of vomiting and possible aspiration. Increasing uterine size increases intraabdominal pressure, whereas pregnancy hormones relax the cardiac sphincter (the valve that prevents reflux of stomach contents). The bladder is displaced superiorly early in pregnancy and then becomes more prone to injury and, when injured, bleeds more heavily.

Increasing uterus and fetal size and weight have several maternal effects that should be considered after trauma. The uterus of a supine patient in late pregnancy may compress the inferior vena cava and reduce venous return to the heart. This may induce hypotension in the uninjured patient and have severe consequences in the

hemorrhaging trauma patient. Increased intraabdominal pressure complicated by inferior vena caval compression (by the large, heavy uterus) raises venous pressures in the pelvic region and lower extremities. This pressure can engorge the vessels and may increase the venous hemorrhage rate from any pelvic fracture or lower-extremity wounds.

The increased maternal vascular volume (up by 45 percent) helps protect the mother from hypovolemia. However, this increase in maternal blood volume does not protect the fetus. (Maternal hypotension will reduce the blood flow to the placenta early in its progression.) In fact, it may take a maternal blood loss of between 30 and 35 percent before changes in maternal blood pressure or heart rate are evident. During this time, reduced placental circulation may endanger the developing fetus. Therefore, it becomes very important to ensure early and aggressive fluid resuscitation of the potentially hypotensive pregnant mother.

In pregnant women, the thick, muscular uterus contains both the developing fetus and amniotic fluid. This uterus is strong and can transmit trauma forces uniformly to the fetus, thereby reducing chances for injury. Significant blunt trauma may cause uterine rupture, and penetrating trauma may perforate or tear it. Here, the dangers of severe maternal hemorrhage and fetal blood supply disruption present life threats to both. The potential release of amniotic fluid into the abdomen is also of great concern. Uterine and fetal injury risk increase with gestational age

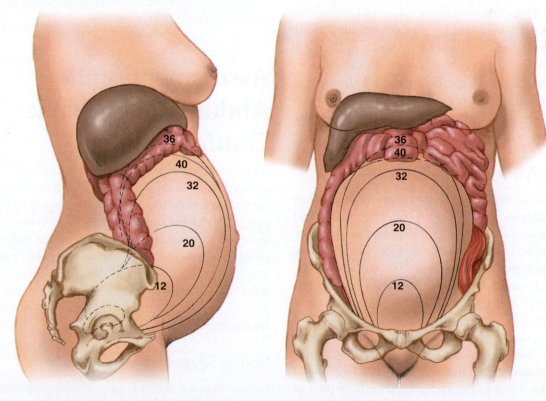

FIGURE 8-11 Changing dimensions of the pregnant uterus. Numbers represent weeks of gestation.

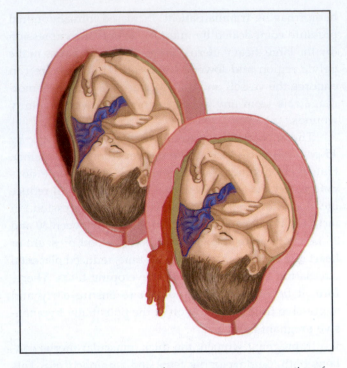

FIGURE 8-12 Blunt trauma to the uterus may cause separation of the placenta from the uterine wall (abruptio placentae), shown at left, or even rupture of the uterus, shown at right.

and are greatest during the third trimester. Frank uterine rupture is a rare complication of trauma but does occur with severe blunt impact, pelvic fracture, and—very infrequently—with stab or shotgun wounds.

Blunt trauma to the uterus can cause forceful uterine flexing possibly causing placental separation from the uterine wall. This is because the placenta is rather inelastic while the uterus is very flexible. This condition, called **abruptio placentae**, presents a life-threatening risk to both mother and fetus because the separation permits both maternal and fetal hemorrhage (Figure 8-12). Abruptio placentae may present with vaginal bleeding although hemorrhage is often contained within the uterus. Blunt trauma may induce preterm labor.

Pediatric Abdominal Trauma

Another special patient affected by abdominal injuries is the child. Children have poorly developed abdominal musculature and a reduced anterior/posterior diameter. The rib cage is more cartilaginous and flexible and more likely to transmit injury to the organs beneath. These factors increase the incidence and seriousness of pediatric abdominal injury, especially to the liver, spleen, and kidneys. Children also compensate very well for blood loss and may not show any signs or symptoms until they have lost more than half their blood volume. This is especially important with abdominal injuries, because a large blood volume may be lost into the abdomen with little pain or noticeable distention.

Assessment of the Abdominal or Pelvic Trauma Patient

Assessment of the abdominal trauma patient is somewhat abbreviated because definitive care for such injury is often surgical intervention. Hence, it is imperative to quickly assess the patient and, if indications of serious abdominal injury exist, package and transport the patient expeditiously. Assessment of the abdominal injury patient is like that for any trauma patient, with pertinent and significant information gained during the scene size-up, primary assessment, rapid or focused trauma assessment, and serial reassessments.[2]

Scene Size-Up

Ensure that the scene is safe. Use appropriate Standard Precautions before approaching the patient. Identify the mechanism of injury and begin to develop an index of suspicion and assess any impact the environment might have on assessment, care, and transport. Also determine the number of expected patients and any need for additional EMS, police, fire, and other service resources, and integrate these with incident oversight.

For a patient who has sustained an abdominal injury, the mechanism of injury analysis is a very important scene size-up element. However, forming an index of suspicion for individual abdominal injuries is critical because the signs and symptoms are, for the most part, limited and nonspecific. In fact, more than 30 percent of patients with serious abdominal injury may initially have no specific signs or symptoms whatsoever. Additionally, other less life-threatening but more painful injuries may overshadow signs and symptoms of an abdominal injury. Furthermore, signs and symptoms that are present may become less specific in nature with time and the progressive nature of peritonitis. Finally, the patient's reporting of his condition may be unreliable, owing to the effects of alcohol or drug ingestion, head injury, or shock.[3] Because of these factors, a well-developed index of suspicion may suggest the presence of injuries that may otherwise be difficult to identify.

If the patient has suffered blunt trauma, identify the possible strength and direction of the forces and the location on the body where they were delivered. Observe and palpate that site during the primary and rapid trauma assessments and develop a suspicion of injury. Begin to develop a list of possible organs injured (the index of suspicion) and the immediate and delayed effects they may have on the patient's condition. In serious blunt trauma or deep penetrating trauma, expect internal and uncontrolled hemorrhage.

If a patient was involved in an auto collision, identify whether seat belts were used and whether they were used properly (Figure 8-13). Remember that improper placement (above the iliac crests) may increase the likelihood of abdominal compression (and lumbar spine) injury. A lack of seat belt use increases the incidence and severity of all types of trauma, including abdominal injury. Examine the vehicle interior for signs of impact, such as deformity of a steering wheel, a deflated air bag, or a structural intrusion into the occupant compartment. Frontal impact is most likely to compress the abdomen, injure the liver and spleen, and possibly rupture distended hollow organs such as the stomach and bladder. A right-side impact may cause liver, kidney, ascending colon, and pelvic injury, whereas a left-side impact may cause splenic, kidney, descending colon, and pelvic injuries. Pedestrians, especially children, are likely to sustain lower abdominal injury, especially if the vehicle impacts the patient's midsection. It is important to determine the impact velocity and the distance the patient was thrown. Motorcyclists and, to a lesser degree, bicyclists are likely to sustain abdominal injury as they are propelled forward while the handlebars restrain the pelvis and lower abdomen. In assaults and other isolated impacts, be observant for left flank impact and splenic or renal damage, and right-side impact causing renal or hepatic (liver) injury. If impact involves the superior abdomen, suspect liver, stomach, spleen, and pancreatic injury. Impact to the middle or lower abdomen will likely damage the small bowel, kidneys, and bladder.

With a patient who has experienced penetrating trauma, determine the nature of the injury. If it is a knife, arrow, or impaled object, determine the probable insertion angle and depth (Figure 8-14). Do not move or remove an impaled object.

With gunshot wounds, try and determine whether the weapon was a handgun, shotgun, or rifle. If possible, determine the gun's caliber and the distance from the gun to the victim. Also try to determine the number of shots fired, if possible, and the angle from which the gun was

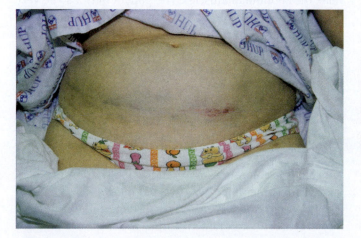

FIGURE 8-13 Use the mechanism of injury to identify where signs of injury might be found—for example, contusions resulting from compression by a seat belt.

(© Edward T. Dickinson, MD)

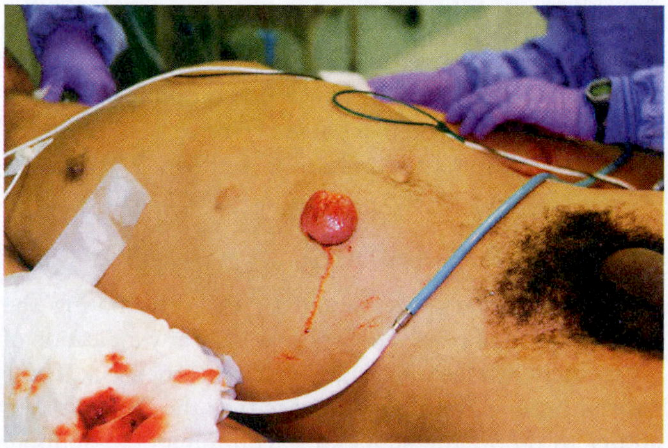

FIGURE 8-14 Analyze the mechanism of a penetrating trauma in an attempt to determine the probable angle and depth of the wound.

(© Edward T. Dickinson, MD)

fired. Expose the patient and examine for wounds carefully. Be prepared to examine the flanks, buttocks, and back for signs of additional or exit wounds. Attempt to estimate blood lost at the scene and communicate this, with the other information previously listed, to the emergency department physician.

Gunshot wounds provide an assessment challenge. Damage done does not correlate well to the wound's external appearance. It is more related to the bullet's kinetic energy (velocity and mass) as it enters the body and to the energy exchange characteristics as it travels into and through tissue. Low-velocity bullets cause little damage beyond the bullet's actual path. However, these projectiles are easily deflected by contact with clothing, bone, or, in some cases, soft tissue. They also can carry pieces of clothing and other debris into the body and do not tend to pass through the body.

High-velocity weapon (rifle) wounds were once seen only in the military setting, Now, civilian trauma centers are seeing similar wounds and internal injuries. These projectiles cause injury well beyond the bullet's path because of the cavitation. The wounding process also draws debris into the wound, where the damaged and devitalized (without circulation) tissue forms a good bacterial growth medium. The wounding process may create secondary projectiles as the bullet hits bone, breaks it apart, and then drives the fragments into adjacent tissue. The high-velocity bullet may also fragment and transmit its injuring potential to several pathways.

Suspect continued and serious internal hemorrhage with either significant blunt or penetrating abdominal trauma. Be especially watchful for signs of hypoperfusion and initiate shock care at the first signs and symptoms. These signs and symptoms include altered mental status, increasing anxiety or restlessness, thirst, increasing pulse rate, decreasing pulse pressure, and increasing capillary refill time.

Information gathered at the scene is invaluable to the attending emergency department physician. That information, however, will be unavailable unless carefully documented and reported on arrival at the hospital. Doing this is essential to ensuring that patients receive the best care in both the prehospital and in-hospital settings.

Primary Assessment

Begin the primary assessment by carefully noting the patient's level of consciousness as well as any indication of impairment by alcohol, drugs, head injury, or shock. These substances and conditions may reduce the patient's reliability to report the signs and symptoms of abdominal trauma. Any decrease in mental status should result in a higher index of suspicion for abdominal injury and the need to perform more careful primary and rapid trauma

assessments. The patient may also complain of dizziness or light-headedness when moving from a supine to a seated or standing position. (Do not ask the patient to move. However, the patient may have moved before your arrival.) Any of these signs and symptoms should increase suspicion for hypovolemia—possibly from an abdominal injury. Use the initial evaluation as a baseline against which to compare any changes in the patient's mental status.

When evaluating the airway, breathing, and circulation, be observant for any associated signs and symptoms of hypovolemia, especially if they appear inconsistent with the obvious or expected injuries. Note any rapid or shallow respirations, diminished pulse pressure, rapid pulse rate, slow capillary refill time, or thirst. Limited chest movement may be due to peritonitis or blood irritating the diaphragm. Shallow respirations may be due to abdominal contents in the thorax from a ruptured diaphragm. Be prepared to protect the airway, because abdominal trauma patients are likely to vomit.

Secondary/Rapid Trauma Assessment

Perform the usual full rapid trauma assessment. However, if there is a high index of suspicion for abdominal injury, pay particular attention to that region. Carefully examine the abdomen for evidence of injury as suggested by the mechanism of injury or by signs or symptoms observed during the primary assessment. If a patient is suspected of having sustained blunt trauma, look carefully over the entire abdominal surface for erythema or minor abrasions associated with superficial soft tissue injury. Remember that any trauma must pass through the abdomen's surface before it can do damage within. Note the patient's positioning, as it may suggest abdominal injury. Often, the patient with abdominal pain will be in the fetal position to relax the abdominal muscles. The patient may also be very quiet and not complaining.

Quickly examine the anterior abdominal surface and then the flanks (Figure 8-15). Then, carefully and gently logroll the patient to examine the back, looking for any signs of injury, erythema, ecchymosis, contusions, or open wounds, including eviscerations and impaled objects. Discoloration of the flank region is called Grey-Turner's sign, and, like most prehospital discoloration due to accumulating blood, it takes some time to develop. If a frank black-and-blue discoloration of an abdominal region is noted, suspect an earlier injury or other pathology.

Look at the abdomen's general shape and examine for any signs of distention. Examine the inguinal area for injury or hemorrhage signs. Jeans or trousers may contain hemorrhage without any external indication, so they should be cut away or removed to assess this region when injury is possible. Remember that the abdominal cavity

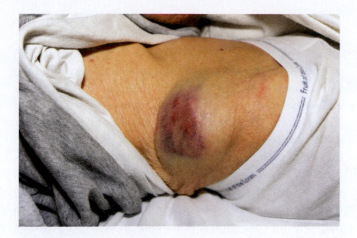

FIGURE 8-15 Examine the abdomen and flanks for signs of injury.
(© Dr. Bryan E. Bledsoe)

can contain a very large volume of blood (on the order of 1.5 liters) before it becomes noticeably distended. In obese patients, the blood volume loss may be even greater before distention is visible. Also be aware that signs and symptoms of peritoneal (hemoperitoneum) or retroperitoneal hemorrhage are limited.

Visualize and palpate the pelvis for signs of injury or instability. Apply gentle pressure directed posteriorly, then medially, on the iliac crests, then place pressure downward on the symphysis pubis. If you note any crepitus or instability, suspect a pelvic fracture and both injury to lower abdominal and pelvic organs and severe internal hemorrhage. If a pelvic injury is suspected or present, do not test or apply any pressure and be very careful during movement to the ambulance and transport to the hospital. Any fracture site manipulation may start, restart, or increase hemorrhage.

Question the patient about pain or discomfort in each quadrant, then palpate the quadrants individually, leaving any quadrant with anticipated injury or patient complaint of pain for last. If the injured quadrant is palpated first, the pain may lead the patient to splint or voluntarily contract the abdominal muscles during any remaining palpation. Feel for any spasm or guarding during palpation. If the abdomen is quite firm to palpation, suspect an injury to the pancreas, duodenum, or stomach—especially if the time since the injury is short. Be observant for any patient pain with patient movement during assessment or care (suggesting peritoneal irritation).

Note any unusual pulsations in the abdomen. Although there will be some pulsing in the thin, young, healthy, athletic patient, most patients will not have any visible or palpable pulses in the abdomen. Abnormal pulsation may suggest arterial injury or aneurysm. Injuries to the thorax or pelvis also suggest abdominal injury, especially if there are lower rib fractures or the pelvic ring is unstable. Auscultation is not beneficial during assessment of the abdominal

trauma patient. It takes a great deal of time to adequately listen for bowel sounds, and their presence or absence neither confirms nor excludes suspected injury.

When evaluating the patient with penetrating abdominal trauma, look carefully at the entrance wound and note its appearance, size, and depth. A "point-blank" discharge of a gun against tissue will introduce barrel exhaust into the open wound created by the bullet, evidenced as powder debris and the crackling of subcutaneous emphysema. Look for contamination and any signs of serious blood loss. Then examine the patient for an exit wound. Exit wounds may look more "blown out" in nature and are generally larger and more serious in appearance than entrance wounds. Exit wounds are more likely to reflect the nature and extent of internal injury. The wounds from a projectile may be very small and difficult to see, while still carrying the potential to cause lethal injury. (It is not advisable to specify entrance and exit wounds on the patient care report, as it is often difficult to distinguish between the two and there are legal ramifications to misidentifying wounds. Instead, simply describe the wound location and characteristics without reference to "entrance" or "exit.")

A new assessment technique now becoming available in the prehospital setting is ultrasonography. This device creates high-frequency sound waves (small and rapid pressure waves oscillating millions of times per second) that are transmitted into the abdomen. They reflect off organs, tissues, and fluids differently, based on density, and form a cross-sectional image. The device creates an image much the same way that radar does. This image can be used to identify the location of pooling blood within the abdomen (e.g., retroperitoneal) after abdominal trauma. Reassessments can also identify if the pooled blood volume is increasing or stable in size. Although sonography use in prehospital care is still new and evolving, it is important to recognize that to be valuable, the sonographic findings must change patient management in some meaningful way. In blunt abdominal trauma, the presence of fluid in the peritoneal cavity suggests blood and could signal the need for transport to a trauma center. Conversely, in penetrating abdominal trauma (e.g., gunshot wound), transport to a trauma center is always indicated and sonography is unlikely to change prehospital management. Consequently, sonographic imaging in penetrating abdominal trauma is not a priority.[4-6]

Anticipate injuries that occurred as the object or bullet went through the body. Remember that it is not uncommon for a bullet to alter its path. Be suspicious of any projectile wound in the proximal extremities because the projectile may travel along the limb and into the body's interior. Also keep in mind that a bullet wound to the thorax may then deflect and penetrate the abdomen, or vice versa.

While performing the rapid trauma assessment, carefully question the patient about the characteristics of any pain he experiences and ask specifically about any abdominal sensations or other symptoms. Serious injury may result while the patient feels limited pain or injury sensation, especially when other, more painful, injuries elsewhere might be distracting him. Abdominal pain evaluation may, however, be subjective, as patients often vary in their response to pain. It may be necessary to watch the patient's response to further assessment or his ease in distraction to accurately gauge his degree of pain. In the male, retroperitoneal pain may be referred to the testicular region. Thirst may be one of the few symptoms of abdominal injury, as significant hemorrhage draws down the body's blood volume. Be sure to record any symptoms in the patient's own words and ensure that these comments and your findings are documented on the prehospital care report and reported to the attending physician.

When determining the patient's history, give special consideration to the last oral intake. The bladder, bowel, and stomach are much more likely to rupture if full and distended. Ask about when the patient last ate or drank and how much he consumed. Relate the intake to the type of impact received—especially blunt trauma to the trunk. Conclude the rapid trauma assessment by gathering a set of baseline vital signs.

At the end of the rapid trauma assessment, reevaluate the patient's priority for transport. The potential for an abdominal injury must factor into this determination. Remember that serious internal hemorrhage from blunt or penetrating trauma frequently occurs with few overt signs and symptoms. Any patient with a history of significant blunt trauma or any penetrating trauma to the torso is a candidate for rapid transport to the trauma center. Always err on the side of providing more patient care and early transport rather than underestimating the seriousness of abdominal trauma.

Special Assessment Considerations with Pregnant Patients

If a patient is pregnant, pay special attention to the abdomen and the possibility of injury. Remember that the maternal blood volume is increased by up to 45 percent in the third trimester and blood loss can exceed 30 percent before the normal signs and symptoms of hypovolemia are seen. Watch for the earliest signs of shock. Ensure that the uterus does not compress the vena cava by placing the noticeably pregnant mother in the left lateral recumbent position. If spinal injury is also suspected, immobilize her firmly to the spine board and, after she is placed on the stretcher, rotate the entire board and patient 15 degrees to the left side. Carefully evaluate the vital signs and remember that the fetus is likely to experience distress before the mother shows any signs of hypotension or hypoperfusion.

Abdominal trauma in late pregnancy may cause several specific uterine injuries and requires careful assessment. The normal uterus will be firm and round to palpation. It will be palpable above the iliac crests after the first 12 weeks of pregnancy and progress upward in the abdominal cavity until it reaches the costal border at about 32 weeks. Palpation of the injured uterus may result in tenderness and muscular contractions that are normal with uterine contusions. These contractions will often be self-limiting. However, any tenderness, pain, or contractions should raise the suspicions of abruptio placentae. The mother may complain of cramping, generally related to palpable uterine contractions and, in some cases, may experience vaginal hemorrhage. Abruptio placentae is a serious fetal and maternal risk and is a true emergency, requiring rapid transport.

Uterine palpation that reveals an asymmetrical uterus may be a sign of uterine rupture. This condition may also present with uterine contractions, but the uterine fundus is not palpable and the mass does not harden with the contractions.

Alert the emergency department well before your arrival if you are transporting a pregnant mother who was injured by trauma. This will allow department personnel to prepare for the special monitoring necessary for both the mother and fetus.

Reassessment

Reassessment is an essential part of the continuing care process for abdominal injury patients. During the reassessment, look for the signs and symptoms of a progressing abdominal injury or continuing hemorrhage. Perform it every 5 minutes in patients with any significant suggestion of abdominal injury. Often, the progressive nature of peritonitis leads to greater and greater patient complaints or may make abdominal signs and symptoms more evident as you care for and reduce the pain of other injuries. Ongoing signs of hemorrhage are equally progressive and may not clearly present until well into patient care.

Pay close attention to the signs of hidden hemorrhage during reassessments of the patient with potential abdominal injury. Watch blood pressure, pulse rate, capillary refill time, oxygen saturation, and the patient's appearance and mental status. A decrease in the difference in the pulse pressure suggests shock compensation. An increasing pulse rate (especially if the pulse strength is diminishing) and an increasing capillary refill time both suggest hypovolemic compensation. Also observe the skin for temperature, clamminess, and color, and watch for pulse oximetry readings that become more erratic. A change in mental status suggests the brain is being hypoperfused. If a source of blood loss cannot be accounted for, suspect internal and continuing abdominal hemorrhage. Subtle changes may be the only apparent signs of gradually worsening shock.

Another sign of continuing blood loss from an abdominal hemorrhage occurs when fluid resuscitation appears ineffective (nonresponder). Note the patient's response to fluid resuscitation. If it takes significant fluid volumes to maintain organ perfusion and all external hemorrhage is controlled, suspect continuing internal hemorrhage.

Management of the Abdominal Trauma Patient

Abdominal injury patient management is supportive, with the major emphasis on getting the patient to surgery as quickly as possible, if necessary. Prehospital care centers on rapid packaging and transport, as needed. Specific care steps for the patient with suspected abdominal injury includes proper positioning, general shock care, fluid resuscitation, and care for specific injuries (open wounds and eviscerations).[7]

The patient with any abdominal pain should be positioned for comfort (unless the positioning is contraindicated by a likely spinal injury). Flex the patient's knees to relax the abdominal muscles. If injuries permit, place the patient in the left lateral recumbent position to maintain knee flexure, relax abdominal muscles, and facilitate clearing the airway of emesis.

Ensure good ventilation and consider early administration of supplemental oxygen if the patient's pulse oximetry values are less than 96 percent. The pain associated with peritonitis or diaphragmatic irritation may reduce respiratory excursion, adding to early shock development in these patients.

Control any moderate or serious external hemorrhage with direct pressure and bandaging. Minor bleeding may be controlled during transport, if at all.

When a serious mechanism of injury is found and the patient does not present with the suspected signs and symptoms of shock, act in anticipation of it. Be prepared to administer fluid boluses if the signs of shock develop and the blood pressure drops below a systolic reading of 80 mmHg. Monitor the pulse rate and blood pressure. If the pulse does not slow and the pulse pressure does not stabilize, consider administering an additional fluid bolus. Do not delay transport to initiate any IV access. Start the IV access en route to the hospital, if necessary. Prehospital infusion is usually limited to 3,000 mL of fluid. Titrate the administration rate to maintain a systolic blood pressure of 80 mmHg and ensure not to exceed this fluid volume limit during field care and transport.[8]

As with all serious trauma patients, communicate frequently with the abdominal injury patient to reduce anxiety and provide emotional support. Also watch for any changes in the patient's description of the pain or injury's character or intensity. Be wary of patient hypothermia, especially when providing fluid resuscitation. Provide ample blankets, keep the patient compartment warm, take patient complaints of being cold seriously, and warm IV fluids when possible. Hypothermia is a special consideration with pediatric patients because they have a disproportionately large body surface area to body volume and will rapidly lose heat to the environment.

Cover any exposed (eviscerated) abdominal organs with a dressing moistened with sterile saline (Procedure 8-1). Be careful to keep the region clean and do not replace any exposed organs. Cover the wet dressing with a sterile occlusive dressing, such as clear plastic wrap, to keep the site as clean as possible and yet retain the moisture. If the transport is lengthy, check the dressing from time to time and remoisten it as necessary.

Another wound that deserves special attention is the impaled object. Try to keep the object from moving and do not remove it. Any motion may cause further injury, disrupt clotting mechanisms, and permit continued hemorrhage. Removal may withdraw the object from a blood vessel, thereby permitting increased internal and uncontrollable hemorrhage. Pad around the object with bulky trauma dressings and wrap around the trunk with soft, self-adherent roller bandaging to secure it firmly. Apply direct pressure around the object if hemorrhage is anything but minor. If the object is too long to accommodate during transport or it is affixed to an immovable object, attempt to cut it. Use a saw, cutter, or torch, but be very careful to ensure that vibration, jarring, and heat are not transmitted to the patient.

Carefully observe and care for penetrating wounds that may involve both the abdominal and thoracic cavities. If the wound is large and may have penetrated the diaphragm or otherwise entered the thoracic cavity, seal the wound with an occlusive dressing taped on three sides to permit air pressure release that occurs in a tension pneumothorax. Be especially cognizant of respiratory excursion and effort.

CONTENT REVIEW

➤ Management of the Abdominal Injury Patient
- Position the patient properly.
- Ensure oxygenation and ventilation.
- Control external bleeding.
- Be prepared for aggressive fluid resuscitation.
- Stabilize impaled objects.

➤ When a serious mechanism of injury is found and the patient does not present with the signs and symptoms of shock, act in anticipation of it.

Procedure 8-1 Eviseration Care

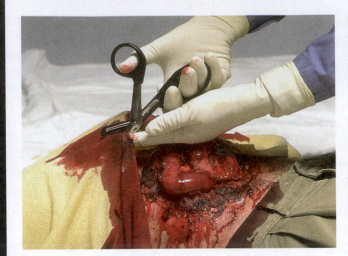

8-1A Remove clothing from around the abdominal wound.

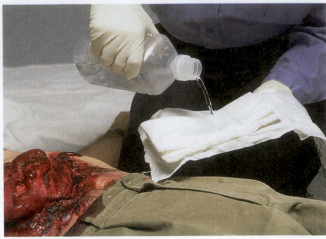

8-1B Cover the wound with a sterile dressing soaked with sterile normal saline.

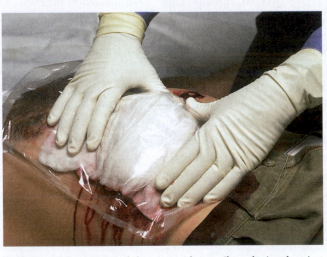

8-1C Cover the moistened dressing with a sterile occlusive dressing to prevent evaporative drying.

Management of the Pregnant Patient

Special care is offered to the pregnant patient because of the anatomic and physiologic changes induced by pregnancy. Place the late-term mother, when possible, in the left lateral recumbent position. If the patient is on a spine board, tilt it 15 degrees to the left to achieve a similar effect. This ensures that the uterus's weight does not compress the vena cava, reduce blood return to the heart, and cause hypotension. It also facilitates airway care. Administer supplemental oxygen early in care. The mother's respiratory reserve volume is diminished because the effort necessary to move air is greater as a result of increased intraabdominal pressure and because the fetus is especially susceptible to hypoxia. If necessary, use positive-pressure ventilation. Also consider aggressive airway care. The pregnant mother is prone to vomiting and aspiration. If she has a significantly reduced level of consciousness, consider rapid sequence intubation.

Maintain a high index of suspicion for internal hemorrhage, as the increased blood volume of the third-trimester mother may permit an increased blood loss before signs and symptoms of hypovolemia become evident. The fetus may be at risk early in the blood loss, well before the mother displays any signs. Initiate IV therapy early, but remember that pregnancy induces a relative anemia and that aggressive fluid resuscitation may further dilute the erythrocyte concentrations and lead to ineffective circulation.

Summary

Blunt or penetrating abdominal trauma can cause serious organ damage and life-threatening hemorrhage. Initially, the signs and symptom of injury are often limited and nonspecific, and do not reflect the seriousness of the injury. It is very important to carefully determine the mechanism of injury and the region of the abdomen affected. This information must be communicated to the emergency department to ensure that personnel acknowledge the significance of the mechanism of injury.

The care for significant abdominal injuries primarily involves rapid transport to the trauma center. Most significant abdominal injuries result in serious internal bleeding or organ injury that can neither be cared for nor stabilized in the prehospital setting. Further, the definitive care for the patient with serious abdominal injury is provided via surgery. The patient must be transported to a facility capable of providing immediate surgical intervention when needed. In most areas, this is a trauma center. Prehospital abdominal injury care is supportive of the airway and breathing, and preventive for shock.

The pregnant patient with abdominal injury deserves special attention because her vascular volume is increased and she will likely not exhibit the signs of shock until the fetus is at risk. Careful observation while preparing for rapid transport to the trauma center is in order. If any of the slightest signs of hypoperfusion are noted, initiate fluid resuscitation.

You Make the Call

You arrive at the scene of a car–pedestrian collision. The victim is a young female about 12 years of age. She is lying on her side, in the fetal position, on the ground. She is conscious and alert, though confused as to where she is and what happened. The patient complains of right shoulder pain, although there is no injury visible in the region. Physical assessment reveals a tender left upper quadrant, just below the margin of the rib cage, with some guarding and no rebound tenderness.

1. Given the signs and symptoms, what is the most likely injury and why?

2. What relation does the right shoulder pain have to the suspected injury?

3. What care will you provide for this patient?

See Suggested Responses at the back of this book.

Review Questions

1. Your patient has a history of trauma to the left flank and complains of pain in that region. Which of the following organs might you suspect to be injured?

   a. Liver   c. Spleen

   b. Heart   d. Gallbladder

2. All of the following statements regarding bile are correct *except* _____

   a. bile is secreted through the bile duct.

   b. bile is released into the gastrointestinal tract in response to fatty foods.

   c. bile aids in the digestion of fats.

   d. bile is produced by the gallbladder.

3. Which of the following is *not* one of the functions of the kidneys?

   a. pH regulation

   b. Blood filtration

   c. Salt/water balance control

   d. Fat emulsification

4. Penetrating trauma to the abdomen most frequently involves which organ?

   a. Liver

   b. Spleen

   c. Kidneys

   d. Small bowel

5. A protrusion of organs from a wound is called an _____
   a. extravasation.
   b. evisceration.
   c. ecchymosis.
   d. exsanguination.

6. One of the functions of the pancreas is _____
   a. destroying spent RBCs.
   b. producing new RBCs.
   c. secreting glucagon.
   d. manufacturing new WBCs.

7. What is the most common cause of death in pregnant women?
   a. Hypertension
   b. Toxemia
   c. Trauma
   d. Sepsis

8. The appendix and portions of the urinary bladder, small bowel, ascending colon, and female genitalia are located in the _____
   a. left lower quadrant.
   b. right upper quadrant.
   c. right lower quadrant.
   d. left upper quadrant.

9. The spleen, though located in the abdominal cavity, is an organ belonging primarily to what system?
   a. Digestive
   b. Respiratory
   c. Cardiovascular
   d. Immune

10. It is very important to ensure early fluid resuscitation of the potentially hypotensive pregnant mother, as it may take a maternal blood loss of between _____ percent before changes in maternal blood pressure or heart rate are evident.
    a. 10 and 15
    b. 20 and 25
    c. 30 and 35
    d. 40 and 45

See Answers to Review Questions at the end of this book.

References

1. Eachempati, S. R., et al. "Factors Associated with Mortality in Patients with Penetrating Abdominal Vascular Injury." *J Surg Res* 108(2) (Dec 2002): 222–228.

2. Collopy, K. T. and G. Friese. "Abdominal Trauma: A Review of Prehospital Assessment and Management of Blunt and Penetrating Abdominal Trauma." *EMS Mag* 39(3) (Mar 2010): 62–66, 68–69.

3. Mulholland, S. A., et al. "Prehospital Prediction of the Severity of Blunt Anatomic Injury." *J Trauma* 64(3) (Mar 2008): 754–760.

4. Heegaard, W., et al. "Prehospital Ultrasound by Paramedics: Results of Field Trial." *Acad Emerg Med* 17(6) (Jun 2010): 624–630.

5. Hoyer, H. X., et al. "Prehospital Ultrasound in Emergency Medicine: Incidence, Feasibility, Indications and Diagnoses." *Eur J Emerg Med* 17(5) (Oct 2010): 254–259.

6. Snaith, B., M. Hardy, and A. Walker. "Emergency Ultrasound in the Prehospital Setting: The Impact of Environment on Examination Outcomes." *Emerg Med J* 28(12) (Dec 2011): 1063–1065.

7. Spaite, D. W., et al. "The Impact of Injury Severity and Prehospital Procedures on Scene Time in Victims of Major Trauma." *Ann Emerg Med* 20(12) (Dec 1991): 1299–1305.

8. Yaghoubian, A., R. J. Lewis, B. Putnam, and C. Virgilio. "Reanalysis of Prehospital Intravenous Fluid Administration in Patients with Penetrating Truncal Injury and Field Hypotension." *Am Surg* 73(10) (2007): 1027–1030.

Further Reading

American College of Surgeons, Committee on Trauma. *Advanced Trauma Life Support Course: Student Manual.* 9th ed. Chicago: American College of Surgeons, 2012.

Bickley, L. *Bates' Guide to Physical Examination and History Taking.* 11th ed. Philadelphia: Wolters-Kluwer, 2012.

Bledsoe, B. E. and D. Clayden. *Prehospital Emergency Pharmacology.* 7th ed. Upper Saddle River, NJ: Pearson/Prentice Hall, 2011.

Bledsoe, B. E., B. J. Colbert, and J. E. Ankney. *Essentials of A & P for Emergency Care.* Upper Saddle River, NJ: Pearson/Prentice Hall, 2010.

Campbell, John E. *International Trauma Life Support for Prehospital Care Providers.* 8th ed. Upper Saddle River, NJ: Pearson/Prentice Hall, 2016.

Ivatury, R. R. and G. C. Cayten, eds. *Textbook of Penetrating Trauma.* Media, PA: Williams & Wilkins, 1996.

Martini, F. *Fundamentals of Anatomy and Physiology.* 10th ed. San Francisco: Pearson, 2014.

Marx, J., R. Hockberger, and R. Walls. *Emergency Medicine: Concepts and Clinical Practice.* 8th ed. St. Louis: Mosby, 2013.

National Association of EMTs. *Prehospital Trauma Life Support.* 8th ed. Burlington, VT: Jones & Bartlett Learning, 2014.

Rosen, P. and R. Barkin, eds. *Emergency Medicine: Concepts and Clinical Practice.* 7th ed. St. Louis: Mosby, 2009.

Tintinelli, J. E., ed. *Emergency Medicine: A Comprehensive Study Guide.* 7th ed. New York: McGraw-Hill, 2012.

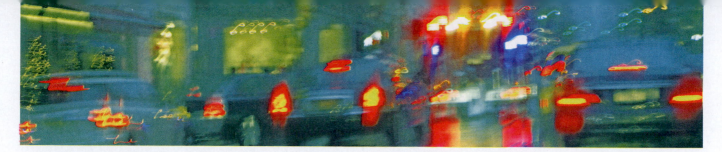

Chapter 9
Orthopedic Trauma

Bryan E. Bledsoe, DO, FACEP, FAAEM, EMT-P

Robert S. Porter, MA, EMT-P

STANDARD
Trauma (Orthopedic Trauma)

COMPETENCY
Integrates assessment findings with principles of epidemiology and pathophysiology to formulate a field impression to implement a comprehensive treatment/disposition plan for an acutely injured patient.

⌄ Learning Objectives

Terminal Performance Objective: After reading this chapter you should be able to assess and manage patients with orthopedic injuries.

Enabling Objectives: To accomplish the terminal performance objective, you should be able to:

1. Define key terms introduced in this chapter.

2. Discuss the basic epidemiology of orthopedic trauma.

3. Describe considerations in preventing orthopedic injuries.

4. Describe the anatomy and physiology of the musculoskeletal system.

5. Describe the pathophysiology of injuries as they occur to muscles, joints, and bones.

6. Describe special considerations in pediatric, geriatric, and sports-related orthopedic injuries.

7. Identify the phases and discuss the steps of assessment followed when encountering orthopedic injuries.

8. Discuss the types of, and indications for, splinting equipment.

9. Identify and discuss any specific management for specific types of injuries such as pelvic, femur, knee, tibia/fibula, ankle, foot, shoulder, humerus, elbow, radius/ulna, wrist, and hand.

10. Given a variety of scenarios, identify and discuss the proper prehospital management of patients with musculoskeletal injuries.

KEY TERMS

Case Study

The dispatch center sends Rescue 201 and its assigned paramedics, Mark and Stephanie, to an adult care center for a patient who has fallen down a flight of stairs. On arrival, the paramedics find the patient lying on the ground. The resident director explains that Mary Herman, a 91-year-old female resident, tripped and fell down three or four steps while walking out of the building on the way to the cafeteria. There are no scene safety issues. After donning gloves, Mark and Stephanie begin the primary assessment. Mrs. Herman seems fully oriented and alert and complains of moderate pain to her right thigh and lower back. She denies any neck pain or spinal symptoms, although her mechanism of injury, age, and distracting injury suggest the need for spinal precautions. The remainder of the primary assessment reveals no significant findings, and Mrs. Herman is classified as a stable (S) patient.

The physical exam, patient history, and chief complaint investigation of the focused trauma assessment concentrate on Mrs. Herman's isolated injury. Mrs. Herman denies dizziness, nausea, or any other symptoms either now or prior to the fall. She denies striking her head or other injury symptoms. Both the patient and nursing staff report that Mrs. Herman has had few medical problems. She has no known allergies, and her medications include a daily vitamin and an aspirin. The focused physical exam evaluates the right lower extremity and finds pain and tenderness to the right thigh, crepitus, the foot externally rotated, and instability to the hip joint. Stephanie performs a quick pulse, motor, and sensory check, revealing an easily palpable posterior tibial pulse, brisk capillary refill (in less than 2 seconds), good foot strength with extension and flexion, and the ability to discern touch. The same tests on the opposing extremity provide equal results.

Vital sign evaluation reveals a blood pressure of 120/90 mmHg, a strong and regular pulse of 90, and respirations of normal depth at a rate of 22 per minute. Mark, the senior paramedic, applies a cervical collar. The pulse oximeter shows a saturation of 97 percent, so Mark and Stephanie withhold oxygen. The ECG shows a regular sinus rhythm at 90.

Next, Mark and Stephanie move Mrs. Herman to a spine board via a scoop stretcher. They place a folded blanket between her legs, maintain her head slightly off the board, pad under the body spaces, and gently but firmly strap her to the spine board. Once they have loaded the patient into the ambulance, they start an intravenous line, hang a normal saline drip, and set it to run at a to-keep-open rate. The paramedics transport her uneventfully to the emergency department. There, X-rays confirm a hip fracture. Because of her age, Mrs. Herman will spend several days in the hospital and then several months in rehabilitation.

Introduction to Orthopedic Trauma

In trauma, the incidence of musculoskeletal injury is second only to that of soft tissue injuries. Musculoskeletal injuries usually result from significant direct or transmitted blunt kinetic forces. Musculoskeletal injuries may also occasionally result from penetrating injuries. Millions of Americans sustain musculoskeletal injuries each year from a variety of sources, including sports, motor vehicle crashes, falls, and acts of violence. These incidents can cause a variety of injuries to the bones, cartilage, ligaments, muscles, or tendons.

Although injuries to the upper extremities can be painful and sometimes debilitating, they rarely threaten life. Lower extremity injuries, however, are generally associated with a greater magnitude of force and greater secondary blood loss and more often constitute threats to life or limb. In addition, the same forces responsible for a musculoskeletal injury can damage the spine, internal organs, nerves, and blood vessels, causing serious problems throughout the body. In fact, most patients (up to 80 percent) who suffer multisystem trauma experience significant musculoskeletal injuries.

Orthopedic injuries are among the most common forms of trauma paramedics encounter. Sprains and strains are certainly the most common injuries encountered. Fractures and dislocations are less common but can be debilitating. Many fractures can be attributed to osteoporosis. Osteoporotic fractures are much more common in women (66 percent) than in men (30 percent).

Prevention Strategies

Stopping injury before it occurs—injury prevention—is the optimal way of dealing with musculoskeletal injuries. Strategies for preventing musculoskeletal injuries include application of modern vehicle and highway designs, as well as safe driving practices, including the use of restraint systems. Auto crashes are the greatest single cause of musculoskeletal injuries, but improved vehicle safety has done much to reduce the incidence and severity of such injuries. Workplace safety standards developed by the National Institute of Safety and Health (NIOSH) and enforced by the Occupational Safety and Health Administration (OSHA) have done much to reduce on-the-job injuries. These standards include criteria for proper footwear, scaffolding, fall-protection devices, and the like.

Sports activities account for a significant number of injuries that most often affect the musculature, joints, and long bones. Although protective gear, improved equipment design, and better athlete conditioning can reduce the number of these injuries, the very nature of contact sports means that they remain a significant cause of injury. Household accidents and falls also account for many musculoskeletal injuries. The use of good safety practices—for example, proper footwear, well-designed railings, and appropriate stepladder use—can reduce injury incidence at home.

With musculoskeletal injuries, severe forces affect the structures of the body. These forces threaten homeostasis by disrupting the tissues responsible for moving the body and by injuring tissues and body systems beyond the muscles and skeleton. To respond properly to musculoskeletal emergencies, paramedics must maintain and build on the knowledge and skills of the EMT. In addition to those fundamentals, there is a need for a deeper understanding of musculoskeletal system structures and functions, a fuller knowledge of the injury progression process, and a complete grasp of assessment and care procedures for these injuries.

Musculoskeletal Anatomy and Physiology

The musculoskeletal system is a complex arrangement of levers and fulcrums powered by biochemical motors that provide motion and support for the body. It has two distinct subsystems: the skeleton and the muscles. The skeleton is the human body's superstructure, and the muscles supply the power of motion to this superstructure, organs, and other body components. These subsystems also produce body heat, store essential salts and energy sources, and create blood cells for transporting oxygen and combating disease. The anatomy and physiology of the musculoskeletal system is discussed in companion anatomy and physiology texts. A review is detailed here.

Skeletal Tissue and Structure

As the body's living framework, the skeleton's structure and design permit it to perform a variety of functions and to repair itself as needed (within limits). The skeleton is a complex, living system of cells, salt deposits, protein fibers, and other specialized elements. It serves five important purposes:

- It gives the body its structural form.
- It protects vital organs.
- It allows for efficient movement despite gravity.
- It stores many salts and other materials needed for metabolism.
- It produces red blood cells used to transport oxygen.

Although the skeleton is not often thought of as alive, it is exactly that. Its cells live within a matrix of protein fibers and salt deposits. These living cells constantly change the structure and dynamics of the skeleton. In fact, 20 percent of the total bone mass (salts, protein fiber, and bone cells) is replaced each year by the remodeling process.

Bone Structure

The typical bone structure consists of numerous aligned cylinders of bone. Minute blood vessels travel lengthwise along the bone through small tubes, called **haversian canals.** Layers of salt deposited in collagen fibers surround these blood vessels. Bone cells called **osteocytes** are trapped within this matrix and maintain collagen and calcium, phosphate, carbonate, and other salt crystals. Other bone cells, osteoblasts and osteoclasts, build or dissolve these salt deposits and protein fibers as necessary. **Osteoblasts** lay down new bone in areas of stress during growth and during the bone repair cycle. **Osteoclasts** dissolve bone structures when they are not carrying pressures of articulation and support, or when the body requires more salts for electrolyte balance. These three types of bone cells maintain a dynamic and efficient structure for supporting and moving the body.

A continuous blood supply brings oxygen and nutrients to bone tissue and removes carbon dioxide and waste products from them. Blood vessels enter and exit the bone shaft through **perforating canals** and distribute blood

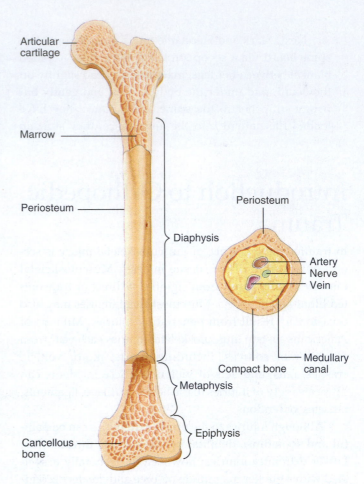

FIGURE 9-1 The internal anatomy of a long bone.

to both bone tissue and structures located within the medullary canal of the shaft and bone ends. As with any other body tissue, if the blood supply is reduced, or ceases, bone tissue becomes ischemic and will eventually die. Bone does not show degeneration evidence for quite some time, and certainly not during prehospital emergency care. However, long-term effects of **devascularization** may result in loss of bony integrity and failure of the bone to support weight or forces.

Long bones, such as those of the forearm (humerus) and thigh (femur), best demonstrate the organization of bone tissue into structural body elements (Figure 9-1). The major areas and tissues of the long bones include the diaphysis, epiphysis, metaphysis, medullary canal, periosteum, and articular cartilage.

The Diaphysis

The **diaphysis** is the central portion or shaft of the long bone. It consists of a very dense and relatively thin layer of compact bone. Because of its tubular structure, the diaphysis efficiently supports weight, yet is relatively light. Although the bone shaft's design enables it to carry weight well, lateral forces may cause the shaft to break rather easily.

CONTENT REVIEW

➤ Functions of the Skeleton
- Gives the body structural form
- Protects vital organs
- Allows for efficient movement
- Stores salts and other materials for metabolism
- Produces red blood cells

The Epiphysis

Long bone structure changes at the bone ends. The bone's diameter increases dramatically, and the underlying thin, hard, compact bone of the shaft changes to a network of skeletal fibers and strands. This network spreads the stresses and pressures of weight bearing over a larger surface. This widened, articular bone end is called the **epiphysis.** Tissue within the epiphysis in cross section resembles a rigid bony sponge and is called spongy or **cancellous** bone. Covering this network of fibers is a very thin layer of compact bone supporting the surface that meets and moves against another bone, the **articular surface.**

The Metaphysis

The **metaphysis** is an intermediate region between the epiphysis and diaphysis. It is where the diaphysis's hollow tube of compact bone makes the transition to the bone-fiber honeycomb of the epiphysis's cancellous bone. In this region is the **epiphyseal plate**, or *growth plate.* During childhood, cartilage is generated here and the plate widens. Osteoblasts from the end of the diaphysis deposit salts within the cartilage's collagen matrix to create new bone tissue. This results in lengthening of the infant's and then the child's bone. During this growth period, the epiphyseal plate is also weaker than the rest of the bone and associated joints and is thus a frequent site of fractures in pediatric patients. If damaged, injury may lead to growth discrepancies between the injured and uninjured extremities or to malunion of the fracture.

The Medullary Canal

The chamber formed within the hollow diaphysis and the cancellous bone of the epiphysis is called the **medullary canal**. The central medullary canal is filled with **yellow bone marrow** that stores fat in a semiliquid form. The fat is a readily available energy source the body can use quickly and easily. **Red bone marrow** fills the cancellous bone chambers of larger long bones, pelvis, and sternum. It is responsible for manufacturing erythrocytes and other blood cells.

The Periosteum

A tough fibrous membrane called the **periosteum** covers the exterior of the diaphysis. With extensive vasculature and innervation, it transmits pain sensation when bones fracture and then initiates the bone repair cycle. Blood vessels and nerves penetrate both the periosteum and compact bone by traveling through small perforating canals. Tendons intermingle with collagen fibers of the periosteum and with collagen fibers of the bony matrix to form strong attachments.

Cartilage

A layer of connective tissue called **cartilage** is a continuous collagen extension of the underlying bone and covers a portion of the epiphyseal surface. It is a smooth, strong, and flexible material that functions as the actual surface of articulation between bones. Cartilage is very slippery and somewhat compressible. It permits relatively friction-free joint movement and absorbs some of the shock associated with activity, such as walking.

Bone Classification

Bones are classified according to their general shape. Those previously described are considered long bones and include the humerus, radius, ulna, tibia, fibula, metacarpals (hand), metatarsals (foot), and phalanges (fingers and toes). The bones of the wrists and ankles—the carpals and tarsals—are short bones. Bones of the cranium, sternum, ribs, shoulder, and pelvis are classified as flat. Irregularly shaped bones include those of the vertebral column and facial bones. Another special type of bone is the sesamoid bone, a bone that grows within tendinous tissue; one example is the kneecap, also called the patella.

Joint Structure

Bones move at, and are held together by, a relatively sophisticated structure called a **joint.** There are three basic types of joints, which are classified by the amount of movement they permit.

Synarthroses are immovable joints, such as the sutures of the skull or the juncture between the jaw and teeth (which is called a *gomphosis*). **Amphiarthroses** are joints that allow some very limited movement. Examples include the joints between vertebrae and between the sacrum and ilium of the pelvis. **Diarthroses**, or **synovial joints**, permit relatively free movement. Such joints include the elbow, knee, shoulder, and hip.

Diarthroses are divided into three joint categories based on movements they allow (Figure 9-2). These are:

- *Monaxial joints* Hinge joints permit bending in a single plane. Examples include the knees, elbows, and fingers.

  Pivot joints are characterized by articulation between the atlas (the first cervical vertebra) and the axis of the spine. They allow the head to rotate through about 180 degrees of motion.

> **CONTENT REVIEW**
>
> ➤ Types of Joints
> - Synarthroses—immovable
> - Amphiarthroses—very limited movement
> - Diarthroses (synovial joints)—relatively free movement
>   - Monaxial
>   - Biaxial
>   - Triaxial

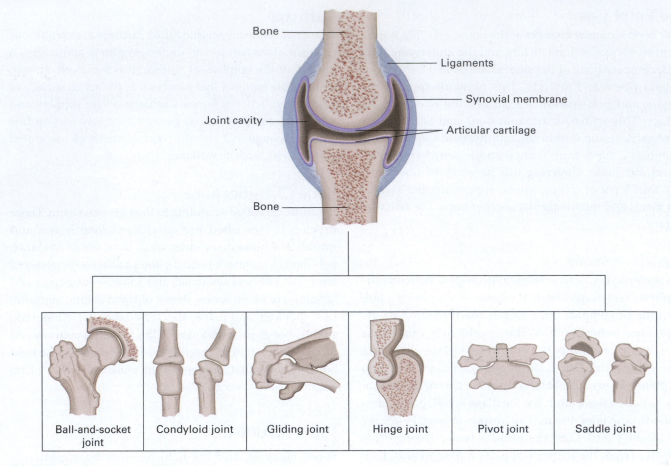

FIGURE 9-2 Types of synovial joints.

- **Biaxial joints** Condyloid, or gliding, joints provide movement in two directions. They are located at the joints of carpal bones in the wrist and between the clavicle and sternum.

  Ellipsoidal joints provide a sliding motion in two planes, as between the wrist and the metacarpals.

  Saddle joints allow for movement in two planes at right angles to each other. Examples are the joints at the bases of the thumbs.

- **Triaxial joints** Ball-and-socket joints permit full motion in a cone of about 180 degrees and allow a limb to rotate. Examples include the hip and shoulder.

These joints permit various types of motion. Flexion/extension is a bending motion that reduces/increases the angle between articulating elements. **Adduction** is the movement of a body part toward the midline; **abduction** is movement away from the midline. **Rotation** refers to a turning along the axis of a bone or joint. **Circumduction** refers to movement through an arc of a circle.

Ligaments

Ligaments are connective tissue bands that hold bones together at joints (Figure 9-3). They stretch and permit

joint motion while holding bone ends firmly in position. Ligament ends attach to the joint ends of each of the associated bones. Ligaments surround the articular region and cross it at many oblique angles. This arrangement ensures that the joint is held together firmly but

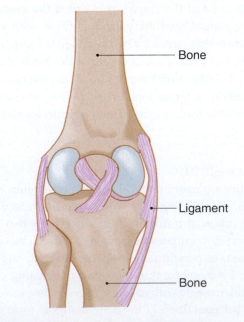

FIGURE 9-3 Ligaments hold bones together at a joint.

flexibly enough to permit movement through a designed range of motion.

Joint Capsule

Ligaments surrounding a joint form what is known as a synovial capsule or **joint capsule** (Figure 9-4). This chamber holds a small amount of fluid to lubricate articular surfaces. This oily, viscous substance, known as **synovial fluid**, facilitates joint motion by reducing friction. Its lubrication reduces friction to about one-fifth that of two pieces of ice sliding together. Small sacs filled with synovial fluid, known as **bursae**, are also located between tendons and ligaments or cartilage in the elbows, knees, and other joints to reduce friction and absorb shock. Synovial fluid flows into and out of articular cartilage as the joint undergoes compression and relaxation and movement. Cartilage acts like a sponge, pushing out fluid as it is compressed and drawing in fluid when it is relaxed. This synovial fluid movement circulates oxygen, nutrients, and waste products to and from joint cartilage.

The joint capsule is a very delicate and sterile environment. If it is opened to the environment and infectious agents during trauma (an open wound), those agents may induce damage that will hinder the joint's future function. Cartilage within the joint also does not have the ability to repair itself. If seriously injured during joint trauma, that injury may require surgical intervention and repair. Anticipate that any open wound in the vicinity of a joint involves the joint capsule and ensure it is evaluated in the emergency department.

Skeletal Organization

The human skeleton is made up of approximately 206 bones (Figure 9-5). These bones form two major divisions: the axial and appendicular skeletons.

The axial skeleton consists of the bones of the head, thorax, and spine. These bones form the axis of the body, protect the central nervous system structures, and make up the thoracic cage, which is the dynamic structure for respiration. The components of the axial skeleton are discussed in the chapters "Head, Neck, and Spinal Trauma" and "Chest Trauma."

The appendicular skeleton consists of the bones of the upper and lower extremities, including the shoulder girdles and pelvis and excluding the sacrum (which is part of the spinal column). These bones provide extremity structure and permit the major joints of the body to function. The extremity long bones are similar in design and structure. Both upper and lower extremities connect with the axial skeleton and articulate with joints supported by several bones. Each of the extremities has a single long bone proximally and paired bones distally. The terminal

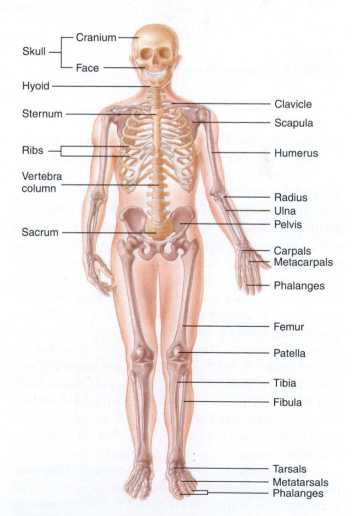

FIGURE 9-5 The human skeleton.

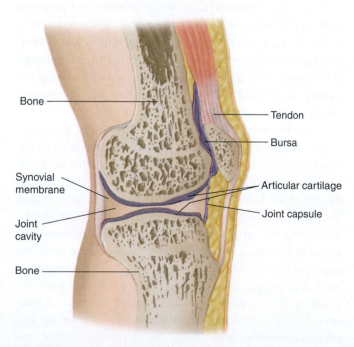

FIGURE 9-4 Structure of a joint.

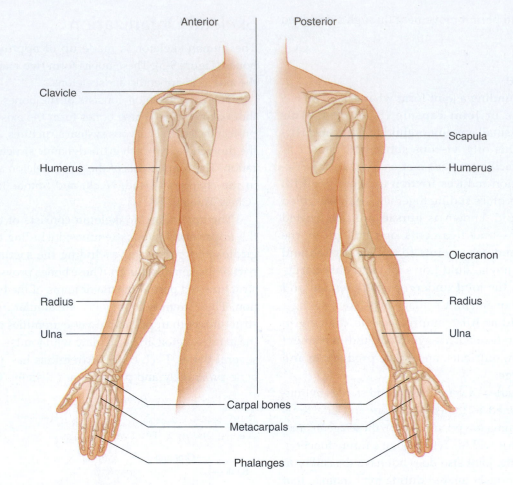

FIGURE 9-6 The upper extremities.

Upper Extremities

member—the hand or foot—is made up of numerous bones with differing purposes, yet parallel designs.

Each upper extremity (Figure 9-6) consists of a shoulder girdle, arm, forearm, and hand. The shoulder is composed of the clavicle and scapula, which are located high on the posterior and lateral thoracic cage. The scapula is a triangular bone buried within the musculature of the upper back. It consists of a flat plate, called the body, and three major irregular outgrowths (processes). The coracoid process and the acromion process are protuberances for muscular attachments. The glenoid process provides the glenoid fossa—the shallow socket that articulates and supports the head of the humerus. The scapula moves freely over the posterior thorax, providing some of the shoulder's large range of motion. The muscular upper back effectively protects the scapula from fracture in all but the most direct and severe trauma.

The clavicle articulates with the acromion of the scapula and the manubrium of the sternum. It is not as well protected as the scapula and is, in fact, the most commonly fractured bone of the human body. It maintans the scapula and shoulder joint at a fixed distance from the sternum. The clavicle permits the shoulder to move up and down (shrug) while somewhat restricting anterior and posterior motion. The shoulder joint is one of the most mobile joints in the body. It permits humeral rotation through about 60 degrees and permits circumduction of the limb through 180 degrees. (For a more complete listing of the ranges of motion associated with the extremities, see the chapter "Secondary Assessment.")

The humerus is the single bone of the proximal upper extremity (the region properly referred to as the arm). Its rounded or surgical head articulates with the scapula's glenoid fossa, proximally. The head is connected to the humeral shaft by the anatomic neck, which also acts as the terminal end of the articular capsule. Two protuberances, the greater and lesser tuberosities, provide places of attachment for tendons and form the superior portion of the humerus. They, and the anatomic neck and surgical head, are connected to the humeral shaft by the surgical neck, a frequent location of fracture. Distally, the humerus shaft widens into lateral and medial condyles and articulates with the radius and ulna at the elbow.

The radius and ulna form the forearm. The radius is on the thumb (lateral) side of the forearm and the ulna is on the little finger (medial) side. They move in conjunction with the humerus and with each other. This biaxial articulation allows the distal forearm to rotate palm up (supination) or palm down (pronation). This articulation also permits folding of the elbow. The ulna's proximal end forms the bump of the elbow, known as the olecranon.

The radius and ulna articulate with carpal bones of the wrist. There are eight carpal bones that form two rows and give the wrist its strength and mobility. The proximal row consists of the scaphoid, lunate, triangular, and pisiform bones. The distal row consists of the trapezium, trapezoid, capitate, and hamate bones. The distal carpal bones, in turn, articulate with the long, thin metacarpals of the palm. The carpal bones, with their saddle, gliding, and ellipsoidal joints, provide the wrist with a high degree of flexibility.

Metacarpals articulate with the phalanges of the fingers. Each of the four fingers consists of three phalanges—the proximal, middle, and distal. The thumb has only two—the proximal and distal. The combination of these hinge, saddle, and ellipsoidal joints in the metacarpals and phalanges allows fine motion and motor control of the hand and fingers.

Lower Extremities

Each lower extremity (Figure 9-7) is similar in structure to the upper extremities and is made up of the pelvis, thigh, leg, and foot. The pelvis is a strong skeletal structure where the lower extremities attach to the body. It consists of two symmetrical structures, called *innominate bones*, and posterior to and joining them is the sacrum. Each innominate is constructed from one large flat bone, the ilium, and two irregular bones, the ischium and pubis, all fused together. Joined anteriorly at the symphysis pubis, the innominates and the sacrum form the pelvic ring. This rigid ring is very strong and provides the basis for support and movement of the lower extremities as well as forming the bony base of the abdomen. Structural pelvic landmarks include the iliac crests (the lateral bony ridges that hold the belt) and ischial tuberosities (bony knobs on which we sit). The pubic bone forms the bony structure at the base of the inguinal area and is divided centrally by the symphysis pubis—the anterior joint between the two innominates. The juncture of the three components of the innominate bones forms the acetabulum, a hollow depression in the lateral pelvis. The acetabulum is the socket and actual articular surface for the femoral head.

The femur is the largest and strongest bone in the body. During the normal stress of walking, it often withstands pressures of up to 1,200 pounds per square inch along its diaphysis. Like the humerus, the femur is not a straight long bone. At its proximal end, where the head meets the acetabulum, the femur makes an almost 50-degree turn. The femoral head is supported by the surgical neck, a narrow shaft at almost a right angle to the uppermost aspect of the widened femoral shaft. This configuration permits the wide range of motion found in the joint and accounts for the femur's great strength. The greater and lesser trochanters, located at the widening of the femur at its upper end, form attachment points for tendons. The long femoral shaft spreads out for articulation as it meets with the tibia and forms a lateral and medial condyle. The patella, or kneecap, is a free-floating bone (sesamoid) within the quadriceps tendon and is located just proximal to the actual knee joint.

The tibia is the only distal bone to articulate with the femur. It pairs with the fibula, a smaller and much more delicate bone, just distal to the knee joint. Because of this arrangement, the tibia bears most of the weight supported by the lower extremity. The fibula's primary function is to add control to foot placement and motion during walking. The tibia and fibula are held together by

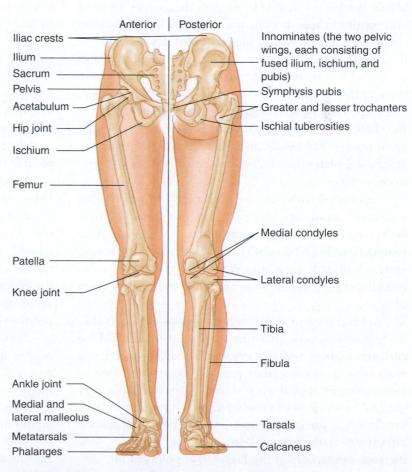

Anterior | Posterior

Iliac crests
Ilium
Sacrum
Pelvis
Acetabulum
Hip joint
Ischium
Femur
Patella
Knee joint
Ankle joint
Medial and lateral malleolus
Metatarsals
Phalanges

Innominates (the two pelvic wings, each consisting of fused ilium, ischium, and pubis)
Symphysis pubis
Greater and lesser trochanters
Ischial tuberosities
Medial condyles
Lateral condyles
Tibia
Fibula
Tarsals
Calcaneus

FIGURE 9-7 The lower extremities.

a fibrous interosseous membrane, and they articulate together to allow the foot to move through about 45 degrees of rotation.

Both the tibia and fibula join the talus and calcaneus to form the ankle. The tibia forms the medial **malleolus** (inner protuberance of the ankle), whereas the fibula forms the lateral malleolus. The calcaneus is the largest foot bone and forms the heel. The talus articulates with the calcaneus and the tarsals. The tarsals, in turn, articulate with the metatarsals and form the arch of the foot. There are actually two arches in the foot, one longitudinal and one transverse. This arrangement distributes stresses of supporting the entire body over all these bones. The metatarsals articulate with the phalanges of the foot in a configuration parallel to that of the bones of the wrist and hand. The great toe has two phalanges (one proximal and one distal), whereas the other four toes each have three (proximal, middle, and distal).

Bone Aging

The bones, like all other body tissues, evolve during fetal development and after birth. Bone initially forms in the embryo as loose cartilaginous tissue. Before birth, the skeletal structure is predominantly cartilage, with very little ossified bone evident. This is one reason that infants are highly flexible yet unable to support themselves. Ossified bone begins to appear along the long bone shafts and then extends to the epiphyseal plates. It also develops within the epiphyses and grows outward to form the articular surfaces. Over time, bone formation becomes complete to the epiphyseal plate, and the epiphysis is fully formed. The epiphyseal plate continues to generate cartilage, with the shaft and epiphyses growing from it. As the young adult reaches full height and the end of skeletal growth, epiphyseal plates narrow, become bony, and cease to produce cartilage.

Associated with bone development and aging is the transition from flexible, cartilaginous bone to firm, strong, and fully ossified bone. Bones of the young child remain flexible and do not reach maximum strength until early adulthood. Each bone matures at a different time, but almost all maturation is complete by 18 to 20 years of age.

Around the age of 40, the body begins to lose its ability to maintain bone structure. It is unable to rebuild the collagen matrix, and salt crystal deposition is reduced from what it was in earlier years (osteopenia). Effects of these changes appear very slowly. They include a very gradual diminution of bone strength, an increase in bone brittleness, a progressive loss of body height, and some curvature of the spine. Bone fracture incidence also increases, especially at the high-stress points of the lumbar spine and the femur's surgical neck. *Osteoporosis* is bone mass loss to the point that strength and function are diminished. This increases fracture incidence in the older patient, may lead to poor healing, and may increase likelihood of refracture.

Age-related changes in the skeletal system also affect other body systems. For example, cartilage of the costochondral joints and costal bones (the ribs) becomes less flexible, which leads to shallower, more energy-consuming respirations. Also, intervertebral disks lose water content and become less flexible, more prone to herniation, and narrower, thus shortening and stiffening the trunk.

Muscular Tissue and Structure

More than 600 muscle groups make up the muscular system (Figure 9-8a and 9-8b). As you might expect, a large number of EMS calls involve injuries to this extensive system. Injuries to it may result from excessive forces indirectly applied to the muscles and their attachments or from direct trauma, either blunt or penetrating.

Skeletal muscles lie directly beneath a protective layer of skin and subcutaneous fat. Because of their oxygen requirements during activity, they have an ample supply of blood vessels. Individual muscle cells layer together to form a muscle fiber, many fibers layer together to form a muscle **fascicle**, and fascicles layer together to form a muscle body, such as the triceps. A muscle body has the strength of about 50 pounds of lift for each square inch of cross-sectional area.

Skeletal muscles attach to bones at a minimum of two locations. These attachment points are called origin and insertion, depending on how the bones move with contraction. An attachment point that remains stationary as the muscle contracts is the **origin**, whereas an attachment point to the moving bone is the **insertion**.

Muscles are usually paired, one on each side of a joint. This configuration is essential because muscles can actively contract, not lengthen. One muscle moves an extremity in one direction by contraction while an opposing (and relaxed) muscle stretches. The opposing muscle, in turn, can then contract, stretching the first muscle and moving the extremity in the opposite direction. This arrangement, called **opposition**, permits limb straightening (extension) and then bending (flexion).

Several muscles attaching to a joint with different origins and insertions give the joint a wide variety of motions. In the shoulder, for example, the humerus can travel through several types and ranges of motion. These include moving the extremity away from the body (abduction) and toward the body (adduction), turning the humerus (rotation) through about 60 degrees, and circling the entire extremity (circumduction) through a 180-degree arc.

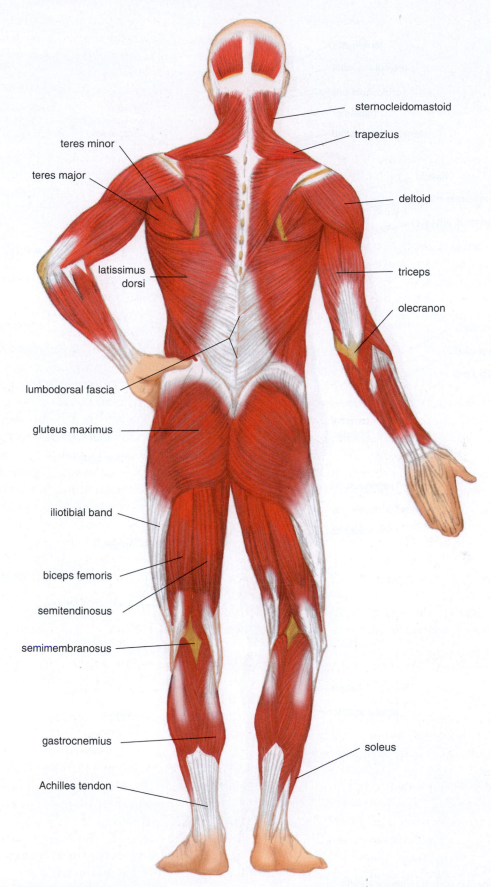

FIGURE 9-8A The muscular system (posterior view).

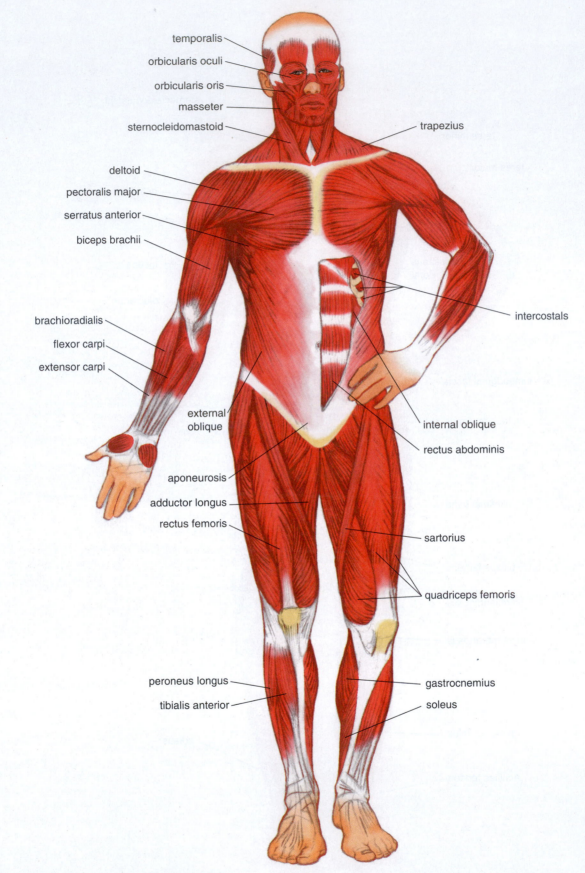

FIGURE 9-8B The muscular system (anterior view).

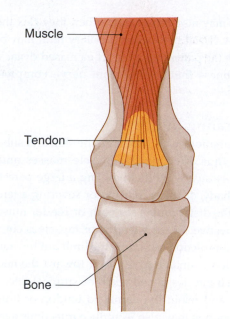

FIGURE 9-9 The tendons are the bands of tissue that connect muscle to bone.

Tendons are specialized bands of connective tissue that accomplish attachment of muscle to bone at the insertion and, in some cases, at the origin (Figure 9-9). These very fibrous ribbons of collagen are extremely strong and do not stretch. They originate at the muscle ends at the musculoskeletal junction that is the transition from muscle to tendon. They are so strong that, in some instances, they will break an area of bone loose rather than tear. The Achilles tendon has a significant amount of strength. It is the band posterior to the malleoli of the ankle. This tendon is the muscle-controlled cord that allows a person to lift the entire body weight when standing on the toes.

The forearm has a similar muscle–tendon relationship. As muscles controlling finger flexion contract, you can feel them tensing in the dorsal forearm. You can also visualize and palpate tendon movement in the distal forearm and wrist as the fingers flex and extend. It is easy to appreciate the damage a deep transverse laceration can cause to these underlying tissues. Tendons are often classified by the action they perform when the muscle associated with them contracts—for example, flexor or extensor, abductor or adductor, and so forth.

Muscle tissue is responsible not only for body movement, but also for heat energy production. A chemical reaction between oxygen and simple sugars produces the energy of motion. Heat, water, and carbon dioxide are byproducts of this reaction. More than half the energy created by muscle motion is heat that helps maintain body temperature. The body dissipates excess heat through the skin via radiation, convection, or evaporation. The body must constantly meet muscle tissue requirements for oxygen and nutrients and eliminate waste products of those tissues, including heat.

Table 9-1 Muscle Strength Scale

Score	Description
5	Active movement against full resistance with no fatigue
4	Active movement against some resistance and gravity
3	Active movement against gravity
2	Active movement with gravity eliminated
1	Barely palpable muscle contraction with no movement
0	No visible or palpable muscle contraction

Muscles are found in a condition of slight contraction called **tone.** Even while the body is at rest, the central nervous system sends some limited impulses to muscle bodies, causing a few fibers to contract. These impulses give the muscles firmness and ensure that they are ready to contract when a need arises. Muscle tone may be very significant in a well-conditioned athlete or absent (flaccid muscle tone) in someone with peripheral motor nerve disruption. Muscle strength is graded from 0 to 5 (Table 9-1).

Musculoskeletal Pathophysiology

The orthopedic injury process is a complicated one, resulting in much more damage than just disruption of a relatively inert structural body element. Remember, bone is alive and requires a continuous supply of oxygenated circulation. Bones lie deep within muscle tissue near major nerves and blood vessels. At points of articulation, there is a complex arrangement of ligaments, cartilage, and synovial fluid that holds joints together while permitting a wide range of movement. Finally, muscles attach and direct skeletal movement through collections of fibers, fasciculi, and muscle bodies connected to the skeletal system by tendons. This complex arrangement of connective, skeletal, vascular, nervous, and muscular tissue is endangered whenever significant kinetic forces are applied to the extremities. If forces are severe enough, they are likely to cause muscular, joint, or skeletal injury.

Muscular Injury

Muscular injuries may result from direct blunt or penetrating trauma, overexertion, or problems with oxygen supply during exertion. These injuries include contusion, compartment syndrome, penetrating injury, fatigue, strain, cramp, spasm, and strain. Muscular problems usually do not contribute significantly to hypovolemia and shock, with the exceptions of severe contusions with large associated hematomas and penetrating injuries with extensive hemorrhage.

Contusion

Severe trauma frequently crushes muscles between a blunt force and skeletal structures beneath. This damages both the muscle cells and blood vessels that supply them. Small blood vessels may rupture, leaking blood into interstitial spaces and causing pain, erythema, and then ecchymosis. Blood in the interstitial spaces and muscle cell damage activate the inflammatory response. Capillary beds engorge with blood and fluid shifts to the interstitial space, leading to tissue edema. Injury may also cause blood to pool beneath or within tissue layers in a hematoma. In more massive body muscles, such as those of the thigh, buttocks, calf, or arm, large blood volumes may accumulate, contributing significantly to hypovolemia. A large hematoma or significant muscular edema will increase the injured limb's diameter, especially as compared to the opposing uninjured limb. For the most part, however, the signs of muscle injury and accumulating blood remain hidden beneath the skin or manifest well after prehospital emergency assessment and care.

Compartment Syndrome

The muscular configuration of the extremities, and especially of the leg and forearm, are prone to a specific injury called *compartment syndrome*. Muscle bodies of these regions are contained in strong inelastic fascial envelopes called compartments. When injured, soft tissues within the compartment swell. Contained by fascia, this swelling increases the pressure within the compartment, thus reducing capillary blood flow to muscle and nerve tissues. Reduced capillary flow causes the release of histamine, which increases capillary permeability and worsens swelling and pressure. As pressure builds, blood flow to tissues slows significantly. However, the pressure necessary to halt capillary blood flow is much less than that needed to stop arterial blood flow to the distal extremity. The patient still has a distal pulse, capillary refill, and venous return from the distal limb. The leg is the most common location associated with this syndrome, although it has also been reported with arm, thigh, and hand injuries.

A patient with compartment syndrome most commonly complains of a deep and burning pain that appears out of proportion to the apparent injury. Pain is not reduced by positioning. An increase in pain when you (not the patient) move the extremity and stretch the muscles involved is a related finding (this is called *passive stretching*).

Patients may also report pain when they flex the affected extremity. Distal pulses and capillary refill may be normal, although the patient may report increased distal sensitivity or numbness that results from nerve compression and injury.[1,2]

Penetrating Injury

Deep lacerations may penetrate the skin and subcutaneous tissues, thus affecting the muscle masses and tendons below. Massive wounds involving a large percentage of a muscle body, or those injuring or severing a tendon, may reduce the distal limb's strength or render muscular control ineffective. When a tendon or muscle is cut, opposing muscle contraction can move the limb but the injured muscle/tendon is unable to return it toward the neutral position. Such injuries usually call for surgical intervention to identify and rejoin the damaged tendon or muscle body. These wounds may also introduce infectious agents, damage muscle tissue, and affect the muscle's blood supply. The resulting infection, ischemia, or a combination of the two may result in further tissue injury and poor healing.

Fatigue

Muscle **fatigue** occurs as muscles reach their performance limit. Exercise uses available muscle oxygen and energy reserves and results in an accumulation of metabolic byproducts, particularly acids. The cell environment becomes hypoxic, acidic, toxic, and energy deprived. Ultimately, fewer and fewer muscle fibers are able to contract. Muscle mass strength diminishes and further exertion becomes painful. Until adequate circulation restores oxygen and muscle cells can replenish energy sources, muscle fibers and the muscle body remain weakened.

Muscle Cramp

Cramping is not really an injury, but a painful muscle tissue spasm. Muscle pain results when exercise consumes available oxygen and energy sources and the circulatory system fails to remove metabolic waste products. Pain begins during or immediately after vigorous exercise or after the limb has been left in an unusual position for a period of time (obstructing circulatory flow). Cramping usually presents with a continuous muscle contraction (spasm). Changing the limb's position or massaging it may help return the circulation and reduce the pain. Once rest and adequate circulation restore metabolic balance, muscle cramp pain usually subsides. Muscle cramp pain can also be caused by electrolyte imbalances, such as hypocalcemia and lactic acid accumulation.

Muscle Spasm

In muscle **spasm**, the affected muscle goes into an intermittent (clonic) or continuous (tonic) contraction. Spasm may be firm enough to feel like deformity associated with a fracture and can confound assessment. As with muscle cramp, muscle spasm usually subsides uneventfully with rest.

Strain

A **strain** occurs when muscle fibers are overstretched by forces that exceed the fiber's strength. Muscle fibers then stretch and tear, causing pain that increases with any further muscle use. The injury may occur with extreme muscle stress, as during heavy lifting or sprinting, or at times of fatigue, when only a limited number of muscle fibers are in contraction. With a strain, the fibers are damaged without significant internal bleeding, edema, or discoloration. The injury site is generally painful to palpation and patients normally report pain that limits affected muscle use.

Joint Injury

Joint injuries include sprain, subluxation, and dislocation. The following sections detail pathologies behind each of these injuries.

Sprain

A **sprain** is a tearing of a joint capsule's connective tissues—specifically a ligament or ligaments. Injury causes acute pain, followed shortly by inflammation and swelling. Ecchymosis occurs over time, but not usually during prehospital care. The tearing of ligaments weakens the joint. Continued joint use when the tear is significant may lead to complete ligamentous failure. Minor tears may actually heal faster if modestly loaded, as in ambulation, as tolerated. Sprains are classified, or graded, according to their severity, using the following criteria:

- *Grade I:* Minor and incomplete tear. The ligament is painful, and swelling is usually minimal. The joint remains stable.
- *Grade II:* Significant but incomplete tear. Swelling and pain range from moderate to severe. The joint is intact but unstable.
- *Grade III:* Complete ligament tear. Because of the severe pain and spasm, the grade III sprain may present as a fracture. The joint is unstable.

Subluxation

Subluxation is a partial bone end displacement from its position within a joint capsule. It occurs as a joint separates under stress, stretching the ligaments. Subluxation differs from a sprain in that it more significantly reduces a joint's integrity. The injured joint is painful and swells quickly, the range of motion is limited, and the joint is unstable. Hyperflexion, hyperextension, lateral rotation beyond the normal range of motion, or application of extreme axial force are common causes of subluxations.

Dislocation

A **dislocation** is a complete displacement of bone ends from their normal joint position (sometimes referred to as a luxation) (Figure 9-10). The joint then fixes in an abnormal position with noticeable deformity. The site is painful, swollen, and immobile. This injury carries with it the danger of entrapping, compressing, or tearing blood vessels and nerves. Dislocation occurs when a joint moves beyond its normal range of motion with great force. By its nature, a dislocation has serious associated ligament damage and may involve joint capsule and articular cartilage injury.

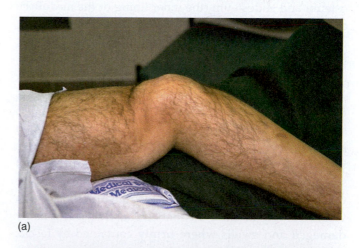
(a)

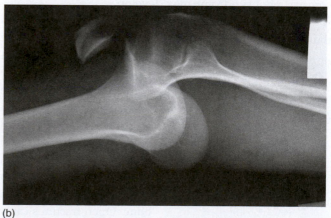
(b)

FIGURE 9-10 Knee dislocation. (a) Presentation of a knee dislocation. (b) X-ray of the dislocation.
(Both: © Edward T. Dickenson, MD)

Bone Injury

A fracture is a complicated process that ultimately disrupts the continuity of a bone. A bone fractures when extreme axial forces or significant lateral forces exceed the bone's tensile strength.

Fractures may be caused by direct injury—for example, an auto bumper strikes a patient's femur or a high-powered rifle bullet slams into a patient's thigh and then into the femur. A fracture cause may also be indirect. This might occur when a bike rider is thrown over the handlebars and braces the fall with an outstretched upper extremity. In this case, the energy of impact is transmitted from the hand to the wrist, to the forearm, to the arm, to the shoulder, to the clavicle. These transmitted forces can ultimately fracture the clavicle and may cause internal injury to blood vessels and the upper chest or shoulder. For this reason, always analyze the mechanism of injury carefully, recognizing that kinetic forces may be transmitted and cause injury far from the impact point. Remember, 80 percent of multisystem trauma cases have associated serious musculoskeletal injury.

As kinetic energy is transmitted to a bone and the bone fractures, collagen, osteocytes, salt crystals, blood vessels, nerves, and medullary canal of the bone, as well as its periosteum and endosteum (the inner lining of the medullary canal), are disrupted. If broken bone ends are displaced, they may further injure surrounding muscles, tendons, ligaments, nerves, veins, and arteries. The result is a serious threat to the limb structure.

Vascular damage may impede blood flow to the limb, thereby increasing capillary refill time, diminishing pulse strength and limb temperature, and causing discoloration and **paresthesia** (a "pins-and-needles" sensation). Nerve injury may result in distal paresthesias, anesthesia (loss of sensation), paresis (weakness), or paralysis (loss of muscle control). Muscle or tendon damage may interfere with a victim's ability to move the limb. If muscle tissue is badly damaged and swells where firmly contained by fascia, compartment syndrome may develop.

If the bone is not significantly displaced and the forces that caused the fracture do not penetrate the skin, the resulting injury is termed a **closed fracture.** If sharp bone ends exit the skin, the result is termed an **open fracture** (Figure 9-11). An open fracture may also occur when an object, such as a bullet, travels through a limb and fractures a bone. Open fractures carry a risk for infection. Such an infection may seriously reduce the bone's ability to

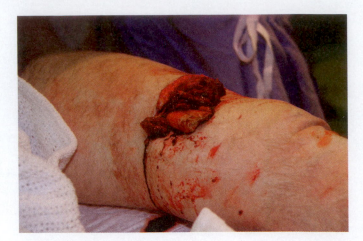

FIGURE 9-11 An open fracture.
(© Edward T. Dickenson, MD)

heal. Where bones are located very close to the skin, as with the tibia, an open fracture can occur with relatively minimal bone displacement. Note that any break in the skin overlying or in close association with a fracture is considered an open fracture.

Surprisingly, some fractures may be relatively stable (Figure 9-12). When a bone suffers a small crack that doesn't disrupt the total structure, the injury is termed a **hairline fracture**. This injury type weakens the bone and is painful, as the bone remains in position and retains some of its strength. Another relatively stable bone injury is the **impacted fracture**. With a compression mechanism of injury, a bone may impact on itself, resulting in a compressed but aligned bone. As in a hairline fracture, an impacted fracture remains in position and retains some of its original strength. The danger with both hairline and impacted fractures is that further stress and movement may complete the fracture and displace the bone ends, increasing both the injury's severity and its healing time.

There are several fracture types whose physical characteristics can be revealed only by X-rays. For example, the **transverse fracture** is a complete break in a bone that runs straight across it at about a 90-degree angle. This is usually a high-energy injury pattern caused by a bending force. A fracture that runs at an angle across the bone is considered an **oblique fracture**. A fracture in which the bone has splintered into several smaller fragments is a **comminuted fracture**. This type of fracture is often associated with crushing injuries or a high-velocity bullet impact. It generally represents a significant energy exchange and is often associated with extensive soft tissue damage. Fractures involving a twisting motion may result in a curved break around the bone shaft known as a **spiral fracture.** Spiral fractures can occur when a child's arm is pulled and rotated by an adult or when an adult's limb is pulled into machinery like an auger.

A **fatigue fracture**, or stress fracture, is associated with prolonged or repeated stress. The bone generally weakens

CONTENT REVIEW

➤ Types of Fractures
- Closed
- Open
- Hairline
- Impacted
- Transverse
- Oblique
- Comminuted
- Spiral
- Greenstick
- Epiphyseal

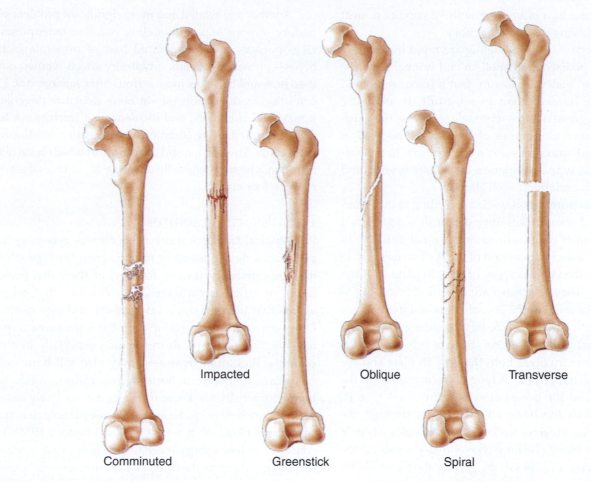

Impacted

Oblique

Transverse

Comminuted

Greenstick

Spiral

FIGURE 9-12 Types of fractures.

and fractures from repetitive application of even modest forces and not through a single great kinetic force. Most stress fractures occur in the lower extremities in association with vigorous aerobic training, such as walking and running. An example is the metatarsal fatigue fracture, also known as a "march fracture."

A very infrequent but serious fracture complication is fat embolism. Bone injury may damage adjacent blood vessels and the medullary canal. Injury may then release fat, stored in a semiliquid form, into the wound site, where it enters the venous system and becomes emboli that may travel to the heart. The heart distributes the emboli to the pulmonary circulation, where they lodge (pulmonary emboli). Fat embolism is usually associated with severe or crush injuries or post-injury manipulation of larger long bone fractures, especially the femur. (See the chapter "Pulmonology" for a discussion of the signs, symptoms, and care of the patient with pulmonary embolism.)

Pediatric Considerations

Physiologically, the bones of infants and children contain a greater percentage of cartilage than those of adults. In addition, they are still growing from the epiphyseal plate.

Because of this, pediatric patients often sustain different types of fractures than do adults.

The flexible nature of pediatric bones is responsible for a **greenstick fracture**, a type of partial fracture. Like a severely bent green twig, the greenstick fracture disrupts only one side of the long bone. It remains angulated and resists alignment due to the disrupted periosteum and bone tissue on the side of the fracture and the intact periosteum and bone tissue on the uninjured side. During the bone repair process, the injured side experiences more rapid growth than the uninjured side. This results in increasing angulation as the bone heals. Surgeons will occasionally complete a greenstick fracture by breaking the bone fully, thereby ensuring proper healing. Another incomplete fracture in pediatric patients is the buckle or torus fracture. This fracture is a buckling of the bone on one side due to increased cartilage and flexibility of the child's bone. Buckle fractures heal very well.

A child's bone grows at the epiphyseal plate and forms a weak spot in the long bone. In pediatric fractures, this is a common site of long bone injury and called an **epiphyseal fracture**. If the growth plate is disrupted, it may lead to a reduction or cessation of bone growth—a condition most commonly involving the proximal tibia.

Fracture repair and remodeling are rapid in children. The increased pediatric metabolism and normal bone tissue replacement generally ensure that a fracture site will stabilize more quickly than in an adult. In pediatric patients, the aggressive bone remodeling process (in which bone is laid down along lines of stress and dissolved in areas of reduced stress) ensures a rapid return to the normal bone shape when circulation to the site is good and injured bones are relatively well aligned.

Pediatric fractures are classified according to the Salter-Harris system. Although definitive diagnosis is determined by X-ray and other diagnostic techniques not available in the ambulance, a short discussion of the system may help in understanding the various types of growth plate (epiphyseal) fractures. These fractures are classified according to degree of involvement in the growth plate and the adjacent bone and joint. A type I fracture traverses the growth plate without affecting either the bone above or below the plate. A type II fracture involves both the growth plate and the bone of the limb (diaphysis). A type III fracture involves the growth plate and the bone below (epiphysis). A type IV fracture involves the bone above, crosses through the growth plate, and involves the bone below. Finally, a type V fracture is generally a crushing type of injury involving the entire distal bone. In general, the greater the Salter-Harris fracture type, the more complex the fracture and the more difficult the healing (Figure 9-13).

Geriatric Considerations

The aging process causes several changes to the musculoskeletal system. A gradual, progressive decrease in bone mass and collagen structure begins around 40 years of age and results in bones that are less flexible, more brittle, and more easily fractured. The bones also heal more slowly. Aging adults also lose some muscle strength and coordination, thus increasing the likelihood of skeletal injury. Lumbar spine and femoral neck fractures occur because of stress—often without a history of significant trauma.

Another age-related and more significant problem secondary to poor bone remodeling is called **osteoporosis.** Osteoporosis is an accelerated loss of minerals in the bones—primarily calcium. It typically affects women more than men and becomes most serious after menopause. The condition leads to increases in bone structure degeneration, spinal curvature, and incidences of fractures. A less significant and more common bone density condition is osteopenia. This is a natural condition, in which bone deterioration with age (generally after age 40) reduces the bone mass and strength.

Pathological Fractures

Pathological fractures result from disease processes that affect bone development or maintenance. Such problems may be caused by tumors (cancer) of the bone, periosteum, or articular cartilage or by diseases that release agents that increase osteoclast activity and osteoporosis. Other diseases and infections can have the same impact on bone tissue and result in fracture, especially in older patients. Radiation treatment may also kill bone cells, resulting in localized bone degeneration, weakened bones, and fractures. These fractures are not likely to heal well, if they heal at all. Be suspicious of pathological fractures in patients with a past medical history (PMH) of cancer or in low-energy mechanisms that cause fractures in young, otherwise healthy, or non-osteoporotic elderly patients.

General Considerations with Musculoskeletal Injuries

The potential effects of trauma can be anticipated when the skeleton and musculature are examined together. It is important to note that long bones are smallest through the diaphysis and largest at the epiphyseal area or joint. However, the external extremity diameter is greatest surrounding the mid-shaft, due to skeletal muscle. This anatomic relationship is significant when looking at the potential for nervous and vascular injury.

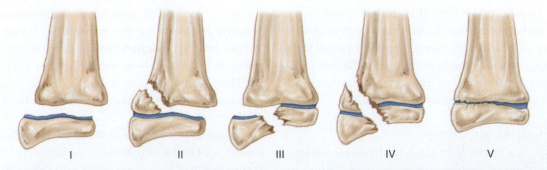

I   II   III   IV   V

FIGURE 9-13 The Salter-Harris system of classifying growth-plate injuries. The likelihood of a permanent growth-plate deformity increases as the classification number increases.

Because there is limited soft tissue surrounding joints, joint fractures, dislocations, and—to a lesser degree—subluxations and sprains may cause severe problems beyond the direct skeletal injury. Any swelling, deformity, or displacement may compromise the nerve and vascular supply to the distal extremity. Fractures near a joint are more likely to compress or sever blood vessels or nerves. With shaft fractures, neurovascular injury is less likely, although manipulation of the fracture site or gross deformity may still endanger blood vessels and nerves running along the bone.

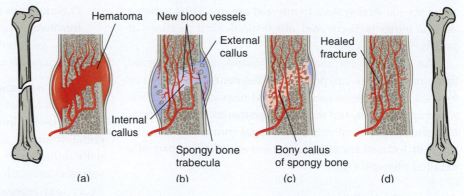

FIGURE 9-14 Bone healing. The bone repair cycle. Presentation of a forearm fracture.

Areas around joints are further at risk because blood vessels supplying the epiphysis enter the long bone through the diaphysis. If a fracture close to the epiphysis displaces the bone ends, it may compromise this blood supply, with devastating results. Distal bone tissue may die without adequate circulation, subsequently destroying the joint and its function.

Once an injury occurs, extremity stability is reduced. Any additional movement can increase pain, damage soft tissues, and injure nerves and blood vessels. Even slight manipulation can cause additional trauma. For example, a fractured femur has bone ends that are about the size of a broken broom handle. If, during extrication, splinting, and patient transport, these bone ends move about within the soft tissue, damage may result and be more severe than the injury that initially caused the fracture. Manipulation and movement of the injury may also increase the likelihood of introducing bone fragments or fat emboli into the venous system—possibly causing a pulmonary embolism.

Another complication associated with long bone fractures is the muscle spasm that results from pain. In a long bone fracture, pain causes surrounding muscles to contract. This contraction can force the broken bone ends to override the fracture site. The result, in the case of the femur, is two broom-handle-sized bones driven into the thigh muscles, causing a cycle of more pain, more spasm, and more damage.

Bone Repair Cycle

The bone repair cycle is a complex process that normally results in complete healing. When a bone is fractured, the periosteum, local blood vessels, soft tissues, and endosteum tear. Blood fills the injured site and clots. The clot mixes with collagen and forms a fracture hematoma. This hematoma stops further hemorrhage and weakly immobilizes the fracture site. Special cartilage-forming cells migrate into

this hematoma from the broken bone ends and begin to repair the site. As cartilage grows, it forms a more significant mass to stabilize the site. This elemental skeletal stabilization is called the **callus**. The osteoblasts migrate into the callus and begin to lay down calcium within protein fibers. This forms spongy bone and a stronger stabilization of the fracture site. The callus becomes rigid and is significantly larger than the bone it is splinting. Eventually (in about four months) the callus will approximate the original strength of the bone it is splinting (Figure 9-14).

With time, bone remodeling occurs. Osteoblasts lay down calcium along stress lines in the bone and osteoclasts remove calcium from areas with limited stress. The result is gradual bone shaping (remodeling) that will eventually resemble the original bone. If a patient is young when a fracture occurs and the bone ends are well aligned, there may be little evidence that an injury ever occurred.

If bone ends are misaligned or if the fracture site experiences stress, infection, or movement before it has a chance to heal properly, it may never return to normal and may leave the person with some disability. Conditions such as smoking, infection, diabetes or poor health, NSAID use, and immunosuppressive drug use may impair the healing process. In some cases, preexisting conditions may disrupt the bone-healing process to a degree that two broken bone ends do not rejoin (nonunion).

Musculoskeletal Injury Assessment

With musculoskeletal trauma patients, fractures, dislocations, or muscular injuries infrequently threaten life or seriously contribute to shock. In most circumstances, a patient with an isolated fracture, dislocation, or muscular or connective tissue injury should receive focused trauma assessment and management at the scene.

However, serious musculoskeletal injuries are common in patients who have other serious injuries. As noted earlier, energy is often transmitted from the impact point along the skeletal system to internal organs. Thus, when a skeletal injury is discovered, always look for indications of possible internal injuries.

As with any trauma patient, assessment progresses through scene size-up, primary assessment, either rapid or focused trauma assessment, detailed physical examination when appropriate, and serial reassessments. Initially, attention should focus on musculoskeletal injuries during the rapid or focused trauma assessment and then as part of a detailed physical exam.

Scene Size-Up

Remember to ensure scene safety and don appropriate personal protective equipment (Standard Precautions) before approaching any scene. Gloves are mandatory when dealing with open wounds, but these wounds do not usually suggest a need for protective eyewear, mask, or gown. (The only exception would be severe arterial hemorrhage.) Analyze the mechanism of injury to anticipate the nature and severity of injuries. Enhance the analysis of the mechanism of injury by talking with the patient, family members, and bystanders to identify what happened and how. Identify any environmental considerations that might have an impact on assessment, care, and transport and integrate these into the incident command structure. Last, ensure that all needed resources are available to secure the scene, access the patient, and extricate him, if necessary.

Primary Assessment

It is imperative that the trauma patient assessment begin with an evaluation of the patient's mental status and ABCs. During this primary assessment, identify any potential for spinal injury and the need for spinal precautions. Remember, any serious musculoskeletal injury suggests kinetic energy forces sufficient to cause spinal injury. Thus, always consider spinal precautions, as directed per local protocols, with such an injury. Remember, too, that a serious fracture is a distracting injury and may mask the symptoms of spinal injury. Proceed with the primary assessment and ensure that any life-threatening injuries are addressed before moving on with the secondary assessment. Never let a gruesome musculoskeletal injury distract from first identifying and caring for life-threatening injuries.

Patients with musculoskeletal injuries are classified into four categories:

- Patients with life- and limb-threatening injuries
- Patients with life-threatening injuries and minor musculoskeletal injuries
- Patients with non–life-threatening injuries but serious limb-threatening musculoskeletal injuries

- Patients with non–life-threatening injuries and only isolated minor musculoskeletal injuries

Perform a rapid trauma assessment for patients with possible life- or limb-threatening injuries. A patient without life threat but with serious musculoskeletal injury may receive a rapid trauma assessment or a focused trauma assessment, depending on the mechanism of injury and information you discover during the primary assessment. Provide patients presenting with isolated and simple musculoskeletal injuries with a focused trauma assessment, yet remain vigilant for any sign or symptom of more serious injury and the need for both a rapid trauma assessment and rapid patient transport to a trauma center.

Secondary Assessment

Secondary assessment includes either a rapid trauma assessment or a focused assessment.

Rapid Trauma Assessment

Rapid trauma assessment is performed on any patient with any sign, symptom, or mechanism of injury that suggests serious injury. Even though musculoskeletal injuries do not often cause life-threatening hemorrhage, remember that 80 percent of patients with serious multisystem trauma have associated musculoskeletal injury. When there is evidence of a serious musculoskeletal injury, maintain a high index of suspicion for serious internal injury.

Perform a rapid trauma assessment in a carefully ordered way, progressing through an evaluation of the head, neck, chest, and abdomen, and arriving at the pelvis. Pay particular attention to possible pelvic fracture because such an injury may account for hemorrhage of more than 2 liters. If there are no signs of pelvic fracture, check pelvic ring stability by directing firm pressure downward, then inward on the iliac crests, and then directing gentle downward pressure on the symphysis pubis. Consider the possibility of a pelvic fracture if pressure reveals any instability or crepitus or elicits a painful response from the patient. If you feel crepitus once, presume that bone injury exists and do not attempt to re-create the sensation, as it represents continued damage to the fractured bone ends and surrounding tissue. It is also quite painful. Consider the patient a possible candidate for rapid transport with fluid resuscitation initiated en route.

In assessing the thighs, look for signs of tissue swelling and femur fracture. Each femur fracture may account for as much as 1,500 mL of blood loss. Evidence of this loss may be hidden within tissue and thigh muscle, so compare one thigh to the other to evaluate swelling. If evidence of either pelvic or bilateral femur fractures is found, consider a pelvic sling or binder and spine board to immobilize the pelvis and the lower extremities. Monitor for any signs that the patient is compensating for blood loss and consider both rapid transport and fluid resuscitation.

Extremity fractures and muscular injuries may or may not cause shock but may significantly contribute to hypovolemia. Consider the effects of these injuries in deciding whether to provide rapid transport or on-scene care. Furthermore, fractures and dislocations may entrap or damage blood vessels or nerves, thus potentially threatening the future use of a limb. Quickly survey each limb and check the distal pulses, capillary refill, temperature, muscle tone, and, if the patient is conscious, sensation and motor function.

Complete the rapid trauma assessment by gathering a patient history and a baseline set of vital signs and Glasgow Coma Scale value (simultaneously with physical assessment). If the rapid trauma assessment reveals a serious threat to life or limb, rapidly transport the patient to the nearest appropriate facility.

Focused Assessment

The focused trauma assessment directs attention to injuries found or suggested during primary assessment, by mechanism of injury, or by the patient's signs and symptoms. This assessment is performed for patients without life-threatening injuries and directs both assessment and care to isolated injuries.

Begin a focused trauma assessment by observing and inquiring carefully for signs and symptoms of fracture, dislocation, or other musculoskeletal injury in each limb with suspected injury (Figure 9-15). Expose and examine the entire limb by removing any restrictive jewelry and clothing or cutting it away carefully. In doing so, avoid any potential injury site manipulation. Inspect the injury site carefully by looking at the medial, lateral, anterior, and posterior surfaces to locate any deformities (angulation or swelling), discolorations (unlikely in the first minutes after the incident), and indications of soft tissue wounds that suggest injury beneath. Any unusual limb placement, asymmetry, or inequality in limb length (when compared to the opposing limb) should also

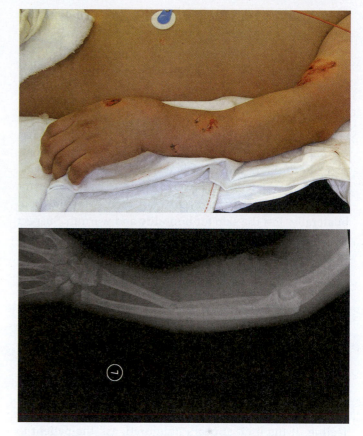

FIGURE 9-15 (a) A fracture will often present with deformity. (b) An X-ray of the fracture.
(Both: © Edward T. Dickenson, MD)

arouse suspicion of musculoskeletal injury. Remember that tendon injury may cause the muscle to contract away from the injury and create a muscle mass near one end of the long bone. Consider that any open wounds may communicate with an associated fracture or dislocation. Observe for any contamination or sign of the bone protruding. Try to question the patient regarding pain, pain with attempted movement, pain on touch, discomfort, or unusual feeling or sensation. Also inquire about weakness, paralysis, paresthesia, or anesthesia. It may be helpful to think of the "six Ps" as a way to remember key elements when evaluating an extremity:[3]

- *Pain:* The patient may report this on palpation (tenderness) or movement.
- *Pallor:* The patient's skin may be pale or flushed, and capillary refill may be delayed.
- *Paralysis:* The patient may have an inability to, or it may be difficult to, move an extremity.
- *Paresthesia:* The patient may report numbness or tingling in the affected extremity.
- *Pressure:* The patient reports a feeling of tension within the extremity.
- *Pulses:* These may be diminished or absent in the distal extremity.

CONTENT REVIEW

➤ The Six Ps in Evaluating Limb Injury
- Pain
- Pallor
- Paralysis
- Paresthesia
- Pressure
- Pulses

➤ An additional "P" sometimes cited is poikilothermia, referring to a limb that is cool to the touch.

An additional "P" sometimes cited is poikilothermia, referring to a limb that is cool to the touch.

If a specific injury is not identified, palpate the extremity for instability, deformity (swelling or angulation), crepitus, unusual motion (joint-like motion where a joint shouldn't exist), muscle tone (normal, flaccid, or spasm), or any regions of unusual warmth or coolness. Palpate the entire anterior and posterior surfaces, then the lateral and medial surfaces. The assessment must be gentle, yet complete. Record any abnormal signs. When assessing the feet, carefully evaluate the distal circulation. Assess pulses for presence and relative strength and then compare them bilaterally. Test the skin for humidity and warmth. Suspect circulatory compromise if capillary refill time is prolonged compared to the uninjured limb. Observe the skin for discoloration, noting any erythema, ecchymosis, or any abnormal hue (pale, ashen, or cyanotic). Approximate the level at which any deficit begins, and note any relation to possible extremity injury.

In a conscious and responsive patient, evaluate sensation and muscle strength distal to the injury (Figure 9-16). Check tactile (touch) response by touching or stroking the bottom of the foot with the blunt end of a bandage scissors or other similar instrument. Ask the patient to describe the feeling. If the limb appears uninjured, ask the patient to push down with the balls of both feet (plantar flexion) against your hands. Then ask the patient to pull upward with the top of both feet (dorsiflexion), again against your hands. If there is any unilateral or bilateral weakness or the patient reports any pain, document these findings on the prehospital care report and look for a cause. Check abnormal sensation and the patient's ability to wiggle the toes or fingers. If the limb appears uninjured, ask the patient to move each joint through its normal range of motion and note any patient symptoms or restrictions to normal movement.

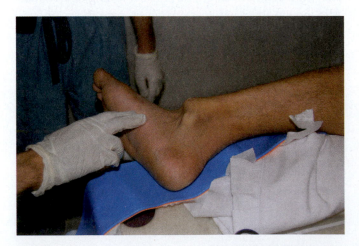

FIGURE 9-16 Evaluate sensation and muscle strength distal to the injury.

(© Edward T. Dickenson, MD)

Assess for potential upper extremity injury in a manner similar to the lower extremity assessment. Expose, examine, question about, and then palpate the limb, as previously described. Determine the tactile response by using the back of the patient's hand. Test muscular strength by having the patient squeeze two of your fingers. Compare strength and sensation bilaterally, identify any deficit, and attempt to locate a cause. Evaluate an upper extremity and ensure it is uninjured before it is used for blood pressure determination.

When extremity assessment suggests injury, treat the limb as though a fracture or dislocation exists. The only definitive way to rule out these injuries is by X-ray evaluation. Also note that splinting protects strains, sprains, and subluxations, as well as fractures and dislocations, from further injury. Treating a soft tissue or muscular injury as a fracture or dislocation produces nothing more harmful than providing slight patient discomfort. Failure to immobilize an injury properly, however, may lead to additional soft, skeletal, connective, vascular, or nervous tissue damage and possibly cause permanent harm.

If possible, find the exact injury site and determine whether it involves a joint area or a long bone shaft. Form a clear visual image of the injury site in order to describe it in the patient care report and to the receiving physician. Remember that a splinting device (e.g., a padded board splint for a wrist fracture) may hide the site from view, leaving the attending physician unable to determine what exists beneath. A good wound description may delay the need to remove a splint to view an injury.

One important complication of musculoskeletal injury to an extremity is compartment syndrome. This condition results from bleeding or edema within a muscle compartment. Increased pressure within the fascia then compresses capillaries and nerves, leading to a reduction in local circulation. This leads to local tissue ischemia and then necrosis, and often some distal sensation loss. A pulse deficit or delayed capillary refill may be late findings in compartment syndrome, as increasing pressure within the fascia may not restrict arterial blood flow early in the syndrome. Suspect compartment syndrome in any patient who has any paresthesia in the webs between medial toes or fingers, who has an extremity injury with a firm mass or increased skin tension at the injury site, or who has pain out of proportion to the injury nature, or pain that increases when you move the limb (passive stretching). Also suspect compartment syndrome in any unconscious patient with a swollen limb. Compartment syndrome most often occurs in the forearm or leg. It takes a long time to develop and may not be recognizable in the prehospital setting. It may be seen in patients well after an emergency department visit for musculoskeletal injuries, in patients with casts in place, and with snake envenomations.

During the physical exam, question the patient about injury symptoms. Ensure that the verbal investigation is detailed and complete. Determine the nature and location of pain, tenderness, or dysfunction. The patient's event description regarding a fracture or dislocation may also be helpful. The patient may state that he felt the bone "snap" or joint "pop out." Determine if the bone snapped, thus causing a fall, or whether a fall caused the fracture. Evaluate for the amount of pain (0 to 10 scale) and discomfort the patient is experiencing with the injury. For example, an elderly patient may present with a fractured hip and limited pain—a presentation usually related to a degenerative disease and secondary fracture. These findings may suggest a less aggressive approach to care for this patient, focusing on patient comfort rather than on traction splinting and shock care. Also identify pertinent patient allergies, medications, past medical history, last oral intake, and events leading up to the incident.

Compare any assessment findings to the index of suspicion for injury developed during scene size-up. If the patient has less significant injuries than suspected, consider reevaluating the patient to ensure that no injury has been overlooked. If a more significant injury is found, suspect that other severe injuries have occurred elsewhere and expand the focused exam.

On conclusion of the focused trauma assessment, identify all injuries found, prioritize them, and establish an order of care. Identify the extent to which each injury may contribute to hemorrhage and shock. Then prioritize the patient for transport. Taking these few moments to sort out what is wrong with the patient and to plan care steps increases the quality and effectiveness of patient care, reduces on-scene time, and ensures that the patient receives proper care in a timely fashion.

Detailed Physical Exam

After potential life threats have been excluded or addressed, attend to any serious problems, and assess any suspected injuries. In some situations, it is necessary to perform a detailed physical exam on a patient who is unconscious or has altered mental status. The exam may be performed at the scene or en route to the hospital. A detailed physical exam is a search for signs and symptoms of further injury not suggested by the mechanism of injury analysis, by patient complaints, or by assessment completed thus far. It is performed in a head-to-toe fashion looking specifically at areas not previously examined in detail. Be alert for signs and symptoms of internal or external injury or hemorrhage. Use the same assessment techniques for evaluating musculoskeletal injuries during a detailed physical exam that you employed during the rapid trauma assessment and focused history and physical exam.

Reassessment

Reassessment focuses on serial measurement of patient vital signs, mental status, and signs and symptoms of major trauma. For patients with musculoskeletal injuries, monitor distal sensation, motor function, capillary refill, and pulses frequently. Remember to ask the patient about how the musculoskeletal injury feels, watching for any change in response. As time passes and the sympathetic response effects wear off, the patient may display more significant and specific injury symptoms. A patient may also begin to complain of other injuries or symptoms, including major and moderate pain or discomfort masked earlier by the chief complaint or complaints. If this occurs, provide a focused trauma assessment for the area of complaint and modify patient priorities as additional injuries are found and evaluated.

Sports Injury Considerations

Many musculoskeletal injuries are associated with sports activities. Activities such as football, basketball, soccer, hockey, baseball, in-line skating, skiing, snowboarding, bicycling, wrestling, hiking, and rock climbing often lead to participant injury. When responding to a sports injury scene, assess the mechanism of injury and determine whether there was a significant kinetic force involved, a hyperextension or flexion injury (or other injury mechanism involving moving a limb beyond its normal range of motion), or a fatigue-type injury. Athletic injuries often affect major body joints such as the shoulder, elbow, wrist, knee, and ankle. Injuries in these areas are especially troublesome for patients because serious ligament damage might preclude future sports participation and limit limb usefulness. It is important to have any potentially significant sports injury evaluated by an emergency physician. The competitive natures of players, teammates, coaches, and athletic trainers may lead them to downplay injuries to keep an injured athlete in competition. Allowing an injured athlete to keep playing places additional stress on the injury and may result in further and more debilitating and/or permanent damage.

Musculoskeletal Injury Management

Musculoskeletal injury management is not normally a high priority in trauma patient care. It usually does not occur until after the primary assessment and the rapid trauma assessment have been completed. Although care focus for a serious trauma patient is for life threats, provide protection for serious musculoskeletal injuries by moving the patient as a unit (with axial alignment) and by packaging the patient for transport (see the chapter "Head, Neck, and Spinal Trauma"). These techniques help to reduce the risks of aggravating musculoskeletal injuries, increasing hemorrhage, and worsening shock. However, do not let gruesome musculoskeletal injury distract from trauma patient management priorities.

Pelvic and femur fractures can significantly contribute to hypovolemia and shock. These injuries deserve a high priority in patient care. Other musculoskeletal injuries that merit a priority for care include those that threaten a limb, such as injuries with loss of distal circulation or sensation (most commonly, joint injuries), and those that cause compartment syndrome (most likely, crushing leg or forearm injuries). Prioritize other injuries by the relative size of the bone fractured or body area involved and by the energy that was required to cause injury, then proceed with splinting and transport.[4]

General Principles of Musculoskeletal Injury Management

Objectives of musculoskeletal injury care are to reduce any further injury during patient care and transport and to reduce patient discomfort. These are accomplished by protecting any open wounds and soft tissues, properly positioning and immobilizing the injured extremity, and monitoring neurovascular function in the distal limb. In some cases, care involves manipulating the injury to reestablish distal circulation and sensation or simply to restore normal anatomic position for the patient expecting prolonged extrication or transport. In most cases, care for musculoskeletal injuries involves application of a splinting device.[4]

Always explain to the patient with musculoskeletal injuries what you are doing, why, and what impact it will have. Alignment and splinting will likely first cause an increase in pain, followed by a significant improvement. If you tell a patient about this in advance, it will increase the patient's confidence in your intent and ability to provide care.

Protecting Open Wounds

If there is any open wound in proximity to the fracture or dislocation, consider the fracture or dislocation to be open. Carefully observe the wound and note any signs of muscle, tendon, ligament, or vascular injury and be prepared to describe it in the report and at the emergency department. Cover the wound with a sterile dressing held in place with bandaging or a splint. Frequently, attempts to align a limb, application of traction, or the splinting process will draw protruding bones back into the wound. This is an expected consequence of proper care but must be brought to the attention of the attending emergency physician.

Positioning the Limb

Proper limb positioning is essential to ensure patient comfort, to reduce chances of further limb injury, and to encourage venous drainage. Proper positioning is different with fractures and dislocations, although splinting a limb in a normal anatomic position—the position of function—is appropriate for both.

Limb alignment is appropriate for any midshaft fracture of the femur, tibia/fibula, humerus, or radius/ulna. Alignment can be maintained by using an air splint, padded rigid splint, vacuum, or traction splint. Proper fracture alignment enhances circulation and reduces the potential for further injury to surrounding tissue. It is also very difficult to immobilize a limb with a fracture in an unaligned, angulated position because fracture segments are short and buried in soft tissue. Perform any limb alignment with great care, so you will not damage tissue surrounding the fracture site. During limb alignment, the proximal limb should remain in position while the distal limb is brought into alignment using gentle axial traction. Stop the process if there is any resistance to movement or if the patient reports any significant increase in pain or discomfort.

Generally, do not attempt alignment of dislocations or fractures within 3 inches of a joint. Manipulate these injury sites only if distal circulation is compromised. Then, try to move the joint while another care provider palpates the distal pulse. If the pulse is restored, if significant resistance to movement is found, or if the patient complains of greatly increasing pain, stop the manipulation and splint the injured limb as it is. Be sure to transport the patient quickly, because a loss of circulation can endanger the limb.

If a possibly dislocated limb will remain dislocated for an extended period, as during lengthy transports or prolonged patient entrapments, consider reducing the dislocation. Apply a firm and progressive traction to the limb that will pull the dislocated ends away from each other and moves the joint toward normal positioning. When (and if) the bone ends "pop" back into anatomic position, ensure

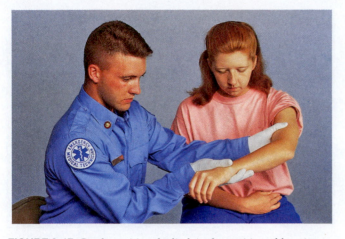

FIGURE 9-17 Gently position the limb in the position of function, unless your attempts meet with resistance or a significant increase in pain or the injury is within 3 inches of a joint.

that there is a distal pulse and immobilize the limb in the position of function.

Proper positioning of injured limbs is important for maintaining distal circulation and sensation and increasing patient comfort. Deformities and extremes of flexion or extension put pressure on soft tissues and may compress nerves and blood vessels. These positions also fatigue surrounding muscles and increase pain associated with injury. By placing uninjured joints halfway between flexion and extension in what is called the position of function, you place the least stress on joint ligaments and muscles and tendons surrounding the injury. Place the limb in the position of function whenever possible (Figure 9-17). Note, however, that some injuries and some splinting devices commonly used for musculoskeletal injuries may preclude this positioning.

When practical, elevate an injured limb. This assists venous drainage and reduces edema associated with musculoskeletal injury.

Immobilizing the Injury

The goal of immobilizing musculoskeletal injuries is to prevent further injury caused by post-injury movement of a strain, sprain, subluxation, dislocation, or fracture. Immobilization restricts fractured bone ends from further lacerating soft tissues, blood vessels, and nerves and from dislodging any clot development and internal hemorrhage control. In dislocations, immobilization prevents movement of dislodged bone ends at a joint where they may entrap or compress nerves and blood vessels and place further stress on ligaments, muscles, or tendons already injured by the injury mechanism. Immobilization of strains, sprains, and subluxations also reduces stress on ligaments, muscles, and tendons and protects the injury from further trauma. Immobilization of an orthopedic injury is also an effective technique to reduce injury pain, especially that likely with limb movement during further care and patient transport. Orthopedic immobilization is usually accomplished using a splinting device.

Checking Neurovascular Function

It is imperative to check circulation, motor function, and sensation status distal to the injury site before, during, and after splinting of all musculoskeletal injuries. A neurovascular check before splinting identifies a baseline condition and establishes whether or not an initial injury disrupts circulation. A neurovascular check during splinting ensures that inadvertent limb movement or circumferential pressure does not compromise distal circulation. The check after splinting identifies any restriction caused by progressive swelling of the injured area against the splinting device. Clearly identify and document these evaluations whenever you apply a splint.

A pulse oximeter can be used to monitor distal pulse during the splint process. Affix a probe to a free finger or toe and ensure a good reading. Then monitor the oximeter, watching for any change, especially if readings become erratic or the device becomes unable to obtain a reading at all. This suggests a compromise in distal circulation (loss of pulsing necessary to obtain a reading) and a need to reassess distal pulse, skin temperature, and capillary refill.

Local Cooling and Gentle Compression

Local cooling and gentle compression are a part of general care principle for orthopedic injuries. Extremity injuries often result in local tissue inflammation and edema, causing pain and swelling with a potential to increase pressure in tissues surrounding the limb (and especially surrounding joints). This swelling may reduce circulation. Immediate local cooling reduces local pain, inflammation, and swelling. Apply cold packs wrapped in a towel, being careful not to apply cold packs or ice directly to skin or a wound, as this may cause further injury. Gentle pressure applied by firm bandaging in conjunction with a splint may also assist in reducing swelling and pain. However, be sure that the pressure does not affect distal circulation. Monitor distal circulation, motor function, and sensation frequently to ensure that they remain adequate.

Splinting Devices

An essential part of managing any musculoskeletal system injury is the use of devices to immobilize a limb and permit patient transport without causing further injury. These devices, called splints, are designed to help reduce or eliminate movement of an injured extremity. Splints come in several forms that can assist in immobilizing common fractures and dislocations associated with musculoskeletal trauma. They include rigid, formable, vacuum, soft, and traction splints, among others.

Rigid Splints

Rigid splints, as the name implies, are firm supports for an injured limb. They can be constructed of plastic, metal, synthetic products, wood, or cardboard. These effectively immobilize injury sites but require adequate padding to lessen patient discomfort. This padding may be built into the splint or may simply be a bulky dressing affixed to the splint with soft bandaging. Several types of commercially available rigid splints are used in prehospital care. They are usually flat, rigid devices and are about 3 inches wide and from 16 to 48 inches long. Cardboard splints are popular, as they store flat, are folded to create a firm splinting surface, are disposable, and are relatively inexpensive (Figure 9-18). A special form of rigid splint is the preformed splint. It is usually a stamped metal or preformed plastic or fiberglass device shaped to limb contours. These splints are usually available for ankles, forearms, and hands.

Formable Splints

Another rigid splint type is the formable, or malleable, splint. It is made up of material that can be easily shaped to match the limb angulation. Apply the formed splint to the limb with circumferential bandaging. Formable splints include both the ladder splint, which is a matrix of soft metal wires soldered together, and the metal sheet splint, which is made up of thin aluminum or another easily shaped metal. The SAM® (structural aluminum malleable)

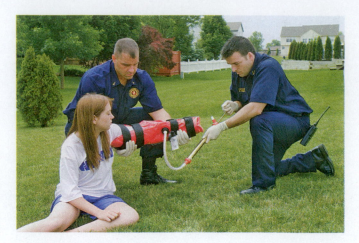

FIGURE 9-19 Suction the air out of a vacuum splint until the device is rigid. Reassess pulse, motor function, and sensation in the extremity after application.

splint is an example of a sheet splint covered with padding and easily formed to a limb's shape.

Vacuum Splints

A vacuum splint is an airtight fabric bag filled with small plastic particles. The splint is placed around an injured limb, conformed to limb shape, and secured around it. As air is removed from the device, the small particles lock into position, firmly maintaining the created shape (Figure 9-19). The splint firmly and comfortably secures a limb in position, although there is a small amount of shrinkage with air evacuation.

Soft Splints

Soft splints use padding or gentle air pressure to immobilize an injured limb. Soft splint varieties include air splints, the pelvic sling or binder, and pillow splints.

Though less frequently used than in the past, some systems continue to use the air splint. Air splints provide immobilization as air pressure fills the splint and compresses a limb. Because the splint is a formed cylinder, it immobilizes the limb in an aligned position. Air splints should not be used with long bone injuries at or above the knee or elbow, because they cannot prevent movement of hip or shoulder joints and are thus unable to immobilize the proximal limb joints. Air splints apply a pressure that may be helpful in controlling both external and internal hemorrhage. Although these devices may limit distal extremity assessment, they do permit observation because they are transparent.

Monitor air splints carefully with any changes in temperature or atmospheric pressure. Increases in ambient heat or decreases in pressure, as during an ascent in a helicopter, increase splint pressure. Conversely, decreases in temperature or a descent in a helicopter decrease splint

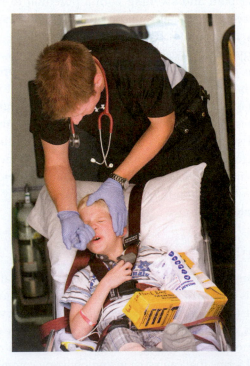

FIGURE 9-18 Cardboard splints are enjoying great popularity. (The medic in this photo is administering nasal fentanyl for pain to the patient with the splinted arm.)

(© Kevin Link)

pressure. Constantly monitor air splint pressure to ensure that it does not rise or fall during care.

Pillow splints are comfortable and effective for ankle and foot injuries. The foot is simply placed on a pillow, while the outer pillow cover fabric is drawn around the foot and pillow. The outer fabric is pinned together or wrapped circumferentially with bandage material (Kling, Kerlix, or cravats) placed tightly around the injury site. This device applies gentle and uniform pressure to effectively immobilize the distal extremity. Using a bulky blanket or two to cradle the ankle and wrapping the blankets firmly may also provide effective immobilization.

Traction Splints

Traction splints were developed during World War I and used extensively during World War II. These splints dramatically reduced both mortality and limb loss from femur fractures caused by projectile wounds, blast injuries, and other battlefield injuries. Today, however, isolated mid-shaft femur fractures are uncommon as is the need for traction splinting.[5]

The traction splint is a frame that applies traction to an injured extremity and against the trunk. Traction application is often necessary when splinting a fractured femur because the bone is surrounded by heavy musculature. Frequently, fracture pain initiates muscle spasm that causes the bone ends to override each other, further aggravating the original injury and increasing pain and muscle spasm. Traction splinting may prevent bone ends from overriding, thus lessening the patient's pain and may help relax any muscle spasm.

There are basically two styles of traction splint, the bipolar frame device and the unipolar device. The bipolar (Fernotrac™, Hare®, or Reel™ splint with ratchet attachment) traction splint has a half ring that fits up and against the ischial tuberosity of the pelvis. A distal ratchet connects to a foot harness and pulls traction from the foot and against the pelvis. The frame lifts and supports the limb and a foot stand holds the injured limb and splint off the ground. This design helps to prevent limb motion during patient movement while elevation supplied by the stand enhances venous drainage. A variation of the bipolar frame device is the Reel Splint. It can be applied to the lower extremity (Figures 9-20a and 9-20b) and to the upper extremity (Figure 9-20c). It has the design features of the bipolar frame traction splint with the added feature that the frame can be bent at the knee. It can accommodate knee dislocations and may provide more comfortable limb positioning for femur fractures.

The unipolar (Sager) traction splint uses a single lengthening shaft to pull a foot harness against pressure applied to the pubic bone. The unipolar splint does not

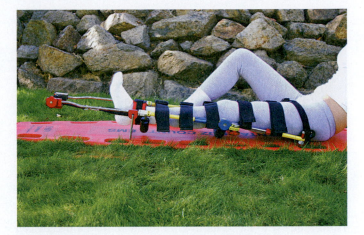

FIGURE 9-20A The Reel™ Splint features of the bipolar frame traction splint.

(© Reel Research and Development)

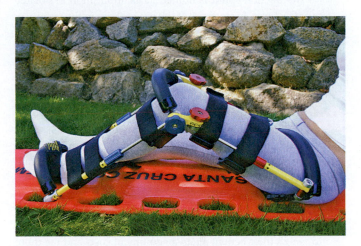

FIGURE 9-20B The Reel™ Splint can be bent at the knee.

(© Reel Research and Development)

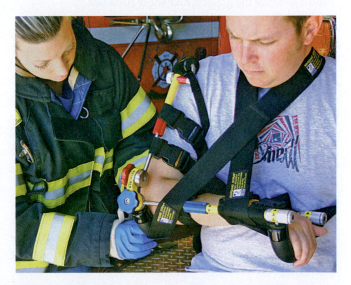

FIGURE 9-20C A pediatric-size Reel™ Splint can be used to splint an adult arm.

(© Reel Research and Development)

elevate or stabilize the extremity, so you must observe greater care whenever you move the patient.

Patho Pearls

The Traction Splint: Past, Present, and Future. The traction splint has been a mainstay of prehospital emergency care ever since J. D. (Deke) Farrington penned the pamphlet titled "Death in a Ditch" and began what is today's modern EMS system. The traction splint was developed in the late 1800s and its worth was proven during the trench warfare of World War I. The old half-ring splint evolved into the "Hare" and then the "Sager"-style splints we find in almost every ambulance today. Surely, everyone who has been in EMS for more than a decade can remember instances when its application turned a patient writhing in pain into someone with only limited discomfort. However, does the traction splint deserve to be a standard of care in the modern EMS system?

The traction splint is limited in its application to isolated femur fractures. In fractures of the hip or those in the vicinity of the knee, traction risks nervous or vascular complications, and the splint is likewise contraindicated in pelvic fractures or any serious skeletal injury to the distal extremity. It may also be contraindicated in multisystem trauma due to the time required for application and the likelihood of contraindicating injuries. Recent research suggests that the incidence of injury requiring the traction splint is about five times in 10,000 prehospital patients. The study further identifies that 40 percent of patients with indications for the traction splint never had it applied, and an equal number of patients (two) had it applied when contraindications existed.

As we examine past, current, and future prehospital care skills, we must evaluate the traction splints' incidence of use and weigh their benefit against equipment costs and the training time necessary to ensure their proper use. As paramedic practitioners, we are aware that we may need to lay aside some mainstays of current prehospital practice as we strive to do the most good for the greatest number of patients.

Other Splinting Aids

Cravats or Velcro straps can augment the effectiveness of rigid splints. These can be used to secure the lower extremities to help stabilize fracture sites. They can also be used as a sling and swathe to help immobilize a splinted upper extremity to the chest. Humerus fractures are difficult to immobilize because the shoulder is such a large and mobile joint. A sling around the neck and across the wrist may hold the elbow at a fixed angle, while a swathe secures the limb against the chest to limit further shoulder motion (cuff and collar sling and swathe). By holding a thumb in the fold of the elbow, the patient can easily reduce any limb motion and complement the splinting process.

In patients with serious multisystem trauma, other injuries preclude splinting individual fractures and dislocations. In such cases, it may be beneficial to splint the extremities to the body with cravats or bandage material and immobilize the patient to a long spine board. Simply strap the body and limbs to the board and transport the patient as a unit. Even though this is not definitive splinting, it will provide reasonable protection for musculoskeletal injuries. If time and patient priorities permit, provide a more definitive splint while transporting the patient.

Fracture Care

A fracture occurring near a joint (generally within 3 inches) carries an increased probability of blood vessel, nerve, and joint capsule involvement. To protect against further complicating this injury, treat any musculoskeletal injury in the proximity of a joint as a joint injury. This requires carefully immobilizing the limb in the position found unless there is a significant circulatory or nervous deficit.

Begin fracture care by ensuring distal pulses, sensation, and motor function. Then align the limb for splinting. Quickly recheck distal circulation and motor and sensory function. If any neurovascular deficit is found, attempt to correct it by gentle repositioning, even if a limb is relatively aligned. If the limb is angulated, proceed with realignment. Remember that most splinting devices are designed to immobilize aligned limbs and that alignment provides the best chance for ensuring good neurovascular function.

To move an injured limb from an angulated position into alignment, use gentle distal traction applied manually. Also consider aligning a limb if a bone end is close to the skin and in danger of converting a closed fracture into an open one. Have an assisting responder immobilize the proximal limb in the position found. Grasp the distal limb firmly and apply traction along and in the direction of the proximal limb's axis, gently moving it from an angulated to an aligned position. Should there be any resistance to movement or a significant increase in patient discomfort, stop alignment and splint the limb as it lies. Once alignment is complete, recheck distal neurovascular function. If it is adequate, proceed with splinting. If function is inadequate, move the limb around slightly while another care provider monitors for a pulse. If one attempt at gentle manipulation does not reestablish a pulse, splint and transport the patient quickly.

Proceed with splinting by selecting an appropriate device and secure the limb to it in a way that ensures that it immobilizes both the fracture site and adjacent joints. Have the second provider, who is holding the limb, apply a gentle traction to stabilize the limb (and monitor the distal pulse) during splinting. If the splint is applied properly, the device may maintain this traction and provide greater limb stabilization and greater patient comfort. Secure the limb to the body (upper extremity) or to the opposite limb (lower extremity) to protect it and to give the patient some control over the limb.

Joint Care

Joint care also begins with assessment for distal neurovascular function. Immobilize the joint in the position found if circulation, sensation, and motor function are adequate. Use a ladder, vacuum, or other malleable splint, shaped to the limb's angle, or cross-wrap with a padded rigid splint to immobilize the joint in place. Ensure that the splint immobilizes the injured joint and both the joint above and the joint below the injury. If not, secure the limb firmly to the body to immobilize these joints.

If circulation or motor or sensory function is lost below the joint injury, consider moving the limb to reestablish it as detailed above in fracture management. When performing a joint **reduction**, attempt to protect the articular surface while directing the bones back to their normal anatomic position. Carefully evaluate distal circulation, sensation, and motor function after reduction. If the procedure does not meet with success within a few minutes, splint the limb as it is and provide rapid patient transport. If reduction is successful, splint the limb in the position of function and transport.

Muscular and Connective Tissue Care

Injuries to musculoskeletal system soft tissues deserve special care. Even though such injuries are not usually life threatening, they can be very painful. Deep contusions, and especially large hematomas, can also contribute to blood loss and hypovolemia. Once more significant injuries have been addressed, assess and treat muscular and connective tissue injuries.

To manage muscle, tendon, and ligament injuries, immobilize the region surrounding them. Doing so reduces associated internal hemorrhage and pain. Provide gentle circumferential bandaging (loose enough to let you slide a finger underneath) to further reduce hemorrhage, edema, and pain, but be sure to monitor distal circulation and loosen the bandage further if there are any signs of neurovascular deficit. Local cooling reduces both edema and patient discomfort. Be careful to wrap any cold or ice pack in a dressing or towel to prevent too drastic a cooling and consequent injury. Consider applying heat to the wound after 48 hours to enhance both circulation and healing. If possible, place the limb in the position of function and elevate the extremity to ensure good venous return, limit swelling, and reduce patient discomfort. Monitor distal neurovascular function to ensure that your actions do not compromise circulation, sensation, or motor function.

Care for Specific Fractures

Pelvis

Pelvic fractures involve either the iliac crest or pelvic ring. Although iliac crest fractures may reflect serious trauma, they are not as serious as pelvic ring fractures. Iliac crest fractures are often isolated and stable injuries that you can care for by simple patient immobilization. The pelvis may also sustain isolated fractures at the symphysis pubis or sacroiliac joint. Pelvic ring fractures are often due to a high-energy event, can carry a high mortality rate, and are considered critical/high-priority injuries.

Pelvic fractures can be divided into four types of fracture. Type I fractures do not involve the pelvic ring and include avulsion fractures and those of the pubis, sacrum, coccyx, ischium, or iliac wing. Type II fractures involve a single break in the pelvic ring, maintain pelvic stability, and include unilateral ring fractures and symphysis pubis and sacroiliac fractures. Type III fractures involve high-energy and multiple ring fractures (and, likely, hypovolemia). Type IV fractures involve the acetabulum.

The pelvic ring shape gives it great strength, but when this ring breaks, the injury often results in fractures at two sites. The kinetic forces necessary to fracture the pelvic ring are significant and are likely to produce fractures and internal injuries elsewhere. Veins in this area are without valves, have limited musculature, and may experience retrograde blood flow when they are torn. Injury to the pelvic ring, therefore, can result in heavy hemorrhage that is likely to empty into the pelvic and retroperitoneal spaces. This blood loss can easily exceed 2 liters. Such an injury may also result in circulation impairment to one or both lower extremities. Pelvic fractures may also be associated with hip dislocations and injuries to the bladder, female reproductive organs, urethra, prostate in the male, and alimentary canal (anus and rectum).

Pelvic injury care objectives include stabilizing the fractured pelvis, supporting the patient hemodynamically, and providing rapid transport to a trauma center. Because of the severe blood loss potential and difficulty in immobilizing a broken pelvic ring, application of a pelvic sling or binder is sometimes recommended for pelvic fractures (Figure 9-21a). The sling or binder is a wide band, either commercially available (Figure 9-21b) or made from a sheet. To make a pelvic sling, fold a sheet to about 10 inches wide and gently negotiate it under a patient, or move the patient to the spine board with the device in place. The band should engage the pelvis with the band's upper border just below the iliac crests. Secure the commercial device or sheet firmly to immobilize the pelvis with firm but not excessive pressure. Place a folded blanket between a patient's lower extremities and tie them together. If necessary for comfort, place a pillow under a patient's knees.[6]

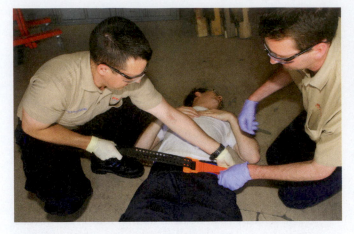

FIGURE 9-21A The SAM® pelvic wrap.

(© Dr. Bryan E. Bledsoe)

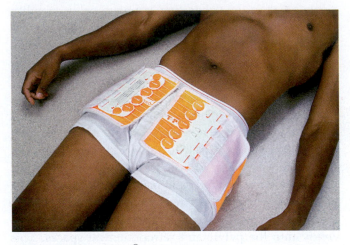

FIGURE 9-21B A T-POD® pelvic splint system.

If the patient is hypotensive, start a large-bore IV and hang one 1,000-mL bag of normal saline. Set up using trauma tubing, and administer fluid boluses as needed to maintain a systolic blood pressure of at least 80 mmHg. Always consider a pelvic fracture patient to be a candidate for rapid transport.

Femur

Femur fractures may be traumatic, resulting from very strong and violent forces, or atraumatic, resulting from degenerative diseases (Figure 9-22). Patients with disease-induced fractures usually are of advancing age and present with a history of a degenerative disease, a clouded or limited trauma history, and only moderate discomfort. The patient often displays some limb shortening, external rotation, and limited deformity. Care for such patients by immobilizing them as found and then providing gentle transport. Generally, effective splinting can be provided by placing the patient on a long spine board and padding with pillows and blankets for patient comfort. A traction splint is not essential because pain does not induce muscle spasms that cause broken bone ends to override.

A patient who has suffered a traumatic femur fracture usually experiences extreme discomfort, and is often

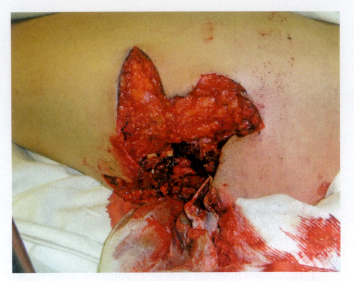

FIGURE 9-22 An open femur fracture.

(© Dr. Bryan E. Bledsoe)

writhing in pain. In such patients, providing distal traction immobilizes both bone ends, relieves muscle spasms, and reduces associated pain. Traction splinting is the best avenue for care of the hemodynamically stable patient with an isolated femur fracture. However, the traction splint is not indicated if the patient has concurrent serious pelvic, knee, tibia, or foot injuries.

Proximal fractures (surgical neck and intertrochanteric fractures) are common—especially in the aged. These proximal femur fractures, commonly referred to as hip fractures, do not benefit from traction splinting. In contrast, mid-shaft fractures often result from high-energy, lateral traumas and are associated with significant blood loss. Injuries to the distal femur (condylar and epicondylar fractures) can be extensive and are likely to involve blood vessels, nerves, and connective tissue. The energy necessary to fracture the femur may be sufficient to dislocate the hip and cause serious internal injuries elsewhere. Mid-shaft femur fractures without associated hip or pelvis injuries gain the most benefit from traction splinting.[7]

It may be difficult to differentiate between proximal femur fractures (hip fractures) and anterior hip dislocations. Generally, a femur fracture presents with the foot externally rotated (turned outward) and the injured limb shortened when compared with the uninjured limb. This difference may be slight and may be unnoticeable if the patient's legs are not straight and parallel. An anterior dislocation presents similarly to the femur fracture, but with the femoral head protruding into the inguinal region. In either case, treat as if it was a dislocation. Traction splints should not be used in either case or if a joint injury (hip or knee) is suspected.

If you suspect an isolated mid-shaft femur fracture, align the limb, determine the circulation and sensory and motor function status, and apply the traction splint. (If you use manual traction to align the femur, maintain it until the splint is applied and continues that traction.) Adjust the splint length against the uninjured extremity, position the device against the pelvis, and secure it in position with the inguinal strap. With a bipolar splint, apply the ankle hitch, provide gentle traction, and elevate the distal limb to place the splint's ring against the ischial tuberosity. With a unipolar splint, position the T-shaped support against the pubic bone and simply apply the ankle hitch. Ensure that the hitch and splint hold the foot and limb in an anatomic position when firm traction is applied. Position and secure the limb to the splint with straps, then gently move the patient and splint to a long spine board. Firmly secure the patient and limb for transport.

Guide traction application by the patient's response. Ask the patient how the limb feels as you initiate and increase the traction. Stop the traction application when the limb is immobilized and patient discomfort eases. Remember, as traction prevents bone end overriding, injury pain should decrease. This reduces muscle spasm strength and lets the limb return toward its initial length. This, in turn, reduces the traction provided by the splint, which may mean that the bone ends are no longer well immobilized. Check the traction frequently to ensure that it does not lessen during care. If the patient reports increasing pain, consider increasing traction gradually until some reduction in pain is noted.

When other patient injuries or need for rapid transport preclude using a traction splint, consider placing the patient on a long spine board for immobilization and transport. Use long, padded rigid splints, one medial and one lateral, to quickly splint the injured limb, and then tie that limb to the uninjured one. Use an orthopedic stretcher or another device or movement technique to transfer the patient to a long spine board and secure the patient firmly on it.[7]

Tibia/Fibula

Fractures of the tibia and fibula can occur separately or together. The tibia is the most commonly fractured leg bone and may be broken by direct force, crushing injury, or twisting forces. A tibial fracture is likely to cause an open wound. Fibular fractures are often associated with injury to the knee or ankle (Figure 9-23). If the tibia is fractured and the fibula is intact, the extremity may not angulate, yet it will not be able to bear weight. If only the fibula is broken, the limb may be relatively stable. Injuries to either bone may result in compartment syndrome. Direct trauma suffered during an auto crash or athletic impact frequently causes these tibia and fibula injuries.

Align the injured limb, assess circulation, sensation, and motor function, and then immobilize the limb with gentle traction. A full-leg air splint (one that accommodates the foot and knee), vacuum, or lateral or medial padded rigid splint provides effective immobilization. A cardboard splint may be used as long as it accommodates the full limb

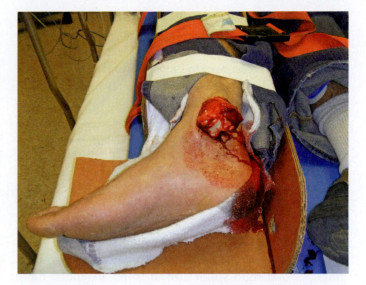

FIGURE 9-23 An open ankle dislocation from a motor vehicle collision. *(© Dr. Bryan E. Bledsoe)*

and is rigid enough to maintain immobilization. After the leg is splinted, secure it to the uninjured leg. This affords some protection against uncontrolled movement and may reassure a patient that he still has some control over the extremity.

Clavicle

The clavicle is the most frequently fractured bone in the human body. Fractures usually result from transmitted forces directed along the upper extremity that cause relatively minor skeletal injury. The clavicle, however, is located adjacent to both the upper reaches of the lung and the vasculature serving the upper extremity and head. The patient with a clavicle fracture often has pain and a shoulder shifted forward, with palpable deformity along the clavicle. Splinting involves simple immobilization with a sling and swathe against the chest. Monitor the patient carefully for any signs of internal hemorrhage or respiratory compromise.

The clavicle may also dislocate with severe forces. A dislocation at the sternum (sternoclavicular) joint can be immobilized with a figure-eight dressing gently pulling the shoulders back. A dislocation at the shoulder (acromioclavicular) joint is best immobilized with a sling and swath.

Humerus

A fractured humerus is very difficult to immobilize. The proximal humerus is buried within the arm and shoulder muscles and the shoulder joint is very mobile. The axillary artery runs through the medial aspect of the shoulder joint (the axilla), making it difficult to apply any mechanical traction to the limb without compromising circulation. Hence, the most effective techniques for splinting this fracture are to apply a sling and swathe to immobilize the bent limb against the chest or to secure the extended and splinted limb against the body.

The preferred technique to secure a fractured humerus is to use a "cuff and collar" sling and swathe. Apply a short, padded rigid splint to the arm's lateral surface to distribute any pressure of the swathing and better immobilize the arm. Sling the forearm with a cravat, catching just the wrist region and not the elbow. This permits some gravitational traction in the seated patient and prevents inadvertent pressure application by the sling, which could flex the limb. Then use several cravats to gently swathe the arm and forearm to the chest. If the patient is conscious, have him place the thumb of the uninjured extremity in the elbow's fold to help control the injured limb's motion. This gives the patient control over the limb, decreases limb movement, and increases patient comfort.

The humerus may also be immobilized by using a long, padded rigid splint affixed to the extended limb. Place the splint along the medial aspect of the upper extremity and ensure that it does not apply pressure to the axilla. Such pressure may disrupt axillary artery blood flow to the limb and is uncomfortable for the patient. Secure the splint firmly to the limb, wrapping from the distal end toward the proximal end. Then secure the splint to the supine patient's body, and move the patient and splint to a long spine board.

Radius/Ulna

The forearm may fracture anywhere along its length and the fracture may involve the radius, ulna, or both. Most commonly, fracture occurs at the distal end of the radius, just above the wrist, and displaces the bone end in a volar (toward the palm) direction. This is known as *Colles' fracture*, which presents with the wrist turned up at an unusual angle. Another term for this injury is "silver fork deformity," because it is contoured like a fork and the distal limb often becomes ashen. As with most joint fractures, a major concern is for distal circulation and innervation. If a neurovascular injury is found, use only slight adjustments to restore nervous or circulatory function, because movement in this area is likely to cause further neurovascular injury.

Splint forearm fractures with a short, padded rigid splint affixed to the forearm and hand. Secure the hand in the position of function by placing a large dressing material wad in the palm to maintain a position like that of holding a large ball. Place a rigid splint along the medial forearm surface and wrap circumferentially from fingers to elbow. Leave at least one digit exposed to permit checking for capillary refill and skin color. Bend the elbow across the chest and use a sling and swathe to hold the limb in position. This provides relative elevation and improves venous drainage in both seated and supine patients.

An air splint, long, formable splint, or padded rigid splint may also adequately immobilize forearm fractures (Figure 9-24). When using these devices, remember to place the hand in the position of function to increase patient comfort.

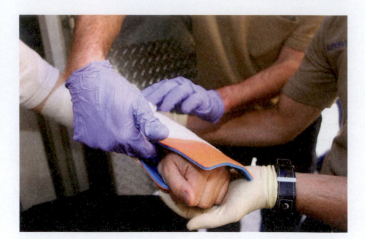

FIGURE 9-24 A "sugar tong" flexible (SAM®) splint can effectively splint a forearm fracture.

(© Dr. Bryan E. Bledsoe)

Care for Specific Joint Injuries

Hip

The hip may dislocate in two directions, anteriorly and posteriorly. Anterior dislocation presents with the foot turned outward and the femur's head palpable in the inguinal area (Figure 9-25). Posterior dislocation is most common and presents with the knee flexed and foot rotated internally. The femur's displaced head is buried in the buttocks muscle and may impinge on the sciatic nerve. Sciatic nerve injury may result in the inability to flex the knee and in reduced sensation in the foot and posterior and lateral leg.

Immobilize the patient with either type of dislocation on a long spine board, using pillows and blankets as padding to maintain patient position and provide comfort. If distal circulation, sensation, or motor function is severely

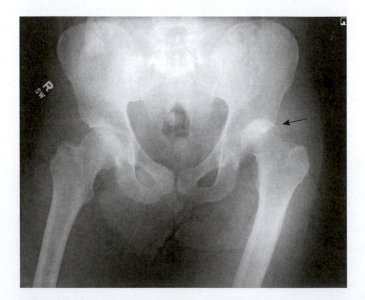

FIGURE 9-25 An anterior hip dislocation (Patient's Left, Reader's Right).

(© Dr. Bryan E. Bledsoe)

compromised, consider one attempt at posterior dislocation reduction. (Consult local protocols and medical direction to identify criteria for reduction attempts.) However, do not attempt reduction if there are other serious injuries, such as a pelvic fracture.

For reduction of a posterior hip dislocation, have a care provider hold the pelvis firmly against a long spine board or other firm surface by placing downward pressure on the iliac crests. Flex both the patient's hip and knee at 90 degrees and apply a firm, slowly increasing traction along the femur's axis. Gently rotate the femur externally (outward). It takes some time for the thigh muscles to relax, but when they do the femoral head will "pop" back into position. If the "pop" is detected or if the patient reports sudden pain relief and is able to easily extend the leg, reduction has likely been successful. Immobilize the patient in a comfortable position, either in flexion (not to exceed 90 degrees) or fully supine with the hip and leg in full extension. Reevaluate sensation, motor function, and circulation. If the femoral head does not move into the acetabulum after a few minutes of your attempted reduction, immobilize the patient as found and consider rapid transport. Because of the strength of the hip joint, posterior and anterior hip dislocation reductions often take several strong providers and possible patient sedation. Again, consult local protocols and medical direction before beginning this procedure.

Knee

Knee injuries may include fractures of the femur, tibia, or both. They also include patellar dislocations and dislocations of the knee. The knee joint contains four major ligaments: the anterior and posterior cruciate and medial and lateral collateral ligaments. Because the knee is such a large joint and bears such a great amount of weight, an injury to it is serious and threatens the patient's future ability to walk. Another concern with knee injury is possible injury to the major blood vessels traversing the area—especially the popliteal artery. This artery is less mobile than blood vessels in other joints, which leaves it more subject to injury and resulting distal vascular compromise.

Immobilize knee joint fractures and patellar dislocations in the position found unless distal circulation, sensation, or motor function is disrupted. If the limb is flexed, splint it with two medium rigid splints, placing one medially and one laterally. Cross-wrap the splint and limb with bandage material to secure the limb in position. Ladder or malleable splints, conformed to the limb's angle and placed anteriorly and posteriorly, can also be used. Vacuum splints can be effective. If the limb is extended, simply apply two padded rigid splints or a full-leg air splint.

Patellar dislocations are more common than actual knee dislocations and usually leave the knee in a flexed position with lateral patella displacement. The injured knee appears significantly deformed.

Anterior knee dislocations produce an extended limb contour that lifts at the knee (moving from proximal to distal), whereas posterior dislocations produce a limb that drops at the knee. (Ensure that the injury is not a patellar dislocation.) If there is neurovascular compromise, have another care provider immobilize the femur firmly in position. Then, grasp the calf muscle just above the ankle and apply firm and progressive traction, first along the axis of the tibia and then pulling the limb toward alignment with the femur. With posterior dislocations, a third care provider may provide moderate downward pressure on the distal femur and upward pressure on the proximal tibia to facilitate reduction. As with most dislocations, success is measured by feeling the bone end "pop" back into place, hearing the patient report a dramatic reduction in pain, and noting freer limb movement at the knee joint. Once a knee dislocation is reduced, immobilize the joint in the position of function and transport the patient. If a dislocation cannot be reduced within a few minutes, immobilize the extremity in the position found and transport quickly. Perform a knee dislocation reduction even if the patient has good distal circulation and nervous function when the time to definitive care will exceed 2 hours.

Ankle

Ankle injuries often produce a distal lower limb that is grossly swollen and deformed as a result of either malleolar fracture, dislocation, or both. Sprains are also common in the ankle, although the limb remains in anatomic position. Splint sprains or nondisplaced fractures with an air splint (shaped to accommodate the foot) or with long rigid splints positioned on either side of the leg and ankle, padded liberally, and wrapped firmly. A pillow splint works well, especially if there is any ankle deformity. Apply local cooling to ease the pain and reduce swelling.

Ankle dislocation may occur in any of three directions: anteriorly, posteriorly, or laterally. An anterior dislocation presents with a dorsiflexed (upward pointing) foot that appears shortened. Posterior dislocations appear to lengthen a plantar flexed (downward-pointing) foot. Lateral dislocations are the most common and present with a foot turned outward with respect to the ankle. If distal neurovascular compromise indicates a need for reduction, have a care provider grasp the calf, hold it in position, and pull against the traction applied. Then grasp the heel with one hand and the metatarsal arch with the other. Pull a distal traction to disengage bone ends and protect articular cartilage during relocation. For anterior dislocations, move the foot posteriorly with respect to the ankle. With lateral dislocations, rotate the foot medially. With posterior dislocations, pull the heel toward you and the foot toward you, and then away. The joint should return to a normal position with a "pop," a reduction in patient pain, and an increase in the mobility of the joint. Apply local cooling and immobilize the limb. If the procedure does not result in joint reduction within a few minutes, splint the joint as found and provide rapid transport.

Foot

Injuries to the foot include dislocations and fractures to calcanei (heel bones), metatarsals, and phalanges. Injuries to calcanei generally result from falls and can cause significant pain and swelling. Injuries to metatarsals and phalanges can result from penetrating or blunt trauma or typical "stubbing" of a toe. Fatigue fractures of metatarsal bones, or "march fractures," are relatively common. These injuries are reasonably stable even though the extremity cannot bear weight. When foot or ankle injury is suspected, anticipate both bilateral foot injuries and lumbar spinal injury.

Immobilize foot injuries in much the same way you do with ankle injuries. Use pillow, vacuum, ladder, or air splints (with foot accommodation). If possible, leave some portion of the foot accessible so you can monitor distal capillary refill or, at least, skin temperature and color.

Shoulder

Shoulder fractures most commonly involve the proximal humerus, lateral scapula, and distal clavicle. Dislocations can include anterior, posterior, and inferior displacement of the humeral head. Anterior dislocations displace the humeral head forward, resulting in a shoulder that appears "hollow" or "squared-off," with a patient holding the arm close to the chest and forward of the mid-axillary line. Posterior dislocations rotate the arm internally. The patient often presents with the elbow and forearm held away from the chest. Inferior dislocations displace the humeral head downward.

Immobilize shoulder injuries (like all joint injuries) as found, unless pulse, sensation, or motor function distal to the injury are absent. Immobilize anterior and posterior dislocations with a sling and swathe and, if needed, place a pillow under the arm and forearm. Immobilization of any inferior dislocation (with the upper extremity fixed above the head) will call for ingenuity in splinting. In such cases, immobilize the extended arm in the position found. Using cravats, tie a long, padded splint to the torso, shoulder girdle, arm, and forearm to immobilize the upper extremity above the head. Gently move the patient to a long spine board and secure both splint and patient to the spine board.

Reduce anterior and posterior shoulder dislocations by placing a strap across the patient's chest, under the affected shoulder (through the axilla), and across the back. Have a care provider prepared to pull countertraction across the chest and superiorly using the strap. Meanwhile, flex the patient's elbow, pulling the arm somewhat away from the body (abduction) and then pull firm traction along the axis of the humerus. Some slight internal and external humerus rotation may facilitate reduction. For reduction of inferior dislocations, have one care provider hold the thorax and then flex the elbow. Gradually apply firm traction

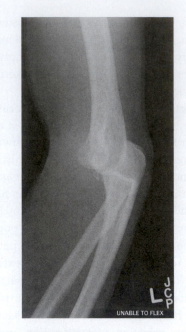

FIGURE 9-26 An elbow dislocation.

(© Dr. Bryan E. Bledsoe)

along the axis of the humerus and gently rotate the arm externally. If the joint does not relocate in a few minutes, immobilize it as it lies and transport the patient. If reduction is successful, immobilize the upper extremity in the normal anatomic position with a sling and swathe.

Elbow

Elbow injuries display a high incidence of nervous and vascular involvement, especially in children (Figure 9-26). As in the knee, blood vessels running through the elbow region are held firmly in place. The possibility that any fracture or dislocation will involve the brachial artery and medial, ulnar, and radial nerves is high. Assess distal neurovascular function and, if a deficit is detected, move the joint very carefully and minimally to restore distal circulation. Then splint the elbow with a single padded rigid splint, providing cross strapping as necessary, or use a ladder splint bent to conform to the limb's angle. Keeping the wrist slightly elevated above the elbow, secure the limb to the chest using a sling and swathe. This position increases venous return and reduces swelling and pain associated with injury.

Wrist/Hand

Hand and wrist fractures are commonly associated with direct trauma. They present with very noticeable deformity and significant pain reported by the patient. These fractures are of serious concern to the patient. Because the hand and wrist bones are small, any fracture is close to a joint. Exercise caution as you care for these injuries because of possible vascular and neural involvement.

Musculoskeletal injuries of the forearm, wrist, hand, or fingers can be effectively immobilized with a padded rigid, vacuum, or air splint. Place a roll of bandaging, a wad of dressing material, or some similar object in the patient's hand to maintain position of function. Then secure the extremity to a padded board with circumferential wrapping or inflate the air splint. Be sure to leave some portion of the distal extremity accessible to monitor perfusion adequacy and sensation. Place the wrist above the elbow to assist venous return and reduce distal swelling.

Hand and wrist injuries are very common, particularly among athletes and children. A particular type of wrist fracture is Colles' fracture, in which the wrist has a "silver fork" appearance (explained earlier). Fortunately, such injuries are seldom serious and can be managed in the pre-hospital setting quite easily.

Finger or Toe

Forces may displace phalanges from their joints, resulting in deformity and pain. Dislocation usually occurs between phalanges or between the proximal phalanx and metacarpal, with the distal bone displaced either anteriorly or posteriorly. (Amputations are multisystem injuries that severely damage the musculoskeletal system. They are addressed in depth in the chapter "Soft-Tissue Trauma.")

Splint finger fractures using tongue blades or small, malleable splints shaped to the injured finger's positioning. The finger may also be taped to adjoining fingers (buddy taping) to limit additional motion. The hand is then placed in the position of function and further immobilized.

Finger dislocations usually involve the proximal joint (and sometimes the distal joint) with the digit commonly displacing posteriorly. If reduction is indicated, grasp the distal finger and apply a firm distal traction. Then direct the digit toward the normal anatomic position by moving its proximal end. You should feel the finger "pop" into place and the digit should resume its normal alignment when compared to an uninjured finger on the other hand. Splint the finger with a slight bend (10 to 15 degrees) and immobilize the hand in the position of function.

Toe fractures and dislocations are generally treated in a fashion similar to finger injuries. Because of their small size and low likelihood of long-term problems, toe injuries are a low-priority problem and should be addressed after all other significant injuries are assessed and treated. Buddy taping and a loose-fitting shoe are an adequate splint for most toe fractures and dislocations of the toes.

Soft and Connective Tissue Injuries

Tendon, ligament, and muscle injuries are rarely, if ever, life threatening. Massive muscular contusions and hematomas can, however, contribute to hypovolemia, whereas ligament and tendon injuries can endanger future limb function. Be careful about permitting the patient to put further stress on a limb, especially with higher grades of sprains. Weakened ligaments may fail completely, resulting in complete joint instability or dislocation. Treat tendon, ligament, and muscle injuries as one would treat dislocations, and immobilize adjacent joints. Monitor distal neurovascular function because tissue swelling and resulting pressure within circumferential wrapping of a splint may compress blood vessels and nerves. Care for muscular injuries with immobilization, gentle compression with snug (but not overly tight) dressings, and local cooling to suppress edema and pain using cold packs or ice wrapped in dressing material or a towel. Be watchful for signs of compartment syndrome, especially in the calf and forearm.

Open wounds involving muscles, tendons, and ligaments can be severe and debilitating. Carefully evaluate such wounds for connective tissue involvement. Be especially watchful with deep open injuries close to joints. With such wounds, tendon and ligament disruption is likely and may adversely affect future use of the joint, muscles controlling the joint, or muscles controlling joint movement proximal or distal to the injury. Carefully evaluate for circulation, sensation, and motor function below these injuries.

Injury to a muscle or tendon may limit its ability to either extend or flex the limb. The opposing muscle moves the limb, but injured muscle cannot return it to a normal position. With limb injuries, note any unusual limb position, especially if the patient is unable to return the limb to a neutral position. At any sign of pain or dysfunction, splint the limb.

Medications

Medications are frequently administered to patients with musculoskeletal injury to relieve pain and to premedicate before relocation of a dislocation. Medications used include diazepam, morphine, and fentanyl. Remember that fentanyl can be given intranasally—especially in children.[8-9]

Pediatric Musculoskeletal Injury

Children are at higher risk than adults for musculoskeletal injuries because of their activity levels and incompletely developed coordination. Special injuries affecting them include greenstick fractures and epiphyseal fractures.

The incomplete nature of the greenstick fracture produces a stable but angulated limb in the young child. The injured limb is painful and will not bear weight. In these cases, do not attempt to realign the limb and understand that the orthopedic specialist will probably complete the fracture to permit proper healing.

Epiphyseal fractures disrupt a child's bone's growth plate and endanger future bone growth. This injury is likely with fractures within a few inches of the joint because the epiphyseal plate is a point of skeletal weakness. Treat these fractures as you would for an adult, but recognize that they are potentially limb-threatening injuries.

Consider the possibility of abuse during evaluation of a pediatric patient with musculoskeletal injuries. Look for injuries inconsistent with the described mechanism of injury or multiple injuries in different stages of healing. Report any suspicions as appropriate under state law and local protocols.

Athletic Musculoskeletal Injuries

Athletes, especially those involved in contact sports such as football, soccer, basketball, and wrestling, have a higher incidence of musculoskeletal injuries than the general public. Injuries to joints—often, serious knee and ankle sprains—are common reasons for calls to EMS. Such injuries are especially important because they occur in individuals who are at least moderately well conditioned and result from significant kinetic force application. When called to evaluate an injured athlete, be especially sensitive to the potential for residual disability caused by the injuries and be predisposed to transport instead of permitting the patient to remain at the scene.

Knowing athletic trainers in your area may help on-scene operations run more smoothly and efficiently. In many cases, athletic trainers work under local physician supervision, much as you work under medical direction. It is important for trainers to understand that once you are called to the scene, an injured athlete becomes an EMS system patient and will be treated under system medical direction and protocols. Also, as a system representative, you are likely to assume responsibility for decisions about patient care and transport. Ensuring that trainers understand these circumstances may eliminate confrontations over care for the injured athlete.

Athletic trainers use the acronym RICE to identify the recommended treatment for sprains, strains, and other soft tissue injuries. RICE stands for *R*est the extremity, *I*ce for the first 48 hours, *C*ompression with an elastic bandage, and *E*levation for venous drainage. This is consistent with standard emergency care for sprains and strains. (Note, however, that the application of the elastic bandage in this case is to strengthen a limb for further activity and is not recommended for pre-hospital care.)

Patient Refusals and Referral

In some situations, you may encounter a patient suffering from an isolated sprain or strain that has no significant mechanism of injury and no other injury signs, symptoms, or complaints. This patient may refuse assistance or be a candidate for on-scene treatment and referral for follow-up medical care. Evaluate the need for immobilization and X-rays and determine whether the patient should seek immediate care in an emergency department or see a personal physician. Any referral to a personal physician or patient refusal must be done in conjunction with medical direction and must follow local protocols.

Psychological Support for the Musculoskeletal Injury Patient

Regardless of the specific type of injury sustained, patients need psychological as well as physiologic support. Too often, we concentrate all efforts on a patient's injuries, forgetting the emotional impact that an incident and emergency care measures employed have on a patient. Keep in mind that patients are not frequently exposed to injuries. They do not know what effects injuries will have on their lives or what to expect from medical care in the prehospital, emergency department, or in-hospital settings. Remember that you can have a significant impact on a patient's emotional response to trauma. Displaying a concerned attitude and a professional demeanor and communicating frequently and compassionately with patients will go far to calm and reassure them. Simple attention paid to a patient may make his experience with prehospital emergency medical service one that is remembered positively.

> **CONTENT REVIEW**
> ➤ RICE Procedure for Strains, Sprains, and Soft Tissue Injuries
> - *R*est the extremity
> - *I*ce for first 48 hours
> - *C*ompress with elastic bandage
> - *E*levate extremity

Summary

Injuries to the bones, ligaments, tendons, and muscles of the extremities rarely threaten the patient's life. Major exceptions to this statement are pelvic and serious or bilateral femur fractures, in which associated hemorrhage can contribute significantly to hypovolemia and shock. In addition, serious musculoskeletal trauma suggests the possibility of other, life-threatening, trauma and, in fact, occurs in about 80 percent of cases of major multisystem trauma. The presence of serious musculoskeletal trauma should increase the index of suspicion for other serious internal injuries.

Care for isolated musculoskeletal trauma is usually delayed until the primary assessment and patient life threats are stabilized. Musculoskeletal care goals are to protect any open wounds, position affected limbs properly, immobilize the injury area, and carefully monitor distal extremities to ensure neurovascular function.

Pelvic and bilateral femur fractures are immobilized using pelvic sling and long spine board application. The pelvic sling immobilizes the unstable pelvis. Manage other fractures by aligning the extremity with gentle traction and immobilizing it by splinting. If there is a loss of distal neurovascular function, move the extremity slightly to restore neurovascular function and then splint.

Joint injuries carry a greater risk of damage to distal circulation, sensation, and motor function. Splint these injuries as found unless there is distal neurovascular compromise. If that is the case, employ gentle manipulation to restore circulation, motor function, or sensation. If gentle manipulation is unsuccessful and transport is to be delayed, attempt dislocation reduction for the hip, knee, ankle, shoulder, or finger, as permitted by local protocol.

Care for injuries to connective and muscular tissues by immobilizing the area of injury in the position of function. Evaluate distal extremities for pulse, capillary refill, color, temperature, sensation, and motor function before, during, and after any immobilization or movement of a limb and provide frequent monitoring thereafter. Consider local cooling, gentle wrapping (most probably associated with splinting), and possibly medication to reduce musculoskeletal injury pain.

You Make the Call

You and your partner are called to 1616 Hampton Avenue for a patient who has tripped in the yard and injured his ankle. Dispatch reports that the patient is a 16-year-old male who is conscious, alert, and breathing; there is no bleeding present. Bystanders are on the scene performing first aid.

On arrival at the scene, you find the patient, Hank Tomlin, leaning against a tree in the front yard of his mother's home. As you interview Hank and bystanders, you discover that he is complaining of pain, swelling, and deformity to his right ankle. Hank tells you that he was running after his dog when his foot twisted in the grass and he fell to the ground. You suspect that the patient has probably dislocated or fractured his ankle.

While your partner continues to obtain a patient history and vital signs, you assess the site of the injury. A third off-duty paramedic is also on the scene to assist.

1. When assessing the injury site, what signs of fracture will you be evaluating?
2. What are the three main factors to consider when evaluating distal neurovascular status?
3. What steps should you take if you determine the patient is suffering from distal neurovascular impairment and choose to realign the injury?
4. How many attempts are permitted when realigning an injury?
5. How would you splint this injury once realignment has taken place?

See Suggested Responses at the back of this book.

Review Questions

1. The skeleton gives the body its structural form. What other purpose does it have?
   a. It protects the vital organs.
   b. It allows for moving and walking.
   c. It stores salts and other materials needed for metabolism.
   d. All of the above.

2. Bones are classified according to their _____
   a. size.
   b. shape.
   c. weight.
   d. diameter.

3. Minute blood vessels, surrounded by layers of salts deposited in collagen fibers, travel lengthwise along the bone through small tubes known as _____
   a. osteocytic pores.
   b. osteoblastic pores.
   c. perforating canals.
   d. haversian canals.

4. The connective tissue(s) that hold bones together at a joint articulation is/are called _____
   a. tendons.
   b. cartilage.
   c. bursal tissue.
   d. ligaments.

5. Biaxial joints allow movement in two planes. An example from this category of joints would be the _____
   a. knee.
   b. wrist.
   c. thumb bases.
   d. fingers.

6. Age-related changes in the skeletal system begin to occur as early as 40 years of age. These changes include _____
   a. calcium retention.
   b. progression in body height.
   c. diminishing ability to maintain bone structure and strength.
   d. an increase in flexibility of costochondral joints.

7. Skeletal muscles provide the ability for voluntary movement associated with the mobility of the body and its extremities. These muscles are controlled by which division of the nervous system?
   a. Somatic
   b. Autonomic
   c. Sympathetic
   d. Musculoskeletal

8. More than half the energy created by muscle motion is _____
   a. heat energy.
   b. chemical energy.
   c. electrical energy.
   d. mechanical energy.

9. If a joint is made to move beyond its normal range of motion as a result of an externally applied force, a displacement of bone ends from their normal position may occur as the ligaments are stretched. This is known as a(n) _____, and is characterized by _____
   a. oblique fracture; pain, edema, and possibly bleeding.
   b. subluxation; pain, edema, and diminished mobility of the joint.
   c. luxation; severe pain and spasm without joint instability.
   d. subluxation; pain, rapid edema, and an unlimited range of motion.

10. The function of the red bone marrow found in the medullary cavities of the sternum, long bones, and pelvis is _____
   a. destruction and recycling of old and fragile blood cells.
   b. manufacturing of erythrocytes and other blood cells.
   c. storage of essential salts and minerals for bone aggregation.
   d. storage of a readily available source of energy generation.

11. A grade _____ sprain may present as a fracture.
   a. I
   b. II
   c. III
   d. IV

12. A small crack in a bone that does not disrupt its total structure is called a(n) _____ fracture.
   a. open
   b. closed
   c. impacted
   d. hairline

13. What type of splinting is recommended for a patient who has palpable instability and pain to the pelvis after being involved in an industrial accident?
   a. Board splints
   b. Pelvic sling or binder
   c. Traction
   d. Vacuum

14. A femur fracture may account for as much as _____ mL of blood loss.
   a. 1,000
   b. 1,500
   c. 2,000
   d. 2,500

15. Your patient has been involved in a motorcycle accident in which he was thrown from his bike onto the road surface and then hit by a car traveling in the opposite direction. You suspect femur, pelvic, and multiple upper extremity fractures. Treatment of this patient would include _____
   a. traction device, long board, transport to trauma center.
   b. long board, one IV line, transport to emergency department.
   c. traction device, PASG, transport to trauma center.
   d. long board, intravenous access, transport to trauma center.

See Answers to Review Questions at the end of this book.

References

1. Badhe, S., et al. "The 'Silent' Compartment Syndrome." *Injury* 40(2) (Feb 2009): 220–222.

2. Flynn, J. M., et al. "Acute Traumatic Compartment Syndrome of the Leg in Children: Diagnosis and Outcome." *J Bone Joint Surg Am* 93(10) (May 18 2011): 937–941.

3. Oprel, P. P., et al. "The Acute Compartment Syndrome of the Lower Leg: A Difficult Diagnosis?" *Open Orthop J* 4 (2010): 115–119.

4. Melamed, E., et al. "Prehospital Care of Orthopedic Injuries." *Prehosp Disaster Med* 22(1) (Jan–Feb 2007): 22–25.

5. Wood, S. P., M. Varhas, and S. K. Wedel. "Femur Fracture Immobilization with Traction Splints in Multisystem Trauma Patients." *Prehosp Emerg Care* 7(2) (Apr–Jun 2003): 241–243.

6. Tan, E. C., S. F. van Stigt, and A. B. van Vugt. "Effect of a New Pelvic Stabilizer (T-POD®) on Reduction of Pelvic Volume and Haemodynamic Stability in Unstable Pelvic Fractures." *Injury* 41(12) (Dec 2010): 1239–1243.

7. Abarbanell, N. R. "Prehospital Midthigh Trauma and Traction Splint Use: Recommendations for Treatment Protocols." *Amer J Emerg Med* 19(2) (Mar 2001): 137–140.

8. Garrick, J. F., S. Kidane, J. E. Pointer, W. Sugiyama, C. Van Luen, and R. Clark. "Analysis of the Paramedic Administration of Fentanyl." *J Opioid Manag* 7(3) (May–June 2011): 229–234.

9. Kanowitz, A., T. M. Dunn, E. M. Kanowitz, et al. "Safety and Effectiveness of Fentanyl Administration for Prehospital Pain Management." *PreHospital Emergency Care* 10(1) (2006).

Further Reading

American College of Surgeons, Committee on Trauma. *Advanced Trauma Life Support Course: Student Manual.* 9th ed. Chicago: American College of Surgeons, 2012.

Bickley, L. *Bates' Guide to Physical Examination and History Taking.* 11th ed. Philadelphia: Wolters-Kluwer, 2012.

Bledsoe, B. E., and D. Clayden. *Prehospital Emergency Pharmacology.* 7th ed. Upper Saddle River, NJ: Pearson/Prentice Hall, 2011.

Bledsoe, B. E., B. J. Colbert, and J. E. Ankney. *Essentials of A & P for Emergency Care.* Upper Saddle River, NJ: Pearson/Prentice Hall, 2010.

Campbell, J. E. *International Trauma Life Support for Prehospital Care Providers.* 7th ed. Upper Saddle River, NJ: Pearson/Prentice Hall, 2016.

Jastremski, M. E., M. Dumas, and L. Penalver. *Emergency Procedures.* Philadelphia: W. B. Saunders, 1992.

Martini, F. *Fundamentals of Anatomy and Physiology.* 10th ed. San Francisco: Pearson, 2014.

Marx, J., R. Hockberger, and R. Walls. *Emergency Medicine: Concepts and Clinical Practice.* 8th ed. St. Louis: Mosby, 2013.

Tintinelli, J. E., ed. *Emergency Medicine: A Comprehensive Study Guide.* 7th ed. New York: McGraw-Hill, 2008.

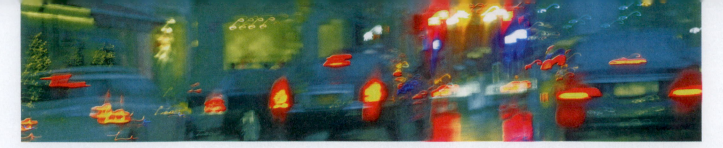

Chapter 10
Environmental Trauma

Bryan Bledsoe, DO, FACEP, FAAEM, EMT-P

Justin Sempsrott, MD

STANDARD
Trauma (Environmental Emergencies)

COMPETENCY
Integrates assessment findings with principles of epidemiology and pathophysiology to formulate a field impression to implement a comprehensive treatment/disposition plan for an acutely injured patient.

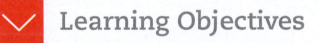

Learning Objectives

Terminal Performance Objective: After reading this chapter, you should be able to assess and manage patients with environmental emergencies.

Enabling Objectives: To accomplish the terminal performance objective, you should be able to:

1. Define key terms introduced in this chapter.

2. Identify factors that place patients at particular risk for environmental emergencies.

3. Describe the physiology of homeostatic mechanisms designed to maintain thermoregulation, including factors that can interfere with thermoregulation

4. Describe the pathophysiology, symptomatology, and prehospital management of heat-related emergencies.

5. Describe the pathophysiology, symptomatology, and prehospital management of cold-related emergencies.

6. Identify measures that can help prevent heat-related and cold-related disorders.

7. Describe the pathophysiology, symptomatology, and prehospital management of drowning emergencies.

8. List and discuss the application of gas laws as they pertain to diving emergencies.

9. Describe the pathophysiology, symptomatology, and prehospital management of diving emergencies.

10. Discuss the role of hyperbaric chambers and the Divers Alert Network as they relate to the prehospital management of diving emergencies.

11. Describe the pathophysiology, symptomatology, and prehospital management of high altitude emergencies.

12. Given a variety of scenarios, describe the assessment and management of typical environmental emergencies.

KEY TERMS

absolute zero, p. 299

acclimatization, p. 302

arterial gas embolism, p. 318

autonomic neuropathy, p. 302

barotrauma, p. 318

basal metabolic rate (BMR), p. 300

conduction, p. 299

convection, p. 299

core temperature, p. 300

decompression sickness, p. 318

deep frostbite, p. 312

drowning, p. 313

environmental emergency, p. 298

evaporation, p. 300

exertional metabolic rate, p. 300

frostbite, p. 312

heat cramps, p. 303

heat exhaustion, p. 304

heat-related illness, p. 301

heatstroke, p. 304

homeostasis, p. 298

hyperbaric oxygen chamber, p. 320

hyperthermia, p. 301

hypothalamus, p. 300

hypothermia, p. 306

J waves, p. 309

mammalian diving reflex, p. 315

negative feedback, p. 300

nitrogen narcosis, p. 318

pneumomediastinum, p. 318

pneumothorax, p. 318

pulmonary overpressure, p. 318

pyrexia, p. 306

pyrogens, p. 306

radiation, p. 300

recompression, p. 320

respiration, p. 300

scuba, p. 316

superficial frostbite, p. 312

surfactant, p. 314

thermal gradient, p. 299

thermogenesis, p. 299

thermolysis, p. 299

thermoregulation, p. 300

trench foot, p. 313

Case Study

Today is Sunday and you and your partner are staffing Medic 7. Because of the bad weather, you pick up your partner from his home in your four-wheel-drive sport utility vehicle and ride together to work at the Thunder Bay station. It is another bitterly cold January day, so you warm up with a mug of hot chocolate, awaiting what the day will bring. Suddenly, central dispatch calls in a "priority A" situation at 1050 Ventura Road, a downtown office building in the bar and nightclub district. Apparently, someone on the way to work found an unconscious man lying in the snow. You and your partner depart immediately.

On arrival you find an approximately 20-year-old man huddled and shivering on the ice-covered ground. His breathing is shallow and irregular. He is quite stuporous and confused but manages to tell you that he had been out celebrating his 21st birthday the night before and early that morning. He thinks he passed out there a couple of hours earlier, but really is not sure.

Your assessment reveals that the patient is bradycardic and mildly hypotensive. His core temperature is 86°F (30°C). While you are speaking with the patient, he stops shivering and his speech becomes unintelligible. You and your partner gently and slowly put him in the ambulance, remove his wet clothing, apply cardiac and core temperature monitors, and then place warm water bottles at his head, neck, chest, and groin. Your partner notes that his core temperature has dropped to 85°F (29.4°C).

En route to Foothills General Hospital, your vehicle passes through a bumpy area of road construction, jostling your patient considerably. The alarms go off, and ventricular fibrillation appears on the monitor. Vitals are absent after checking for 2 minutes. Your partner administers a single 200 J biphasic shock without success. You intubate the patient, ventilate with warmed oxygen, and begin chest compressions. You give no medications through the IV.

In the emergency department, the patient is gradually rewarmed, using active techniques. Once the core temperature is above 86°F (30°C), the usual hypothermia protocol is initiated. The patient is converted from ventricular fibrillation, slowly regains vital signs, and is eventually admitted to the ICU. Following admission, he does well and is discharged five days later. The day before his discharge, you and your partner stop by to check his progress. He reports that he is doing very well but does not remember the prehospital care or the ambulance ride. The patient is adamant about one thing, however: He vows never to drink alcohol again.

Introduction

The *environment* can be defined as all of the surrounding external factors that affect the development and functioning of a living organism. Human beings obviously depend on the environment for life, but they also must be protected from its extremes. When factors such as temperature, weather, terrain, and atmospheric pressure act on the body, they can create stresses for which the body is unable to compensate. A medical condition caused or exacerbated by such environmental factors is known as an **environmental emergency**.

Environmental emergencies include a variety of conditions, such as heatstroke, hypothermia, drowning, diving accidents or barotrauma, and altitude sickness. Such emergencies often call for special rescue resources.

Although environmental emergencies can affect anyone, several risk factors predispose certain individuals to developing environmental illnesses. These factors include:

- Age—especially very young children and older adults who do not tolerate environmental extremes very well
- Poor general health
- Fatigue
- Predisposing medical conditions
- Certain medications—either prescription or over-the-counter

Environmental factors must also be considered when determining the risk for environmental emergencies. For example, weather in a particular place may vary greatly from moment to moment. Areas where change in temperature can be drastic over the course of the day may catch unwary individuals off guard. For example, desert areas can have temperatures of 105°F during the day but drop below freezing at night, placing unprepared travelers in a difficult situation. As another example, temperatures in parts of southern Alberta can change drastically when the Chinook winds kick up. Other considerations include the current season, local weather patterns, atmospheric pressures (high altitude or underwater), and the type of terrain, which can cause injury or hinder rescue efforts.

As a paramedic, you will frequently be called on to treat medical emergencies related to environmental conditions. It is critical that you understand the particular conditions that prevail in your region. If you live in a mountainous area, near large caves, in an area with swift-moving water, or in a resort area where diving is prominent, you need to be familiar with the specialized rescue resources these situations may require and the particular environmental emergencies they may cause. Understanding their causes and underlying pathophysiology can help you recognize these emergencies promptly and manage them effectively.

Although many environmental factors can result in medical emergencies, this chapter will focus primarily on problems related to temperature extremes, drowning, diving emergencies, and high-altitude illness.

Homeostasis

For the human body to function properly, it must interact with the environment to obtain oxygen, nutrients, and other necessities, but it must also avoid being damaged by extreme external environmental conditions. The process of maintaining constant suitable conditions within the body is called **homeostasis**. Various body systems respond in an effort to maintain the correct core and peripheral temperature, oxygen level, and energy supply to maintain life.

The following sections address how the body attempts to maintain these normal settings and what happens when certain environmental conditions exceed the ability of the body to compensate.

Pathophysiology of Heat and Cold Disorders
Mechanisms of Heat Gain and Loss

The body gains and loses heat in two ways: from within the body itself and by contact with the external environment.

The body receives heat from, or loses it to, the environment via the thermal gradient. The **thermal gradient** is the difference in temperature between the environment (the ambient temperature) and the body. The ambient temperature is usually different from body temperature. If the environment is warmer than the body, heat flows from the environment to the body. If the body is warmer than the environment, heat flows from the body to the environment. Other environmental factors, including wind and relative humidity (the percentage of water vapor in the air), also affect heat gain and loss.

The mechanisms by which heat is generated within the body and by which heat is gained or lost to the environment are discussed in more detail in the following sections.

Thermogenesis (Heat Generation)

In the science of physics, heat is created by molecules in motion. The faster the molecular motion, the higher the heat. Only when molecular motion comes to a stop does the object in question fall to a temperature of **absolute zero** (–273°C or –459°F).

The amount of heat in the body continually fluctuates as a result of the heat generated or gained and the heat lost. The body gains heat from both external and internal sources. In addition to the heat the body absorbs from the environment, the body also generates heat through energy-producing chemical reactions (metabolism).

The creation of heat is called **thermogenesis**. There are several types of thermogenesis. One is *work-induced thermogenesis*, which results from exercise. Our muscles need to create heat because warm muscles work more effectively than cold ones. One way muscles can produce heat is by shivering. Another type, *thermoregulatory thermogenesis*, is controlled by the endocrine system. Hormones from the thyroid gland, or the hormones norepinephrine and epinephrine from the adrenal gland, can cause an immediate increase in the rate of cellular metabolism, which, in

turn, increases heat production. The last type of thermogenesis, metabolic thermogenesis or *diet-induced thermogenesis,* is caused by the processing of food and nutrients. When a meal is eaten, digested, absorbed, and metabolized, heat is produced as a byproduct of these activities.

Thermolysis (Heat Loss)

The loss of heat is called **thermolysis**. Heat always flows from the warmer substance to the cooler substance. The heat generated by the body is constantly lost to the environment. This occurs because the body is usually warmer than the surrounding environment. The transfer of heat into the environment occurs through the following mechanisms (Figure 10-1):

- *Conduction.* Direct contact of the body's surface to another, cooler object causes the body to lose heat by **conduction**. Heat flows from higher-temperature matter to lower-temperature matter.

- *Convection.* Heat loss to air currents passing over the body. Heat, however, must first be conducted to the air before being carried away by **convection** currents.

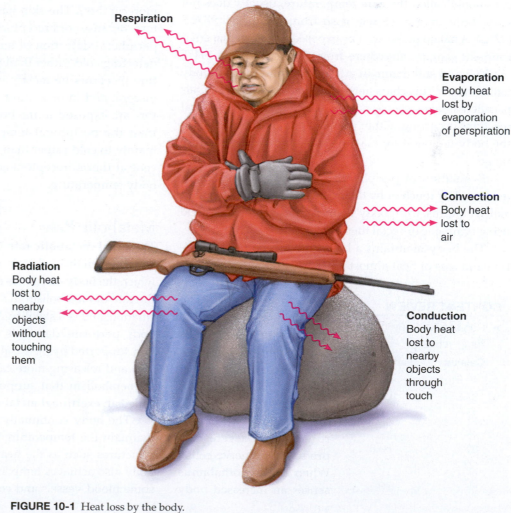

Respiration

Evaporation
Body heat lost by evaporation of perspiration

Convection
Body heat lost to air

Radiation
Body heat lost to nearby objects without touching them

Conduction
Body heat lost to nearby objects through touch

FIGURE 10-1 Heat loss by the body.

- *Radiation.* An unclothed person will lose approximately 60 percent of total body heat by **radiation** at normal room temperature. This heat loss is in the form of infrared rays. All objects not at absolute zero temperature will radiate heat into the atmosphere.

- *Evaporation.* The change of a liquid to vapor. Evaporative heat loss occurs as water or sweat evaporates from the skin. Additionally, a great deal of heat loss occurs through **evaporation** of fluids in the lungs. Water evaporates from the skin and lungs at approximately 600 mL/day.

- *Respiration.* Combines the mechanisms of convection, radiation, and evaporation. **Respiration** accounts for a large proportion of the body's heat loss. Heat is transferred from the lungs to inspired air by convection and radiation. Evaporation in the lungs humidifies the inspired air (adds water vapor to it). During expiration, this warm, humidified air is released into the environment, creating heat loss.

Thermoregulation

Thermoregulation is the maintenance or regulation of temperature. The body temperature of the deep tissues, commonly called the **core temperature**, usually does not vary more than a degree or so from its normal 98.6°F (37°C). A naked person can be exposed to an external environment ranging anywhere from 55°F (12.8°C) to 144°F (62.2°C) and still maintain a fairly constant internal body temperature. This characteristic of warm-blooded animals is called *steady-state metabolism.* The various biochemical reactions occurring within the cell are most efficient when the body temperature is within this narrow temperature range.

Evaluation of peripheral body temperature can be measured by touch or by taking the temperature by oral or axillary means. Core body temperatures can be measured using tympanic or rectal thermometers.

The body maintains a balance between the production and loss of heat almost entirely through the nervous system and negative feedback mechanisms. The **hypothalamus**, located at the base of the brain, is responsible for temperature regulation. It functions as a thermostat, controlling temperature through the release of neurosecretions (secretions produced by nerve cells). When the hypothalamus senses an increased body temperature, it shuts off the mechanisms designed to create heat, for example, shivering. When it senses a decrease in body temperature, the hypothalamus shuts off mechanisms designed to cool the body, for example, sweating. Because the action involved requires stopping, or negating, a process, it is called a **negative feedback** system.

When the heat-regulating function of the hypothalamus is disrupted, the result can be an abnormally high or low body temperature. At the extremes, such abnormal temperatures can result in death (Figure 10-2).

Thermoreceptors

Although the hypothalamus plays a key role in body temperature regulation, temperature receptors in other parts of the body also help to moderate temperatures. There are thermoreceptors in the skin and certain mucous membranes (peripheral thermoreceptors), as well as in certain deep tissues of the body (central thermoreceptors). The skin has both cold and warm receptors. Because cold receptors outnumber warm receptors, peripheral detection of temperature consists mainly of detecting cold rather than warmth. Deep body temperature receptors lie mostly in the spinal cord, abdominal viscera, and in or around the great veins. These receptors are exposed to the body's core temperature rather than the peripheral temperature. They also respond mainly to cold rather than warmth. Both peripheral and central thermoreceptors act to prevent lowering of the body temperature.

Metabolic Rate

The **basal metabolic rate (BMR)** is the metabolism that occurs when the body is completely at rest. It is the rate at which the body consumes energy just to maintain itself—the rate of metabolism that maintains brain function, circulation, and cell stability. Any additional activity that the body performs demands energy consumption beyond that supported by the basal rate, metabolizing more nutrients and releasing more calories (units of heat). The rate of metabolism that supports this additional activity is called an **exertional metabolic rate**.

The body continually adjusts the metabolic rate to maintain the temperature of the core (where the crucial structures such as the heart and brain are located). The body also achieves temperature maintenance by dilating some blood vessels and constricting others so the blood

CONTENT REVIEW

➤ Comparative Body Temperatures

Celsius	Fahrenheit
40.6°	105°
37.8°	100°
37°	98.6°
35°	95°
32°	89.6°
30°	86°
20°	68°

CONTENT REVIEW

Thermoregulation

➤ Mechanisms of Heat Dissipation
  - Sweating
  - Vasodilation
➤ Mechanisms of Heat Conservation
  - Shivering
  - Vasoconstriction

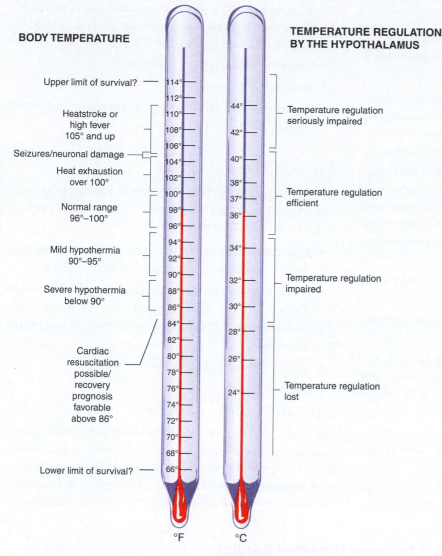

BODY TEMPERATURE

TEMPERATURE REGULATION BY THE HYPOTHALAMUS

Upper limit of survival? — 114°

Heatstroke or high fever 105° and up — 110°, 108°

Seizures/neuronal damage — 106°, 104°

Heat exhaustion over 100° — 102°

Normal range 96°–100° — 100°, 98°, 96°

Mild hypothermia 90°–95° — 94°, 92°, 90°

Severe hypothermia below 90° — 88°, 86°

Cardiac resuscitation possible/ recovery prognosis favorable above 86° — 84°, 82°, 80°, 78°, 76°, 74°, 72°, 70°, 68°

Lower limit of survival? — 66°

°F   °C

44° — Temperature regulation seriously impaired

42°, 40°

38°, 37°, 36° — Temperature regulation efficient

34°, 32°, 30° — Temperature regulation impaired

28°, 26°, 24° — Temperature regulation lost

FIGURE 10-2 Temperature regulation by the hypothalamus.

carries the excess heat from the core to the periphery, where it is close to the skin. This allows heat to dissipate through the skin into the environment.

Conversely, when the environment is too cold, *countercurrent heat exchange* is used to shunt warm blood away from the superficial veins near the skin and back into the deep veins near the core to keep vital structures warm. Another body response that counters a cold environment is shivering, a physical activity that increases metabolism and generates heat.

It is important to note that these various mechanisms can create a difference between the core body temperature and the peripheral body temperature. Core temperature is the crucial measurement because, as noted, the core is where the major organs are located. Therefore, it is important in any heat-related or cold-related emergency to obtain a core temperature reading, such as from the rectum. Oral and axillary temperatures may provide convenient approximations in some situations but may lead

to incorrect interventions if relied on for treatment of the patient with an environmental illness.

Heat Disorders

Disruption of the body's normal thermoregulatory mechanisms can produce a number of heat illnesses, such as hyperthermia and fever. **Heat-related illness** is increased core body temperature (CBT) resulting from inadequate thermolysis (heat loss).[1]

Hyperthermia

Hyperthermia is a state of unusually high body temperature, specifically the core body temperature. Hyperthermia is usually caused by heat transfer from the external environment for which the body cannot compensate. Additionally, it can be caused by excessive generation of heat within the body. Hyperthermia can also occur in conjunction with the use and/or abuse of certain medications (malignant hyperthermia).

As the body attempts to eliminate this excessive heat, you will see the general signs of thermolysis. These signs are caused by the body's two chief methods of heat dissipation, sweating (which leads to evaporative heat loss) and vasodilation (which allows the blood to carry heat to the periphery for dissipation through the skin). These include:

- Diaphoresis (sweating)
- Increased skin temperature
- Flushing

As heat illness progresses, you will also note signs of thermolytic inadequacy (the failure of the body's thermoregulatory mechanisms to compensate adequately):

- Altered mentation
- Altered level of consciousness

Hyperthermia can range from minor heat cramps to heat exhaustion or life-threatening heatstroke, which will be discussed in later sections.

CONTENT REVIEW

➤ Heat Disorders
  - Hyperthermia
  - Heat cramps
  - Heat exhaustion
  - Heatstroke
➤ Heatstroke is a true environmental emergency.

Predisposing Factors

Age, general health, and medications are predisposing factors in hyperthermia. Factors that may contribute to a susceptibility to hyperthermia include:

- *Age of the patient*—Pediatric and geriatric populations can tolerate less variation in temperature, and their heat-regulating mechanisms are not as responsive as those of young adult and adult populations.

- *Health of the patient*—Diabetics can become hyperthermic more easily because they develop **autonomic neuropathy.** This condition damages the autonomic nervous system, which may interfere with thermoregulatory input and with vasodilation and perspiration, which normally dissipate heat.

- *Medications*—Various medications can affect body temperature in the following ways:

  - *Diuretics* predispose to dehydration, which worsens hyperthermia.

  - *Beta-blockers* interfere with vasodilation and reduce the capacity to increase heart rate in response to volume loss, and may also interfere with thermoregulatory input.

  - *Psychotropics and antihistamines,* such as antipsychotics and phenothiazines, interfere with central thermoregulation.

- *Level of acclimatization*—**Acclimatization** is the process of becoming adjusted to a change in environment.

In response to an environmental change, reversible changes in body structure and function take place that help to maintain homeostasis.

- *Length of exposure*
- *Intensity of exposure*
- *Environmental factors* such as humidity and wind (Figure 10-3).

Preventive Measures

Ideally, prevention of heat disorders is preferable to treating an illness already in progress. Measures to prevent hyperthermia include the following:

- Maintain adequate fluid intake, remembering that thirst is an inadequate indicator of dehydration.

- Allow time for gradual acclimatization to being out in the heat. Acclimatization results in more perspiration with lower salt concentration and increases body-fluid volume.

- Limit exposure to hot environments.

Specific Heat Disorders

Inevitably, you will be required to respond to heat-related emergencies: heat cramps, heat exhaustion, or heatstroke. Heat cramps and heat exhaustion result from dehydration and depletion of sodium and other electrolytes. Heatstroke—a far more serious, life-threatening condition—

NOAA's National Weather Service
Heat Index
Temperature (°F)

Relative Humidity (%)	80	82	84	86	88	90	92	94	96	98	100	102	104	106	108	110
40	80	81	83	85	88	91	94	97	101	105	109	114	119	124	130	136
45	80	82	84	87	89	93	96	100	104	109	114	119	124	130	137	
50	81	83	85	88	91	95	99	103	108	113	118	124	131	137		
55	81	84	86	89	93	97	101	106	112	117	124	130	137			
60	82	84	88	91	95	100	105	110	116	123	129	137				
65	82	85	89	93	98	103	108	114	121	128	136					
70	83	86	90	95	100	105	112	119	126	134						
75	84	88	92	97	103	109	116	124	132							
80	84	89	94	100	106	113	121	129								
85	85	90	96	102	110	117	126	135								
90	86	91	98	105	113	122	131									
95	86	93	100	108	117	127										
100	87	95	103	112	121	132										

Likelihood of Heat Disorders with Prolonged Exposure or Strenuous Activity

☐ Caution ☐ Extreme Caution ☐ Danger ☐ Extreme Danger

FIGURE 10-3 The Heat Index. The Heat Index factors in both temperature and relative humidity and provides information about the condition of the environment and problems related to the duration of exposure.

results from the failure of the body's thermoregulatory mechanisms.

Signs and symptoms and emergency care procedures for heat cramps, heat exhaustion, and heatstroke are discussed in the following sections and summarized in Procedure 10-1.

Heat (Muscle) Cramps

Heat cramps are muscle cramps caused by overexertion and dehydration in the presence of high atmospheric temperatures. Sweating occurs as sodium (salt) is transported to the skin. Because "water follows sodium," water is deposited on the skin surface, where evaporation occurs,

Procedure 10-1 Heat Disorders

Condition	Muscle Cramps	Mental Status	Respirations	Pulse	Blood Pressure	Body Temperature	Other Possible
Heat Cramps	Yes	Alert	Normal	Normal	Normal	Normal	Weakness, dizziness, faintness
Heat Exhaustion	Sometimes	Anxiety to possible loss of consciousness	Rapid, shallow	Weak	Normal	Somewhat elevated	Headache, paresthesia, diarrhea
Heatstroke	No	Confusion, disorientation, or loss of consciousness	Deep, rapid; later shallow, slowing	Rapid, full; later slowing	Low	Very high	Seizures

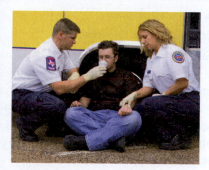

10-1A Heat cramps.

Heat Cramps: Emergency Care

- Remove the patient from hot environment. Place in a cool, shaded, or air-conditioned area.
- Administer oral fluids if patient is alert and able to swallow, or administer an IV of normal saline.

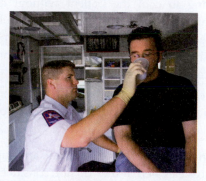

10-1B Heat exhaustion.

Heat Exhaustion: Emergency Care

- Remove the patient from hot environment. Place in a cool, shaded, or air-conditioned area.
- Administer oral fluids if the patient is alert and able to swallow, or administer an IV of normal saline.
- Place the patient in a supine position.
- Remove some clothing and fan the patient. Be careful not to cool to the point of chilling or causing shivering.
- Treat for shock, if suspected; however, do not cover the patient to the point of overheating.

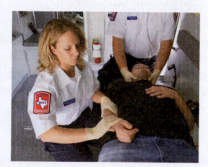

10-1C Heatstroke.

Heatstroke: Emergency Care

- Remove the patient from hot environment. Place in a cool, shaded, or air-conditioned area.
- Initiate rapid active cooling en route to the hospital. Remove the patient's clothing and cover the patient with sheets soaked in tepid water. Lower body temperature to 102°F (39°C). Avoid cooling to a lower temperature.
- Administer supplemental oxygen as needed to correct hypoxia.
- If patient is alert and able to swallow, administer oral fluids. Begin one or two IVs of normal saline, wide open.
- Monitor the ECG.
- Avoid vasopressors and anticholinergic drugs.
- Monitor the body temperature.

aiding in the cooling process. Because sweating involves not only the loss of water but also the loss of electrolytes (such as sodium), intermittent cramping of skeletal muscles may occur. Heat cramps are painful but are not considered to be an actual heat illness.

SIGNS AND SYMPTOMS The patient with heat cramps will present with cramps in the fingers, arms, legs, or abdominal muscles. The patient will generally be mentally alert, with a feeling of weakness, and may feel dizzy or faint. Vital signs will be stable. Body temperature may be normal or slightly elevated. The skin is likely to be moist and warm.

TREATMENT Treatment of the patient with heat cramps is usually easily accomplished:

1. *Remove the patient from the environment.* Place the patient in a cool environment, such as a shaded area or the air-conditioned back of the ambulance.

   In the case of severe cramps:

2. *Administer water or a sports drink.* Do NOT administer salt tablets, which are not absorbed as readily and may cause stomach irritation and ulceration or hypernatremia. *If the patient is unable to take fluids orally, an IV of normal saline may be needed.* Antiemetic medications, such as ondansetron, can be effective in assisting the patient with oral intake.

3. *Educate.* Educate the patient that heat cramps may indicate that he is at risk for heat exhaustion or heatstroke if he continues his current activity without appropriate cooling or hydration.

Some EMS systems recommend massaging the painful muscles. Application of moist towels to the patient's forehead and over the cramped muscles may also be helpful.

Heat Exhaustion

Heat exhaustion, which is considered to be a mild heat illness, is an acute reaction to heat exposure. It is the most common heat-related illness seen by prehospital personnel. An individual performing work in a hot environment will lose 1 to 2 liters of water an hour. Each liter lost contains 20 to 50 milliequivalents of sodium. The resulting loss of water and sodium, combined with general vasodilation, leads to a decreased circulating blood volume, venous pooling, and reduced cardiac output.

Dehydration and electrolyte loss from sweating often account for the presenting signs and symptoms. However, these signs and symptoms are not exclusive to heat exhaustion. Instead, they mimic those of an individual suffering from fluid and sodium loss from any of a number of other causes. A history of exposure to high environmental temperatures is needed to obtain an accurate assessment.

If not treated, heat exhaustion may progress to heatstroke.

SIGNS AND SYMPTOMS Signs and symptoms that you may encounter include increased body temperature (over 100°F, or 37.8°C), skin that is cool and clammy with heavy perspiration, breathing that is rapid and shallow, and a weak pulse. There may be signs of active thermolysis, such as diarrhea and muscle cramps. The patient will feel weak and, in some cases, may lose consciousness. If the patient shows any signs of central nervous system (CNS) symptoms, such as headache, anxiety, paresthesia, impaired judgment, and even psychosis, then the patient should be treated for heatstroke.

TREATMENT Prehospital management of the patient with heat exhaustion is aimed at immediate cooling and fluid replacement. Steps include:

1. *Remove the patient from the environment.* Place the patient in a cool environment, such as a shaded area or the air-conditioned ambulance.

2. *Place the patient in a supine position.*

3. *Administer water or a sports drink.* Do NOT administer salt tablets, which are not absorbed as readily and may cause stomach irritation and ulceration or hypernatremia. Antiemetic medications, such as ondansetron, can be effective in assisting the patient with oral intake. *If the patient is unable to take fluids orally, an IV of normal saline may be needed.*

4. *Remove some clothing and fan the patient.* Remove enough clothing to cool the patient without chilling him. Fanning increases evaporation and cooling. Again, be careful not to cool the patient to the point of chilling. If the patient begins to shiver, stop fanning and perhaps cover the patient lightly.

5. *Treat for shock, if shock is suspected.* However, be careful not to cover the patient to the point of overheating him.

Symptoms should resolve with fluids, rest, and supine posturing with knees elevated. If they do not, consider that the symptoms may be due to an increased core body temperature, which is predictive of impending heatstroke and should be treated aggressively, as outlined in the following section. The decision to transport the patient should be based on local protocols. The range of heat exhaustion is wide—some patients may respond quickly to cooling and fluids, requiring no additional treatment, whereas others progress rapidly to heatstroke despite aggressive measures.

Heatstroke

Heatstroke is a true environmental emergency that occurs when the body's hypothalamic temperature regulation is lost, causing uncompensated hyperthermia. This, in turn, causes cell death and damage to the brain, liver, and kidneys. There is no arbitrary core temperature at which heatstroke begins. However, heatstroke is generally characterized by a body temperature of at least 105°F (40.6°C), CNS disturbances, and usually the cessation of sweating.

SIGNS AND SYMPTOMS Sweating is thought to stop because of destruction of the sweat glands or when sensory overload causes them to dysfunction temporarily. However, the patient's skin may be either dry or covered with sweat that is still present on the skin from earlier exertion. In either case, the skin will be hot.

The patient may present with the following signs and symptoms:

- Cessation of sweating
- Hot skin that is dry or moist
- Very high core temperature
- Deep respirations that become shallow; rapid at first but may later slow
- Rapid, full pulse; may slow later
- Hypotension with low or absent diastolic reading
- Confusion or disorientation or unconsciousness
- Central nervous system (CNS) symptoms such as headache, anxiety, paresthesia, impaired judgment, or psychosis
- Possible seizures

Classic heatstroke commonly presents in those with chronic illnesses, with the increased core body temperature caused by deficient thermoregulatory function. Predisposing conditions include age, diabetes, and other medical conditions. In this type of heatstroke hot, red, dry skin is common.

Exertional heatstroke commonly presents in those who are in good general health, with the increased core body temperature caused by overwhelming heat stress. There is excessive ambient temperature, as well as excessive exertion with prolonged exposure and poor acclimatization. In this type of heatstroke you will find that, although sweating has ceased and the skin is hot, moisture from prior sweating may still be present.

If the patient develops heatstroke from exertion, he may go into severe metabolic acidosis caused by lactic acid accumulation. Hyperkalemia (excessive potassium in blood) may also develop because of the release of potassium from injured muscle cells, renal failure, or metabolic acidosis.

TREATMENT Prehospital management of the heatstroke patient is aimed at immediate cooling and replacement of fluids. Steps include:

1. *Remove the patient from the environment.* This first step is essential. If you do not remove the patient from the hot environment, any other measures will be only minimally useful. Move the patient to a cool environment, such as the air-conditioned ambulance.

2. *Initiate rapid active cooling.* Body temperature must be lowered to 102°F (39°C). (A target of 102°F [39°C] is used to avoid an overshoot.) This can be accomplished en route to the hospital. Remove the patient's clothing and cover the patient with sheets soaked in tepid water. Fanning and misting may also be used, if necessary. Refrain from overcooling, as this may cause reflex hypothermia (low body temperature). This results in shivering, which can raise the core temperature again. Tepid water is used because ice packs and cold-water immersion may affect peripheral thermoreceptors, producing reflex vasoconstriction and shivering.

3. *Administer oxygen if the patient is hypoxic.* Administer supplemental oxygen as needed to correct hypoxia. If respirations are shallow, assist with a bag-valve-mask unit supplied with supplemental oxygen. Utilize pulse oximetry.

4. *Administer fluid therapy if the patient is alert and able to swallow.*
   - *Oral fluids.* If the patient can tolerate oral fluids, these may be administered initially. Sports drinks are preferred. Antiemetics, such as ondansetron, can be used to treat nausea and vomiting.
   - *Intravenous fluids.* Begin one or two IVs, using normal saline. Initially infuse them wide open.

5. *Monitor the ECG.* Cardiac arrhythmias may occur at any time. ST segment depression, nonspecific T wave changes with occasional PVCs, and supraventricular tachycardias are common.

6. *Avoid vasopressors and anticholinergic drugs.* These agents may potentiate heatstroke by inhibiting sweating. They can also produce a hypermetabolic state in the presence of high environmental temperatures and relatively high humidity.

7. *Monitor body temperature.* EMS systems operating in extremely warm climates should carry some device to record the body temperature, whether a simple rectal thermometer or a sophisticated electronic device. Simple glass thermometers generally do not measure above 106°F (41°C) or below 95°F (35°C). This may become significant during long transport when it is essential to detect changes in the patient's condition.

Role of Dehydration in Heat Disorders

Dehydration often goes hand in hand with heat disorders because it inhibits vasodilation and, therefore, thermolysis. Dehydration leads to orthostatic hypotension (increased pulse and decreased blood pressure on rising from a supine position). The following symptoms may occur along with the signs and symptoms of heatstroke:

- Nausea, vomiting, and abdominal distress
- Vision disturbances
- Decreased urine output
- Poor skin turgor
- Signs of hypovolemic shock

When these signs and symptoms are present, rehydration of the patient is critical. Oral fluids may be administered if the patient is alert and not nauseated. Administration of IV fluids may be necessary, especially if the patient has an altered mental status or is nauseated. It is not uncommon for the adult patient with moderate to severe dehydration to require 2 to 3 liters of IV fluids (occasionally more!).

Fever (Pyrexia)

A fever (**pyrexia**) is the elevation of the body temperature above the normal temperature for that person. (An individual person's normal temperature may be one or two degrees above or below 98.6°F, or 37°C.) The body develops a fever when pathogens enter and cause infection, which in turn stimulates the production of pyrogens.

Pyrogens are any substances that cause fever, such as viruses and bacteria or substances produced within the body in response to infection or inflammation. They reset the hypothalamic thermostat to a higher level. Metabolism is increased, which produces the elevation of temperature. The increased body temperature fights infection by making the body a less hospitable environment for the invading organism. The hypothalamic thermostat will reset to normal when pyrogen production stops or when pathogens end their attack on the body.

Fever is sometimes difficult to differentiate from heatstroke, and neurologic symptoms may present with either, but there is usually a history of infection or illness with a fever. The heatstroke patient usually has a history of exertion and exposure to high ambient temperatures, but this is not always the case. In some cases, heatstroke can be caused by impaired functioning of the hypothalamus without exertion or exposure to ambient heat. Treat for heatstroke if you are unsure which it is.

Although fever may be beneficial, it can be disconcerting to the parents of children with fever. In addition, fever can be uncomfortable for the patient. If the patient is uncomfortable, measures should be taken to treat the fever. Also, if a child has a history of febrile seizures, the fever should be treated. Parents will often have their febrile children wrapped in several layers of clothing or blankets because the child is "cold." These should be

removed, leaving only the diaper or underclothes, exposing the child to the ambient air. This will allow a controlled cooling.

Sponge baths and cool-water immersion should not be used. These cause a rapid drop in the body core temperature and result in shivering. This again elevates the core temperature, which complicates the process. Several medications are good antipyretics (that is, they lower body temperature in fever). These include acetaminophen (Tylenol) and ibuprofen (Motrin). Many EMS systems will utilize an antipyretic in the treatment of fever, particularly in pediatric patients. Liquid acetaminophen and ibuprofen are easy to administer and effective. Acetaminophen is also available in a suppository form for patients with active vomiting. These antipyretics are typically dosed based on the patient's weight:

- *Acetaminophen*—15 mg/kg for pediatric patients; adult dose is typically 650–1,000 mg
- *Ibuprofen*—10 mg/kg for pediatric patients; adult dose is typically 600–800 mg

These liquid medications should be dosed with syringes, as teaspoons are inaccurate measuring devices. EMS services with prolonged transport times should consider the use of antipyretics for patient comfort as well as for the prevention of febrile seizures.

Cold Disorders

Disruption of the body's normal thermoregulation may produce cold-related disorders such as hypothermia, frostbite, and trench foot.

Hypothermia

Hypothermia is a state of low body temperature—specifically, low core temperature. When the core temperature of the body drops below 95°F (35°C), an individual is considered to be hypothermic. Hypothermia can be attributed to inadequate thermogenesis, excessive cold stress, or a combination of both. It is now a common practice to initiate induced therapeutic hypothermia (ITH) following resuscitation of cardiac arrest victims. Because of this, it is important to differentiate ITH from accidental hypothermia. Although much of this discussion relates to both, we will primarily address accidental hypothermia.

> **CONTENT REVIEW**
> ➤ Cold Disorders
> • Hypothermia
> • Frostbite
> • Trench foot
> ➤ Do not thaw frozen flesh if there is any possibility of refreezing. Do not massage the frozen area or rub it with snow.

Mechanisms of Heat Conservation and Loss

Exposure to cold normally triggers compensatory mechanisms designed to conserve and generate heat to maintain a normal body temperature. One such mechanism is piloerection (hair standing on end, "goose bumps") to impede airflow across the skin. Shivering and increased muscle tone occur, resulting in increased metabolism. Peripheral vasoconstriction occurs, with an increase in cardiac output and respiratory rate. When these mechanisms can no longer adequately compensate for heat lost from the body surface, the body temperature falls. As the body temperature falls, so do the metabolic rate and cardiac output.

As discussed, the major mechanisms of body heat loss are conduction, convection, radiation, evaporation, and respiration. Heat loss can be increased by the removal of clothing (decreased insulation, increased radiation), the wetting of clothing by rain or snow (increased conduction and evaporation), air movement around the body (increased convection), or contact with a cold surface or cold-water immersion (increased conduction).

Predisposing Factors

Several factors can contribute to the risk of developing hypothermia. They also contribute to the severity of damage if cold injury occurs. Risk factors that increase the danger of developing hypothermia include:

- *Age of the patient*—Pediatric or geriatric patients cannot tolerate cold environments and have less responsive heat-generating mechanisms to combat cold exposure. Elderly persons often become hypothermic in environments that seem only mildly cool to others.

- *Health of the patient*—Hypothyroidism suppresses metabolism, preventing patients from responding appropriately to cold stress. Malnutrition, diabetes, Parkinson's disease, fatigue, and other medical conditions can interfere with the body's ability to combat cold exposure.

- *Medications*—Some drugs interfere with proper heat-generating mechanisms. These include narcotics, alcohol, phenothiazines, barbiturates, antiseizure medications, antihistamines and other allergy medications, antipsychotics, sedatives, antidepressants, and various pain medications such as aspirin, acetaminophen, and NSAIDs.

- *Prolonged or intense exposure*—The length and severity of cold exposure have a direct effect on morbidity and mortality (Figure 10-4).

- *Coexisting weather conditions*—High humidity, brisk winds, or accompanying rain can all magnify the effect of cold exposure on the human body by accelerating the loss of heat from skin surfaces.

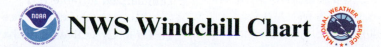

NWS Windchill Chart

Wind (mph)	Temperature (°F)																	
Calm	40	35	30	25	20	15	10	5	0	-5	-10	-15	-20	-25	-30	-35	-40	-45
5	36	31	25	19	13	7	1	-5	-11	-16	-22	-28	-34	-40	-46	-52	-57	-63
10	34	27	21	15	9	3	-4	-10	-16	-22	-28	-35	-41	-47	-53	-59	-66	-72
15	32	25	19	13	6	0	-7	-13	-19	-26	-32	-39	-45	-51	-58	-64	-71	-77
20	30	24	17	11	4	-2	-9	-15	-22	-29	-35	-42	-48	-55	-61	-68	-74	-81
25	29	23	16	9	3	-4	-11	-17	-24	-31	-37	-44	-51	-58	-64	-71	-78	-84
30	28	22	15	8	1	-5	-12	-19	-26	-33	-39	-46	-53	-60	-67	-73	-80	-87
35	28	21	14	7	0	-7	-14	-21	-27	-34	-41	-48	-55	-62	-69	-76	-82	-89
40	27	20	13	6	-1	-8	-15	-22	-29	-36	-43	-50	-57	-64	-71	-78	-84	-91
45	26	19	12	5	-2	-9	-16	-23	-30	-37	-44	-51	-58	-65	-72	-79	-86	-93
50	26	19	12	4	-3	-10	-17	-24	-31	-38	-45	-52	-60	-67	-74	-81	-88	-95
55	25	18	11	4	-3	-11	-18	-25	-32	-39	-46	-54	-61	-68	-75	-82	-89	-97
60	25	17	10	3	-4	-11	-19	-26	-33	-40	-48	-55	-62	-69	-76	-84	-91	-98

Frostbite Times ■ 30 minutes ■ 10 minutes ■ 5 minutes

Wind Chill (°F) = $35.74 + 0.6215T - 35.75(V^{0.16}) + 0.4275T(V^{0.16})$

Where, T= Air Temperature (°F)   V= Wind Speed (mph)   *Effective 11/01/01*

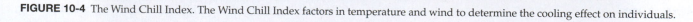

FIGURE 10-4 The Wind Chill Index. The Wind Chill Index factors in temperature and wind to determine the cooling effect on individuals.

Preventive Measures

Certain precautions can decrease the risk of morbidity related to cold injury.

- Dress warmly.
- Get plenty of rest to maximize the ability of heat-generating mechanisms to replenish energy supplies.
- Eat appropriately and at regular intervals to support metabolism.
- Limit exposure to cold environments.

Degrees of Hypothermia

There are several hypothermia classification schemes. The two-tiered hypothermia classification system classifies the patient as having mild or severe hypothermia, as follows:

- *Mild hypothermia*—a core temperature greater than 90°F (32°C) with signs and symptoms of hypothermia
- *Severe hypothermia*—a core temperature less than 90°F (32°C) with signs and symptoms of hypothermia

The three-tiered hypothermia classification system classifies the patient as having mild, moderate, or severe hypothermia, as follows:

- *Mild hypothermia*—a core temperature between 90°F and 95°F (32°C to 35°C) with signs and symptoms of hypothermia:
  - Tachycardia
  - Shivering
  - Vasoconstriction
  - Tachypnea
  - Fatigue
  - Impaired judgment
- *Moderate hypothermia*—a core temperature between 82°F and 90°F (28°C to 32°C) with signs and symptoms of hypothermia:
  - Cold-induced arrhythmia (bradycardia, Osborn wave)
  - Hypotension
  - Respiratory depression
  - Altered mental status
  - Loss of shivering
- *Severe hypothermia*—a core temperature less than 82°F (28°C) with signs and symptoms of hypothermia:
  - Coma
  - Apnea
  - Ventricular arrhythmias or asystole

Initially, some patients may exhibit *compensated* hypothermia. In this case, signs and symptoms of hypothermia will be present but with a normal core body temperature, temporarily maintained by thermogenesis. As energy stores from the liver and muscle glycogen are exhausted, the core body temperature will drop.

The onset of symptoms may be *acute*, as occurs when a person suddenly falls through ice into a frigid lake. *Subacute* exposure can occur in situations such as when mountain climbers are trapped in a snowy, cold environment. Finally, *chronic* exposure to cold is a growing problem in our inner cities, where homeless people endure frequent and prolonged cold stress without shelter.

In some cases, cold exposure is the primary cause of hypothermia, but in others, hypothermia may develop secondary to other problems, such as medical problems. For example, hypothyroidism depresses the body's heat-producing mechanisms. Brain tumors or head trauma can depress the hypothalamic temperature control center, causing hypothermia. Other conditions, such as myocardial infarction, diabetes, hypoglycemia, drugs, poor nutrition, sepsis, or old age, can also contribute to metabolic and circulatory disorders that predispose to hypothermia. Any patient thought to have hypothermia, but with no history of exposure to a cold environment, should be assessed for any predisposing factors. Evaluate the patient for level of consciousness, cool skin, and shivering. Also, evaluate the rectal temperature. A rectal temperature of less than 95°F (35°C) indicates hypothermia. Key findings at different degrees of hypothermia are summarized in Table 10-1.

Patients who experience body temperatures above 86°F (30°C) will usually have a favorable prognosis. Those with temperatures below 86°F (30°C) show a significant increase in mortality rate. Remember that most thermometers used in medicine do not register below 95°F (35°C). EMS systems in colder areas should carry special thermometers for recording subnormal temperature readings because there is no reliable correlation between signs and symptoms and actual core body temperature.

Assessment and Management of Hypothermia

Signs and Symptoms

Signs and symptoms of hypothermia are summarized in Table 10-2. Patients experiencing mild hypothermia (core temperature >90°F or 32°C) will generally exhibit shivering. The patient may be lethargic and somewhat dulled mentally. (In some cases, however, the patient may be fully oriented.) Muscles may be stiff and uncoordinated, causing the patient to walk with a stumbling, staggering gait.

Table 10-1 Key Findings at Different Degrees of Hypothermia

C°	F°	Clinical Findings
37.6	99.6	Normal rectal temperature
37	98.6	Normal oral temperature
36	96.8	Metabolic rate increased
35	95	Maximum shivering seen
		Impaired judgment
34	93.2	Amnesia
		Slurred speech
33	91.4	Severe clouding of consciousness/apathy
		Uncoordinated movement
32	89.6	Most shivering ceases
		Pupils dilate
31	87.8	Blood pressure may no longer be obtainable
30	86	Atrial fibrillation/other arrhythmias develop
		Pulse and cardiac output decreased by 33 percent
29	84.2	Progressive decrease in pulse and breathing
		Progressive decrease in level of consciousness
28	82.4	Pulse and oxygen consumption decreased by 50 percent
		Severe slowing of respiration
		Increased muscle rigidity
		Loss of consciousness
		High risk of ventricular fibrillation
27	80.6	Loss of reflexes and voluntary movement
		Patients appear clinically dead
26	78.8	No reflexes or response to painful stimuli
25	77	Cerebral blood flow decreased by 66 percent
24	75.2	Marked hypotension
22	71.6	Maximum risk for ventricular fibrillation
19	66.2	Flat electroencephalogram (EEG)
18	64.4	Asystole
16	60.8	Lowest reported adult survival from accidental exposure
15.2	59.2	Lowest reported infant survival from accidental exposure
10	50	Oxygen consumption 8 percent of normal
9	48.2	Lowest reported survival from therapeutic exposure

Table 10-2 Hypothermia: Signs and Symptoms

Mild	Severe
Lethargy	No shivering
Shivering	Arrhythmias, asystole
Lack of coordination	Loss of voluntary muscle control
Pale, cold, dry skin	Hypotension
Early rise in blood pressure, heart, and respiratory rates	Undetectable pulse and respirations

indicated for anyone experiencing hypothermia. The ECG will frequently show pathognomonic (indicative of a disease) **J waves**, also called *Osborn waves*, associated with the QRS complexes (Figure 10-5), but these are not useful diagnostically. Atrial fibrillation is the most common presenting arrhythmia seen in hypothermia. As the body cools, however, the myocardium becomes progressively more irritable and may develop a variety of arrhythmias. In severe hypothermia, bradycardia is inevitable.

Ventricular fibrillation becomes more probable as the body's core temperature falls below 86°F (30°C). The severely hypothermic patient requires assessment of pulse and respirations for at least 30 seconds every 1 to 2 minutes.

Treatment

All victims of hypothermia should have the following care (Figure 10-6):

1. *Remove wet garments.*
2. *Protect against further heat loss and wind chill.* **Use passive external warming** methods such as application of blankets, insulating materials, and moisture barriers.
3. *Maintain the patient in a horizontal position.*
4. *Avoid rough handling,* which can trigger arrhythmias.
5. *Monitor the core temperature.*
6. *Monitor the cardiac rhythm.*

ACTIVE REWARMING Victims of mild hypothermia may also be rewarmed using *active external methods.* This

Patients experiencing severe hypothermia (core temperature <90°F or 32°C) may be disoriented and confused. As their temperatures continue to fall, they will proceed into stupor and complete coma. Shivering will usually stop, and physical activity will become uncoordinated. Muscles may be stiff and rigid. Continuous cardiac monitoring is

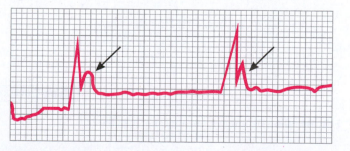

FIGURE 10-5 ECG tracing showing J wave following the QRS complex as seen in hypothermia.

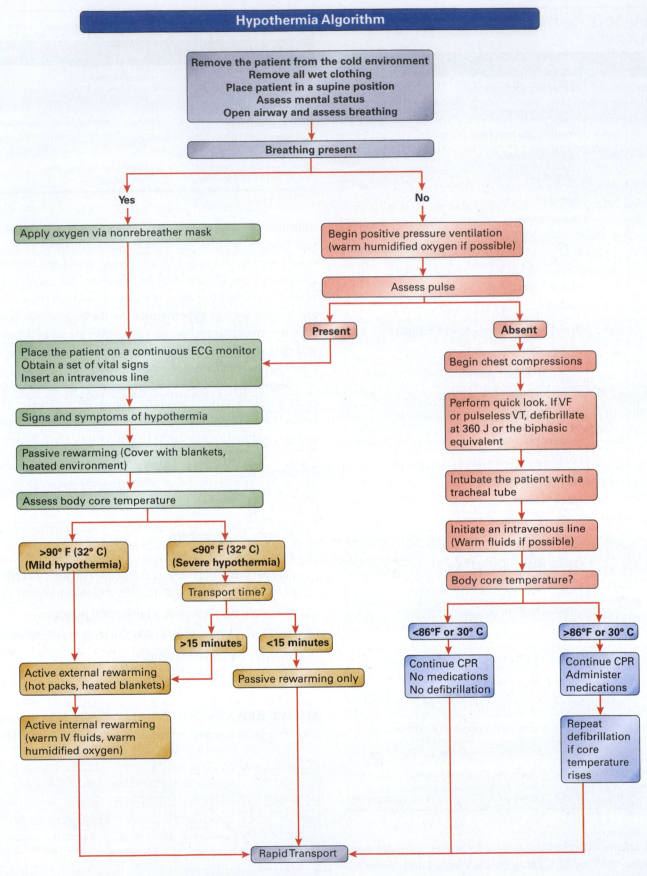

FIGURE 10-6 Algorithm for treatment of hypothermia.

includes the use of warmed blankets and/or heat packs placed over areas of high heat transfer with the core: the base of the neck, the axilla, and the groin. Be sure to insulate between the heat packs and the skin to prevent burning. Intravenous fluid heaters can be used to heat the IV fluid to 95°F to 100°F (35°C to 38°C). If not available, use warmed IV fluids. Heat guns and lights may also be used, but this will most likely take place in the emergency department. Warm-water immersion in water between 102°F and 104°F (39°C to 40°C) may be used, but can induce rewarming shock (see the next section), so this method also has little application in an out-of-hospital setting.

Active rewarming of the severely hypothermic patient is best carried out in the hospital using a prearranged protocol. Most patients who die during rewarming die from ventricular fibrillation, the risk of which is related to both the depth and the duration of hypothermia. Rough handling of the hypothermic patient may also induce ventricular fibrillation (Figure 10-7). Active rewarming should not be attempted in the field unless travel to the emergency department will take more than 15 minutes.

If such is the case, *active internal rewarming* methods may also be used, including the use of warmed (102°F to 104°F or 39°C to 40°C) humidified oxygen and administration of warmed IV fluids (also warmed to 102°F to 104°F, or 39°C to 40°C). This is crucial to prevent further heat loss, but actual heat transferred is minimal, so there is limited contribution to the rewarming effort.

REWARMING SHOCK Although application of warmed blankets is a safe and effective means of rewarming the hypothermic patient, application of external heat, as with heat packs, is usually not recommended in the prehospital setting. For effective rewarming, more heat transference is

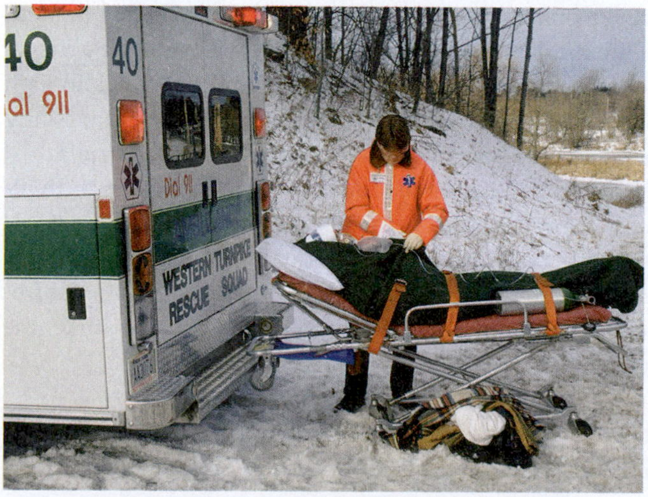

FIGURE 10-7 The hypothermia patient should be handled gently because of myocardial irritability.

generally required than is possible with prehospital methods. Additionally, application of external heat may result in *rewarming shock* by causing reflex peripheral vasodilation. This reflex vasodilation causes the return of cool blood and acids from the extremities to the core. This may cause a paradoxical "afterdrop" core temperature decrease and further worsen core hypothermia. This, in turn, may cause the blood pressure to fall, especially when there is also volume depletion.

If active rewarming is necessary in the prehospital setting (e.g., when transport is delayed), administration of warmed IV fluids during rewarming can prevent the onset of rewarming shock.

COLD DIURESIS Volume depletion can occur as a result of *cold diuresis*. Core vasoconstriction causes increased blood volume and blood pressure, so the kidneys remove excess fluid to reduce the pressure, thus causing diuresis. A warmed IV volume expander (e.g., normal saline) should be used both to prevent rewarming shock and to replace fluid lost from cold diuresis.[2]

The conscious patient who is able to manage his airway may be given warmed, sweetened fluids. Alcohol and caffeine should be avoided.

Resuscitation

There are certain resuscitation considerations when handling cardiac arrest victims with core temperatures below 86°F (30°C).

BASIC CARDIAC LIFE SUPPORT BLS providers should start cardiopulmonary resuscitation (CPR) immediately, although pulse and respirations may need to be checked for longer periods to detect minimal cardiopulmonary efforts. Use normal chest compression and ventilation rates and ventilate with warmed, humidified oxygen. If an AED is available and ventricular fibrillation is detected, a single shock at 360 joules (or the biphasic equivalent) may be given. Further shocks should be avoided until after rewarming to above 86°F. CPR, rewarming, and rapid transport should immediately follow the three defibrillation attempts.

ADVANCED CARDIAC LIFE SUPPORT Because there is no increased risk of inducing ventricular fibrillation from orotracheal or nasotracheal intubation, ALS providers may intubate the patient and ventilate with warmed, humidified oxygen. Drug metabolism is reduced, however, so administered medications such as epinephrine and amiodarone may accumulate to toxic levels if used repeatedly in the severely hypothermic patient. In addition, administered drugs may remain in the peripheral circulation. When the patient is rewarmed and perfusion resumes, large, toxic boluses of these medications may be delivered to the central circulation and target tissues.

Patho Pearls

Some Cautions about Rewarming. It is important to remember that rewarming of a hypothermic patient must occur in conjunction with resuscitation. In addition, rewarming is most effective if active internal warming techniques are used (warmed IV fluids; warmed, humidified oxygen). It is virtually impossible to rewarm a hypothermic patient in the prehospital setting using external rewarming techniques alone.

During rewarming, as the patient's external surfaces (skin) begin to warm, blood vessels within the skin and extremities dilate. When this occurs, cool blood from the skin and extremities is shunted toward the core of the body. In addition, metabolic acids, such as lactic acid and pyruvic acid, which may have accumulated in the skin and extremities as a result of poor perfusion, are also shunted to the body's core structures. The influx of cool blood from the extremities can activate temperature sensors in the core and cause the hypothalamus to attempt to warm the body. This can lead to "rewarming shock" and can actually make the patient worse.

So if you do not have the capability of providing active internal rewarming for the severely hypothermic patient, simply try to prevent additional heat loss and transport the patient emergently to a facility where effective rewarming can take place.[3]

The American Heart Association recommends that, if the patient fails to respond to initial defibrillation attempts or initial drug therapy, subsequent defibrillations or boluses of medication should be avoided until the core temperature is about 86°F (30°C). This is because it is generally impossible to electrically defibrillate a heart that is colder than 86°F. Active core rewarming techniques are the primary modality in hypothermia patients who are either in cardiac arrest or unconscious with a slow heart rate.

Techniques that may be used include the administration of heated, humidified oxygen and warmed intravenous fluids, preferably normal saline, infused centrally at rates of 150 to 200 mL/hour to avoid overhydration. Peritoneal lavage with warmed potassium-free fluid administered 2 L at a time may be used, as may extracorporeal blood warming with partial cardiac bypass. Obviously, some of these techniques may be carried out only in a hospital setting.

Transportation

When transporting a hypothermic patient, remember that gentle transportation is necessary because of myocardial irritability and that the patient should be kept level or slightly inclined with head down. Contact the receiving hospital for general rewarming options. When determining your destination, consider the availability of cardiac bypass rewarming.

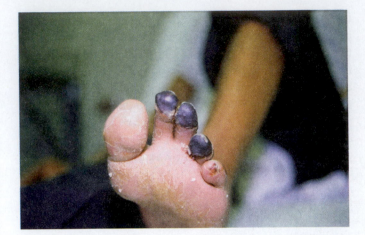

FIGURE 10-8 Frostbite.

(© Edward T. Dickinson, MD)

Frostbite

Frostbite is environmentally induced freezing of body tissues (Figure 10-8). As the tissues freeze, ice crystals form within and water is drawn out of the cells into the extracellular space. These ice crystals expand, causing the destruction of cells. During this process, intracellular electrolyte concentrations increase, further destroying cells. Damage to blood vessels from ice crystal formation causes loss of vascular integrity, resulting in tissue swelling and loss of distal nutritional flow.

Superficial and Deep Frostbite

Generally, there are two types of frostbite: superficial and deep. **Superficial frostbite** (also called *frostnip*) exhibits some freezing of epidermal tissue, resulting in initial redness, followed by blanching. There will also be diminished sensation. **Deep frostbite** affects the epidermal and subcutaneous layers. There is a white appearance and the area feels hard (frozen) to palpation. There is also loss of sensation in deep frostbite.

Frostbite mainly occurs in the extremities and in areas of the head and face exposed to the environment. Subfreezing temperatures are required for frostbite to occur, although they are not necessary to produce hypothermia. Many patients who have frostbite will also have hypothermia.

There can be tremendous variation in how an individual can present with frostbite. For example, some patients feel little pain at onset. Others will report severe pain. A certain degree of compliance may be felt beneath the frozen layer in superficial frostbite, but in deep frostbite, the frozen part will be hard and noncompliant.

Treatment

In treating frostbite, take the following recommended steps:

- Do not thaw the affected area if there is any possibility of refreezing.

- Do not massage the frozen area or rub with snow. Rubbing the affected area may cause ice crystals within the tissues to damage the already injured tissues more seriously.

- Administer analgesia prior to thawing.

- Transport to the hospital for rewarming by immersion. If transport will be delayed, thaw the frozen part by immersion in a 102°F to 104°F (39°C to 40°C) water bath. Water temperature will fall rapidly, requiring additions of warm water throughout the process.

- Cover the thawed part with loosely applied dry, sterile dressings.

- Elevate and immobilize the thawed part.

- Do not puncture or drain blisters.

- Do not rewarm frozen feet if they are required for walking out of a hazardous situation.

Trench Foot

Trench foot (also called *immersion foot*) is similar to frostbite, but it occurs at temperatures above freezing. It is rarely seen in the civilian population. It received its name in World War I, when troops confined to trenches with standing, cold water developed progressive symptoms over days. Symptoms are similar to those of frostbite, but there may be pain. Blisters may form on spontaneous rewarming.

Treatment

Treatment of trench foot requires early recognition of developing symptoms and immediate steps to warm, dry, aerate, and elevate the feet. Measures to prevent trench foot are most effective, such as avoiding prolonged exposure to standing water, changing wet socks frequently, and never sleeping in wet boots or socks.

Drowning

Drowning is defined as the *process* of experiencing respiratory impairment as the result of submersion or immersion in a liquid. There are three possible outcomes from a drowning incident:

- Mortality (death)

- Morbidity (having medical problems)

- No morbidity (no problems)

Before 2002, there were many different definitions and terms related to "drowning." These varied definitions created confusion about the best techniques for prevention, rescue, and treatment. When the new definition was adopted in 2005 by the World Health Organization (WHO), American Heart Association (AHA), and other agencies,

they recommended abandoning previous definitions and outdated terms. These outdated terms include "near drowning," "dry drowning," and "wet drowning." The next paragraph briefly discusses these terms in their historical context.[4]

"Near drowning" was loosely used to identify persons who survived the initial drowning incident—yet who later either survived or died. "Dry drowning" and "wet drowning" were used to describe whether the patient experienced laryngospasm during the drowning process. We now understand that this phenomenon is not clinically relevant.

It is estimated that annually more than 4,500 persons in the United States die from drowning. However, it is difficult to know the actual number of persons who die each year from drowning in the United States, because disaster-related drowning deaths (e.g., from floods or hurricanes) are considered natural-disaster deaths. Similarly, drowning incidents that occur from boats are counted as boating injuries. Additionally, for every drowning death in the United States, two people drown and survive with no morbidity, whereas an additional two people survive with some morbidity (usually severe neurologic impairment).

Altogether, these make drowning the third most frequent cause of accidental death in the United States. Approximately 40 percent of these deaths occur in children under five years of age, making it the leading cause of death in this age group. There is a second peak incidence in teenagers, usually occurring during summer months and in a recreational setting. Finally, a third peak is noted in the elderly as a result of accidental bathtub drownings. Approximately 85 percent of drowning victims are male, two-thirds of whom did not know how to swim. Most commonly, these drownings result from freshwater submersion—especially in swimming pools. Commonly, alcohol use by the victim or momentary lapses in attention by the supervising adult are associated with this type of accident.

It is important to note that other emergency conditions are often associated with drowning. If the cause of the submersion is unknown, consider the possibility of trauma and treat the patient accordingly.

In some instances the submersion occurs in cold water, causing hypothermia. Hypothermia slows the body's metabolic processes, thereby decreasing the need for oxygen. If the water is near freezing, this can have a protective effect on organs and tissues that become hypoxic (low in oxygen). If it is just cold, it can complicate the resuscitation.

Pathophysiology of Drowning

As a paramedic, you need to understand the sequence of events that occur in drowning. Following submersion, if the patient is conscious, there will be an initial struggle, with attempted breath holding. This panicked struggle may include stereotypical loud splashing, such as with a teen caught in a river current, or the silent submersion of a three-year-old whose water-wing floats have slipped off. During this stage, the patient makes violent inspiratory and swallowing efforts, often allowing water to enter the mouth, posterior oropharynx, and stomach. If the patient is unconscious when he reaches the water, he will become apneic from an involuntary reflex. During this time, blood is shunted to the heart and brain because of the mammalian diving reflex, which is described later in this chapter.

Thus, with either mechanism (conscious or unconscious), the patient is apneic and not taking in oxygen. When the patient is apneic, the $PaCO_2$ in the blood rises to more than 50 mmHg. Meanwhile, the PaO_2 of the blood falls, often below 50 mmHg. The stimulus from the hypoxia ultimately overrides the sedative effects of the hypercarbia, resulting in central nervous system stimulation. This, in turn, triggers the patient to gasp. Water in the hypopharynx, either from water in the mouth during the struggle or from the final gasp before unconsciousness, often causes reflexive laryngospasm and resultant bronchospasm (Figure 10-9). Because of these mechanisms, usually less than 30 mL of water actually enters the lungs.

The laryngospasm that keeps water out of the lungs further aggravates the hypoxia, ultimately resulting in coma. Persistent anoxia results in a deepening of the coma. Following unresponsiveness, reflex swallowing continues, resulting in gastric distention and increased risk of vomiting and aspiration. If untreated, hypotension, bradycardia, and death result in a short period. The water that enters the lungs—either before laryngospasm or after

laryngeal relaxation—can cause respiratory problems through mechanisms that are critical to understanding the appropriate treatment of drowned persons. First, the presence of water blocks gas exchange at the alveolar level. Secondly, even a small amount of fluid washes away the surfactant, causing atelectasis (alveolar collapse).

Surfactant is the substance in alveoli that is responsible for keeping the alveoli open. In drowning, some surfactant is lost when the capillaries of the alveoli are damaged. Plasma proteins then leak back into the alveoli, resulting in the accumulation of fluid in the small airways. This in turn leads to multiple areas of atelectasis—areas of alveolar collapse. Atelectasis causes shunting, which is the return of deoxygenated blood from the damaged alveoli to the bloodstream. In other words, blood is traveling through the lungs without being oxygenated. The result is hypoxemia (inadequate oxygenation of the blood) (Figure 10-10).

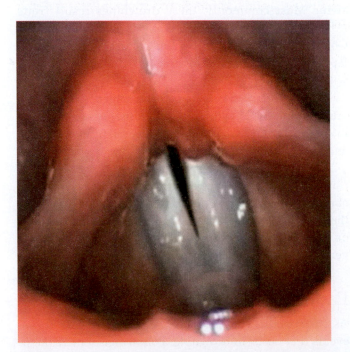

FIGURE 10-9 Laryngospasm as seen in drowning.

(© Dr. Bryan E. Bledsoe)

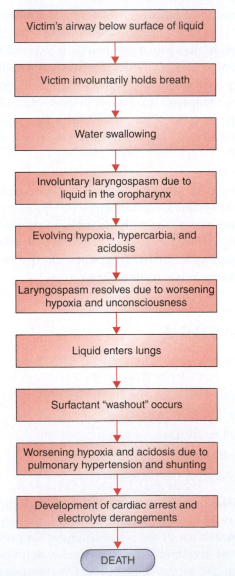

PATHOPHYSIOLOGY OF DROWNING

Victim's airway below surface of liquid

Victim involuntarily holds breath

Water swallowing

Involuntary laryngospasm due to liquid in the oropharynx

Evolving hypoxia, hypercarbia, and acidosis

Laryngospasm resolves due to worsening hypoxia and unconsciousness

Liquid enters lungs

Surfactant "washout" occurs

Worsening hypoxia and acidosis due to pulmonary hypertension and shunting

Development of cardiac arrest and electrolyte derangements

DEATH

FIGURE 10-10 The pathophysiology of drowning.

Drowning morbidity and mortality are primarily due to anoxic brain injury caused by airway obstruction from laryngospasm or aspirated water. If the drowning process is interrupted at any time and does not end in death, the lungs are resilient and generally recover. The patient's outcome is determined by the amount of anoxia that the brain has suffered, and treatment should be directed at reversing anoxia.[5]

Freshwater versus Saltwater Drowning

Based on studies of dogs in the 1960s, it was previously believed that the type of water aspirated would cause different physiologic responses. These studies used massive amounts of water (up to 22 mL/kg), which would be the equivalent of 1,850 mL in a 185-pound adult or 330 mL in a 33-pound child. However, as previously discussed, the amount of water that actually enters the lungs is a low volume (<30 mL) and does not cause hemodilution, electrolyte shifts, or metabolic abnormalities.[6] The prehospital treatment for all drowning persons is the same, regardless of the type of water.

Factors Affecting Survival

A number of factors have an impact on drowning and drowning survival rates. These include the cleanliness of the water, the length of time submerged, and the age and general health of the patient. Children have a longer survival time and a greater probability of a successful resuscitation. The most important factor affecting survival is immediate initiation of bystander CPR. This is why many organizations emphasize that pool owners and other persons around water learn CPR.

There are numerous case reports of adults and children being successfully resuscitated after prolonged (30–60 minutes) periods in cold or near-freezing water. If the patient falls into water that is near freezing (≥10°C/34°F), there may be some protective effect from the mammalian diving reflex. The concept of developing brain death after 4 to 6 minutes without oxygen is not applicable in cases of drowning in near-freezing water. Some patients in cold water (below 68°F) can be resuscitated after 30 minutes or more in cardiac arrest. However, the slower induction of hypothermia generally does not trigger the mammalian diving reflex and leads to a worse outcome. Unfortunately, it is not possible for prehospital providers to predict the outcome, and all persons submerged for less than 60 minutes should be resuscitated. Persons underwater for 60 minutes or longer usually cannot be resuscitated.

A possible contribution to survival in near-freezing water may be the **mammalian diving reflex**. When a person dives into cold water, he reacts to the submersion of the face. Breathing is inhibited, the heart rate becomes bradycardic, and vasoconstriction develops in tissues relatively resistant to hypoxia. Meanwhile, cerebral and cardiac blood flow is maintained. In this way, oxygen is sent and used only where it is immediately needed to sustain life. The colder the water, the more oxygen is diverted to the heart and brain. A common saying in emergency medicine is, "The cold-water drowning patient is not dead until he is warm and dead." In other words, a person who has been submerged in cold water may only seem to be dead, but because of the continued supply of oxygen to the heart and brain that person may indeed still be alive.

Treatment for Drowning

The primary insult of drowning is anoxic brain injury, and treatment should be directed at reversing it. Your approach to a drowning patient should be directed toward reversing his profound hypoxia. Think about your "usual" arrest situation—an adult patient with coronary artery disease who has a sudden myocardial infarction, resulting in ventricular fibrillation and unconsciousness. Even though this patient has poor health, he still has circulating oxygen and will respond to chest compressions and defibrillation. Now think about a drowning patient—an otherwise healthy child or young adult unable to oxygenate or ventilate. The heart continues circulating blood to the brain until nearly all the oxygen has been extracted, then cardiac arrest occurs. The person's blood is now depleted of oxygen and full of waste products (carbon dioxide and metabolic acids).

Take the following steps to correct the hypoxia:

- Remove the patient from the water as soon as possible. This should be performed **ONLY** by a trained rescue swimmer.

- If possible, initiate ventilation while the patient is still in the water. Rescue personnel should wear protective clothing if water temperature is less than 70°F. In moving or open water, it is essential to use personnel specifically trained for this type of rescue.

- Position the patient. Many drowning resuscitations begin on sloped beaches, riverbanks, or boat ramps. The patient should be placed on a flat surface parallel to the water (perpendicular to the slope), so that blood does not pool at the head or the feet (Figure 10-11).

- Administer oxygen at 100 percent concentration.

- Examine the patient for airway patency, breathing, and pulse. If indicated, begin CPR and defibrillation.

- Manage the airway using proper suctioning and airway adjuncts.

- Anticipate vomitus and laryngospasm. Based on your protocols, use suction for vomitus and positive-pressure ventilation, jaw thrust, or RSI (rapid sequence induction) for laryngospasm. Note that many drowning patients will have significant foaming from the mouth and nose. Copious secretions should be cleared,

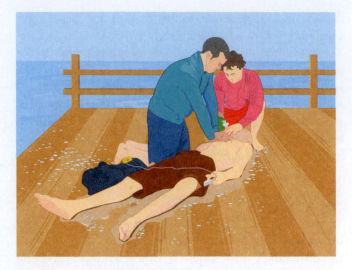

FIGURE 10-11 Proper positioning of the drowning victim parallel to the water and perpendicular to any detected slope.

but focus on oxygenation and ventilation rather than suctioning foam.

- Routine C-spine stabilization is unnecessary unless you suspect a significant mechanism of injury (axial loading). Suspect a head and neck injury if the patient experienced a fall or was diving. Rapidly place the patient on a long backboard before removing him from the water and use C-spine precautions throughout care.

- Protect the patient from heat loss. Avoid laying the patient on a cold surface. Remove wet clothing and cover the body to the extent possible.

- Use respiratory rewarming, if available, and if transport time is longer than 15 minutes.

- Establish an IV of lactated Ringer's or normal saline for venous access and run at 75 mL/hr. If indicated, carry out defibrillation.

- Follow ACLS protocols if the patient is normothermic. If the patient is hypothermic, treat him according to the hypothermia protocol presented earlier in the chapter.

- Resuscitation is not indicated if immersion has been extremely prolonged (unless hypothermia is present) or if there is evidence of putrefaction (decomposition).

Special Considerations

COMPRESSION-ONLY CPR   As previously discussed, drowning causes a hypoxic arrest, and the priority should be oxygenation and ventilation. There is no role for compression-only CPR in drowning resuscitation.

AIRWAY MANAGEMENT   The drowning process inherently makes airway management difficult for BLS and ALS providers. In addition to vomitus and laryngospasm, atelectasis and bronchospasm decrease pulmonary compliance, which translates to more resistance to air entering the lungs. You should anticipate that you will need increased positive

pressure (PEEP or CPAP) while ventilating these patients with a BVM, supraglottic airway, or endotracheal airway.

ABDOMINAL THRUSTS   Previous discussions on drowning resuscitation incorporated the use of abdominal thrusts to "clear" water from the airway. This should never be done. Abdominal thrusts delay oxygenation and ventilation, while increasing the risk of aspiration.

ADULT RESPIRATORY DISTRESS SYNDROME   All drowning patients with respiratory symptoms (cough, foam, crackles [rales], and/or rhonchi) should be transported to the hospital for observation, as some complications may not appear for 24 hours.

Adult respiratory distress syndrome (ARDS) is one of the more severe postresuscitation complications, with a high rate of mortality. The physiologic stress of drowning causes the lungs to leak fluid into the alveoli. This fluid is loaded with chemical factors that cause severe inflammation of the tissues and subsequent failure of the respiratory system. In addition, some of these patients have problems with pulmonary parenchymal injury, destruction of surfactant, aspiration pneumonitis, or pneumothorax. A number require an extended hospital stay because of renal failure, hypoxia, hypercarbia, and mixed metabolic and respiratory acidosis. The resultant effects of cerebral hypoxia are often profound and require treatment throughout hospitalization and beyond.

Diving Emergencies

Scuba diving has become an extremely popular recreational sport. Divers wear portable equipment containing compressed air, which allows the diver to breathe underwater. Although scuba diving accidents are fairly uncommon, inexperienced divers have a higher rate of injury. Scuba diving emergencies can occur on the surface, in 3 feet of water, or at any depth. The more serious emergencies usually occur following a dive. To better assess and care for diving injuries, it is important to understand a few principles of pressure.

The Effects of Air Pressure on Gases

Water is an incompressible liquid. Freshwater has a density, or weight per unit of volume, of 62.4 pounds per cubic foot. Saltwater has a density of 64 pounds per cubic foot. This density can be equated to pressure, which is defined as the weight or force acting on a unit area. Thus, a cubic foot of freshwater exerts a pressure ("weight") of 62.4 pounds over an area of 1 square foot. This measurement is typically stated in pounds per square inch (psi).

Humans at sea level live in an atmosphere of air, which is a mixture of gases. These gases weigh and exert a pressure of 14.7 pounds per square inch (760 mmHg). This pressure, however, may vary within the environment. For example, ascending to an altitude of 1 mile will decrease the atmospheric pressure by 17 percent, to approximately 12.2 pounds.

To understand how air pressure affects diving accidents, we look at three physical laws: Boyle's law, Dalton's law, and Henry's law.

Boyle's Law

Boyle's law states that the volume of a gas is inversely proportional to its pressure if the temperature is kept constant. As pressure increases, the gas is compressed into a smaller space. For example, doubling the pressure of a gas mixture will decrease its volume by one-half. The pressure of air at sea level is 14.7 lb/in^2, or 760 mmHg. This pressure is called 1 "atmosphere absolute" or 1 "ata." Two ata occur at a depth of 33 feet of water, 3 ata occur at a depth of 66 feet of water, and so on. Therefore, 1 L of air at the surface is compressed to 500 mL at 33 feet. At 66 feet, 1 L of air would be compressed to 250 mL.

Dalton's Law

Dalton's law states that the total pressure of a mixture of gases is equal to the sum of the partial pressures of the individual gases. The air we breathe is a mixture of nitrogen (about 78 percent), oxygen (about 21 percent), and carbon dioxide plus traces of argon, helium, and other rare gases (about 1 percent). Because the pressure of air at sea level is 760 mmHg, the pressure of nitrogen is about 593 mmHg, the pressure of oxygen is about 160 mmHg, and the pressure of carbon dioxide is somewhat less than 4 mmHg—each gas exerting its proportion of the total pressure of the mixture.

At different altitudes above sea level or depths below sea level, the pressure of air will change (less at higher altitudes, more at greater depths), but the component gases will still account for the same proportion of whatever the total pressure is at that level: nitrogen 78 percent, oxygen 21 percent, and carbon dioxide less than 1 percent.

Henry's Law

Henry's law states that the amount of gas dissolved in a given volume of fluid is proportional to the pressure of the gas above it. When we descend below sea level, and the pressure bearing down on us increases, the gases that make up the air we breathe tend to dissolve in the liquids (mainly blood plasma) and tissues of the body.

Let us compare what happens to the two chief components of the air we breathe—oxygen and nitrogen—when a person descends to greater and greater depths below sea level. Much of the oxygen is used up in the normal metabolism of the cells, leaving only a small amount to be dissolved in the blood and tissues. Nitrogen, however, is an inert gas and, as such, is not used by the body. Therefore, a far greater quantity of nitrogen is available to dissolve in the blood and tissues as a person descends below sea level. In brief, at depths below sea level, oxygen metabolizes but nitrogen dissolves.

When the person ascends toward sea level again, the gases that are dissolved in the blood and tissues, being under less and less pressure, come out of the blood and tissues and, if the ascent is too rapid, form bubbles. To understand this phenomenon, compare the human body to a bottled carbonated soft drink—that is, a liquid in which carbon dioxide gas is dissolved. The gas is kept dissolved in the liquid by the cap on the bottle and a high-pressure gas under the cap, on top of the liquid. When the cap is removed and the pressure is released, the gas bubbles out of the liquid, causing a fizz that will sometimes rise completely out of the bottle.

In the following sections, we will discuss how the phenomena of gases and pressure can cause serious problems for divers.

Pathophysiology of Diving Emergencies

As noted, gases are dissolved in the diver's blood and tissues under pressure. As the diver goes deeper into the water, pressure increases, causing more gas to dissolve in the blood (Henry's law). According to Boyle's law, these gases will have a smaller volume because of the increased ambient pressure. During *controlled* ascent, with decreasing pressure, dissolved gases come out of the blood and tissues slowly, escaping gradually through respiration.

If ascent is *too rapid*, however, the dissolved gases, mostly nitrogen, come out of solution and expand quickly, forming bubbles in the blood, brain, spinal cord, skin, inner ear, muscles, and joints. Once bubbles of nitrogen have formed in various tissues, it is difficult for the body to remove them. The ascending diver who comes to the surface too rapidly, not adhering to safety measures, is at risk of becoming a veritable living bottle of soda.

Classification of Diving Injuries

Scuba diving injuries are the result of barotrauma, pulmonary overpressure, arterial gas embolism, decompression sickness, cold, panic, or a combination of these. Accidents generally occur at one of the following four stages of a dive:

- On the surface
- During descent
- On the bottom
- During ascent

Injuries on the Surface

Surface injuries can involve any of several factors. One such factor can be entanglement of lines or entanglement in kelp fields while swimming to the area of the dive. Divers in these situations may panic, become fatigued, and even drown. Another factor may be cold water that produces shivering and blackout. Boats in the area are another potential source of injury to the diver. To prevent such accidents, divers will usually mark the area of their dive with a flag. Maritime rules require boat operators to stay clear of a flagged area.

Injuries during Descent

Barotrauma means injuries caused by changes in pressure. Barotrauma during descent is commonly called "the squeeze." It can occur if the diver cannot equilibrate the pressure between the nasopharynx and the middle ear through the eustachian tube. The diver can experience middle ear pain, ringing in the ears, dizziness, and hearing loss. In severe cases, rupture of the eardrum can occur. A diver who has an upper respiratory infection, and who therefore cannot clear the middle ear through the eustachian tube, should not dive. A similar lack of equilibration can occur in the sinuses, producing severe frontal headaches or pain beneath the eye in the maxillary sinuses.

Injuries on the Bottom

Major diving emergencies while at the bottom of the dive often involve **nitrogen narcosis** (a state of stupor), commonly called "raptures of the deep." This is due to the effect on cerebral function of nitrogen or any gas in high concentration (similar to the altered mental status that high carbon dioxide causes in asthmatics). The diver may appear to be intoxicated and may take unnecessary risks. Other emergencies occur when a diver runs low on or out of air. The diver who panics will use more energy and exacerbate this situation by consuming even more oxygen and producing even more carbon dioxide.

Injuries during Ascent

Serious and life-threatening emergencies, many involving barotrauma, can occur during the ascent. For example, as during descent, an ascending diver may be unable to equilibrate inner ear and nasopharyngeal pressure.

Dives below 33 feet may require staged ascent to prevent **decompression sickness**, also called *the bends* or *dysbarism*. This condition develops in divers subjected to rapid reduction of air pressure while ascending to the surface following exposure to compressed air, with formation of expanding nitrogen bubbles causing severe pain, especially in the abdomen and the joints.

The most serious barotrauma that occurs during ascent is injury to the lung from **pulmonary overpressure**. This can occur with a deep dive, or it can occur with a dive of as little as 3 feet below the surface. The injury results from the diver holding his breath during the ascent. As the diver ascends, the air in the lung, which has been compressed, expands. If it is not exhaled, the alveoli may rupture. If this occurs, the result will be structural damage to the lung and, possibly, **arterial gas embolism (AGE)**, an air bubble or air embolism that enters the circulatory system from the damaged lung. Another result may be **pneumomediastinum**, the release of gas (air) through the visceral pleura into the mediastinum and pericardial sac around the heart, as well as into the tissues of the neck. **Pneumothorax** is possible if the alveoli rupture into the pleural cavity. Air embolism can occur if the air ruptures into the pulmonary veins or arteries and returns to the left atrium and finally into the left ventricle and out into the systemic circulation.

General Assessment of Diving Emergencies

In the early assessment of diving accidents, all symptoms of air embolism and decompression sickness are considered together. Early assessment and treatment of a diving injury is of more importance than trying to distinguish the exact problem. One of your most important tasks in a diving-related injury is elicitation of a diving history or profile.[7] The essential factors to consider are as follows:

- Time at which the signs and symptoms occurred
- Type of breathing apparatus utilized
- Type of hypothermia protective garment worn
- Parameters of the dive:
  - Depth of dive(s)
  - Number of dives
  - Duration of dive(s)
- Aircraft travel following a dive (in a pressurized cabin)
- Rate of ascent
- Associated panic forcing rapid ascent
- Experience of the diver, for example, student, inexperienced, or "pro"
- Properly functioning depth gauge
- Previous medical diseases
- Old injuries
- Previous episodes of decompression sickness

- Use of medications
- Use of alcohol

From a quick assessment of the patient's diving profile, you can rapidly determine whether the diver is a likely candidate for a pressure disorder.

Pressure Disorders

Injuries caused by pressure, as noted earlier, are known as *barotrauma*. In the case of diving accidents, most barotrauma results from a pressure imbalance between the external environment and gases within the body. The following sections describe some of the most common forms of barotrauma involved in diving accidents.

Decompression Sickness (Dysbarism)

Decompression sickness develops in divers subjected to rapid reduction of air pressure after ascending to the surface following exposure to compressed air. A number of general and individual factors can contribute to the development of decompression sickness, or the bends (Table 10-3). Decompression sickness results as nitrogen bubbles come out of solution in the blood and tissues, causing increased pressure in various body structures and occluding circulation in the small blood vessels. This occurs in joints, tendons, the spinal

Table 10-3 Factors Related to the Development of Decompression Sickness

General Factors
Cold-water dives
Diving in rough water
Strenuous diving conditions
History of previous decompression dive incident
Overstaying time at given dive depth
Dive at 80 ft or greater
Rapid ascent—panic, inexperience, unfamiliarity with equipment
Heavy exercise before or after dive to the point of muscle soreness
Flying after diving (24-hour wait is recommended)
Driving to high altitude after dive

Individual Factors
Age—older individuals
Obesity
Fatigue—lack of sleep prior to dive
Alcohol—consumption before or after dive
History of medical problems

Table 10-4 Signs and Symptoms of Decompression Sickness

Type	Signs and Symptoms

I	Musculoskeletal symptoms:
	• Joint pain ("bends")
	  • Myalgias
	• Dermatologic symptoms:
	  • Rash (*cutis marmorata*)
	• Lymphatic symptoms:
	  • Swollen or painful lymph nodes

II	Neurologic symptoms: • Numbness • Paresthesias • Mental status change Inner ear symptoms ("staggers"): • Tinnitus (ears ringing) • Hearing loss • Vertigo • Dizziness • Ataxia • Nausea/vomiting Cardiopulmonary symptoms ("chokes"): • Chest pain (worse with inspiration) • Cough • Tachypnea • Pulmonary congestion • Circulatory collapse

cord, skin, brain, and inner ear. Symptoms develop when a diver rapidly ascends after being exposed to a depth of 33 feet or more for a time sufficient to allow the body's tissues to be saturated with nitrogen.

SIGNS AND SYMPTOMS Decompression sickness is commonly classified as Type I or Type II. The signs and symptoms of the two classes of decompression sickness are detailed in Table 10-4. The principal signs and symptoms of decompression sicknesses are joint and abdominal pain, fatigue, paresthesias, and CNS disturbances. A rash is sometimes seen (Figure 10-12). The most common symptom is

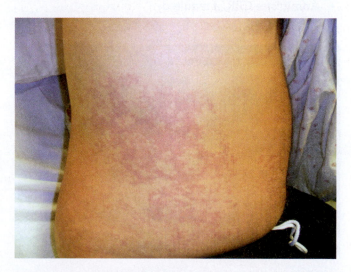

FIGURE 10-12 Rash sometimes seen with decompression sickness (dysbarism).

(© Dr. Bryan E. Bledsoe)

joint pain, and the most concerning is ataxia or any other CNS disturbance. The nitrogen bubbles produced by rapid decompression are thought to produce obstruction of blood flow, which leads to local ischemia, subjecting tissues to anoxic stress. In some cases, this stress may lead to tissue damage.

TREATMENT Initial treatment includes oxygen. Patients with decompression sickness usually seek medical treatment within 12 hours of ascent from a dive. Some patients may not seek treatment for as long as 24 hours after the last dive. It is generally safe to assume that signs or symptoms developing more than 36 hours after a dive cannot reasonably be attributed to decompression sickness.

Decompression sickness may require urgent definitive care through **recompression**. This can be accomplished by placing the patient in a **hyperbaric oxygen chamber** (Figure 10-13). There, the patient is subjected to oxygen under greater-than-atmospheric pressure to force the nitrogen in the body to redissolve, then gradually decompressed to allow the nitrogen to escape without forming bubbles. However, prompt stabilization at the nearest emergency department should be accomplished before transportation to a recompression chamber.[8]

Early oxygen therapy may reduce symptoms of decompression sickness substantially. Divers who are administered high-concentration oxygen have a considerably better treatment outcome. Many diving emergencies occur a significant distance from definitive care. Prehospital providers should administer high-concentration oxygen until their supplies are exhausted. Do not attempt to "ration" oxygen by maintaining a lower flow rate. The following list outlines some of the steps in the prehospital management of decompression sicknesses:

- Perform a primary assessment.
- Check for, and treat, pneumothorax.
- Administer CPR, if required.

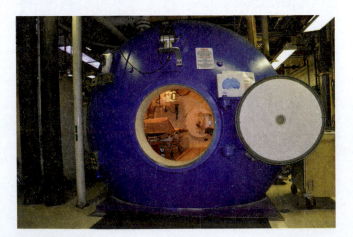

FIGURE 10-13 Hyperbaric oxygen chamber used in the treatment of decompression illness.

(© Edward T. Dickinson, MD)

- Administer oxygen at 100 percent concentration with a nonrebreather mask (consider CPAP if no pneumothorax). An unconscious diver should be intubated.
- Consider contacting DAN (Divers Alert Network).
- Keep the patient in the supine position.
- Protect the patient from excessive heat, cold, wetness, or noxious fumes.
- Give the conscious, alert patient nonalcoholic liquids such as fruit juices or sports drinks.
- Evaluate and stabilize the patient at the nearest emergency department prior to transport to a recompression chamber. Begin IV fluid replacement with electrolyte solutions for unconscious or seriously injured patients. You may use lactated Ringer's or normal saline. Do not use 5 percent dextrose in water.
- If there is evidence of CNS involvement, consider dexamethasone, heparin, or diazepam if ordered by medical direction.
- If air evacuation is used, do not expose the patient to decreased barometric pressure. Cabin pressure must be maintained at sea level, or fly at the lowest possible safe altitude.

Send the patient's diving equipment with the patient for examination. If that is impossible, arrange for local examination and gas analysis.

Pulmonary Overpressure Accidents

Lung overinflation caused by rapid ascent is the common cause of a number of emergencies, particularly at shallow depths of less than 6 feet. Air can become trapped in the lungs by mucus plugs, bronchospasm, or simple breath holding. With rapid ascent, ambient pressure drops quickly, causing the trapped air to expand. Air expansion can rupture the alveolar membranes. This can result in hemorrhage, reduced oxygen and carbon dioxide transport, and capillary and alveolar inflammation. Air can also escape from the lung into other nearby tissues and cause pneumothorax and tension pneumothorax, subcutaneous emphysema, or pneumomediastinum.

SIGNS AND SYMPTOMS Divers with this type of condition will complain of substernal chest pain. Respiratory distress and diminished breath sounds are common findings on examination.

TREATMENT Treatment for this condition is the same as for pneumothorax caused by any other mechanism. Rest and supplemental oxygen are important, but hyperbaric oxygen is not usually necessary.

Arterial Gas Embolism

As described, a pressure buildup in the lung can damage and rupture alveoli. This can allow air, in the form of a large bubble, to escape into the circulation. This air embolism, or arterial gas embolism (AGE), can travel to the left atrium and ventricle of the heart and out into various parts of the body, where it may lodge and obstruct blood flow, causing ischemia and possibly infarct. Such obstruction of blood flow can have devastating effects triggered by cardiac, pulmonary, and cerebral compromise.

SIGNS AND SYMPTOMS   Signs and symptoms of AGE include onset within 2 to 10 minutes of ascent; a rapid and dramatic onset of sharp, tearing pain; and other symptoms related to the organ system affected by blocked blood flow. The most common presentation mimics a stroke, with confusion, vertigo, visual disturbances, and loss of consciousness. Although rare, you may also encounter paralysis on one side of the body (hemiplegia), as well as cardiac and pulmonary collapse. If any person using scuba equipment presents with neurologic deficits during or immediately after ascent, AGE should be suspected. Prompt medical treatment is crucial because death or serious disability can result.

TREATMENT   Management of air embolism includes the following steps:

- Perform a primary assessment.
- Check for, and treat, pneumothorax.
- Administer oxygen by nonrebreather mask at 100 percent (consider CPAP, if no pneumothorax).
- Consider contacting DAN (Divers Alert Network).
- Place the patient in a supine position.
- Monitor vital signs frequently.
- Place a saline lock.
- Administer a corticosteroid agent, if ordered by medical direction.
- Transport to a recompression chamber as rapidly as possible. If air transport is used, it is very important to use a pressurized aircraft or to fly at a low altitude.

Pneumomediastinum

As noted earlier, a pneumomediastinum is the release of gas (air) through the visceral pleura into the mediastinum and pericardial sac around the heart. It can result from a pulmonary overpressure accident during rapid ascent from a dive.

SIGNS AND SYMPTOMS   Signs and symptoms of a pneumomediastinum include substernal chest pain, irregular pulse, abnormal heart sounds, reduced blood pressure and narrow pulse pressure, and a change in voice. There may or may not be evidence of cyanosis.

TREATMENT   The field management of pneumomediastinum includes the following:

- Administer high-concentration oxygen via nonrebreather mask.

- Check for, and treat, pneumothorax.
- Consider contacting DAN (Divers Alert Network).
- Start an IV of lactated Ringer's or normal saline per medical direction.
- Transport to the emergency department.

Treatment generally ranges from observation to recompression for relief of acute symptoms. The patient should be observed for 24 hours for any other signs of lung overpressure. He should not be recompressed unless air embolism or decompression sickness is also present.

Nitrogen Narcosis

Nitrogen narcosis develops during deep dives and contributes to major diving emergencies while the diver is at the bottom. With an elevated partial pressure, more nitrogen dissolves in the bloodstream. With higher concentrations of nitrogen in the body, including the brain, the result is intoxication and altered levels of consciousness similar to the effects of alcohol or narcotic use. Between 70 and 100 feet, these effects become apparent in most divers, but at 200 feet, most divers become so impaired that they cannot do any useful work. At 300 to 350 feet, unconsciousness occurs. The main concern with nitrogen narcosis is the same as with any person who is intoxicated while in a situation requiring alertness and common sense. Impaired judgment during a deep dive can cause accidents and unnecessary risk taking.

SIGNS AND SYMPTOMS   Signs and symptoms include altered levels of consciousness and impaired judgment.

TREATMENT   Treatment simply requires a return to a shallow depth, as this condition is self-resolving on ascent. To prevent this problem altogether in deep dives, oxygen mixed with helium is used, as helium does not have the anesthetic effect of nitrogen.

Other Diving-Related Conditions

There are less frequent problems that can occur as a result of scuba diving. For example, oxygen toxicity caused by prolonged exposure to high partial pressures of oxygen can cause lung damage or even convulsions. Hyperventilation caused by excitement or panic may lead to a decreased level of consciousness or muscle cramps and spasm. This will impair the diver's ability to function properly, possibly leading to injury. Inadequate breathing or faulty equipment may lead to increased CO_2 levels, or *hypercapnia*. This also may cause unconsciousness. Finally, poorly prepared air tanks may be contaminated with other gases, which can increase the risk of hypoxia, narcosis, and accidental injury.

Hyperbaric Chambers

Although many diving emergencies are treated in a hyperbaric chamber, many of these patients first require emergent stabilization at the closest appropriate emergency department. Recompression often does not take place immediately on arrival to the emergency department, and the patient can usually be stabilized, then transferred to a hyperbaric center. Understand your local transport protocols with regard to special transport considerations in diving-related emergencies.

Divers Alert Network

Clearly, scuba diving has a unique set of potential problems. With the popularity of this activity rising so dramatically, it is important for EMS personnel in popular diving areas to become familiar with recognition and treatment of these problems. If assistance is needed, the Divers Alert Network (DAN) operates a nonprofit consultation and referral service in affiliation with Duke University Medical Center. For all emergency and non-emergency consultations, contact (919) 684-9111. DAN has a worldwide presence and can be consulted for any and all diving emergencies. Think of it as the poison control center for diving emergencies. Consultations are free, and DAN always has a physician trained in dive medicine available 24 hours a day. You can call DAN collect or from anywhere in the world, and it is better to involve it sooner rather than later.

High-Altitude Illness

In contrast to illnesses related to diving and high atmospheric pressure, high-altitude illnesses are caused by a decrease in ambient pressure. Essentially, high altitude is a low-oxygen environment. As noted in the discussion of Dalton's law, oxygen concentration in the atmosphere remains constant at 21 percent. Therefore, as you go higher and barometric pressure decreases, the partial pressure of oxygen also decreases (it is 21 percent of a lower total pressure). Oxygen becomes less available, triggering a number of related illnesses as well as aggravating preexisting conditions such as angina, congestive heart failure, chronic obstructive pulmonary disease, and hypertension.

Even in healthy individuals, ascent to high altitude, especially if it is very rapid, can cause illness. It is difficult to predict who will be affected and to what degree. The only predictor is the hypoxic ventilatory response.

Every year, millions of visitors to mountains expose themselves to altitudes greater than 2,400 m (8,000 ft), the altitude at which high-altitude illnesses start to become manifest. For reference purposes, Denver, Colorado, is at 1,610 m, where there is 17 percent less oxygen than at sea level. Aspen, at 2,438 m, has 26 percent less oxygen, and at the top of Mount Everest (8,848 m or 29,028 ft) there is 66 percent less oxygen than at sea level. At *high altitude* (4,900 to 11,500 ft), the hypoxic environment causes decreased exercise performance, although without major disruption of normal oxygen transport in the body. However, if ascent is very rapid, altitude illness will commonly occur at 8,000 ft and beyond. *Very high altitude* (11,500 to 18,000 ft) will result in extreme hypoxia during exercise or sleep. It is important to ascend to these altitudes slowly, allowing for acclimatization to the environment. *Extreme altitude* beyond 18,000 ft will cause severe illness in almost everyone.

Some of the signs and symptoms of altitude illness are malaise, anorexia, headache, sleep disturbances, and respiratory distress that increases with exertion.

Prevention

Acclimatization, exertion, sleep, diet, and medication are key considerations in preventing or limiting high-altitude medical emergencies.[9] A description of each follows.

Gradual Ascent

To avoid developing high-altitude medical problems, it is important to allow a period of acclimatization. Slow, gradual ascent over days to weeks gives the body a chance to adjust to the hypoxic state caused by high altitudes. A person who would normally become short of breath, dizzy, and confused by a rapid drop in oxygen can function quite well if the oxygen level is decreased to the same level gradually over a long period of time. Acclimatization occurs through several mechanisms. They are:

- *Ventilatory changes.* The *hypoxic ventilatory response (HVR)* is triggered by decreased oxygen. When oxygen is decreased, ventilation increases. This hyperventilation causes a decrease in CO_2, but the kidneys compensate by eliminating more bicarbonate from the body. In essence, the body resets its normal ventilation and operating level of CO_2. The process takes four to seven days at a given altitude.

- *Cardiovascular changes.* The heart rate increases at high altitude, allowing more oxygen to be delivered to the tissues. In addition, peripheral veins constrict, increasing the central blood volume. In response, the central receptors, which sense blood volume, induce a diuresis, which causes concentration of the blood. Unfortunately, pulmonary circulation also constricts in a hypoxic environment. This causes or exacerbates preexisting hypertension and predisposes to developing high-altitude pulmonary edema.

- **Blood changes.** Within 2 hours of ascent to high altitude, the body begins making more red blood cells to carry oxygen. Over time, this mechanism will significantly compensate for the hypoxic environment. It is this mechanism that fostered the idea of "blood-doping" during athletic competition, especially at high altitudes. Athletes donate their own blood long in advance of a competition at high altitude. This allows them time to rebuild their red blood cells. Just before the competition, they receive a transfusion of their own blood to increase their oxygen-carrying capacity. Most athletic governing bodies frown on this practice.

Limited Exertion

Clearly, one of the easiest ways to avoid some effects of high altitude is to limit the amount of exertion. By limiting the body's need for oxygen, the effects of oxygen deprivation will be minimized.

Sleeping Altitude

Sleep is often disrupted by high altitude. Hypoxia causes abnormal breathing patterns and frequent awakenings in the middle of the night. Descending to a lower altitude for sleep improves rest and allows the body to recover from hypoxia. This practice will, however, interfere with the process of acclimatization.

High-Carbohydrate Diet

Carbohydrates are converted by the body into glucose and rapidly released into the bloodstream, providing quick energy. The theory that this is helpful in acclimatizing to high altitude is controversial.

Medications

Two medications will limit or prevent the development of medical conditions related to high altitude. They are:

- **Acetazolamide.** Acetazolamide (Diamox) acts as a diuretic. It forces bicarbonate out of the body, which greatly enhances the process of acclimatization, as discussed earlier. The hypoxic ventilatory response reaches a new set point more quickly. This improves ventilation and oxygen transport with less alkalosis. In addition, the periodic breathing that occurs at high altitude is resolved, thereby preventing sudden drops in oxygen.
- **Nifedipine.** Nifedipine (Procardia, Adalat) is a medication used to treat high blood pressure. It causes blood vessels to dilate, preventing the increase in pulmonary pressure that often causes pulmonary edema.

Other treatments are currently under evaluation. Phenytoin (Dilantin), for example, is being studied because of its membrane stabilization effects. Steroids are commonly used, but their efficacy is still controversial.

Types of High-Altitude Illness

A variety of symptoms occur when the average person ascends rapidly to high altitude. These may range from fatigue and decreased exercise tolerance to headache, sleep disturbance, and respiratory distress. The following section will deal with some of the specific syndromes that will occur (Table 10-5).

Acute Mountain Sickness

Acute mountain sickness (AMS) usually manifests in an unacclimatized person who ascends rapidly to an altitude of 2,000 m (6,600 ft) or greater.

SIGNS AND SYMPTOMS The mild form of acute mountain sickness presents with the following symptoms:

- Light-headedness
- Breathlessness
- Weakness

CONTENT REVIEW

➤ Types of High-Altitude Illness
- Acute mountain sickness
- High-altitude pulmonary edema
- High-altitude cerebral edema

Table 10-5 Definitions of Altitude Illness (Lake Louise Consensus)

Disease	Criteria
Acute mountain sickness (AMS)	In the setting of a recent increase in altitude, the presence of a headache and at least one of the following symptoms: • Gastrointestinal problems (anorexia, nausea, or vomiting) • Fatigue or weakness • Dizziness or light-headedness • Difficulty sleeping
High-altitude cerebral edema (HACE)	*Can be considered "end-stage" or severe AMS.* In the setting of a recent increase in altitude, either: • The presence of a change in mental status and/or ataxia in a person with AMS. *OR* • The presence of both mental status changes *and* ataxia in a person without AMS.
High-altitude pulmonary edema (HAPE)	In the setting of a recent increase in altitude, the presence of the following: **Symptoms** (at least 2 of): • Dyspnea at rest • Cough • Weakness or decreased exercise performance • Chest tightness or congestion **Signs** (at least 2 of): • Crackles or wheezing in at least one lung field • Central cyanosis • Tachypnea • Tachycardia

- Headache
- Nausea and vomiting

These symptoms can develop from 6 to 24 hours after ascent. More severe cases can develop, especially if the person continues to ascend to higher altitudes. These symptoms include:

- Weakness (requiring assistance to eat and dress)
- Severe vomiting
- Decreased urine output
- Shortness of breath
- Altered level of consciousness

Mild AMS is self-limiting and will often improve within one to two days if no further ascent occurs.

TREATMENT   Treatment of AMS consists of halting ascent, possibly lowering altitude, using acetazolamide (Diamox) and antinauseants such as ondansetron (Zofran) as necessary. It is not usually necessary to descend to sea level. Supplemental oxygen will relieve symptoms but is usually used only in severe cases. In severe cases oxygen, if available, will help. In addition, immediate descent is the definitive treatment. For very severe cases, hyperbaric oxygen may be necessary.

High-Altitude Pulmonary Edema

High-altitude pulmonary edema (HAPE) develops as a result of increased pulmonary pressure and hypertension caused by changes in blood flow at high altitude. Children are most susceptible, and men are more susceptible than women.

SIGNS AND SYMPTOMS   Initially, symptoms include dry cough, mild shortness of breath on exertion, and slight crackles in the lungs. As the condition progresses, so will the symptoms. Dyspnea can become quite severe and cause cyanosis. Coughing may be productive of frothy sputum, and weakness may progress to coma and death.

TREATMENT   In the early stages, HAPE is completely and easily reversible with descent and the administration of oxygen. It is therefore critical to recognize the illness early and initiate appropriate treatment. If immediate descent is not possible, supplemental oxygen can completely reverse HAPE, but requires 36 to 72 hours. Such a supply of oxygen is rarely available to mountain climbers. In this situation, the portable hyperbaric bag can be very useful. This is a sealed bag that can be inflated to 2 psi, which simulates a descent of approximately 5,000 feet. Acetazolamide can be used to decrease symptoms. Medications such as morphine, nifedipine (Procardia), and furosemide (Lasix) have been used with some success, but they carry complications such as hypotension and dehydration and should be used with caution.

High-Altitude Cerebral Edema

The exact cause of high-altitude cerebral edema (HACE) is not known. It usually manifests as progressive neurologic deterioration in a patient with AMS or HAPE. The increased fluid in the brain tissue causes a rise in intracranial pressure.

SIGNS AND SYMPTOMS   The symptoms of high altitude cerebral edema include:

- Altered mental status
- Ataxia (poor coordination)
- Decreased level of consciousness
- Coma

Headache, nausea, and vomiting are less common. Occasionally, actual focal neurologic changes may occur.

TREATMENT   As in all altitude illnesses, definitive treatment is descent to lower altitude. Oxygen and steroids may also help to improve recovery. The phosphodiesterase inhibitor sildenafil (Viagra) has shown some benefit in selected patients. In most cases, the use of oxygen with steroids (dexamethasone) and a hyperbaric bag may be sufficient, although these are often unavailable. If coma develops, it may persist for days after descent to sea level but usually resolves, although sometimes leaving residual disability.

Summary

Our environment provides us with all that we need to survive and prosper. The extremes of our environment, however, can have significant impact on human metabolism. Our bodies will, of course, compensate for these extremes, but sometimes this is not enough. Sometimes the heat gain or loss is too much. Sometimes the pressure change is too much. As a result, medical illnesses and emergencies arise. These can range from abnormal core body temperatures to decompensation, shock, and even death.

Basic knowledge of common environmental, recreational, and exposure emergencies is necessary for you to administer prompt and proper treatment in the prehospital setting. It is not easy to remember this type of information because these problems are not usually encountered on a daily basis. Remember the general principles involved: Remove the environmental influence causing the problem. Support the patient's own attempt to compensate. Finally, select a definitive care location and transport the patient as rapidly as possible.

In every case, remember that you must maintain your own safety. In too many cases, paramedics have lost their lives as a result of attempting a rescue for which they were not properly trained. Rapid action is always necessary when performing an environmental rescue; however, common sense must prevail.

You Make the Call

You and your partner, Christina, are paramedics stationed at Mike Leigh General Hospital in Lake Dulce, Colorado. You have enjoyed working at this beautiful mountain ski resort (elevation 8,815 ft) for the past year. This morning you are expecting a busy day, as this is the first day of spring break and hundreds of visitors have been arriving daily for their weeklong romp in the snow.

Shortly after 10 A.M., a call comes in from the first-alert ski patrol. A skier on Mount Giulio is in unspecified distress. You and Christina hasten to your snowmobiles and proceed immediately to the slope. On arrival you find a 25-year-old man crouched in the snow, surrounded by curious onlookers. The ski patrol informs you that he is a scuba diving expert, Biff Western. Biff arrived yesterday with his wife Muffy to try skiing for the first time. Biff did not sleep well last night, despite taking one sleeping pill he had brought with him. This morning he felt very tired, a condition that was aggravated by a dry cough he seemed to have developed. Now on his second run down the slope, the exertion has exhausted him. The ski patrol thinks he is becoming confused and disoriented. He is short of breath, weak, and dizzy, and his cough has become productive of white frothy sputum.

On examination, you find that Biff is breathing very rapidly. His heart is racing and his lips are tinged blue. Listening to his chest, you note coarse diffuse crackles on inspiration. You and Christina share a momentary knowing glance then spring into action.

1. What illness are you probably dealing with?

2. What predisposing factors lead to this illness?

3. What is the definitive treatment for this condition?

4. If definitive treatment is not possible, what other measures can be used?

See Suggested Responses at the back of this book.

Review Questions

1. The type of thermogenesis that results from exercise is _____
   a. metabolic.
   b. diet induced.
   c. work induced.
   d. thermoregulatory.

2. Through the mechanism called evaporation, how much water is lost by the body per day?
   a. 200 mL
   b. 400 mL
   c. 600 mL
   d. 800 mL

3. Of the following, if a core temperature is needed in a patient with a cold-related emergency, it should be obtained from which location?
   a. Ear   c. Rectum
   b. Mouth   d. Axilla

4. Which of the following factors may contribute to a patient's susceptibility to hyperthermia?
   a. Prescription medications
   b. Environmental temperature the patient is in
   c. Health of the patient
   d. All of the above

5. Treatment of the patient with heat cramps and nausea includes all of the following *except* _____
   a. administer salt tablets.
   b. administer an IV antiemetic.
   c. place the patient in a cool environment.
   d. if the patient is unable to take fluids orally, consider an IV of normal saline.

6. When the core temperature of the body drops below _____, an individual is considered to be hypothermic.
   a. 95°F
   b. 90°F
   c. 85°F
   d. 80°F

7. In what degree of hypothermia is a patient found to be hypotensive with an altered mental status, no shivering, and respiratory depression?
   a. Mild
   b. Moderate
   c. Severe
   d. Chronic

8. The third most common cause of accidental death in the United States is _____
   a. heatstroke.
   b. snake envenomation.
   c. drowning.
   d. hypothermia.

9. What physiologic structure either ceases to function or is significantly diminished in a patient with a water emergency/near drowning that results in shunting of deoxygenated blood back to the arterial bloodstream?
   a. Surfactant
   b. Bronchiole smooth muscle
   c. Alveolar phagocytes
   d. Blood glucose levels

10. All symptomatic drowning patients should be transported to the hospital for observation because complications may not appear for up to how long after the incident?
    a. 10 minutes
    b. 16 hours
    c. 20 minutes
    d. 24 hours

11. Which gas law states that the volume of a gas is inversely proportional to its pressure if the temperature is kept constant?
    a. Henry's
    b. Boyle's
    c. Dalton's
    d. Starling's

12. Which diving injury may occur if a scuba diver rapidly ascends to the surface without sufficiently exhaling while ascending?
    a. Nitrogen narcosis
    b. Nitrogen rapture
    c. Decompression sickness
    d. Pulmonary underpressure

13. What emergency may develop in a patient who has not been acclimatized to high altitudes achieves a high altitude and develops respiratory distress and other findings consistent with pulmonary edema?
    a. AMS
    b. HACE
    c. HAPE
    d. AGE

14. You are treating a patient whom you suspect is suffering from acute mountain sickness following a trail hike high in the mountains, to which he has not acclimated. For this patient, which of the following interventions would *least* likely be part of your treatment plan?
    a. Diamox
    b. Zofran
    c. Move to a lower altitude
    d. Proventil

See Answers to Review Questions at the back of this book.

References

1. Becker, J. A. and L. K. Stewart. "Heat-Related Illness." *Am Fam Physician* 83 (2011): 1325–1330.

2. Polderman, K. H. "Mechanisms of Action, Physiological Effects, and Complications of Hypothermia." *Crit Care Med* 37 (7Suppl) (2009): S186–S202.

3. Imray, C., A. Grieve, and S. Dhillon. "Cold Damage to the Extremities: Frostbite and Non-Freezing Injuries." *Postgrad Med J* 85 (2009): 481–488.

4. Idris, A. H., R. Berg, J. Bierens, et al. "Recommended Guidelines for Uniform Reporting of Data from Drowning: The 'Utstein Style.'" *Circulation* 108 (2003): 2565–2574.

5. Layon, A. J. and J. H. Modell. "Drowning: Update 2009." *Anesthesiology* 110 (2009): 1390–1401.

6. Modell, J. H., M. Gaub, F. Moya, B. Vestal, and H. Swarz. "Physiologic Effects of Near-Drowning with Chlorinated Freshwater, Distilled Water, and Isotonic Saline." *Anesthesiology* 27 (1966): 33–41.

7. Salahuddin, M., L. A. James, and E. Bass. "SCUBA Medicine: A First Responder's Guide to Diving Injuries." *Curr Sports Med Rep* 10 (2011): 134–139.

8. Vann, R. D., F. K. Butler, F. J. Mitchell, and R. E. Moon. "Decompression Illness." *Lancet* 377 (2011): 153–164.

9. Luks, A. M., S. E. McIntosh, C. K. Grissom, et al. "Wilderness Medical Society Consensus Guidelines for the Prevention and Treatment of Acute Altitude Illness." *Wilderness Environ Med* 21 (2010): 146–155.

Further Reading

Auerbach, P. S., ed. *Wilderness Medicine*. 6th ed. St. Louis: Mosby Year Book, 2012.

Bierens, J. L., ed. *Drowning: Prevention, Rescue, Treatment*. 2nd ed. New York: Springer, 2012.

Bledsoe, B. E. and D. E. Clayden. *Prehospital Emergency Pharmacology*. 7th ed. Upper Saddle River, NJ: Pearson/Prentice Hall, 2012.

Guyton, A. C., and J. E. Hall. *Textbook of Medical Physiology*. 13th ed. Philadelphia: Elsevier, 2015.

Sutton, J. R., G. Coates, and C. S. Houston, eds. "The Lake Louise Consensus on the Definition and Quantification of Altitude Illness." *Hypoxia and Mountain Medicine*. Burlington, VT: Queen City Printers, 1992.

Tintinalli, J. E., et al., eds. "Environmental Injuries," in *Emergency Medicine: A Comprehensive Study Guide*. 7th ed. New York: McGraw-Hill, 2011.

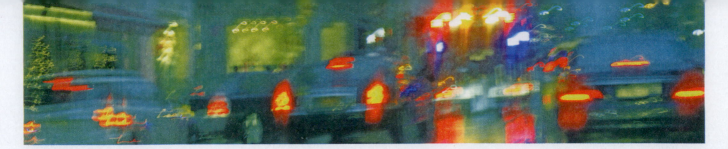

Chapter 11
Special Considerations in Trauma

Bryan E. Bledsoe, DO, FACEP, FAAEM, EMT-P

Robert S. Porter, MA, EMT-P

STANDARD
Trauma (Trauma Overview; Multisystem Trauma)

COMPETENCY
Integrates assessment findings with principles of epidemiology and pathophysiology to formulate a field impression to implement a comprehensive treatment/disposition plan for an acutely injured patient.

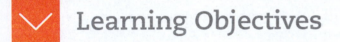

Learning Objectives

Terminal Performance Objective: After reading this chapter, you should be able to integrate principles of trauma management, injury prevention, and care of special patient populations into professional decision making to affect trauma morbidity and mortality.

Enabling Objectives: To accomplish the terminal performance objective, you should be able to:

1. Define key terms introduced in this chapter.

2. Describe the importance of an organized system of trauma care to reducing trauma morbidity and mortality, and how EMS can participate in injury prevention programs.

3. Describe the key actions and decisions paramedics must be aware of during each phase of trauma assessment.

4. Briefly discuss the steps of the primary assessment as it relates to traumatically injured patients.

5. Briefly discuss the steps of the secondary assessment as it relates to traumatically injured patients.

6. Briefly discuss the steps of the reassessment phase as it relates to traumatically injured patients.

7. Understand and be able to apply numeric scoring systems for traumatized patients.

8. Given a variety of trauma patient scenarios, identify signs and symptoms of injury.

9. Given a variety of trauma patient scenarios, discuss assessment-based decision making, including treatment and transport decisions.

10. Describe the importance of recognizing, preventing, and treating hypothermia in trauma patients.

11. Describe the differences in anatomy, physiology, pathophysiology, assessment, and management of special population patients.

12. Discuss the paramedic's role relative to interacting with other EMS and ED health care providers as it relates to traumatized patients.

13. Identify the purpose and describe the use of air medical transport in the traumatized patient.

KEY TERMS

hypoperfusion, p. 348

hypotension, p. 348

hypothermia, p. 349

hypovolemia, p. 347

Case Study

At 2:30 A.M., County Dispatch calls ALS 21 to the scene of an auto collision on Highway 192. Once en route, ALS 21, and paramedic Alex Dalburg, receive an update on the crash. An OnStar dispatcher reports a serious frontal impact with air bag deployment at the GPS coordinates of Highway 192, one mile south of Bronson Road. The OnStar dispatcher is unable to communicate with the vehicle occupants. County Dispatch reports that Emerson Police, Fire Rescue, and their BLS Ambulance units are responding as well.

As ALS 21 arrives at the scene, Alex notes that the police and fire services have secured the scene and have routed traffic safely around the collision site. Two vehicles have collided head-on in the northbound lane of the divided highway. A sedan and a pickup truck have sustained severe front-end damage, the front windows are broken out, and it appears that the air bags have deployed. An EMT from the Emerson Fire Department ambulance reports that the driver of the pickup truck is conscious, alert, and apparently uninjured. The driver of the sedan appears unconscious. Both drivers wore lap and shoulder belts.

Alex reports to the sedan to find a woman in her early 20s who is unresponsive to his initial introduction and his query "Are you OK?" He directs the EMT to enter the vehicle from the other side and initiate spinal precautions. Alex notes some snoring airway sounds that clear as the EMT brings her head and neck from flexion to the neutral position. A quick check of her radial pulse reveals a rapid and strong pulse, but no response as he asks the woman to grasp his fingers. Capillary refill is at about 3 seconds. Alex places his hand on her upper chest and notes modest chest rise at

a slightly rapid rate. Further examination of the passenger compartment reveals that the steering wheel and dash have been pushed inward and are trapping the woman against the seat. Alex categorizes her as unstable because of her unresponsiveness and asks fire rescue to extricate her quickly.

While they prepare the equipment, Alex begins a rapid trauma assessment. Using a penlight to illuminate the woman's face, neck, and left arm, Alex notices a bit of air bag dust, but the facial features and assessment are otherwise unremarkable. Her skin is slightly pale in color. The left pupil is slowly reactive to light and Alex cannot access the right pupil. The neck appears symmetrical, with flat jugular veins. Palpation of the upper chest notes a "crackling-like" feeling with skin that moves under his fingers, and quick auscultation picks up only very quiet breath sounds on the right and somewhat louder sounds on the left. Alex notes that her respiratory rate appears to have increased and is now about 26 breaths per minute. Alex cannot continue his rapid trauma assessment while the woman remains trapped in the car.

Emerson Fire Rescue has its equipment ready and begins disentanglement. After about 45 seconds, they have removed the roof and have pushed the dash forward and seat back, freeing the woman. Rapid extrication ensues and the woman is moved to the waiting stretcher, where a cervical collar is applied and she is firmly secured. A quick look at the abdomen defines that this woman is pregnant and probably in the late second or early third trimester. Both lower extremities appear deformed; Alex suspects bilateral femur fractures and a possible pelvic fracture. Alex continues his assessment while the EMTs place a splint between the patient's legs and firmly immobilize the lower extremities. Alex notices a grating feeling as he compresses the ribs inward (indicating probable rib fractures) and confirms reduced breath sounds over the entire left thorax. The left thorax is hyperresonant to percussion.

An EMT reports the blood pressure is 66 by palpation and the pulse is at a rate greater than 140. Pulse oximetry intermittently reads about 84 percent and displays a pulse rate of about 146. Alex calls for high-concentration oxygen via nonrebreather mask and prepares for needle decompression of the chest. Chest decompression appears to release some air and the woman's breathing rate slows and depth increases. Alex decides to rapidly transport the patient to the ambulance, then to the trauma center with IVs started en route.

Once in the ambulance, Alex tilts the entire spine board 15 degrees, elevating the right side. Alex starts one IV with normal saline, a nonrestrictive three-way valve, and trauma tubing. He administers a quick 500 mL bolus of fluid and rechecks vital signs. The automatic BP cuff displays 72/46 and a pulse rate of 148. Oxygen saturation is 92 and the pregnant woman does not respond to painful stimuli as Alex squeezes the fleshy skin between the thumb and first finger. Alex reassesses respiration and notes that the breath sounds on the left and right are now equal. Because of the pregnancy and the MOI, Alex inspects for vaginal bleeding and finds a small amount of hemorrhage.

On arrival at the emergency department, the trauma team takes Alex's report and performs a quick assessment. They place a chest tube in the fifth intercostal space along the left midaxillary line and then arrange for a CT scan of the head, neck, chest, and abdomen, and an ultrasound of the uterus and fetus. While waiting for the scans, the emergency department staff administers packed red blood cells and more fluids, the blood pressure rises to 86/62, and the pulse slows a bit. Fetal heart tones are not found by auscultation or by Doppler.

Shortly after returning to headquarters, ALS 21 receives a call from the trauma center. The woman had an apparent placental abruption and miscarried about 30 minutes after arrival. She has regained consciousness from an apparent concussion and is in serious condition but is expected to recover.

Introduction to Shock Trauma Resuscitation

In the mid-1960s, trauma was identified as the neglected disease of a modern society. At that time, more than 150,000 persons died each year from trauma, and even greater numbers suffered some level of disability. Health care leaders, recognizing that no organized system existed to care for these victims, took the first steps toward forming what has grown into today's emergency medical services system. Fifty years later, EMS has become a highly sophisticated system, yet 193,000 lives are still lost yearly to trauma (Figure 11-1).[1] Most of these lives are taken not at the end of a progressive disease in the later years of life, but from young and active members of society. Today, research has indicated that the skills that have been mainstays of prehospital trauma care often do not improve patient outcome—and, worse, they occasionally increase patient mortality and morbidity.

As professionals in the field of prehospital emergency care, we need to look carefully and honestly at our practices and ensure that they best serve our patients. We must do several things to secure a future for prehospital emergency care and to ensure that our patients receive the best chances for survival. We must reduce the incidence of trauma at its source by supporting and promoting injury prevention in our society. We need to ensure that our practices are current and truly benefit those who receive our care. Finally, we need to function as an integrated component of the health care system serving our patients and our communities. To help accomplish these objectives, this chapter examines injury prevention, trauma assessment, shock/multisystem trauma resuscitation, care for special patients (pediatric, pregnant, bariatric, geriatric, and cognitively impaired), care provider interaction, air medical service, and trauma research.

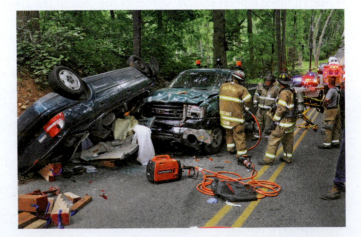

FIGURE 11-1 Motor vehicle crashes account for about 30 percent of trauma fatalities in the United States.

(© Edward T. Dickinson, MD)

Injury Prevention

Of all the care procedures and advanced interventions available to treat the trauma patient, none has more promise for reducing mortality and morbidity than prevention. We in emergency medical services can learn a great deal from the fire service. The efforts of the fire service in encouraging smoke and carbon monoxide detector use, promoting more rigorous fire codes and inspections, and educating the public—especially children—about both the dangers of fire and the techniques to preserve life during fire are credited with greatly decreasing fire incidence, morbidity, and mortality. These fire service efforts are a valuable model for programs aimed at reducing death and disability from trauma.

If EMS is to maintain a leadership role in prehospital emergency care, we must place a new and continuing emphasis on injury prevention. The "Let's Not Meet by Accident" program, developed jointly by a trauma system and prehospital providers, is just one example of a prevention program. It aims both to acquaint high school students with EMS and to alert them to trauma hazards in our society. Other citizen groups have formed to help increase public awareness of social behaviors that lead to trauma. One such group, Mothers Against Drunk Driving (MADD), brings attention to the motor vehicle death toll associated with driving while alcohol or substance impaired. To fulfill its responsibilities to the community, the EMS system must encourage or conduct programs like these with active participation from prehospital care providers.

A new program, sponsored by EMS and modeled after the fire service approach to prevention, is the home inspection (Figure 11-2). After a significant event, such as the birth of a child, local EMS personnel perform a voluntary home inspection. The inspectors survey the home for potential hazards, notify the family of their findings, and suggest changes that would increase home safety. For example, inspectors might check the temperature of the hot water tank (and suggest lowering it when necessary) to prevent scalding injury to children; examine infant cribs to ensure that the slats are close enough together to prevent strangulation and other injuries; and test child auto seats for proper fit and instruct parents in their proper use. They might also check for ground fault outlets in bathrooms, overloaded electrical sockets or circuits, electrical cords under rugs, and other improper electrical connections. The inspectors can recommend installation of railings or replacement of treads on stairways, porches, and other potential fall locations. While in the home, the crew also ensures that there are adequate smoke and carbon monoxide detectors with fresh batteries. While carrying on the inspection, the EMS crew can also promote other safe practices, such as the use of helmets and other protective equipment for motorcycling, skateboarding, in-line skating, and bicycling. In addition, they can instruct the family on the best way to access police, fire, and medical services in the event of emergency. Widespread adoption of programs like these carries a tremendous potential to reduce trauma mortality and morbidity by reducing trauma in the home. These programs also introduce family members to the EMS team before an emergency strikes, thus helping to foster a good public image for the EMS system.

Currently, the Occupational Safety and Health Administration (OSHA) and other governmental agencies have developed and are enforcing workplace safety standards. Their efforts ensure that the workplace is reasonably safe and that workers are provided both with training in safe practices and with protective equipment appropriate to their work environment. The Department of Transportation is constantly improving motor vehicle safety through encouragement of better highway and vehicle design, testing, and inspection. These DOT programs ensure that the highways are safer and crashes are more survivable. Other governmental and quasigovernmental agencies monitor the safety of various products such as children's toys, electronic equipment, and other consumer products.

An important consideration to keep in mind regarding any safety education program is the impact serious trauma has on the young male population. Males between 11 and 35 years of age account for about 27 percent of all serious trauma injuries and more than 30 percent of all trauma deaths (Figure 11-3).[2] At the same time, this group represents less than 20 percent of the total population. Thus, trauma among young males represents an epidemic of serious proportions. It is probable that the risk-taking nature of young males and an associated disregard for safe practices (for instance, failure to use seat belts and motorcycle helmets and a willingness to drink and drive) contribute to this mortality. Encouraging behavioral changes in this population would likely have a marked effect on the overall incidence of trauma and the associated death and disability. Because many people entering EMS are of this gender and age group, we need to both speak to the problem and demonstrate safe practices by example to our peers.

Trauma Assessment

Trauma patient assessment is essential both to determining patient transport priority and identifying and prioritizing patient injuries for care. In the previous chapters, we discussed trauma related to body regions or systems. During these discussions, we examined how assessment elements are applied to each system or region. In this chapter, we

Healthy Homes

Healthy Homes > Tips by Topic

Injury Prevention

Many unintentional injuries and deaths are related to the home and its environment. Within the home, more than 11,000 people are estimated to die each year from preventable unintentional injuries, including falls, fires, drownings, and poisonings.

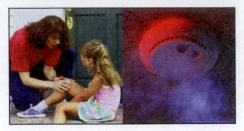

Health and Safety Tips

- Prevent falls in <u>older adults</u> and in <u>children</u>:
    - Install grab bars in showers and tubs.
    - Use nonslip mats in bathtubs and showers.
    - Install stair rails.
    - Have good lighting.
    - Keep stairs in good repair.
    - Keep stairs free of clutter.
    - Use safety gates in homes with young children.
- <u>Prevent fire-related deaths and injuries</u>:
    - Keep flammable objects away from the stove.
    - Make sure every bedroom has two exits in case of fire.
    - Practice your fire escape plan.
    - Install smoke alarms on every floor, including basements, and change the batteries at least once a year.
- <u>Prevent drowning</u>:
    - Supervise young children in bathtubs.
    - Always watch young children while they are swimming or playing in or around water.
    - Teach your children to swim and about water and pool safety rules.

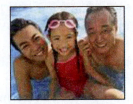

FIGURE 11-2 An EMS Injury-Prevention Home Inspection might include surveying the home for the injury hazards listed in this document from the Centers for Disease Control and Prevention. Go to http://www.cdc.gov/healthyhomes/bytopic/injury.html and click on the links to find further information.

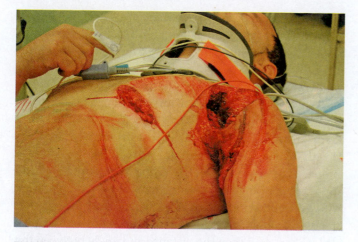

FIGURE 11-3 Young men account for a disproportionate representation of mortality and morbidity among trauma victims.

(© Edward T. Dickinson, MD)

review trauma assessment in a comprehensive way, much as you would when presented with a seriously injured trauma patient.

Trauma assessment progresses through the scene size-up, the primary assessment, and the secondary assessment (either the rapid or focused trauma assessment), and is then followed by serial reassessments. However, your first opportunity to begin the assessment process is through a review of the dispatch information.

Dispatch Information

Dispatch information provides critical information that you can evaluate while responding to the scene. This information provides the nature of the call. Often, it specifies the mechanism of injury (e.g., a fall, shooting, or auto crash) or the nature of the injury (e.g., a broken leg, head injury, or deep laceration). This information permits you to prepare for patient care and to contemplate your approach to the scene. Occasionally, the dispatch information may suggest that the scene is too dangerous to approach until it is secured by the police (such as cases of violence like shootings, stabbings, or domestic altercations with injuries). In such cases, you should remain at a distance from the scene until police arrive and notify you that it is safe to enter. At other times, dispatch information may alert you to potential hazards, such as a toxic gas release or downed electrical wires, for which you may need to request specialized response teams to secure the scene. This information also can cause you to be wary of the dangers as you approach the scene.

Use dispatch information to anticipate and prepare for your injury care. To speed your response at the scene, locate any equipment you will be likely to use. If

appropriate, lay the equipment out on the stretcher so it can be taken immediately to the patient. (It is always easier to have a first responder or bystander return a piece of equipment to the ambulance than it is to ask the person to go to the ambulance, find it, and bring it to the patient's side.) Inspect the equipment, check to see that it is working properly, and review its application and use. If you expect severe injuries, set up an IV bag and administration set in the ambulance for later use on the patient. This saves time that would otherwise be taken from patient care to assemble the administration equipment. Finally, review the assessment and care you intend to provide and, as necessary, review your protocols to ensure you are ready to respond to the emergency. These actions help you move quickly through the required care steps and to offer the optimum patient care in the shortest span of time.

Scene Size-Up

Trauma scene size-up involves several major elements (Figure 11-4): identifying scene hazards including the need for Standard Precautions, determining the mechanism of injury, accounting for and locating all patients, requesting any additional resources, identifying any environmental factors that might affect patient assessment and care, and establishing or linking up with scene oversight. The mechanism of injury analysis is also essential to help you anticipate and identify all scene hazards.

Analysis of the Mechanism of Injury

Analyze the mechanism of injury by re-creating the incident in your mind and, from that, anticipating the cause,

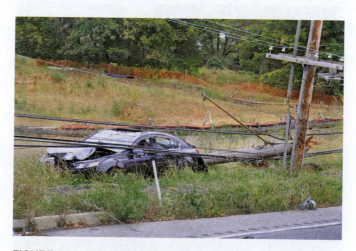

FIGURE 11-4 Assess the emergency scene quickly and carefully, looking for scene hazards, possible mechanisms of injury, the location of patients, and the possible need for additional resources.

(© Edward T. Dickinson, MD)

nature, and severity of your patient's injuries (the index of suspicion). Take any evidence available to you as you arrive at, and first view, the scene, and use that evidence to determine exactly how the forces were expressed to the patient. If two autos came together, for example, determine what vehicle surfaces collided, from which direction the vehicles were traveling, and which patient surfaces were impacted (Figure 11-5). Use the amount of internal compartment vehicular damage to approximate the impact energy delivered and then determine whether restraints or air bags were deployed that may have reduced the injury potential. Frontal and rear impacts afford the vehicle occupants the most protection, especially if seat belts are properly worn and air bags deploy. (Air bags deploy only in frontal and lateral impacts.) Lateral and rollover impacts are likely to cause the most serious injuries. (Remember, modern vehicle design has the ability to absorb great amounts of energy while protecting the patient. Confirm any suspicion of serious injury with the physical signs and symptoms gathered during the assessment.) In motorcycle, bicycle, and pedestrian-versus-vehicle collisions, identify the relative speed of impact and appreciate the lack of protection afforded the victim. In other nonvehicular blunt trauma, examine the height of the fall or other indications of impact energy and the point of impact, as well as the transmission path of those forces through the body.

When assessing the mechanism of injury for penetrating trauma, look at the relative velocity of the offending agent or projectile. Remember that an increase in mass directly increases the force's energy, whereas an increase in speed greatly increases (a squared relationship) the impact energy and the potential for serious patient injury. With gunshot wounds, identify the nature of the weapon (handgun, shotgun, or rifle), the relative power and profile (caliber), and then the distance and angle between the gun barrel and the impact point. Visualize the pathway taken by the bullet and its destructive power as it travels through human tissue. Head, central chest, and upper abdominal injuries are most lethal. Remember, however, that the bullet's path is frequently deflected from a straight line. In other penetrating trauma, mentally re-create the injury process and use kinetic energy principles to analyze the nature, process, and severity of the injury. Try to determine the object length and the depth and angle of insertion.

From your re-creation of the injury process, identify the individual organs affected and the extent of the injury to them. Approximate what significance their injury will have on the patient's condition and how it will affect the patient as time progresses. Assign each suspected injury a priority for both assessment and care. Finally, approximate the seriousness of your patient's overall condition and the potential need for either (1) rapid transport with most care provided en route or (2) on-scene care and then transport or (3) treatment and release (as permitted by protocol). Remember that patients with preexisting medical conditions, patients of advanced age, and the very young are at greatest risk when seriously injured. If there is more than one patient, identify the most seriously injured and order your patient assessment and care accordingly.

Hazard Identification

The mechanism of injury analysis helps you to identify many possible hazards at the scene. Search out all hazards and protect yourself, your patient, bystanders, and fellow rescuers from them. These hazards include the mechanism that injured your patient and may range from traffic associated with the auto crash to the assailant who is still holding a handgun. Search for additional sources of blunt and penetrating trauma, such as the broken glass and jagged metal at an auto crash scene or moving machinery at an industrial injury site. Also search out and exclude any hazards from fire, heat,

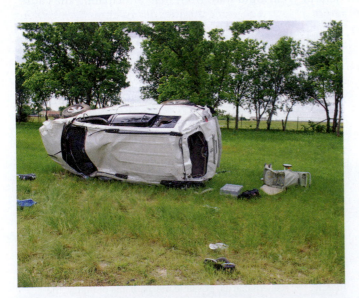

FIGURE 11-5 Analyze the forces of a vehicle collision and, based on that analysis, anticipate possible patient injuries.

(© Dr. Bryan E. Bledsoe)

explosion, electricity, toxic chemicals, radiation, or deadly gas at each and every scene. It is important to rule out these hazards rather than just to note them when they are obvious. Otherwise you risk injury to yourself, fellow rescuers, the patient, and bystanders. Look for hazardous material placards. Your ambulance should carry the most current Department of Transportation's *Emergency Response Guidebook,* which will help you identify the type of material and the level of risk. (However, it is not the role of EMS to directly address the risks of hazardous materials. That responsibility lies with the hazardous material team or fire department.)

Be aware of the presence and mood of family members, bystanders, and crowds at the emergency scene. These people may welcome your assistance, obstruct your ability to assess and care, or possibly represent a serious threat of violence.

Analyze the scene carefully to identify each of these hazards and exclude them from the scene or be prepared to deal with each before you approach the patient. Your well-being and that of your patient depend on it.[3] If you are injured at the scene, you will be less able to help your patient and may, in fact, become a patient yourself rather than a caregiver. For the paramedic, safety must be a lifestyle.

Standard Precautions

A special type of hazard existing at almost every emergency scene is the presence of body fluids and substances with the potential to spread infection (Figure 11-6). Realize that infection risk extends to both you and your patient, especially when dealing with trauma. A patient's open wound releases blood that poses an infection threat to you and others, but it also presents a pathway through which infection can enter your patient's body. The use of gloves and other Standard Precautions protects both you

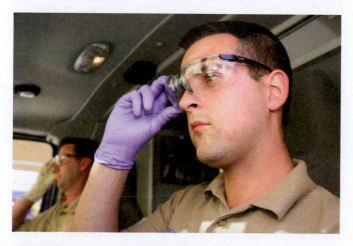

FIGURE 11-6 Use Standard Precautions at all scenes.

(© Dr. Bryan E. Bledsoe)

and your patient. Ensure that all rescuers who may come into contact with the patient also employ appropriate Standard Precautions as you prepare to approach the scene.

In all patient contacts, it is essential to don gloves in anticipation of contact with blood, saliva, mucus, urine, or fecal material. If the scene size-up reveals multiple patients, put on two or three sets of gloves, one over the other. Then peel gloves off as you move from one patient to another. If you prefer not to double-glove, be sure to carry additional glove pairs and change them with each patient contact or whenever they become contaminated. Remember that body fluids from one patient are potentially as infectious to another patient as they are to you. Also remember that with any open wound, the risk of infection transmission increases.

Your analysis of the mechanism of injury may also suggest airway or chest trauma or possible external arterial hemorrhage. These injuries may result in spurting blood or in blood or other fluids being propelled or coughed into the air. In such cases, wear both eye protection and splatter protection for your clothing. A mask may also be advisable. Consider wearing a mask if you have any type of respiratory infection, again to protect your patient. Ensure that all rescuers use the appropriate personal protective equipment (PPE). Once at the patient's side, your continuing patient evaluation may reveal the need for higher levels of protection than the scene size-up suggested; for this reason, always have goggles, gowns, masks, and additional gloves handy.

Accounting for and Locating All Patients

During your scene size-up, identify the number of likely patients and their locations around the emergency scene. During a collision, patients may be thrown from an auto or trapped within a twisted wreck and completely out of sight (this most frequently occurs with infants). A patient may also leave the vehicle and mill about the scene with bystanders, leave in an attempt to find help, or simply wander from the scene in confusion. Search for evidence that suggests the number and types of patients. Consider the number of vehicles involved in a crash; the number of spiderwebs on the windshields; purses or articles of clothing; and child seats, clothing, or toys. As you arrive at the scene, question the apparent patients and bystanders to better determine the number and locations of any additional patients.

Determining Resource Needs

Once you determine the likely number of patients and their injuries, estimate the type and nature of any other

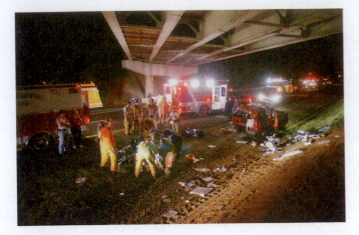

FIGURE 11-7 Assess the emergency scene to determine the need for any additional resources.

(© Mark C. Ide/Science Source)

emergency medical resources that will be needed at the scene (Figure 11-7). This may include additional ambulances—one for each seriously injured patient— and air medical service for patients who meet trauma triage criteria at a scene more than 45 minutes from the nearest trauma center (or as otherwise established by your system's protocols).

In addition, determine the resources needed to control hazards identified in your scene analysis. These resources may include police for traffic control or for scene security with gathering crowds, a heavy rescue unit for extrication, the hazardous material team for fuel and oil spill cleanup, the power company for downed electrical lines, or the fire service for potential fire control at vehicle crashes. It is essential that you contact dispatch early so needed equipment and trained personnel are quickly en route to the scene. Waiting until later in the call delays their arrival and may hinder your ability to access and care for patients.

Environmental Considerations

Vehicle collisions and other trauma-causing events do not always occur on bright sunny days in 70-degree weather. View the scene and consciously note any impact weather might have on your ability to access, assess, care for, and move your patient. Rain-soaked grassy surfaces or those covered with ice or snow may make patient movement more risky. Weather extremes like excessive heat or cold may give you less time at the scene to assess and care. Wind and driving rain may make obtaining vital signs and bandaging and splinting less practical outside the ambulance. Evaluate the ambient lighting to determine any special needs for scene and patient lighting.

Scene Oversight

At the end of the scene size-up, you should have the information necessary to organize an overall incident response and determine the special focus of your assessment for each patient. Take a few seconds to organize how you will address the scene and coordinate additional resources as they arrive. Identify in your mind what you wish each respective service to accomplish and how these functions can best work together to meet your patient's needs. Then think through your primary assessment and what specific problems you might expect to find with each element of that evaluation for each patient (Figure 11-8).

Define roles and assign tasks to the members of your crew. If you find that you are responding to an incident that will require many different services (police, fire, rescue, and otherwise), ensure that scene oversight or incident command is established. If not, do a scene walk-around, report your findings to dispatch, and report yourself as incident commander. (This will be temporary, as your skills are best applied to assessment [or triage] and patient care.) If incident command is established, ensure that you integrate with it to report the number and seriousness of patient injuries and communicate your needs.

Primary Assessment

The primary assessment is intended to identify immediate patient life threats and correct them before a more detailed assessment continues. It consists of determining a general patient impression, applying spinal precautions when needed based on local protocols, and assessing the patient's airway, breathing, and circulatory status. If any serious or life-threatening problem is found, correct it immediately. As you carry out these steps, you add to the information you gathered during the scene size-up and continue to refine your general patient impression. Finally, you determine your patient's priority for assessment, care, and transport.

General Impression

The mechanism of injury analysis and the index of suspicion for injuries begin the development of a general patient impression. You continue to refine that impression as you arrive at your patient's side. Include any information you gather as you determine the need for spinal precautions based on local protocols and as you evaluate the patient's mental status, airway, breathing, and circulation. Add to it the general appearance and mental status you observe during these first few minutes at the patient's side. This general patient

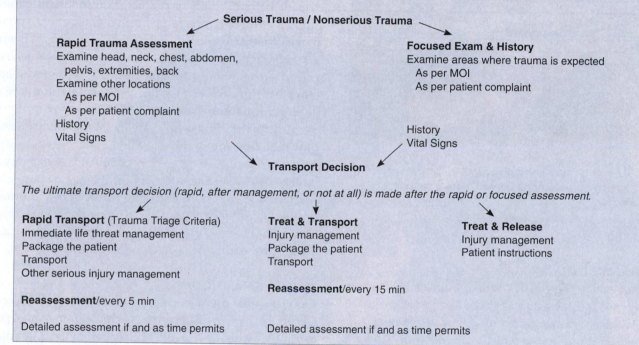

Trauma Assessment Format

Scene Size-Up
Body substance isolation
Scene safety
Mechanism of injury
Locate all patients
Request additional resources

Primary Assessment
Spinal precautions
General patient impression
Mental status
Airway
Breathing
Circulation

The decision to employ rapid trauma assessment is based on an evaluation of the forces of trauma and the results of the primary assessment. Here you will also make a preliminary decision on priority of transport.

Serious Trauma / Nonserious Trauma

Rapid Trauma Assessment
Examine head, neck, chest, abdomen,
  pelvis, extremities, back
Examine other locations
  As per MOI
  As per patient complaint
History
Vital Signs

Focused Exam & History
Examine areas where trauma is expected
  As per MOI
  As per patient complaint

History
Vital Signs

Transport Decision

The ultimate transport decision (rapid, after management, or not at all) is made after the rapid or focused assessment.

Rapid Transport (Trauma Triage Criteria)
Immediate life threat management
Package the patient
Transport
Other serious injury management

Reassessment/every 5 min

Detailed assessment if and as time permits

Treat & Transport
Injury management
Package the patient
Transport

Reassessment/every 15 min

Detailed assessment if and as time permits

Treat & Release
Injury management
Patient instructions

FIGURE 11-8 A trauma assessment form can help you organize priorities at any emergency scene.

impression (Figure 11-9) grows to include the seriousness of the patient's injuries and your patient's priority for care and transport. These determinations are very challenging to make early in your career; however, with experience, your level of comfort in judging patient severity and identifying the need for either rapid transport or on-scene care will grow.

In some cases, your general patient impression will not necessarily match the seriousness of trauma suggested by the mechanism of injury or with the signs and symptoms you gather during the primary assessment. Remember, however, that you attend your patient very soon after trauma. Often, enough time has not passed for

hemorrhage to draw down the blood supply. The body is not yet required to employ the most extreme compensatory mechanisms and does not yet display the most noticeable signs and symptoms of shock. Remain suspicious of developing hypovolemia and observe carefully for even the most subtle and early signs and symptoms of shock. On the other hand, the mechanism of injury may not reflect the actual injury severity and the patient may appear (and be) in a worse condition than expected. In all cases, base your patient management on the worst-case scenario. As time and further assessment continue, modify your general patient impression and the care it suggests.

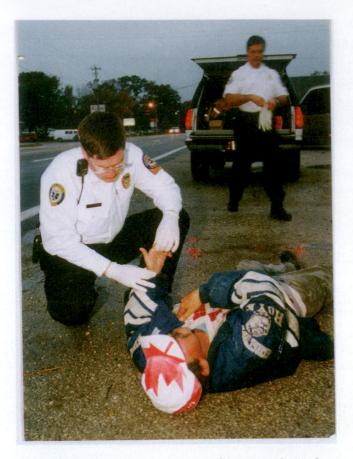

FIGURE 11-9 Form a general impression of the patient during the primary assessment and refine it during the rest of your time at the patient's side.

(© Craig Jackson/In the Dark Photography)

Mental Status

As you develop the general patient impression, evaluate the patient's mental status. Begin by introducing yourself, identifying your level of training, and explaining your desire to offer care to the patient. Extend your hand and offer to shake hands with the patient. While asking the patient what happened and what is bothering him the most, palpate the patient's radial pulse. This permits the patient to refuse care, ensures that he knows who you are and that your intentions are helpful, and calls for a physical reaction and a verbal response. By using this or a similar approach, you evaluate a conscious patient's mental status and airway, respiratory, and cardiac status—all in less than 30 seconds. Listen carefully to any responses as you continue your primary and secondary assessments.

At a minimum, identify the patient's level of consciousness using the AVPU mnemonic (*A*lert; responsive to *V*erbal stimuli; responsive to *P*ain; or *U*nresponsive). A more discerning approach is to evaluate the patient's degree of orientation by asking a few simple questions. Does the patient know the day and time of day (orientation to time); recognize what happened or where he is (orientation to event or place); and recognize who he is, as well as recognizing friends and family (orientation to person)? (Patients will usually lose orientation in this order.) Orientation is scored from 3 to 0, with the alert and completely oriented patient being alert and oriented times 3 (A + O × 3). Determining a patient's level of orientation provides a baseline reading of the patient's mental status against which improvement or deterioration can be trended in reassessments.

When your patient is not responsive to verbal stimuli, check for the specific response to noxious stimuli. For example, if you apply a noxious stimulus (usually by squeezing the fleshy region between the thumb and first finger or the trapezius muscle of the shoulder), does the patient move away from the stimulus (purposeful); move, but not effectively, away from the stimulus (purposeless); or does he not move at all? Some patients move toward a specific body position, or posture, in response to painful stimuli. With decorticate posturing, the patient's body moves toward extension with elbows flexing, whereas decerebrate posturing occurs when the body and elbows extend. Determining a baseline response permits you and other care providers to track patient deterioration or improvement throughout the course of care.

A helpful technique to evaluate the trauma patient is the Simplified Motor Score (SMS). It involves assessing only two factors—ability to obey commands and ability to localize pain, is a reliable test of potential brain injury and, because of its quickness and simplicity, can be performed during the primary assessment. Review the discussion of SMS in the chapter "Head, Neck, and Spinal Trauma" and see the further discussion later in this chapter.

Spinal Precautions

Employ spinal precautions as dictated by local protocols. Generally, many patients can be excluded from spinal precautions by using the NEXUS criteria, the Canadian C-Spine Rule, or similar protocols. Spinal precautions can range from neutral positioning of the head, neck, and spine to full spinal stabilization. When in doubt, err on the side of using spinal precautions (as dictated by local protocols) for your patient. In children and the elderly, signs and symptoms of spinal injury may be nonspecific or not obvious, and you should maintain a high index of suspicion.

Airway

It is easy to evaluate the airway in the conscious patient by listening to him speak. If the patient can talk clearly, you know that he has control over an open airway, is breathing adequately enough to speak in full sentences, and has cerebral oxygenation enough to support conscious thought. If the speech is broken or forced, there are unusual airway sounds, or the statements are confused or unintelligible, suspect and further evaluate the airway and breathing for problems.

In the unconscious patient, watch to see whether the chest rises and falls. Listen for the sound of air moving during respirations and feel for escaping air during exhalation. Reposition the patient's head and jaw with the head-tilt/chin-lift or the jaw thrust as needed. If repositioning improves air movement, then consider inserting an oral airway. If the patient does not have protective airway reflexes, consider early airway protection with an extraglottic airway or intubation, either now (if the airway is at immediate risk) or at the end of the primary assessment.

If you note airway sounds such as stridor, snoring, gurgling, or wheezing, presume a partial airway obstruction that will get worse during assessment and care. Trauma to airway soft tissue will likely cause swelling and progressive airway restriction. Expect swelling to seriously obstruct respiration and, again, consider early airway protection.

Breathing

Apply a pulse oximeter and then administer only enough supplemental oxygen to maintain the SpO_2 above 96 percent. Avoid hyperoxia. Watch for symmetrical chest and abdominal movement with each breath. If necessary, expose the chest for a better assessment. Rule out flail chest, or stabilize the flail segment and provide overdrive ventilation (bag-valve masking the breathing patient). Rule out diaphragmatic breathing (associated with cervical spine injury) or provide overdrive ventilation. If the patient complains of dyspnea or if chest excursion or tidal volumes seem limited, auscultate the lung fields to identify unilateral diminished or absent breath sounds. Percuss the chest for resonance: A dull sound indicates blood in the pleural space, whereas hyperresonance indicates air, under pressure, in the pleural space. If you cannot rule out a building tension pneumothorax, consider needle decompression. If you note pneumothorax or decompress a tension pneumothorax, monitor the chest carefully for the development or redevelopment of tension pneumothorax.

If respirations are less than 10 per minute and/or the tidal volume appears less than a normal breath in the unconscious patient, consider overdrive ventilation. If the patient is breathing rapidly but ineffectively, you should also consider overdrive ventilation. If the patient is not breathing, ventilate at 10 to 12 times per minute with full breaths (500 mL) with high-concentration oxygen using the bag-valve mask and reservoir. Ensure good chest rise in the patient and maintain an oxygen saturation of greater than 96 percent. Use capnography to guide your ventilation (35 to 45 mmHg of carbon dioxide), especially in the head injury patient (30 to 40 mmHg of carbon dioxide) (Figure 11-10).

Circulation

Quickly check the radial pulse for strength, regularity, and rate. A strong tachycardia suggests excitement, whereas a weak and thready pulse suggests shock compensation. If a

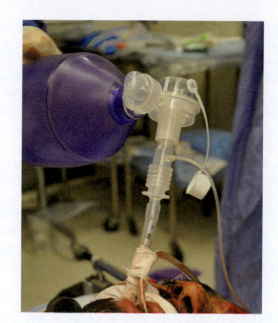

FIGURE 11-10 Monitor capnography as you ventilate the patient.
(© Edward T. Dickinson, MD)

radial pulse cannot be palpated, check for a carotid pulse. A rapid, weak carotid pulse suggests serious compensation for hypovolemia, the presence of severe hemorrhage (possibly internal), and the probable need for aggressive fluid resuscitation.

During the pulse check, also note the patient's skin condition. Cool, clammy, ashen, or pale skin suggests shock compensation. Perform a capillary refill check. If refill takes more than 3 seconds, that finding supports a possible diagnosis of hypovolemia and compensation. (Note that other conditions, such as smoking, low ambient temperatures, preexisting disease, and use of medications, may delay capillary refill as well. Using a central location to measure capillary refill and avoiding the extremities avoid the effects of these conditions.)

Make a quick visual sweep of the body, looking for any signs of serious and continuing hemorrhage. Using your mechanism of injury analysis, identify probable locations of bleeding and view them or, if the site is hidden from view, carefully pass a gloved hand under the area, looking for evidence of blood loss on your gloves. Also use the mechanism of injury analysis to identify likely locations of internal injury and any associated internal hemorrhage. Use this information to approximate the rate of probable blood loss and the priority for rapid transport.

A critical element of the primary assessment is detecting the earliest signs of shock. Remember that internal hemorrhage is the greatest killer of patients who survive the initial impact of trauma. Look carefully at your patient for any early signs of shock. These include a decreased level of consciousness or orientation, or increasing anxiety, restlessness, or combativeness. If the patient has consumed alcohol or is otherwise affected by drugs, be especially watchful and wary.

As internal hemorrhage continues, the body employs more drastic measures to compensate for the blood loss, and signs and symptoms become more obvious with the passage of time. The sooner the signs or symptoms develop, the more rapid the internal blood loss and the more quickly a patient is moving through compensated, then uncompensated, then irreversible shock. However, do not wait for signs and symptoms of later stages of shock to appear. At the first signs of hypovolemic compensation, prioritize the patient for immediate transport to the trauma center. If the patient demonstrates any early shock signs or the mechanism of injury suggests serious internal injury, initiate the steps of aggressive shock care that are described later in this chapter.

Concluding the Primary Assessment

As you complete the primary assessment, modify your mechanism of injury analysis based on additional evidence gained at the scene, such as a bent steering wheel or intrusion into the passenger compartment. Continue to monitor the scene for safety, remaining alert to any alterations in conditions at the scene and ensuring that all providers, patients, and bystanders are protected from scene hazards (including the use of personal protective equipment).

At the conclusion of the primary assessment for the trauma patient, you must determine whether the patient merits a rapid trauma assessment or is best served by a focused trauma exam. The rapid trauma assessment aims to identify other life threats not revealed during the primary assessment, to provide appropriate rapid intervention, and to ensure that the seriously injured trauma patient receives quick transport to the trauma center. The focused physical exam is used for less seriously injured patients and focuses on the probable injury, or injuries, and their care. With both these categories of patients, you will also make a preliminary decision about priority for transport. If the patient meets any of the trauma triage criteria—either a mechanism of injury recognized during the scene size-up, a recognized anatomic injury, or a physical condition identified during the primary assessment—consider the patient for rapid transport.

Blunt trauma patients found in cardiac arrest in the prehospital setting rarely, if ever, survive. This has prompted many EMS systems to institute trauma arrest protocols that permit paramedics to halt resuscitation when presented with a pulseless, nonbreathing blunt trauma patient who displays asystole on the ECG (in two leads). This action prevents the consumption of valuable resources by the EMS system and the generation of anxiety and expense for the family for what would be a fruitless effort. Consult your local protocols and medical director for your system's position on trauma arrest resuscitation.

Using the "CUPS" criteria, place your patient into the Critical, Unstable, Potentially unstable, or Stable category. Any patient who does not move out of the primary assessment because you cannot stabilize airway, breathing, or circulation is considered critical. The unstable patient is one with signs and symptoms that suggest shock or who has a potential problem with airway or breathing. A stable patient has relatively limited signs of injury, no major complaints, and no mechanism of injury to suggest serious injury. The potentially unstable patient is one who fits between stable and unstable. Early in your career, you will place a large majority of patients into the potentially unstable category. With experience, the number of patients you place in this category will shrink.

Finally make your preliminary decision regarding the patient's priority for care and transport, using the Centers for Disease Control and Prevention's Guidelines for Triage of Injured Patients, as discussed in the chapter "Trauma and Trauma Systems and as further discussed under "Transport Decision" later in this chapter.

Secondary Assessment

The secondary assessment employs the general examination techniques of questioning, inspection, palpation, auscultation, and percussion. It is either provided as the focused trauma assessment, in which assessment is directed to a specific body area to assess a specific and isolated injury, or as the rapid trauma assessment, in which assessment focuses where serious injuries are expected and to where serious injury might have occurred. Both the rapid and focused trauma assessments conclude with a quick, abbreviated patient history and the gathering of a set of baseline vital signs.

Questioning

Before you inspect or palpate a body region, question the patient about any symptoms. Symptoms may include sensations of discomfort, pain, pain on movement, tingling, a pins-and-needles sensation (paresthesia), numbness or lack of feeling (anesthesia), weakness, inability to move, or other unusual sensations. Also note the patient's response to the complaint. Patient complaints are subjective, and different people have different levels of pain tolerance. Watch how the patient responds to the pain and how easy it is to distract him from it. This gives you a good approximation of how significant the pain or sensation is to

CONTENT REVIEW
➤ Secondary Assessment Techniques
• Questioning
• Inspection
• Palpation
• Auscultation
• Percussion

the patient. Report and record any patient complaint in the patient's own words.

Inspection

As you continue inspecting the patient, look first at the skin color. The skin of a Caucasian with normal circulation will appear light pink. Note any ashen (gray or dusky), cyanotic (bluish), or pale (very light pink or white) colorations. In people of color, look at the coloration of the lips, the conjunctiva of the eyes, the palms of the hands, or the soles of the feet. Any discoloration indicates a possible generalized problem such as hypovolemia, hypoventilation, or hypothermia. Use the initial coloration you observe as a baseline when you examine specific regions of the body for injury. Look at those regions for erythema, a general reddening of the skin and the first sign of injury. The discoloration of ecchymosis (the "black and blue" normally associated with a contusion) is delayed because it takes the erythrocytes some time to migrate into injured tissue, lose their oxygen, and turn a deeper red or bluish color. A portion of a limb may also change color as a result of problems with distal circulation. The limb may turn pale (and cold) when arterial circulation is reduced or dark red, dusky, or ashen as circulation stagnates or venous return is halted.

The second element of inspection is looking for deformities. These become most recognizable if you carefully examine and compare limb to limb or one side of the body to the other. Deformity can be either an enlargement of the dimensions of a limb or body region or an abnormal angle or position of a limb or region. Enlargement is usually due to the accumulation of fluid—blood, as in a hematoma, or plasma and interstitial fluid (edema), as in inflammation associated with a contusion—but it may also be associated with the accumulation of air associated with subcutaneous emphysema. Angulation is the unusual positioning of a limb, as with a bend in a bone where a bend would not be expected. Such a condition is most likely associated with a fracture. An unusual bend in a joint, meanwhile, suggests either a fracture or dislocation. Muscle spasm or abnormal retraction of a muscle caused by tendon rupture may also cause deformity. Compare any apparent deformity to the opposite limb to better determine the nature and extent of the variance from normal.

The third element of inspection is an examination for disruption of the skin (wounds). Examine for any abrasion of the skin's surface, any tearing of the skin (laceration), or any signs of skin damage that may be associated with a burn, such as erythema, blistering or gross disruption of the skin, and discoloration. Also look for any penetrations and determine whether they are superficial or deep. Remember that deep wounds that close encourage infection and are often more serious than more grotesque superficial open wounds.

Palpation

After inspection, palpate any area for additional signs of injury. Gently touch the entire surface of the area being evaluated, feeling for general skin and muscle tone, any unusual or warm masses, any grating sensation, or the "Rice Krispies" feel of subcutaneous emphysema. You should also note any muscle spasm (guarding) or pain on palpation (tenderness) that may reflect injury. Determine if that pain is pain on touch (tenderness), pain on movement, or pain on rapid release of pressure (rebound tenderness). (Do not seek out rebound tenderness, but note it if it occurs during your assessment and care.) Also palpate for relative muscle tone—normal, flaccid, or in spasm.

Auscultation

Auscultate the chest carefully to evaluate for the presence and quality of breath sounds. Note side to side, upper lobe to lower lobe, anterior to posterior, or regional differences. Crackles may represent pulmonary edema, most commonly related to pulmonary contusion and associated edema in trauma, whereas side-to-side inequality suggests pneumothorax or tension pneumothorax. Also listen for heart sounds, noting muffled sounds, as in pericardial tamponade. Abdominal auscultation is not merited in trauma because of the time required to adequately assess for bowel sounds and their poor correlation to injury.

Percussion

Percuss each lobe of the chest for resonance. A dull response suggests fluid or blood accumulating in the pleural space. Hyperresonant response suggests air under pressure in the pleural space.

Rapid Trauma Assessment

Use the rapid trauma assessment when you suspect that a patient has a serious injury to the body and are inclined to transport him quickly to the trauma center. Such a patient is one who meets the trauma triage criteria: vital signs, anatomic signs of trauma, and mechanism of injury. Also consider consulting with medical direction regarding the transport of seriously injured patients to the trauma center if they are elderly (patients over 55 years of age); children; patients taking anticoagulants, with bleeding disorders, or with end-stage kidney disease; patients with burns; patients in the later stages of pregnancy; or those who, in your judgment, need the services of a trauma center. During the rapid trauma assessment, quickly scan the body, looking for hemorrhage or evidence of significant injury, and examine the patient's head, neck, chest, abdomen, pelvis, extremities, and back. (Order your assessment to minimize the movement of the patient. For example, if the patient is found lying face down, quickly assess the back before turning the patient for further assessment and care.)

Check the distal function in each limb by noting distal pulse strength, skin temperature and color, capillary refill time, and—as appropriate—sensation and grip strength. If you suspect specific injuries, provide a focused evaluation of the body region using the considerations for that region as specified in the detailed physical exam, discussed later in this chapter. Conclude the rapid trauma assessment by taking a quick patient history and a set of vital signs.

Focused Trauma Assessment

The focused trauma assessment is performed on a patient whom you suspect has limited injuries. This is unlikely to be a patient who meets trauma triage criteria. Direct your examination to the location of the patient's complaint or to any region of injury suggested by the mechanism of injury or by any signs and symptoms noted during the primary assessment. The actual focused trauma assessment uses the examination criteria for the body region as specified in the detailed exam. Like the rapid trauma assessment, it concludes with a quick patient history and vital signs.

Detailed Physical Exam

The detailed physical exam is a comprehensive examination of the entire body to locate and identify signs of injury. It is rarely used in the prehospital setting, as seriously injured patients receive attention directed at their life-threatening injuries and time becomes a premium as they are rushed to a trauma center. The patient with moderate or minor injuries receives assessment and care directed just at those injuries (the focused trauma assessment). The only case in which a complete detailed exam may be necessary is in a patient with an altered level of consciousness, limited apparent minor injuries, and a mechanism of injury that suggests possible multiple injury sites. Perform the detailed exam only after you have concluded the primary assessment and have stabilized or corrected any life-threatening conditions discovered during it.

The detailed physical exam is an organized and intensive evaluation of each body area: the head, neck, chest, abdomen, back, pelvis, and each extremity. When performing the detailed exam, use the physical assessment techniques of questioning, inspection, palpation, auscultation, and percussion discussed earlier in the chapter. (Using DCAP-BTLS or some other mnemonic or system may help you remember most of the important aspects of the evaluation of a body region.)

HEAD When evaluating the head, inspect and palpate its entire surface, looking for any deformity, asymmetry, or hemorrhage. In addition to looking for the obvious signs of trauma, direct special attention to the eyes, auditory canal, nose and mouth, and facial region.

Evaluate the eyes for pupillary response. Shade the eyes in a bright environment (or shine a light into them in a dark environment) and note their response. They should dilate (or constrict) briskly, equally, and consensually (together). Check eye movement by having the patient follow your finger as you trace an "H" pattern in front of him; any deficit in the patient's ability to follow your finger suggests either cranial nerve injury or orbital fracture and muscle entrapment.

Move your head to where you can visualize the length of the external auditory canal. The auditory canal should be clear of fluid and the tympanic membrane should be intact. The nose and mouth should be free of hemorrhage and physical obstruction. Any drainage of fluid from the mouth or nose endangers the airway, and nasal drainage suggests skull fracture and the possible leakage of cerebrospinal fluid. Notable signs of basilar skull fracture include bilateral periorbital ecchymosis (raccoon eyes) or retroauricular ecchymosis (Battle's sign), although both are late signs. (If you see them, suspect an earlier episode of trauma.) Gently palpate the upper jaw and feel for any crepitus or instability, indicative of a Le Fort-type fracture.

NECK Evaluate the neck for signs of injury, for the position of the trachea, and for the status of the jugular veins. The trachea should be midline in the neck and not moving to one side or tugging with respiration. Displacement to one side suggests tension pneumothorax, although this is a very late sign and not as distinguishable as the other signs of the condition. The jugular veins should be distended in the supine, normovolemic patient and flatten as the patient's torso and head are raised to a 45-degree angle. Extremely distended jugular veins (or ones distended beyond 45 degrees) suggest tension pneumothorax, pericardial tamponade, or traumatic asphyxia. Flat jugular veins in the supine patient suggest hypovolemia. It may be helpful to shine a flashlight across the jugular veins to better visualize their state of fill. Examine the neck and head for the progressive distortion and crepitus associated with subcutaneous emphysema that may accompany tension pneumothorax. Examine for any open wounds, control any hemorrhage, and cover open wounds with occlusive dressings to prevent air embolism. Anticipate tracheal (airway) compromise that may result from swelling or hemorrhage and consider early extraglottic airway insertion, intubation, or possibly rapid sequence intubation if serious neck trauma is present.

CHEST In addition to the standard elements of the physical assessment, examine the chest for intercostal or suprasternal retractions, air moving through any open wounds, and paradoxical chest wall motion. Carefully observe the chest's surface for erythema mirroring the structure of the rib cage. When the skin is trapped between an impacting force and the ribs, it contuses and may demonstrate this sign. Auscultate all lung fields of the chest, both anteriorly and posteriorly. Also listen for heart sounds. If rib injury is not obvious and the patient does not complain of rib pain, apply pressure to the lateral aspect of the rib cage and direct it medially. This will help identify any fracture site along the ribs. The pressure flexes the ribs, moves the fracture site slightly, and creates local pain. You may feel a grating sensation (crepitus) that also suggests rib or sternal fracture. Palpation may reveal a crackling sensation associated with air under the skin (subcutaneous emphysema).

ABDOMEN   Observe the abdomen for any asymmetry or apparent pulsing masses. Also look for any indication of compression by the lap belt or other signs of impact. Palpate each quadrant, with one hand placing pressure on the other while you sense any unusual masses or muscle spasm (guarding). Quickly release the pressure of palpation to detect any rebound tenderness, only if no other sign of abdominal injury is present. Always palpate the quadrant with the suspected injury last. Finally, observe and palpate the flanks.

PELVIS   In the absence of any indication of pelvic fracture, evaluate the pelvis by placing firm pressure on the iliac crests directed medially and on the pubic bone directed downward. Suspect fracture and serious internal hemorrhage if you notice any crepitus and/or any instability of the pelvis. Examine the inguinal and buttock areas, as these locations are often sites of serious injury and hemorrhage. It is essential that you expose these areas if the mechanism of injury suggests injury there, because hemorrhage is frequently hidden in jeans or other articles of clothing. Examine the underwear or other clothing for blood staining often caused by urethral injury.

EXTREMITIES   Examine each extremity and evaluate its muscle tone, distal pulse, temperature, color, and capillary refill time. Also evaluate for motor response, sensory response, and limb strength. Compare your findings in one limb to those of the opposing limb.

BACK   Examine the patient's back during your assessment or when using movement techniques such as a logroll. If spinal injury is suspected, be sure to maintain manual stabilization of the head or promptly place a cervical collar as you position the patient for examination. Examine the total surface of the back, and palpate the spine from top to bottom. Look carefully for any slight deformities, minor reddening, very subtle pain, or tenderness; these may be the only sign or symptom indicative of spinal injury.

At the conclusion of the rapid trauma assessment, the focused trauma assessment, or the detailed assessment, mentally inventory all the suspected injuries you have found. Place them in descending order of priority for care and note the contribution they make to the patient's shock state.

Trauma Patient History

During the rapid trauma assessment or the focused trauma assessment (or, in some cases, the detailed physical exam), conduct an abbreviated patient history.

SIGNS AND SYMPTOMS   The elements of the *S* component of the SAMPLE history assessment, signs and symptoms, are extensively addressed as you perform the physical assessment. Gather the remaining elements of the SAMPLE history—*A*llergies, *M*edications, *P*ast medical history, *L*ast oral intake, and *E*vents leading up to the incident—either while performing your physical examination of the patient or immediately after it.

ALLERGIES   Question the patient about allergies, especially those to medications used commonly in emergency medicine. Such allergies include those to antibiotics, the "-caine" family, analgesics, and tetanus toxoid. If any of these are noted, pass this information on to the emergency department staff.

MEDICATIONS   Investigate the patient's use of prescription and nonprescription medications, as such use may affect the patient's response to care or suggest underlying medical problems or disease. For example, drugs such as beta-blockers reduce the heart's ability to respond to hypovolemia with an increased rate. Be especially watchful for use of aspirin and clopidogrel (Plavix), which interfere with clotting; anticoagulants such as warfarin (Coumadin), rivaroxaban (Xarelto), and dabigatran (Pradaxa); and antibiotics.

PAST MEDICAL HISTORY   Question the patient about any significant medical history that may affect either his response to shock, your care, or the medications the emergency department is likely to use during treatment. Current medical problems may limit the body's ability to compensate for shock from trauma and may affect the presentation of signs and symptoms. For example, a heart condition may limit the heart's ability to increase its rate in response to a reduced preload, confounding your assessment. A normally hypertensive patient may present with a normal blood pressure that, in fact, represents hypotension.

LAST ORAL INTAKE   The quantity and time since the patient's last fluid and solid oral intake should affect your index of suspicion for abdominal injury and the care a

CONTENT REVIEW

➤ Elements of a Trauma History
  • Signs and symptoms
  • Allergies
  • Medications
  • Past medical history
  • Last oral intake
  • Events leading to the incident

patient will receive in the emergency department. If the patient's bladder, stomach, or bowel was full and strong forces of deceleration or compression were directed to the abdomen, the risk of rupture and peritonitis is increased. You should be concerned if the trauma patient has recently had anything to eat or drink, because vomiting and aspiration may complicate your prehospital airway care. Food and liquid in the stomach also pose serious risks should the patient need surgery. This is because anesthesia may precipitate vomiting, result in aspiration, and increase mortality and morbidity.

EVENTS LEADING UP TO THE INCIDENT   The events immediately preceding the incident are very important. They may suggest that the patient's trauma was caused by a medical or other problem, such as falling asleep while driving or becoming dizzy just before a fall. (Seeing no skid marks at a scene where an auto has collided with a tree is an important finding and suggests an intentional impact [attempted suicide] or some other contributing factor.)

VITAL SIGNS   Complete the rapid trauma assessment or focused exam by collecting a baseline set of vital signs. You can do this either at the scene or during transport as the patient's condition and circumstances allow. These vital signs include pulse rate and quality, blood pressure, respiration rate and quality, and skin temperature and condition. Watch for increasing pulse rate and decreasing pulse strength, increasing respiratory rate and decreasing volume, decreasing pulse pressure, and the patient's skin becoming cool and clammy. These changes all suggest increasing compensation for blood loss and shock.[4]

Glasgow Coma Scale Score

At the end of the primary assessment or concurrent with the rapid trauma assessment or focused assessment and history, determine your patient's Glasgow Coma Scale score. (Review the discussion of the GCS in the chapter "Head, Neck, and Spinal Trauma," in which Table 6–6 details the adult GCS and Table 6–7 the pediatric GCS.) Record the best eye opening, verbal response, and motor response individually (e.g., e4, v4, m6) along with the initial vital signs. Then track any changes during subsequent reassessments.

Research is demonstrating that two components of the Glasgow Coma Scale—obeying verbal commands and localizing pain—are as reliable predictors of traumatic brain injury and patient severity as is the complete GCS. These two factors make up the Simplified Motor Score (SMS), as shown in Table 6–3 of the chapter "Head, Neck, and Spinal Trauma." If the patient obeys verbal commands (SMS 2), he is considered normal. If a patient cannot obey commands but can localize pain (SMS 1), the need for airway protection is indicated.[5] If the patient can neither obey

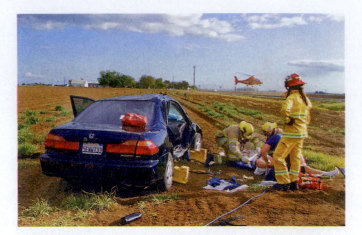

FIGURE 11-11 At the end of the rapid trauma assessment or the focused assessment, make the final decision on whether to provide stabilization on the scene or to expedite transport of the patient.
(© REACH Air Medical Services)

commands nor localize pain, there is likely to be serious traumatic brain injury.

Transport Decision

The transport decision is made in a preliminary way at the end of the primary assessment and finalized at the end of the rapid or focused trauma assessment (Figure 11-11). You will decide whether to provide rapid transport to the trauma center, treat at the scene and then transport to the nearest emergency department, or treat and release as permitted by local protocols.

The Centers for Disease Control and Prevention (CDC) has prepared a four-step process (trauma triage criteria) to make the final determination as to where the trauma patient should be transported. (Review the discussion and the CDC Guidelines for Field Triage of Injured Patients, United States 2011, which appeared in the chapter "Trauma and Trauma Systems." For review and emphasis, the CDC guidelines, which were shown in Figure 1–8 of that chapter, are shown again here, in Figure 11-12. Step 1 considers the Glasgow Coma Scale score and vital signs, as they are the most dependable predictor of trauma seriousness and outcome. Step 2 examines anatomic signs of injury, such as evidence of penetrating trauma, serious extremity injuries, flail chest, or open or depressed skull fracture. Step 3 looks at mechanism of injury to identify collisions or events that are most likely to produce serious injury. Finally, step 4 recognizes special patients who might be served by the services of a trauma center and patients who, in the paramedic's judgment, are in serious condition when the other three steps of trauma triage criteria might not suggest it.

You will notice that the steps presented here do not mirror the assessment process defined in this text. Obviously you should not defer evaluating the mechanism of

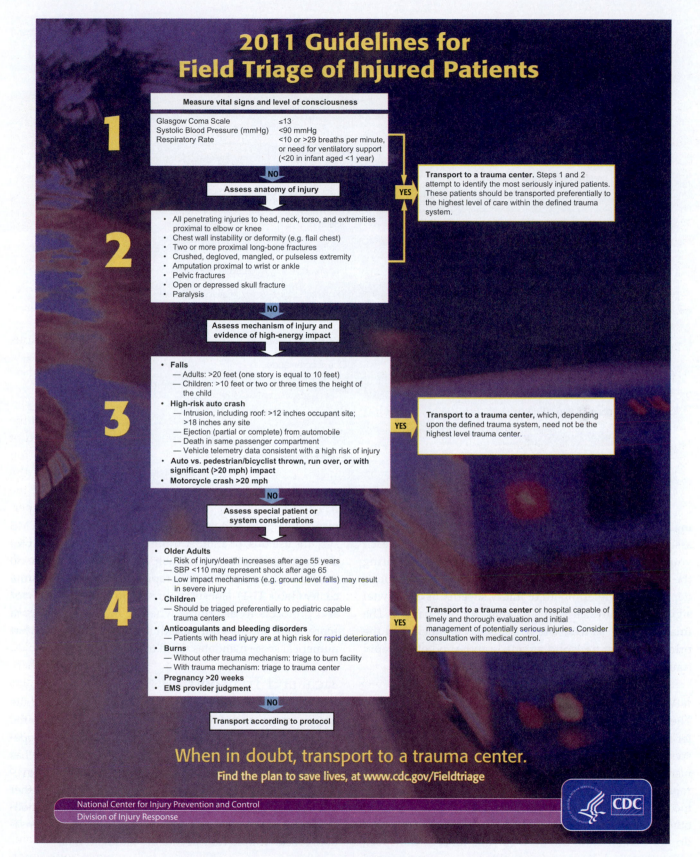

FIGURE 11-12 Centers for Disease Control and Prevention Guidelines for Field Triage of Injured Patients.

Table 11-1 Revised Trauma Score and Glasgow Coma Scale

Revised Trauma Score		Glasgow Coma Scale Score	
Respiratory Rate		**Eye Opening**	
10 to 29 breaths per minute	4	Spontaneous	4
More than 29 breaths per minute	3	To voice	3
6 to 9 breaths per minute	2	To pain	2
1 to 5 breaths per minute	1	None	1
No respiration	0	**Verbal Response**	
Systolic Blood Pressure		Oriented	5
Greater than 89 mmHg	4	Confused (cries, consolable)	4
76 to 89 mmHg	3	Inappropriate words (persistently irritable)	3
50 to 75 mmHg	2	Incomprehensible words (restless, agitated)	2
1 to 49 mmHg	1	None	1
No blood pressure	0	**Motor Response**	
Glasgow Coma Scale		Obeys commands	6
GCS score of 13 to 15	4	Localizes pain	5
GCS score of 9 to 12	3	Withdraws to pain	4
GCS score of 6 to 8	2	Flexes to pain	3
GCS score of 4 or 5	1	Extends to pain	2
GCS score of less than 4	0	None	1

injury until after you have determined the vital signs. MOI assessment occurs, to some degree, even before you reach your patient, whereas vital signs are determined during the rapid trauma assessment. Note that MOI is not as dependable a determinant of injury severity as either vital signs or the physical signs of injury on the patient. The final decisions as to where to transport a patient and the priority for that transport are made at the end of the rapid trauma assessment using the trauma triage criteria.

Rapid Transport

The decision to provide rapid transport to the trauma center is predicated on the trauma triage criteria. If any of the specified vital signs, anatomic signs of injury, or mechanisms of injury are present, the patient is a candidate for rapid transport. If the patient demonstrates a significant mechanism of injury but the signs and symptoms and the other results of your primary and rapid trauma assessment do not demonstrate the need for this level of transport, contact medical direction to possibly transport to a general hospital emergency department instead.

Revised Trauma Score

The revised trauma score is a numeric evaluation of the patient using the elements of the GCS and the patient's

respiratory rate and systolic blood pressure. Some EMS systems use this, or another trauma scoring system, to predict patient outcome and help make the decision on whether the patient requires rapid transport to a trauma center (Table 11-1). Consult your system's medical director and protocols to determine whether the revised trauma score is in use in your jurisdiction and to learn what numerical score mandates rapid transport.

Treat and Transport

Provide on-scene care to any patient who does not meet the trauma triage criteria and then transport the patient to the nearest emergency department. Manage the patient's specific injuries on the scene, and transport once your care has stabilized the injuries and the patient is packaged so movement to the ambulance and hospital will not cause further harm. If at any time during your care the patient demonstrates any signs of more serious injury or shock compensation, consider rapid transport to the trauma center.[6]

Treat and Release

Some EMS systems permit care providers to treat patients with minor injuries and then release them to see their personal physician. Provide this service only to the patient with very minor and isolated injuries. Ensure that you carefully explain to the patient what care is needed for the injury. Describe the signs that may develop indicating that the injury requires immediate attention and advise the patient that he should call your service again if those signs appear. Finally, tell the patient that he should seek care from a family physician. If possible, provide this information in written form, approved by your system of medical direction, and have the patient acknowledge in writing the receipt of these instructions. If you have any questions about treatment or release of a patient, contact your medical direction physician.

Patient Care Refusals

Some patients suffering trauma will refuse assessment, care, and transport. Although this is the patient's right, the situation represents a dilemma for prehospital care providers. The patient may not understand the significance of his injuries, and the early signs of trauma may not clearly reflect its nature or seriousness.

When confronted with a patient refusing care, advise the patient that serious injury may not present with overt or painful symptoms. Try to convince the patient to permit you to perform an assessment and provide on-scene care. If you are not successful, attempt to have the patient talk with the medical direction physician. Be sure that the patient is an adult and is fully conscious, oriented, and able to make a rational decision. Try to use family members to help you encourage the patient to accept your assessment and care. If your attempts to convince the patient fail, suggest that he see a personal physician at the earliest opportunity. Stress that the patient should feel free to call for emergency medical service if additional signs or symptoms develop or existing ones worsen. Be sure to document the refusal thoroughly. Include your recommendation that the patient receive assessment, care, and transport; your warning of the dangers of refusing assessment, care, and transport; your suggestion that the patient see a family physician; and your recommendation to contact EMS again if the problem persists or worsens. Should the patient refuse to sign this documentation, have someone else review your documentation and sign to witness it.

CONTENT REVIEW

➤ Steps to Follow If a Patient Refuses Treatment
- Suggest strongly that the patient should receive assessment, care, and transport
- Warn the patient of the dangers of refusing assessment, care, and transport
- Suggest that the patient see a family physician
- Encourage the patient to contact EMS again if the problem persists or worsens

Reassessment

Periodic trauma patient reassessment is important to monitoring and guiding the care you provide. It is performed every 5 minutes with critically or seriously injured patients and every 15 minutes with other patients. Also perform a reassessment whenever you note any change in the patient's condition or you institute any significant intervention.

During the reassessment, perform the mental, airway, breathing, and circulation status checks of the primary assessment and recheck any significant findings of the rapid or focused trauma assessment. Reassess vital signs—blood pressure; rate, regularity, and strength of the pulse; respiratory rate, volume, and regularity; skin condition; and GCS score. With any limb injury, recheck the distal pulse, capillary refill, muscle strength, and sensation.

Pay particular attention to an increasing pulse rate, decreasing pulse strength (pulse pressure), increasing respiratory rate, decreasing respiratory volume, increasing capillary refill time, decreasing level of consciousness or orientation, change in skin color or temperature, or increasing anxiety or restlessness. Any of these signs may indicate patient deterioration. Compare results of each reassessment to baseline findings and those from previous reassessments to identify any deterioration or improvement in the patient's condition. Record the results serially so that trending of the patient's signs can continue after arrival at the emergency department.

CONTENT REVIEW

➤ Signs of Deterioration during Reassessment
- Increasing pulse rate
- Decreasing pulse strength
- Narrowing pulse pressure
- Increasing respiratory rate
- Decreasing respiratory volume
- Increasing capillary refill time
- Decreasing level of consciousness or orientation
- Changes in skin color or temperature
- Increasing anxiety or restlessness

Shock/Multisystem Trauma Resuscitation
Hypovolemia/Hypotension/ Hypoperfusion

Three very important terms are used to describe the status of the cardiovascular system in trauma: hypovolemia, hypotension, and hypoperfusion. **Hypovolemia** refers to a reduced volume in the cardiovascular system, caused by hemorrhage, by an excess of fluid loss against inadequate fluid intake, or by losses into third spaces, as with plasma into burns. A relative hypovolemia may occur as the vascular system expands (with spinal injury) and the normal vascular volume is inadequate to fill it. **Hypotension** simply refers to a reduction in blood pressure caused by cardiac, vascular, neurogenic, or volume problems to a level that is lower than normal for the patient. **Hypoperfusion** is a low or inadequate distribution of blood to body organs and tissues caused by cardiac, vascular, neurogenic, or volume problems.

In serious trauma, it is likely that more than one body system will be involved. This multisystem trauma often involves the central nervous, respiratory, and cardiovascular systems. Shock trauma resuscitation is care for multisystem trauma to rapidly support the seriously injured trauma patient while he is rushed to the trauma center (Figure 11-13). These include:

- Providing airway protection with extraglottic airway insertion, endotracheal intubation, or rapid sequence intubation

- Ensuring adequate oxygenation and ventilations

- Halting any serious external hemorrhage

- Providing appropriate fluid resuscitation with isotonic solution

- Performing pleural decompression

Whenever serious trauma is expected or the signs of shock compensation are evident, consider protecting the airway with an extraglottic airway. If that is unsuccessful, consider introducing an endotracheal tube using the

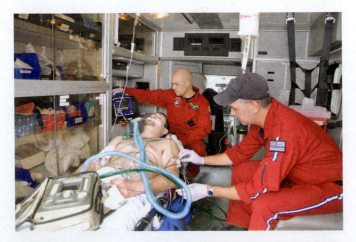

FIGURE 11-13 With a seriously injured trauma patient, employ the aggressive care steps of shock trauma resuscitation.

(© Edward T. Dickinson, MD)

orotracheal method of insertion. Anticipate that the seriously injured patient will deteriorate and be prepared to protect the airway early. Consider using rapid sequence intubation in the extremely agitated or combative patient when shock is evident and the patient demonstrates a steady deterioration. Recent studies are demonstrating that endotracheal intubation, and especially rapid sequence intubation, are not without risks. It may be prudent to focus on placing an extraglottic airway as a first choice and considering intubation only if that airway choice proves ineffective.[7]

If oxygen saturation is below 96 percent, apply supplemental oxygen immediately. Consider ventilating the patient (overdrive ventilation with bag-valve mask) if the respirations move less than 500 mL of air or respirations occur fewer than 10 or more than 29 times per minute. Rapidly control significant hemorrhage with direct pressure. Consider tourniquet use if you are providing care in a hazardous environment or direct pressure does not quickly control the bleeding.

Initiate a large-bore intravenous site in a large vein and connect a nonrestrictive (either trauma or blood tubing) administration set and a 1,000-mL bag of normal saline.[8] If traditional IV sites are not available, consider the humoral (or other) intraosseous site. If shock is present or expected, choose large veins for cannulation (the antecubital veins). Veins in the forearm or hand are secondary choices. Run the fluid at a to-keep-open rate as long as the patient maintains his blood pressure (pulse pressure) and pulse rate. Be ready to rapidly infuse fluids quickly should the patient begin to show increasing signs and symptoms of serious compensation and shock. Generally, the maximum prehospital fluid volume is 3,000 mL of isotonic solution administered in boluses. You may adjust this volume based on the size of the patient and the patient's response to infusion (slowing pulse, increasing pulse strength, increasing level of consciousness). Titrate your infusion rate to ensure a systolic blood pressure of 80 mmHg (or 90 mmHg for the suspected head injury patient). Auscultate the lung fields for signs of edema and halt or reduce the rate of fluid administration with the development of any crackles.[9]

Be sure to seek signs and symptoms of tension pneumothorax during your assessment. If the patient displays the appropriate signs and has significant dyspnea, decompress the affected side of the chest with a large-bore catheter inserted in the second or third intercostal space, midclavicular line. These steps of shock care are essential to maintain the patient until further, possibly invasive, procedures occur at the hospital.

There are several general considerations to keep in mind in shock/multisystem trauma resuscitation situations. These include preventing hypothermia, providing rapid body splinting, providing rapid transport, and reducing the effects of the fight-or-flight response.

Cultural Considerations

Beliefs about Blood Loss and Transfusion. Many religions and cultures have specific beliefs about blood loss and transfusions. It is important for EMS personnel to understand and respect these beliefs. For example, large numbers of Hmong immigrated to the United States and Canada after the Vietnam conflict. The Hmong are among the oldest groups of people in Asia and are often referred to as the "Hill People." They put great faith in folk medicine and sometimes will trust a shaman more than a Western medical practitioner. Many Hmong believe that the body has a limited amount of blood, and any blood loss can cause permanent problems. Furthermore, many Hmong believe that any injuries or surgical procedures sustained in life will remain with them when they enter the spirit world. Thus, many Western practices, such as surgery and autopsy, may be forbidden by members of this culture.

The Jehovah's Witnesses are a religious group that has specifically forbidden blood transfusions. This belief comes from their interpretation of a Bible verse (Acts 15:29) that states "That ye abstain from meats offered to idols, and from blood, and from things strangled, and from fornication, from which if ye keep yourselves, ye shall do well. Fare ye well." Although some have interpreted this verse to mean the literal "eating of blood," the Jehovah's Witnesses have interpreted it to include the transfusion of blood. The beliefs will vary from individual to individual. Some Jehovah's Witnesses will allow the administration of crystalloid fluids, whereas others will allow the actual administration of some blood components (plasma, globulins, and platelets). However, many will refuse all blood or similar products. Regardless of the severity of the patient's condition, the paramedic must respect this wish and adjust treatment plans accordingly.

Hypothermia

Hypothermia is a relatively unappreciated complication of serious trauma and shock. Lessons from the wars in Iraq and Afghanistan, however, have highlighted the need for attention to trauma-induced hypothermia and its consequences. Trauma often initiates the fight-or-flight response, which causes the body to direct its energy away from the internal organs and to the skeletal muscles. When a patient stops his flight (as during your care), the body's energy and heat production decrease dramatically. The problem is further compounded as the body directs its remaining blood volume to critical organs and not to temperature regulation activities. The result is a patient who is very susceptible to hypothermia (Figure 11-14). Caregivers contribute to this problem when they provide rapid fluid resuscitation with fluids that are often at ambient, rather than body, temperature. The result is a rapid infusion of hypothermic fluid and a further lowering of the body's core temperature. In addition, care providers

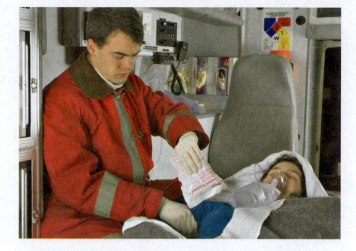

FIGURE 11-14 Hypothermia poses a serious threat to trauma patients. Ensure that your care helps the patient maintain body temperature.

frequently disrobe patients during assessment and fail to re-cover them adequately with warm blankets. In all but the warmest environments, this behavior only compounds hypothermia.

Hypothermia can have several negative effects on a patient suffering from injury and shock. The body's natural response to heat loss is increased skeletal muscle activity, specifically shivering. This heat generation consumes the body's energy reserves and increases the impact of injury and shock. A decrease in body temperature also affects blood clotting by inhibiting the clotting cascade and prolonging clotting times. The colder temperature also causes the platelets to release a heparin-like anticoagulant agent that further slows the clotting process. Critical body enzymes, too, do not function efficiently at subnormal body temperature. This can disrupt oxygen use, decrease metabolism, and exacerbate acidosis.

It is essential to recognize the negative impact a lowering of body temperature has on the patient during shock. Always try to administer fluids that are as close to body temperature as possible, especially in colder environments. Use fluid warmers as necessary. Use more blankets to cover an injured patient than you would use with an uninjured patient in the same environmental conditions. A number of commercial high-efficiency passive and active external rewarming devices are available and should be considered for any lengthy transports or cold-weather operations. Keep your ambulance warmer than is comfortable for you with a target of 85 degrees Fahrenheit.

Body Splinting

The seriously injured trauma patient is likely to have suffered internal injury, life-threatening hemorrhage, and long-bone and possible spinal fractures. To ensure rapid transport to the trauma center while not compounding the patient's injuries, splinting must be effective, yet must be done quickly. For the seriously injured trauma patient, you can best accomplish this splinting by gently aligning all the limbs and firmly securing the entire patient to a long spine board or orthopedic stretcher. Movement onto the movement device should occur in one coordinated move from the patient's initial location. Body splinting ensures that if there is any movement of the limbs while packaging, loading, or transporting the patient, the movement will be limited, thus reducing the chances of aggravating existing injuries.[10]

Rapid Transport

Research has clearly demonstrated that the best way to reduce trauma mortality is to bring the seriously injured patient to surgery as quickly as possible. This presumes that the greatest risk to life is from internal hemorrhage and the only definitive remedy for that risk may be surgical repair. Care providers can help meet this objective by providing rapid on-scene assessment, extrication, patient packaging, and transport while maintaining the patient through airway, ventilatory, and circulatory support. Make every effort to reduce the time at the emergency scene, and limit your actions there so that on-scene time is no more than 10 minutes (the "platinum 10 minutes" of prehospital care). Perform procedures such as IV insertion while applying spinal stabilization based on local protocols, ensuring and supporting the airway and breathing, or controlling hemorrhage, or while preparing to move the patient. Otherwise, carry out these procedures in the ambulance during transport. Use air medical service only when it will substantially reduce transport time to definitive care. Be sure to alert the trauma center of the nature of your patient's injuries, the mechanism of injury that caused those injuries, the care you are providing, the patient's response to that care, and any trending in vital signs you note. Always provide detailed and complete documentation of these items in your prehospital care report.

Fight-or-Flight Response

When a person is under extreme stress or in fear of bodily harm, the autonomic nervous system responds with a release of adrenaline and an increase in several body functions. These actions induce an increase in heart rate, stroke volume, blood pressure, respiratory rate and volume, and a release of glucose and insulin into the bloodstream. The result is a rapid expenditure of body resources that might be otherwise used for repair and recovery. To reduce the effect of the fight-or-flight response and to make the patient more comfortable with the emergency medical care, try to be calming and reassuring. Clearly tell the patient who you are and that you are there to help. Listen carefully to what the patient says, and describe what will happen during care

and why. Let the patient see that you are confident in the care you are about to provide and that your sincere desire is to attend to his injuries. Maintain continuous communication with the patient and try to distract him from concerns over the injuries and the impact they may have on the patient's life. Doing these things will help reduce patient anxiety and the effects of the fight-or-flight response.

It should be noted that four critical factors are directly related to preventable trauma death. They are controllable airway obstruction, external hemorrhage, pneumothorax, and hypothermia. Ensure that any patient you are treating for serious injury and possible shock has a clear airway and no significant dyspnea. Ensure that all significant external hemorrhage is controlled. Rule out tension pneumothorax, and maintain the patient's body temperature.

Noncritical Patients

Patients needing the services of a trauma center represent only about 10 percent of all trauma patients.[11] Although we "overtriage" around twice this number to ensure that we do not miss individuals with subtle or concealed injuries, noncritical patients account for about 80 percent of trauma responses and receive the largest part of prehospital trauma care.[11] These are patients who do not demonstrate the vital signs, anatomic signs, or mechanisms of injury detailed in trauma triage criteria and who receive the focused trauma assessment.

Noncritical trauma patients receive care directed at their specific injuries. These patients normally require dressing, bandaging, and immobilization of the wound or skeletal injury site and comfortable (and slow) transport to the emergency department of their choice (within reason). With these patients, be careful to monitor distal sensation, motor function, pulses, temperature, and capillary refill to ensure that there is no neurologic or vascular compromise from the injury or from the bandaging or splinting provided. Should you detect any deficit or any signs or symptoms of developing hypovolemia or shock, increase the patient's priority for transport and consider rerouting to the trauma center.

Special Patients

Two categories of trauma patients who require special attention are the very young and the old. The pediatric patient is small, growing, and somewhat different anatomically from the adult. The geriatric patient often has preexisting medical problems and body systems that are not as responsive to the effects of trauma as those of their younger adult counterparts. Three other categories of special patients are pregnant, bariatric (obese), and cognitively impaired patients. These five categories of special patients respond differently to trauma than average adult patients and must be assessed, prioritized, and cared for accordingly.

Pediatric Patients

Pediatric patients are, in many ways, just small adults. They have the same basic anatomy and, for the most part, the same physiology. Because of their smaller size and the dynamics of their growth, however, the effects of trauma on pediatric patients are different from the effects on adults (Figure 11-15). Further, damage to the child's rapidly growing body may have significant, long-lasting effects.

Trauma is the greatest cause of death and disability among pediatric patients after the first year of life. The pediatric patient is most likely to suffer blunt trauma. The most commonly experienced forms of blunt trauma in pediatric patients are auto impacts (including vehicle crashes and pedestrian-versus-auto and bicycle-versus-auto collisions), falls, and abuse (in that order). Penetrating trauma (gunshot and knife wounds) is also on the rise in the pediatric population over age 14.[12] Contributing factors to the mortality and morbidity of pediatric trauma are the child's limited life experience and undeveloped recognition of and respect for trauma hazards and their consequences.

The smaller size and weight of infants and children mean that they have a larger ratio of body surface area to volume than adults do. This means that infants and children lose or gain heat from the environment much more quickly than adults do. Extensive body surface injuries (such as abrasions and burns) become more devastating because of the proportionally greater fluid loss to the injury and the environment. Because of their smaller size, the organs of pediatric patients are closer together, and multisystem trauma is thus more frequent. In pediatric pedestrian-versus-auto impacts, the energy causing injury is delivered higher on the anatomy. The initial impact is likely to affect the pelvis, abdomen, and chest, resulting in greater internal injuries and a smaller incidence of extremity trauma. The impact is also more likely to propel the child ahead of the car, where he may be struck again by it or run over.

Some aspects of pediatric anatomy differ significantly from those of adults. The limbs are proportionally shorter than those of the mature adult and are less able and effective in protecting children from trunk trauma. Infants and young children have less subcutaneous fat and less-developed

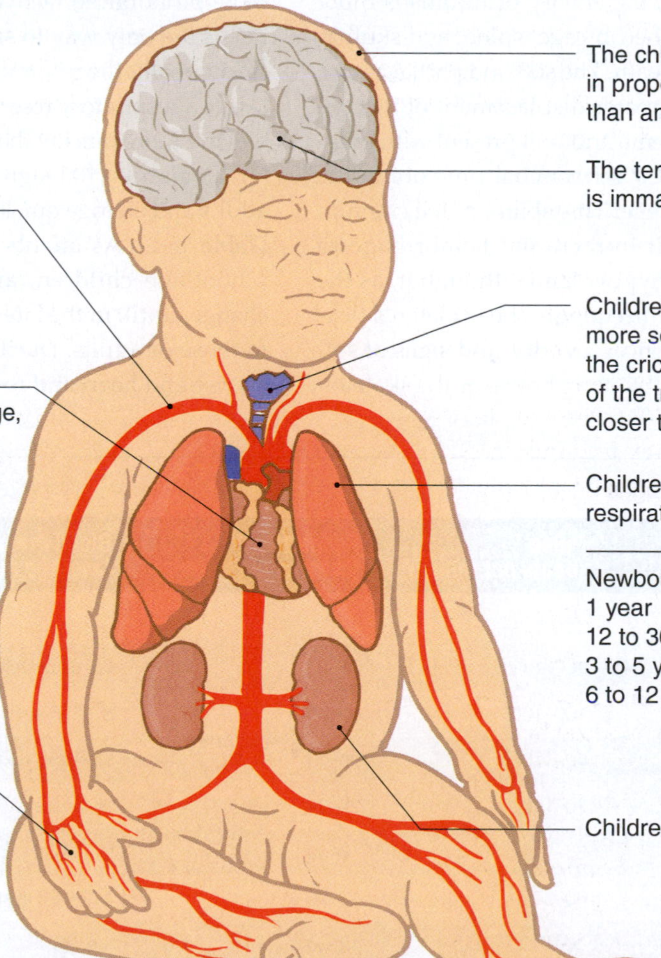

Children have less blood and are therefore in greater danger of developing shock from a relatively minor wound.

Children have faster heart rates:

Normal range, pulse per minute	
Newborn	100–180
1 year	100–160
12 to 36 months	80–110
3 to 5 years	70–110
6 to 12 years	65–110

Perfusion to extremities markedly decreases in shock. Testing capillary refill is useful in assessment.

The child's head is larger in proportion to the body than an adult's head.

The temperature control mechanism is immature in infants.

Children have smaller airways with more soft tissue and a narrowing at the cricoid cartilage. The openings of the trachea and esophagus are closer together.

Children have faster respiratory rates:

Breaths per minute	
Newborn	30–60
1 year	30–60
12 to 36 months	24–40
3 to 5 years	22–34
6 to 12 years	18–30

Children dehydrate easily.

FIGURE 11-15 Anatomic and physiologic considerations with infant and child patients.

muscle masses to protect the internal organs. The heads of infants and children are proportionally larger than those of adults, which results in a greater incidence of blunt head trauma and the application of proportionally greater forces to the neck during acceleration or deceleration. The increased head size also means that when infants or young children are supine the neck is flexed, which may contribute to airway obstruction. The tongues of infants and children fill more of the oral cavity and are more likely to obstruct the airway than in adults. Infants' anatomy also means they must breathe through the nose (obligate nasal breathers), thus providing only one airway with no detour around its obstruction. The trachea in infants and children is shorter, more delicate, more prone to kinking, and more prone to intubation of the right mainstem bronchus and soft tissue trauma. The mediastinum is more mobile in pediatric patients, which permits greater displacement during tension pneumothorax, resulting in an earlier development of the pathology and a greater restriction of venous return to the heart than in adults.

The pediatric skeletal system grows rapidly. It begins as cartilage and becomes more rigid and stronger with age. This development permits great flexibility and protects the skeleton from fracture. However, the energy of trauma is more easily transmitted through the rib cage, spine, and skull to injure the vital structures beneath. The soft and partial nature of the skull also permits a greater displacement of its contents with hemorrhage or edema and will present with bulging fontanelles with increased intracranial pressure in the child less than 18 months of age. This ability of the cranium to expand may also permit intracranial hemorrhage to substantially contribute to hypovolemia, though it, as the sole cause of shock, is very infrequent. The skeleton's flexibility also lessens the incidence, severity, and signs of soft tissue injury. When injured, the long bones of the skeleton frequently resist fracture until just one side of the bone gives way. The resulting fracture, called a greenstick fracture, provides a relatively stable, though somewhat deformed, limb. However, this type of fracture promotes increased growth on the uninjured side, causing further angulation of the limb. For this reason, a surgeon sometimes completes a greenstick fracture later in the process of care. Long-bone injury is also likely to occur at the site of bone growth, the epiphyseal plate. This type of injury may damage the growth potential of the limb and create a lifelong disability.

The components of the cardiovascular systems of infants and children are much more vibrant than those in adults. They are very able to compensate for blood loss secondary to trauma and do not show overt signs of compensation as quickly. In fact, pediatric patients may lose up to 25 percent of their blood volume before any signs appear and may lose 50 percent of their blood volume before compensation fails. However, once pediatric patients can no longer compensate for blood loss, they move very quickly toward irreversible shock. The heart of a pediatric patient cannot increase its stroke volume as the heart of an adult does. In hypovolemia and shock, this results in an earlier and more pronounced tachycardia because an increase in heart rate is the only way to significantly increase cardiac output. Additionally, the respiratory system in a pediatric patient has less of a respiratory reserve, is less able to tolerate stress, and will tire more quickly than an adult's respiratory system.

Pediatric vital signs are very different from those of adults and change quickly during the developmental years (Table 11-2). As infants grow into toddlers, preschoolers, school-age children, and adolescents, their vital signs change, until, in the late teens, their ranges are very similar to those of adults. During these years, blood pressure levels rise and heart and respiratory rates fall. These changing

Table 11-2 Normal Vital Signs

	Pulse (beats per minute)	Respiration (breaths per minute)	Blood Pressure (average mmHg)	Temperature	
Infancy					
At Birth	100–180	30–60	60–90 systolic	98°–100°F	36.7°–37.8°C
At 1 Year	100–160	30–60	87–105 systolic	98°–100°F	36.7°–37.8°C
Toddler (12 to 36 months)	80–110	24–40	95–105 systolic	96.8°–99.6°F	36.3°–37.9°C
Preschool Age (3 to 5 years)	70–110	22–34	95–110 systolic	96.8°–99.6°F	36.3°–37.9°C
School Age (6 to 12 years)	65–110	18–30	97–112 systolic	98.6°F	37°C
Adolescence (13 to 18 years)	60–90	12–26	112–128 systolic	98.6°F	37°C
Early Adulthood (19 to 40 years)	60–100	12–20	120/80	98.6°F	37°C
Middle Adulthood (41 to 60 years)	60–100	12–20	120/80	98.6°F	37°C
Late Adulthood (61 years and older)	+	+	+	98.6°F	37°C

+ Depends on the individual's physical health status.

vital signs make accurate assessment of pediatric patients more difficult because you must accurately determine the child's age and vital signs and then compare them to the normal rates for that age. It is helpful to keep a pediatric vital sign table handy when responding to a pediatric trauma emergency.

Psychologically and socially, pediatric patients respond very differently both to injury and to care providers than do adults. The responses also change dramatically with the child's growth and development. Refer to the chapter "Pediatrics" for a fuller discussion of pediatric growth and development.

As with adults, calculation of a trauma score can help to predict patient outcome and form transport decisions. However, the criteria for pediatric patients are different from the criteria for adults, as shown in Table 11-3.

Table 11-3 Pediatric Trauma Score and Glasgow Coma Scale Score

Pediatric Trauma Score			
Score	**+2**	**+1**	**−1**
Weight	> 44 lb (> 20 kg)	22–44 lb (10–20 kg)	< 22 lb (< 10 kg)
Airway	Normal	Oral or nasal airway	Intubated, tracheostomy, invasive airway
Blood pressure	Pulse at wrist > 90 mmHg	Carotid or femoral pulse palpable 50–90 mmHg	No palpable pulse or < 50 mmHg
Level of consciousness	Completely awake	Obtunded or any loss of consciousness	Comatose
Open wound	None	Minor	Major or penetrating
Fractures	None	Closed fracture	Open or multiple fractures

Pediatric Glasgow Coma Scale				
		>1 Year	**<1 Year**	
Eye opening	4	Spontaneous	Spontaneous	
	3	To verbal command	To shout	
	2	To pain	To pain	
	1	No response	No response	
		>1 Year	**<1 Year**	
Best motor response	6	Obeys		
	5	Localizes pain	Localizes pain	
	4	Flexion—withdrawal	Flexion—withdrawal	
	3	Flexion—abnormal (decorticate rigidity)	Flexion—abnormal (decorticate rigidity)	
	2	Extension (decerebrate rigidity)	Extension (decerebrate rigidity)	
	1	No response	No response	
		>5 Years	**2–5 Years**	**0–23 Months**
Best verbal response	5	Oriented and converses	Appropriate words and phrases	Smiles, coos, cries appropriately
	4	Disoriented and converses	Inappropriate words	Cries
	3	Inappropriate words	Cries and/or screams	Inappropriate crying and/or screaming
	2	Incomprehensible sounds	Grunts	Grunts
	1	No response	No response	No response

MANAGEMENT OF THE PEDIATRIC PATIENT Shock/multisystem trauma resuscitation for pediatric patients follows the same basic processes of assessment and care used with adults, but makes allowances for differences in pediatric anatomy and physiology. Maintain the airway in a neutral position with padding under the shoulders for an infant and limited or no padding under the shoulders or head of a child (depending on the child's anatomic size). This avoids kinking the relatively soft trachea, avoids blocking the airway, and helps align the structures of the posterior pharynx, the larynx, and the trachea to ease intubation. To secure the airway, use an appropriately sized oral airway or intubate. Insert the oral airway using a tongue blade, as the normal insertion technique with a 180-degree turn used in adults may injure the delicate soft tissue of the infant or very young child's oral pharynx. Be sure to keep the nasal passage clear in pediatric patients under six months of age, as they are obligate nasal breathers. If intubation is considered, use a tube that approximates the diameter of the patient's little finger. Insert the tube gently and pass it only a couple of centimeters beyond the glottis because the pediatric patient is prone to soft tissue injury and (because of the short trachea) to right mainstem bronchus intubation. Secure the endotracheal tube firmly and carefully monitor the tube's location and the breath sounds because uncuffed tubes, if used, may easily be dislodged from the very short trachea.

Initiate intravenous access as with an adult, and be certain to use catheters sized to the patient's veins because you will infuse reduced volumes of fluid. If you cannot obtain normal venous access, consider using the intraosseous site for administration of both medications and fluid (Figure 11-16). Fluid boluses for volume replacement are usually given as 20 mL/kg boluses. Administer this volume sooner in the pediatric patient than you would in the adult. This is because infants and children compensate more effectively for fluid loss and you are likely to recognize hypovolemia late in its development. This bolus may be given up to three times, for a total of 60 mL/kg.

Consider less significant mechanisms of injury and more minimal signs of injury than you would with adults as grounds for transporting pediatric patients to the trauma center. Pediatric patients have less protection for internal body organs and are more likely to show fewer signs and symptoms of injury. They have a greater incidence of serious and multisystem trauma than adults. If possible, consider transport to a facility able to accommodate the special needs of pediatric trauma patients—the pediatric trauma center.

Pregnant Patients

Trauma in pregnancy represents an injury endangering the life and health of both the mother and developing fetus. Pregnancy represents physiologic changes to the mother

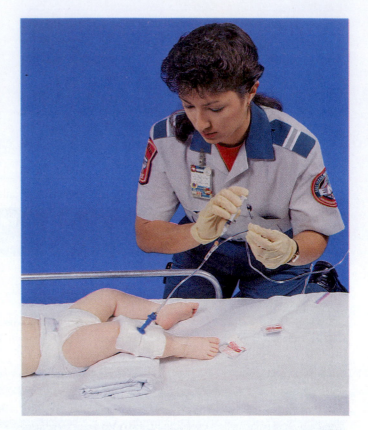

FIGURE 11-16 Consider intraosseous placement in the tibia when administering fluids and medications in children under age 6 if you cannot obtain normal intravenous access.

that alter the way she responds to injury and blood loss. It also represents a second patient, the fetus. The fetus is completely dependent on the health of the mother and her ability to provide oxygen and nutrients and remove carbon dioxide and waste products from the fetal circulation through the placenta/uterine wall. This exchange is at risk early in the development of hypovolemia and shock in the mother. It is important for us to look at the incidence of trauma in pregnancy, physiologic changes to the mother during pregnancy, and factors that change the assessment and management of the pregnant female.

Trauma in pregnancy is the most common cause of both maternal and fetal mortality. Trauma in pregnancy is most frequently related to motor vehicle collisions, violence (most frequently domestic violence), and falls. Seat belt use is the most modifiable risk factor and has a significant influence on both maternal and fetal mortality and morbidity. Proper seat belt use for the pregnant mother should be a target of the EMS system's efforts at prevention.

PHYSIOLOGY OF THE PREGNANT PATIENT The blood volume of a pregnant woman increases throughout gestation to about 150 percent of normal (an increase of 50 percent). Most of this increased volume consists of increased plasma volume. Because red blood cell production does not match the vascular fluid increase, there is a relative anemia (that is, the number of red blood cells remains the same, but the plasma volume is increased). The heart rate increases by 10 to 15 beats per minute, with an associated increase in cardiac output. Blood pressure falls by 5 to 15 mmHg during the second trimester but then returns to normal near term. Because of the size and placement of the near-term uterus, it may compress the inferior vena cava and result in supine hypotension. Displacement by the pregnant uterus can push the heart upward in the chest and may demonstrate a leftward 15-degree axis shift on the 12-lead ECG. Pregnancy induces an increased oxygen demand. To accommodate this increased demand, maternal tidal volume increases, resulting in a greater minute volume. The increased respiratory minute volume produces a slight hypocapnia at end of term.

The thickening uterus and developing fetus are well protected within the pelvic cavity during the first trimester. During the second trimester they are equally protected by the pelvic ring and the lower abdomen. However, by the third trimester the pregnant uterus is much thinner, the fetus much larger, and they displace the abdominal contents upward. This more directly exposes the uterus and fetus to direct trauma and places the abdominal contents much higher anatomically than they would be in the nonpregnant woman.

PATHOPHYSIOLOGY OF THE PREGNANT PATIENT

During gestation, the developing fetus is well protected by the pelvic ring, the muscular uterine wall, and the amniotic fluid that surrounds it and fills the uterus. However, because the fetus receives its nourishment from the maternal circulation through the placenta and umbilical cord, it is at risk whenever the mother is at risk. Any hypovolemia, shock, or hypoxia endangers the fetus well before it endangers the mother. It is said that the best fetal care is to care for the mother. The fetus is also at risk from blunt trauma that may occur as the mother strikes the auto dash during a crash or when struck by an object like a baseball bat during an assault. These mechanisms may cause direct or indirect (contrecoup) injuries to the fetus or cause the placenta to shear and separate from the uterine wall—abruptio placentae.

The abdomen is dynamic as the pregnancy progresses. In the first trimester and early second trimester, the abdominal contents remain in their normal position and are subject to trauma as with those organs for the nonpregnant patient. As the pregnancy progresses, however, the increasing size of the pregnant uterus displaces most abdominal organs laterally and superiorly. This generally protects the organs and puts the uterus and developing fetus more at risk for injury. Pelvic fractures, when they occur in very late pregnancy (as when the head is engaged), may result in fetal head injury, but this is rare. Cardiac arrest occurs no more frequently in the pregnant

mother than in nonpregnant women of the same age. When it does occur, it represents a threat to two lives and special energies toward resuscitation should be initiated. However, remember that arrest resulting from hypovolemia has a very poor prognosis.

Seat belts reduce the incidence of premature delivery, abruptio placentae, and fetal death. The use of a lap belt alone, though, permits forward motion of the pregnant mother, compressing the uterus and its contents. This may lead to uterine rupture or abruptio placentae. A lap belt used alone and placed too high may compress the pregnant uterus and result in the same pathologies. The shoulder belt should be moved to the side of the pregnant uterus in the late pregnancy female.

Domestic violence is a major cause of trauma in pregnancy.[13] Be suspicious if you note the explanation of what happened does not fit with the injuries found, there is a series of unexplained injuries, the patient has a lowered self-image, or the domestic partner attempts to monopolize the conversation. Report any suspected abuse to the emergency department or as called for by your protocols or state statutes.

ASSESSMENT OF THE PREGNANT PATIENT   Progress through your primary assessment as you would with any trauma patient, observing the following differences for the pregnant woman. During the general impression, ask the mother about the length of pregnancy and the trimester she is in. Visualize the abdomen and, from the size and placement of the uterus, approximate the gestational age. If spinal precautions are required, rotate the patient at least 15 to 30 degrees to take the uterine weight off the vena cava. Ensure that the airway is adequate and provide supplemental oxygen if needed to maintain an oxygen saturation of at least 96 percent. Remember, the fetus is often first affected by inadequate oxygen levels.

Quickly evaluate respiratory rate and depth. They should be slightly faster than normal and a bit deeper. If the respiratory rate is less than 20 it is possible that respirations are not adequate. Seek other respiratory signs and symptoms such as dyspnea and low oxygen saturation. Carefully look for signs of hemorrhage and be very watchful for signs of shock. They develop later in the blood loss process than for nonpregnant patients, yet the fetus is at risk very early as shock develops. The third-trimester pregnant patient may not display a significantly elevated pulse rate until late in the shock process. It is critical to stop bleeding early and stabilize the circulatory system with fluid resuscitation, as needed. If a late-term pregnant patient is found in cardiac arrest, resuscitation efforts should be considered, as the fetus may be viable. Note, however, that the heart may be displaced somewhat higher and to the left in the chest and the normal landmarks for CPR may not provide for proper hand positioning.

Categorize the pregnant patient one category more serious in the CUPS system at the end of the primary assessment. If you find your patient to be either U (unstable) or P (potentially unstable), perform the rapid trauma assessment. Otherwise, provide a focused trauma assessment while being watchful for any signs of maternal distress or early signs of shock.

If the patient is noticeably pregnant and a victim of a serious vehicle crash, and especially if a lap belt was worn without the shoulder strap, palpate the fundus of the uterus in the lower abdomen. It should be firm and round. If you feel significant irregularity, and any features of the fetus, suspect a ruptured uterus. Also maintain a high index of suspicion for abruptio placentae with any significant blunt trauma to the abdomen. Examine for vaginal hemorrhage.

MANAGEMENT OF THE PREGNANT PATIENT

Management of the pregnant woman subjected to trauma must place special emphases on ensuring an adequate airway, ventilation, and circulation. It is important to apply supplemental oxygen to ensure an oxygen saturation of at least 96 percent or higher. Remember that oxygen must travel through the mother's circulation to reach the uterine wall, then traverse the wall to the placenta and enter the fetal circulation. Then it must be circulated by the fetal circulation to the target tissues. Place a special emphasis on ensuring a good airway and ventilation for the mother because any hypoxia may have profound effects on the fetus.

The mother in late stages of pregnancy should be positioned not supine, but rather in the left lateral recumbent position. If the patient is secured to a spine board, tilt the board 15 degrees. This prevents the uterus from compressing the inferior vena cava against the sacral spine, slowing venous return to the heart, and inducing hypotension. When blood loss is suspected, consider aggressive fluid resuscitation. Remember that pregnancy increases the vascular volume, and the pregnant mother may lose a great deal of blood and endanger the baby while displaying limited signs and symptoms of hypovolemia. A significant trauma risk to the mother and fetus is abruptio placentae. It should be considered when the patient complains of abdominal pain and there is any uterine bleeding (in about 70 percent of abruptio placentae cases).

Bariatric Patients

Society as a whole is getting heavier, and it estimated that more than 25 percent of the population is obese. This is, in part, associated with greater access to higher-caloric food and a more sedentary lifestyle. The pathophysiology of obesity is explained elsewhere in this series, but these patients present problems for assessment and care when trauma is involved (Figure 11-17).[14]

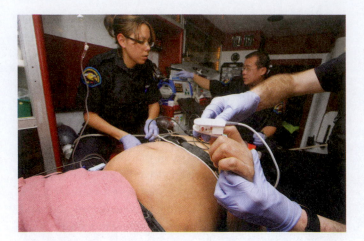

FIGURE 11-17 Obese trauma patients present numerous challenges for assessment and care.

(© Kevin Link/Science Source)

The obese patient is likely to have increased blood volume and increased cardiac output as a result of increased oxygen demand caused by an increase in body tissue. Over time, this can lead to systemic hypertension and myocardial hypertrophy and a higher risk of arrhythmias, cardiac failure, and cardiac arrest. In trauma, it can leave the obese patient less able to accommodate the stresses of injury, hypovolemia, and shock. Obesity also increases the work of breathing as a result of increased intraabdominal pressure and increased chest wall resistance. Often, the patient will exhibit reduced tidal volume, vital capacity, and total lung capacity. He may, however, have an increased respiratory rate and minute volume to accommodate increased metabolic needs. Obesity in trauma leads to an increase in multiple organ involvement, more serious pulmonary complications, and a mortality of up to six times greater than a normal-weight patient. Obese patients are more likely to suffer pulmonary contusions and pelvic, rib, and extremity fracture, with slightly less incidence of head injury.[15] (Obese patients may also have multiple disease pathologies, such as diabetes, and may be on multiple medications—all of which may make assessment and care of the bariatric patient more complicated.)

The obese patient's primary assessment follows the standard primary assessment process and priorities. However, the patient's normal blood volume is more closely associated with ideal body weight, and any hemorrhage is likely to be more severe than it appears. Carefully assess for shock and remember that the cardiovascular system is already stressed by the excess weight.

During the rapid trauma assessment, pay special attention to the thorax and pelvic ring because of the increased incidence of rib fractures, pulmonary contusions, and pelvic fractures. Carefully assess vital signs, as they may be more difficult to palpate and hear because of greater body fat in the limbs and surrounding the chest cavity.

Management of the heavy patient presents hazards to the care provider. The increased weight makes lifting more hazardous and may stress equipment beyond its safe limits. Be careful to bring in enough people to provide a safe lift for you, your crew, and the patient. Splinting equipment may need to be modified or used in innovative ways to accommodate obese patients with fractures. Be careful to plan all moves through hallways, narrow spaces, over rough terrain, and up or down stairways very carefully.

Geriatric Patients

The geriatric population is one of the fastest-growing demographics in the country. Healthier lifestyles and modern medicine advances are extending life and increasing the older population (Figure 11-18). As this population grows over the next few decades, it will account for more and more trauma emergency responses. Currently, trauma accounts for 25 percent of all geriatric mortality and, with the expected growth of this population, will become an even greater proportion of EMS responses.

The geriatric trauma patient often has coexisting problems associated with aging and chronic disease. Aging affects virtually every body system. Reduced reflexes, hearing, and eyesight result in more injuries in this population, and brittle bones produce fractures with less force than with younger patients. This is especially true of the cervical spine, where the vertebral column becomes more fragile and calcification narrows the spinal

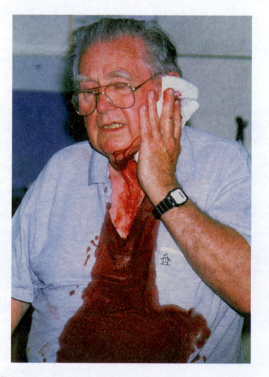

FIGURE 11-18 Geriatric patients are one of the fastest-growing groups requiring emergency medical services.

(© Science Photo Library)

foramen, predisposing the geriatric patient to spinal injury. The brain loses mass after middle age and results in a greater incidence of injury because the brain is freer to move about within and impact the interior of the cranium. Smaller cardiac reserves leave older patients less able to respond to hypovolemia with increases in heart rate or cardiac stroke volume. Reduced fluid reserves limit the amount of fluid the cardiovascular system can draw from body tissues to compensate for fluid lost through burns or hemorrhage. The system also cannot accommodate great fluctuations in fluid volume and is more prone to problems of overhydration with resulting pulmonary edema. The vascular system, especially the venous system, is less able to constrict in response to hypovolemia and restore cardiac preload. In addition, reduced respiratory reserves reduce the ability of older patients to accommodate the problems of diaphragmatic respiration associated with spinal injury, pneumothorax or tension pneumothorax, and even the reduction in respiratory movement associated with the pain of rib fractures. A higher pain tolerance and reduced pain perception may also mask the symptoms of serious injury, and poorer temperature regulation may predispose the geriatric patient to hypothermia.

Preexisting diseases are more prevalent in the geriatric population and reduce these patients' abilities to handle the physiologic stress of trauma. Cardiovascular disease limits the heart's ability to assist with shock compensation. Chronic respiratory diseases (such as emphysema) increase the cardiac workload and reduce respiratory efficiency and reserves. Many other chronic diseases likewise affect geriatric patients by reducing their ability to compensate for hypovolemia and respond to the stresses of shock. Because of aging and chronic disease, geriatric patients are likely to move more quickly into compensation, then more quickly to uncompensated shock, and then to irreversible shock. They are less able to tolerate the shock state, and they experience a mortality rate from hypovolemia that is much greater than that of average adults.

Assessment of the geriatric patient is often difficult because the problem that led to the call to EMS is often masked or confused by signs and symptoms of preexisting disease or by a diminished response to pain. However, accurate assessment of these patients is critical because they are less able to tolerate hypovolemia and the stress of shock.

MANAGEMENT OF THE GERIATRIC PATIENT Initiate shock care early with geriatric patients. Provide that care conservatively, however, to avoid the possibility of fluid overload. Intravenous catheters should be smaller than for normal adults, as the catheters must be inserted through rather thin, yet tough, skin and then through veins that tend to be smaller and more delicate than normal adult veins and that also roll more. During any infusion, auscultate the chest frequently for breath sounds and halt fluid flow at the first signs of crackles. Keep the patient warm and watch carefully for any progression of the signs of shock. The use of ECG monitoring is indicated because hypovolemia and shock may initiate arrhythmias in patients with preexisting cardiac disease. Administer oxygen early to geriatric patients to increase the effectiveness of respirations. Artificial ventilation may be met with greater resistance because of lung stiffness, but excessive ventilation pressures are more likely to lead to pneumothorax. Carefully adjust the bag-valve-mask volume to obtain gentle chest rise. Remember that the elderly are prone to hypothermia, so ensure they are well covered in a cool or cold environment.

Cognitively Impaired Patients

Caring for the patient who has been subjected to trauma and is cognitively impaired presents some special challenges to prehospital assessment. These patients, by definition, have a lower intelligence quotient (IQ) and are less able to communicate and describe what has happened to them or how they feel. Often, they have an atypical presentation of symptoms and a decreased threshold to pain. They are often unable to process information in a way that permits informed consent and may tend to be uncooperative. They may have anatomic abnormalities, but they are assessed and managed as most other trauma patients.

The cognitively impaired patient often has a lower developmental grade level than an individual of the same age without cognitive impairment. It may benefit your assessment to initially use simple, open-ended sentences to help you determine at what level you can communicate. Try to identify any caregiver and use that person to reduce anxiety and increase communications. And be patient. Otherwise, prehospital care should follow that provided to other trauma patients.

Autism (autism spectrum disorder) is a prevalent subset of impaired patients. Incidence is about 1 in 100 and is four to five times more common in males.[16,17] The autism patient handles information differently than other patients do and has difficulty in understanding information, resulting in abnormal social interactions, behavior, and communication. The autistic patient is treated as any other trauma patient.

Interaction with Other Care Providers

Emergency medical services often have a tiered structure consisting of progressive levels of care providers

CONTENT REVIEW

➤ Key Elements for the Patient Care Report
- Mechanism of injury
- Results of assessment
- Interventions
- Results of interventions

attending to the needs of patients. These care providers include the trained or untrained bystanders, certified Emergency Medical Responders, Emergency Medical Technicians, Advanced EMTs, and other Paramedics. Other members of the system include air medical personnel and the physicians, nurses, and technical personnel in the hospital emergency department, intensive care unit, or surgery. Appropriate interactions among all these members of the EMS system are essential to ensure a good continuum of care for the patient. Your interactions with these members also determine how you are perceived as a care provider and as a professional within the health care system. The information exchanged during these interactions is essential to an effective EMS system and, most importantly, to appropriate patient care (Figure 11-19).

The initial information you receive from emergency medical responders and EMTs about the patient's condition and the care he received as you assume assessment and care responsibilities is vital. This information is essential for developing your initial patient impression and then formulating a patient management plan. This information, supplemented by your assessment findings, is equally essential to the emergency department physician or nurse as he assumes responsibility for patient care from you. This information should include a description of the mechanism of injury, the results of your assessment, the interventions performed, and the results of those interventions.

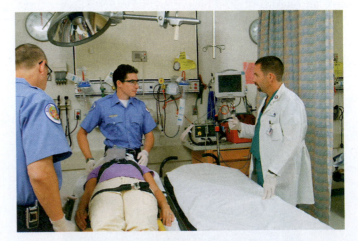

FIGURE 11-19 It is essential that information exchange among care providers be rapid, thorough, and accurate.

Mechanism of Injury

Concisely describe the mechanism of injury with enough detail to identify the nature and severity of the energy exchange. An example might be "a high-speed frontal impact with severe vehicle deformity and passenger compartment intrusion of about 10 inches" or "a head-on collision while two football players were running full speed." Also indicate what the patient was doing when the incident occurred—for example, "was the driver." Give the approximate time of the incident (or time since the incident), if known.

Results of Assessment

Communicate the results of your assessment, describing the injuries and relating any abnormal or unusual history, vital signs, and other assessment findings to the emergency department staff. Describe any wounds covered by bandages or splints in significant detail so those items need not be removed for immediate assessment. Include in your statement all pertinent patient information such as the patient's age, sex, and weight. Also include any allergies, significant medications, significant medical history, last oral intake, and up-to-date vaccinations, such as the last tetanus booster. Finally, identify the last set of vital signs, the Glasgow Coma Scale score, and any trends in patient condition noted from your serial ongoing assessments.

Interventions

Identify the care provided by others, then by you, and the results of that care on the patient's condition. Include the size of IV catheters and location of placement; the rate, volume, and type of fluid administered; the dosages, routes, and times of medications administered; and the size and depth of insertion of any advanced airway that has been used.

You should get this information from care providers as you accept responsibility for patient care. If necessary, question the care provider to obtain this information. This information exchange should take only a few moments, and rarely more than a minute. Use this same format and communicate this information to the receiving physician or nurse when you present your patient to the emergency department. If you receive a patient care report from a previous care provider in another format, convert it to this order of information. As you continue to assess and provide care, you will quickly identify whether the information obtained from previous care providers is valid or the patient needs reassessment of both his condition and the care offered up to that point.

It is essential that the information exchange between care providers is rapid and complete, or care will suffer. If a care provider does not use a standard, organized format to communicate information, organizing and using the information quickly and efficiently will be difficult. If this happens, talk with the care provider about it after the call and suggest a format to help future exchanges. Be careful to compliment the provider on skills that were performed well and suggest ways that "both of us" could improve the information exchange and patient care. Also appreciate the role of the emergency department physician as he applies this process to your report and patient care.

As you receive your patient report and begin to assume patient care responsibilities, use available basic and advanced life support providers to assist in your patient care. Have them perform manual cervical immobilization, use the bag-valve mask on the patient, and take vital signs. You can also use these personnel to bring equipment from the ambulance and help with patient movement procedures. This leaves you freer to oversee care, provide advanced interventions, and communicate with medical direction. It also makes the other providers feel a part of the response and the overall system. Again, compliment the providers on what they do well and offer constructive and supportive comments on ways to improve their performance. It is rare that you can accomplish all aspects of patient care alone. Having assistance from other providers who feel comfortable working with you improves the coordination and quality of the care at the scene.

Air Medical Transport

In recent years, the helicopter has become widely available to EMS systems throughout the country. Helicopters transport patients rapidly (at about 100 to 140 mph), bypassing traffic and flying directly to the nearest trauma center (Figure 11-20). Recent studies, however, have demonstrated that medical helicopters may not improve trauma outcomes to the degree once thought, especially in patients above the age of 55 years.[18,19] However, because trauma care is often a race against time, air medical service can provide a welcome, lifesaving addition to the prehospital care system. To better interact with this EMS and trauma resource, consider the indications for its use, the criteria for establishing a landing zone, the elements of flight physiology, and how to prepare a patient for air medical transport.

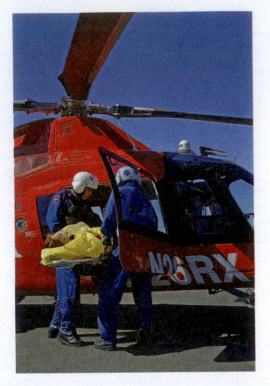

FIGURE 11-20 In recent years, use of helicopters has become widely available to EMS systems throughout the country.

Indications for Air Medical Transport

Your system will have its own protocols and procedures for air medical transport, but the following are common considerations. (Table 11-4 lists the guidelines of the American College of Emergency Physicians.) Consider summoning a helicopter when its use will significantly reduce transport time for severely injured trauma patients or when air medical service can provide care not otherwise available.[20] In making this decision, consider the normal activation and warm-up time for the helicopter (3 to 5 minutes) and the flight time to the scene (about 1 minute for each 2 miles). It is counterproductive to wait 15 minutes at the scene for a helicopter when it will reduce transport time by 10 minutes. However, if the helicopter arrives during a prolonged extrication or during rush hour, the time saved may be worthwhile. As a general rule, if transport by ground will exceed 45 minutes, request the helicopter. Also consider an intercept en route to the hospital if it will significantly reduce patient transport time. Air medical response times can be reduced if flight crews are placed on stand-by for serious trauma calls. This permits the crew to get ready and the pilot to warm up the helicopter. If the seriousness of the call is confirmed by police or first responders, you may ask to have the helicopter begin its response. If you arrive at the scene and find that the mechanism of injury and the apparent injuries are less serious than expected, you can then cancel the flight.

Although helicopter transport is a very valuable medium for trauma care, it is very expensive and not always available. The service area of a helicopter is rather large and the number of helicopters is usually limited because of their high operational costs. If the helicopter is on a flight, it will not be available for other responses. Weather conditions such as fog, heavy rain, or snow may obscure visibility, making it dangerous to take off, fly, or land at an emergency scene. Icing conditions on the ground or at altitude may also endanger the aircraft and restrict its flight. The helicopter is also a maintenance-intensive vehicle and can be out of service for scheduled repairs. These factors may reduce the availability of the service, so be prepared to use ground transport if the helicopter is unavailable.

The helicopter may be able to offer additional services to EMS (Figure 11-21). It can help search rough terrain and can cover great distances quickly when trying to find lost hikers or walkaways from nursing homes. It can provide vertical patient lift services and help transport patients out of remote areas. With special equipment, the helicopter may also be able to illuminate the scene or use infrared optics to locate patients in wilderness or remote areas at night. Contact your local EMS and police helicopter services to learn what support activities they can provide.

Table 11-4 American College of Emergency Physicians (ACEP) Guidelines for Appropriate Use of Air Medical Transport in the Out-of Hospital Setting

Appropriate reasons to use an air medical helicopter in the out-of-hospital setting include:

1. Patient has a significant potential to require high-level life support available from an air medical helicopter, which is not available by ground transport.

2. Patient has a significant potential to require a time-critical intervention, and an air medical helicopter will deliver the patient to an appropriate facility faster than ground transport.

3. Patient is located in a geographically isolated area, which would make ground transport impossible or greatly delayed.

4. Local EMS resources are exceeded.

The air ambulance should be recognized as a regional resource that is available to every person needing care, at any time (weather permitting), regardless of the ability to pay. The patient should have initial stabilization and preparation for flight, then be expeditiously transported to the closest appropriate facility.

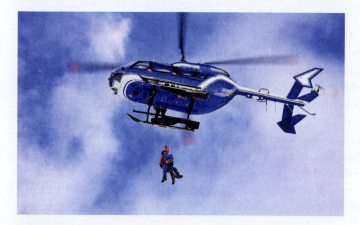

FIGURE 11-21 Helicopters can provide special services like search and rescue, vertical lifting, and specialized transport.

(© Mikaudin/Shutterstock)

Research and Trauma

Over the past few years, research has looked carefully at several assessment and care procedures used by prehospital emergency care. These include the pneumatic anti-shock garment (PASG), capillary refill, and rapid isotonic infusion.

On its introduction, the PASG was thought to be a great weapon in the fight against shock. It compressed the lower portion of the body, reducing hemorrhage there. It displaced blood from the abdomen and lower extremities into the critical circulation of the chest and head. And it reduced the size of the total vascular space by compressing the venous vessels beneath it. The end result is a relatively reduced hypovolemia and an increase in blood pressure that was thought to benefit the patient in shock. Although these effects occur, they do not occur to the degree once thought and, in many circumstances, are counterproductive to shock patient survival. A relatively large study in Houston, Texas, and supported by other studies thereafter, demonstrated that the application of the PASG and the resulting increase in blood pressure also increased the rate and total volume of blood loss in cases of penetrating chest trauma. Since then, numerous studies have determined that the PASG's use in many situations in which it was thought to be beneficial is, in fact, detrimental or does not positively affect patient survival.[21]

The value of capillary refill evaluation has also come into question with recent research. This research points out that refill times by themselves are poor indicators of a patient's circulatory status. Preexisting conditions such as caffeine intake, smoking, cold environmental temperatures, COPD, and many chronic conditions delay refill times well beyond what was previously thought to reflect normal distal skin perfusion. However, capillary refill remains an important diagnostic technique for the status of distal perfusion, guides the administration of oxygen, and is especially useful for trending distal perfusion or for comparing circulation from one limb to another. Increasing capillary refill times reflect a decreasing perfusion, whereas decreasing capillary refill times equate to an increase in distal perfusion.

For reasons similar to the concerns raised about PASG use, the value of rapid infusion of isotonic solutions to the hypovolemic patient in the prehospital setting is being questioned. As with application of the PASG, restoration of fluid volume may increase patient mortality, as the increase in blood pressure may dislodge clots and increase the rate and volume of internal hemorrhage. This problem is compounded because isotonic fluid replaces blood, effectively thinning the clotting factors and red blood cells that remain. The guideline for fluid resuscitation still remains at up to 3 liters of fluid for the adult during the normal prehospital care time period. However, the end point of fluid resuscitation is a blood pressure significantly subnormal—80 mmHg systolic and 90 mmHg systolic for the head injury patient with the signs of herniation (Cushing's triad).

Research must continue to ensure that EMS personnel use care procedures that contribute to patient survival. This research may lead to adoption of new techniques that support the chances of trauma patient survival or may reveal that other currently used skills and equipment do not benefit patients. In the future, research will change the way we deliver prehospital emergency care.

Summary

Trauma has remained the number-one killer of those below the age of 44 for the past three decades, often taking lives during their most productive years. The EMS system as a whole, and you as a paramedic member of it, must expend resources toward supporting and encouraging injury prevention programs. These programs may be the most effective way to reduce trauma mortality and morbidity. Once serious injury occurs, you must anticipate the nature and severity of the trauma, based on the mechanism of injury analysis, then assess and stabilize the cervical spine, airway, breathing, and circulation during the primary assessment. You provide directed assessment and care during the rapid trauma assessment and quickly transport the seriously injured patient to the trauma center. With trauma patients, shock is a critical concern.

You must anticipate shock and look for its earliest signs on your arrival at the scene and then monitor the patient for any progressive signs or symptoms of hypovolemia compensation during the remainder of your assessment, care, and reassessments. If you suspect shock, you must intervene quickly with rapid fluid infusion, aggressive airway care, and pleural decompression, as needed. Ensure that your patient is directed to the trauma center as quickly as possible.

You Make the Call

You arrive at an auto collision to find one car significantly deformed around a large tree. Inside, there is a young woman draped against the steering wheel. She appears to be unconscious.

1. Your scene survey determines the answers to what questions?

   Your questions answered, you move to the patient's side and find her conscious but very confused. She has a weak pulse of 110 beats per minute; her skin is cool, clammy, and ashen in color; and her respirations are 28 and shallow. She complains of general chest pain and speaks in short phrases because she is having "great difficulty breathing." Auscultation of her chest reveals diminished breath sounds on the right and a hyperinflated right hemithorax.

2. You suspect which immediately life-threatening problem?

3. Given your suspicions, what immediate actions should you take with this patient?

See Suggested Responses at the back of this book.

Review Questions

1. All of the following are considered reasons to conduct research in prehospital trauma care *except* _____

   a. to ensure that EMS is best serving its patients.

   b. to help ensure a future for prehospital emergency care.

   c. to ensure that the research evidence justifies mainstay treatments.

   d. to identify areas in which injury prevention programs may be beneficial.

2. The demographic group most prone to traumatic injuries and deaths is _____

   a. females over the age of 65.

   b. males under the age of 12.

   c. females between the ages of 15 and 20.

   d. males between the ages of 11 and 35.

3. Which of the following groups of criteria is used when developing the revised trauma score?

   a. Systolic blood pressure, respiratory rate, GCS

   b. GCS, heart rate, and best motor response

   c. Best motor response, eye opening, and verbal response

   d. Respiratory rate, blood pressure, and capillary refill rate

4. While on the scene of a motor vehicle collision in a rural location, you may want to use helicopter transport of the patient if ground transport time exceeds _____ minutes.

   a. 15

   b. 25

   c. 35

   d. 45

5. All of the following are appropriate steps for shock trauma resuscitation *except* _____
   a. maintaining adequate ventilations.
   b. splinting major long-bone fractures.
   c. providing airway maintenance.
   d. providing rapid fluid resuscitation with hypertonic crystalloid solutions.

6. Of all the care procedures and advanced interventions available to treat the trauma patient, none has more promise for reducing mortality and morbidity than _____
   a. early transport.
   b. injury prevention programs.
   c. oxygen therapy.
   d. air medical transport.

7. All of the following are terms that could be used to describe the status of the cardiovascular system in a multisystem trauma patient *except*
   _____
   a. hypovolemia.   c. hypotension.
   b. hypothermia.   d. hypoperfusion.

8. Generally, the maximum prehospital fluid volume administered by the paramedic is _____
   a. 2,000 mL.
   b. 3,000 mL.
   c. 1,000 mL.
   d. 2,500 mL.

9. Noncritical patients account for about _____ percent of trauma responses and receive the largest part of prehospital trauma care.
   a. 40
   b. 60
   c. 70
   d. 80

10. In the pediatric trauma patient, fluid boluses for volume replacement are usually given at what dosage?
    a. 10 mL/kg
    b. 15 mL/lb
    c. 20 mL/kg
    d. 25 mL/lb

See Answers to Review Questions at the back of this book.

References

1. Centers for Disease Control and Prevention. *Deaths: Final Data for 2012*, Table 18. (Available at www.cdc.gov/nchs/fastats/injury.htm.)

2. Centers for Disease Control and Prevention, National Center for Injury Prevention and Control. *Leading Causes of Death 2009* (WISQARS). Atlanta, GA, 2012. (Available at www.cdc.gov.)

3. Reichard, A. A., S. M. Marsh, and P. H. Moore. "Fatal and Nonfatal Injuries among Emergency Medical Technicians and Paramedics." *Prehosp Emerg Care* 15(4) (Oct–Dec 2011): 511-517.

4. Chen, L., A. T. Reisner, A. Gribok, and J. Reifman. "Exploration of Prehospital Vital Sign Trends for the Prediction of Trauma Outcomes." *J Spec Oper Med* 10(3) (Summer 2010): 55–62.

5. Davis, D. P., et al. "The Relationship between Out-of-Hospital Airway Management and Outcome among Trauma Patients with Glasgow Coma Scale Scores of 8 or Less." *Prehosp Emerg Med* 15(2) (Apr–Jun 2011): 184–192.

6. Gonzalez, R. P., et al. "On-Scene Intravenous Line Insertions Adversely Impacts Prehospital Time in Rural Vehicle Trauma." *Am Surg* 74(11) (Nov 2008): 1083–1087.

7. Hubble, M. W., et al. "A Meta-Analysis of Prehospital Airway Control Techniques Part II: Alternative Airway Devices and Cricothyrotomy Success Rates." *Prehosp Emerg Care* 14(4) (Oct–Dec 2010): 515–530.

8. Merlin, M. A., et al. "Study of Placing a Second Intravenous Line in Trauma." *Prehosp Emerg Med* 15(2) (Apr–Jun 2011): 208–213.

9. Pepe, P. E., et al. "Prehospital Fluid Resuscitation of the Patient with Major Trauma." *Prehosp Emerg Care* 6 (2002): 81.

10. Wood, S. P., M. Varhas, and S. K. Wedel. "Femur Fracture Immobilization with Traction Splints in Multisystem Trauma Patients." *Prehosp Emerg Care* 7(2) (Apr–Jun 2003): 241–243.

11. Hubble, M. and J. Hubble. "Overview of Trauma Care." In *Principles of Advanced Trauma Care*. Albany: Delmar, 2002.

12. Hutson, H. and D. Anglin. "Youth and Gang Violence." In *Emergency Medicine: Concepts and Clinical Practice*, 4th ed. St. Louis: Mosby, 1998.

13. Bradley, W. "Trauma in Pregnancy." In *International Trauma Life Support for Prehospital Care Providers*. 6th ed. Upper Saddle River, NJ: Pearson/Prentice Hall, 2008.

14. Holmberg, T. J., et al. "The Association between Obesity and Difficult Prehospital Tracheal Intubation." *Anesth Analg* 112(3) (May 2011): 1132–1138.

15. Brown, C. B. and G. C. Velahos. "The Consequences of Obesity on Trauma, Emergency Surgery, and Surgical Care." *World J Emerg Surg* 1 (2006): 27.

16. National Institute for Child Health and Human Development. *Autism Overview: What We Know*. US Department of Health and Human Services. National Institute of Health. Washington, DC. Government Printing Office, 2008.

17. Centers for Disease Control and Prevention, *Facts about Autism Spectrum Disorders*" (NCBDDD). Atlanta, GA, 2012. (Available at www.cdc.gov.)

18. Sullivent, E. E., M. Faul, and M. M. Wald. "Reduced Mortality in Injured Adults Transported by Helicopter Emergency Medical Services." *Prehosp Emerg Care* 15(3) (Jul–Sep 2011): 295–302.

19. Talving, P., et al. "Helicopter Evacuation of Trauma Victims in Los Angeles: Does It Improve Survival?" *World J Surg* 33(11) (Nov 2009): 2469–2476.

20. American College of Emergency Physicians. "Appropriate Utilization of Air Medical Transport in the Out-of-Hospital Setting." ACEP, 2008.

21. Dickenson, K. and I. Roberts. "Medical Anti-Shock Trousers (Pneumatic Anti-Shock Garments) for Circulatory Support in Patients with Trauma." Unpublished study (PubMed).

Further Reading

American College of Surgeons, Committee on Trauma. *Advanced Trauma Life Support Course: Student Manual*. 9th ed. Chicago: American College of Surgeons, 2012.

American College of Surgeons, Committee on Trauma. *Resources for Optimal Care of the Injured Patient*. Chicago: American College of Surgeons, 2007.

Bickley, L. *Bates' Guide to Physical Examination and History Taking*. 11th ed. Philadelphia: Wolters-Kluwer, 2012.

Bledsoe, B. E., B. J. Colbert, and J. E. Ankney. *Essentials of A & P for Emergency Care*. Upper Saddle River, NJ: Pearson/Prentice Hall, 2010.

Bledsoe, B. E. and D. Clayden. *Prehospital Emergency Pharmacology*. 7th ed. Upper Saddle River, NJ: Pearson/Prentice Hall, 2011.

Campbell, J. E. *International Trauma Life Support for Prehospital Care Providers*. 8th ed. Upper Saddle River, NJ: Pearson/Prentice Hall, 2016.

Martini, F. *Fundamentals of Anatomy and Physiology*. 10th ed. San Francisco: Pearson, 2014.

Marx, J., R. Hockberger, and R. Walls. *Emergency Medicine: Concepts and Clinical Practice*. 8th ed. St. Louis: Mosby, 2013.

National Association of EMTs. *Prehospital Trauma Life Support*. 8th ed. Burlington, VT: Jones & Bartlett Learning, 2014.

National Association of EMS Physicians Position Paper. Guidelines for Air Medical Dispatch. *Prehospital Emergency Care* 7(2) (2003): 265–271.

Tintinalli, J. E., ed. *Emergency Medicine: A Comprehensive Study Guide*. 7th ed. New York: McGraw-Hill, 2012.

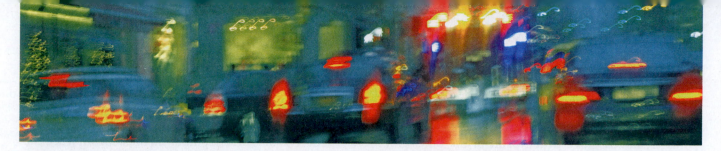

Precautions on Bloodborne Pathogens and Infectious Diseases

Prehospital emergency personnel, like all health care workers, are at risk for exposure to bloodborne pathogens and infectious diseases. In emergency situations it is often difficult to take or enforce proper infection control measures. However, as a paramedic, you must recognize your high-risk status. Study the following information on infection control carefully.

Infection control is designed to protect emergency personnel, their families, and their patients from unnecessary exposure to communicable diseases. Laws, regulations, and standards regarding infection control include:

- *Centers for Disease Control and Prevention (CDC) Guidelines.* The CDC has published extensive guidelines on infection control. Proper equipment and techniques that should be used by emergency response personnel to prevent or minimize risk of exposure are defined.
- *The Ryan White Act.* The Ryan White Act of 1990 allows emergency personnel to find out if they were exposed to an infectious disease while rendering patient care. Employers are required to name a "designated officer" to coordinate communications with the treating hospital.
- *Americans with Disabilities Act.* This act prohibits discrimination against individuals with disabilities, including those with contagious diseases. It guarantees equal employment opportunities and job protection if the infected individual can perform essential job functions and does not pose a threat to the safety and health of patients and coworkers.
- *Occupational Safety and Health Administration (OSHA) Regulations.* OSHA has enacted a regulation entitled Occupational Exposure to Bloodborne Pathogens that classifies emergency response personnel as being at the greatest risk of occupational exposure to commu-

nicable diseases. This regulation requires employers to provide hepatitis B (HBV) vaccinations free of charge, maintain a written exposure control plan, and provide personal protective equipment. These requirements primarily apply to private employers. Applicability to local and state governmental employees varies by locality. Many states have developed their own OSHA plans.

- *National Fire Protection Association (NFPA) Guidelines.* This is a national organization that has established specific guidelines and requirements regarding infection control for emergency response agencies, particularly fire departments and EMS services.

Standard Precautions and Personal Protective Equipment

Emergency response personnel should practice Standard Precautions by which ALL body substances are considered to be potentially infectious. To practice Standard Precautions, all emergency personnel should utilize personal protective equipment (PPE). Appropriate PPE should be available on every emergency vehicle. The minimum recommended PPE includes the following:

- *Gloves.* Disposable gloves should be donned by all emergency response personnel BEFORE initiating any emergency care. When an emergency incident involves more than one patient, you should attempt to change gloves between patients. When gloves have been contaminated, they should be removed as soon as possible. To properly remove contaminated gloves, grasp one glove approximately 1 inch from the wrist. Without touching the inside of the glove, pull the glove halfway off and stop. With that half-gloved hand, pull the glove on the opposite hand completely off. Place the removed glove in the palm of the other glove, with the inside of the removed glove exposed. Pull the second glove completely off with the ungloved hand, only touching the inside of the glove. Always wash hands after gloves are removed, even when the gloves appear intact.

- *Masks and Protective Eyewear.* Masks and protective eyewear should be present on all emergency vehicles and used in accordance with the level of exposure encountered. Masks and protective eyewear should be worn together whenever blood spatter is likely to occur, such as during arterial bleeding, childbirth, endotracheal intubation, invasive procedures, oral suctioning, and cleanup of equipment that requires heavy scrubbing or brushing. Both you and the patient should wear masks whenever the potential for airborne transmission of disease exists.

- *HEPA and N-95 Respirators.* Due to the resurgence of tuberculosis (TB), prehospital personnel should protect themselves from TB infection through use of an N-95 or a high-efficiency particulate air (HEPA) respirator, as approved by the National Institute of Occupational Safety and Health (NIOSH). It should fit snugly and be capable of filtering out the tuberculosis bacillus. An N-95 or HEPA respirator should be worn when caring for patients with confirmed or suspected TB. This is especially true when performing "high-hazard" procedures such as administration of nebulized medications, endotracheal intubation, or suctioning on such a patient.

- *Gowns.* Gowns protect clothing from blood splashes. If large splashes of blood are expected, such as with childbirth, wear impervious gowns.

- *Resuscitation Equipment.* Disposable resuscitation equipment should be the primary means of artificial ventilation in emergency care. Such items should be used once, then disposed of.

Remember, the proper use of personal protective equipment ensures effective infection control and minimizes risk. Use ALL protective equipment recommended for any particular situation to ensure maximum protection.

Consider ALL body substances potentially infectious and ALWAYS practice Standard Precautions.

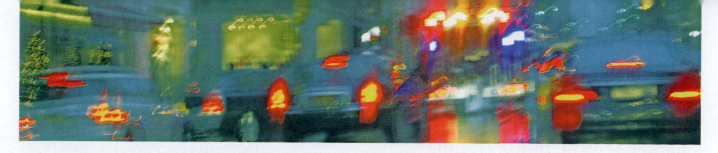

Suggested Responses to "You Make the Call"

The following are suggested responses to the "You Make the Call" scenarios presented in each chapter of Volume 4, Trauma. Each represents an acceptable response to the scenario but should not be interpreted as the only correct response.

Chapter 1—Trauma and Trauma Systems

1. *What authority does Janet have regarding the decision to transport her daughter?*

Janet is the mother and legal authority over her child. She has full authority to make decisions for the child. In the case where parents or guardians are present, they are capable of making the decisions for the patient as if they were the patient.

2. *What will you tell her regarding your choice for a hospital destination?*

Explain to the mother your concern for the injuries and the need for specialized treatment that the trauma center can provide. By explaining your rationale and letting the mother know that this is what you feel is truly in the best interest of the patient, you should be able to persuade the mother and get her to agree to transport to the trauma center.

Chapter 2—Mechanism of Injury

1. *What scene hazards would you expect on this call?*

Typical scene hazards would include leaks and spills of vehicle fluids such as oil, antifreeze, and gasoline. If extrication is necessary, watch for additional hazards such as an undeployed driver's air bag in the vehicle that was struck in the side, broken glass, and sharp metal edges.

2. *What injuries would you suspect?*

Lateral injuries for the driver in the vehicle that was struck. Injuries such as a fractured arm, ribs (suspect pneumohemothorax), pelvis, or femur (all on the side of impact). Additional injuries to suspect include spinal injuries and head injuries (coup and contrecoup).

3. *What care would you expect to provide?*

Care would include rapidly assessing the airway and breathing, stabilizing the cervical spine, and stabilizing any fractures. Perform extrication as necessary to begin rapid transport to the nearest trauma facility. Provide ALS care as your protocols outline, to include oxygen and IV therapy.

Chapter 3—Hemorrhage and Shock

1. *What signs suggest hypovolemia and early shock?*

Agitation and anxiousness, cool and moist skin, and increased pulse rate.

2. *Does the blood pressure suggest shock? Why or why not?*

The blood pressure alone does not indicate shock. However, when coupled with all the other signs and symptoms, the pressure can be explained. The increased blood pressure indicates an excited state and is currently compensating well for the blood loss.

3. *What progressive steps would you take to control the hemorrhage?*

The first step is to firmly bandage a dressing over the wound. If this does not control the hemorrhage, include finger pressure through the dressing to the site of the leaking vessel. If the bleeding is persistent and life-threatening and cannot be controlled by direct pressure, as a last resort apply a commercial tourniquet or, if a commercial tourniquet is not available, a wide cravat, belt, or blood pressure cuff. Leave the tourniquet in place until the patient is in the emergency department or other facility where blood replacement is available and the negative effects of reperfusion can be addressed. Be sure to notify personnel at the receiving facility that a tourniquet has been applied.

4. *What supportive care measures would you employ?*

Provide oxygen therapy and IV therapy, maintain body temperature, and calm and reassure the patient.

Chapter 4—Soft Tissue Trauma

1. *What type of wound is this and what significance does it have for infection?*

This is a puncture wound that is vulnerable to a variety of infections. The most concerning complication would be tetanus.

2. *What elements of history and specifically vaccinations will be important in assessing this patient?*

Are the child's vaccinations up to date and when was his last tetanus shot?

3. *What direction would you give this patient if his parents do not wish to have him transported to the local emergency department?*

Depending on whether or not the patient has an updated tetanus, advise the patient to be seen by his doctor for a tetanus shot or simply watch for signs of infection, including increased pain, redness, and swelling around the injury site. Especially watch for signs of tetanus, including muscle stiffening, especially in the muscles of the face and jaw.

Chapter 5—Burns

1. *What severity are the burns of the forearm and hand and of the upper arm?*

The forearm and hand are most likely third-degree burns.

2. *What percentage of the body surface area is burned?*

Nine percent or less. (The entire arm is estimated as 9 percent BSA. If the entire arm is burned, you are looking at a total of 9 percent BSA.)

3. *What level of acuity would you assign this patient?*

This is a severe/critical burn that should be treated rapidly and transported urgently. It involves the patient's hands and bends of the arm, making this a potentially debilitating injury.

Chapter 6—Head, Neck, and Spinal Trauma

1. *What structures are most likely injured?*

The bubbling with expiration indicates her trachea has been perforated along with several major vessels in the neck.

2. *What care would you employ?*

Immediately cover the bleeding areas with occlusive dressings and attempt to control the hemorrhage. An ET tube could be placed into the trachea through the neck if the wound is large enough; otherwise, securing her airway with a conventional ET tube would be acceptable.

3. *What are serious life threats associated with this injury?*

The serious life threats include airway compromise, air embolus to the brain, and hemorrhagic shock.

Chapter 7—Chest Trauma

1. *Considering the mechanism of injury and what is known about the patient, what thoracic pathophysiology may explain the patient's presentation?*

The patient struck his chest on the steering wheel of the vehicle, resulting in a "flail" segment of chest which has also caused a tension pneumothorax.

2. *As the treating paramedic, what is your next step in stabilizing this patient?*

Secure the airway as necessary. Then provide for more effective ventilatory support by securing the flail segment. Finally, determine which side (if not both) needs to be decompressed and provide a chest decompression.

3. *What further emergency treatment is likely indicated by the absence of breath sounds on the left side and a relatively normal abdominal exam?*

A chest decompression is likely to be indicated along with a chest tube to help remove any blood and air caught in the pleural space.

Chapter 8—Abdominal and Pelvic Trauma

1. *Given the signs and symptoms, what is the most likely injury and why?*

Splenic injury is most likely because of the level of the vehicle in relation to her size when she was struck.

2. *What relation does the right shoulder pain have to the suspected injury?*

The right shoulder pain is most likely caused by being thrown to the ground following the injury. Referred pain from the spleen, Kehr's sign, is pain in the left shoulder region.

3. *What care will you provide for this patient?*

You will provide immediate spinal immobilization, oxygen, IV therapy, and rapid transport to the nearest trauma center.

Chapter 9—Orthopedic Trauma

1. *When assessing the injury site, what signs of fracture will you be evaluating?*

You are looking for instability, deformity such as swelling or angulation, crepitus, unusual motion, abnormal muscle tone, and regions of unusual warmth or coolness. Consider the "six Ps"—pain, pallor, paralysis, paresthesia, pressure, and pulses.

2. *What are the three main factors to consider when evaluating distal neurovascular status?*

Circulation, motor function, and sensation.

3. *What steps should you take if you determine the patient is suffering from distal neurovascular impairment and choose to realign the injury?*

Have your partner immobilize the proximal limb in the position found. Grasp the distal limb firmly and apply traction along the axis. If you feel resistance to movement or great increase in patient discomfort, stop and splint the limb as it lies. Once you complete alignment, recheck distal neurovascular function. If function is inadequate, move the limb around. If one attempt at gentle manipulation does not reestablish a pulse, splint and transport the patient quickly.

4. *How many attempts are permitted when realigning an injury?*

This should only be attempted once.

5. *How would you splint this injury once realignment has taken place?*

Splinting the injury in a "position of function" or natural position is the best method for splinting and maintaining distal function. A manufactured splint will accomplish this. Another very effective method for splinting an ankle is with a pillow.

Chapter 10—Environmental Trauma

1. *What illness are you probably dealing with?*

High altitude pulmonary edema (HAPE).

2. *What predisposing factors lead to this illness?*

The victim, being a SCUBA instructor, had recently flown to a dramatically different, higher altitude.

3. *What is the definitive treatment for this condition?*

Oxygen administration and descent to lower altitudes.

4. *If definitive treatment is not possible, what other measures can be used?*

Oxygenation over 36 to 72 hours or a hyperbaric treatment with a portable hyberbaric bag that can simulate a descent of approximately 5,000 feet can be used. Additionally, acetazolamide can be used to decrease symptoms. Morphine, nifedipine, and furosemide are sometimes used but carry complications such as hypotension and dehydration, so they should be used with caution.

Chapter 11—Special Considerations in Trauma

1. *Your scene survey determines the answers to what questions?*

Is the scene safe?

What is the mechanism of injury?

How many patients do I have?

What additional resources do I need?

What environmental factors might impact assessment and care?

2. *You suspect which immediately life-threatening problem?*

Pneumothorax.

3. *Given your suspicions, what immediate actions should you take with this patient?*

Administration of supplemental oxygen and pleural decompression should be performed to relieve the pressure inside the chest and allow the patient to begin breathing better.

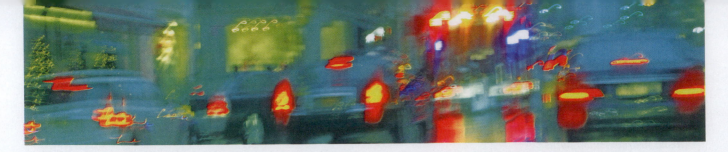

Answers to Review Questions

Below are the answers to the Review Questions presented in each chapter of Volume 4.

Chapter 1—Trauma and Trauma Systems

1. c
2. b
3. c
4. b
5. a
6. a
7. b
8. c
9. d
10. c

Chapter 2—Mechanism of Injury

1. b
2. b
3. a
4. d
5. d
6. a
7. b
8. c
9. a
10. b
11. b
12. a
13. c
14. b
15. c
16. a
17. a
18. b

Chapter 3—Hemorrhage and Shock

1. a
2. a
3. d
4. b
5. d
6. c
7. b
8. b
9. c
10. d

Chapter 4—Soft-Tissue Trauma

1. d
2. b
3. c
4. c
5. c
6. d
7. a
8. a
9. b
10. d
11. a
12. b
13. d

Chapter 5—Burns

1. b
2. b
3. c
4. b
5. d
6. a
7. c
8. d
9. a
10. b
11. a
12. b

Chapter 6—Head, Neck, and Spinal Trauma

1. a
2. b
3. d
4. c
5. c
6. b
7. c
8. a
9. b
10. d
11. c

14. b
15. a

12. a
13. d
14. a
15. a
16. d
17. a
18. d
19. a
20. c
21. d
22. d
23. b
24. d
25. a
26. a
27. b
28. d
29. b
30. c

Chapter 7—Chest Trauma

1. d
2. c
3. a
4. c
5. d
6. a
7. d
8. a
9. b
10. c

Chapter 8— Abdominal and Pelvic Trauma

1. c
2. d
3. d
4. a
5. b
6. c
7. c
8. c
9. d
10. c

Chapter 9—Orthopedic Trauma

1. d
2. b
3. d
4. d
5. b
6. c
7. a
8. a
9. b
10. b
11. c
12. d
13. b
14. b
15. d

Chapter 10— Environmental Trauma

1. c
2. c
3. c
4. d
5. a
6. a
7. b
8. c
9. a
10. d
11. b
12. c
13. c
14. d

Chapter 11—Special Considerations in Trauma

1. b
2. d
3. a
4. d
5. d
6. b
7. b
8. b
9. d
10. c

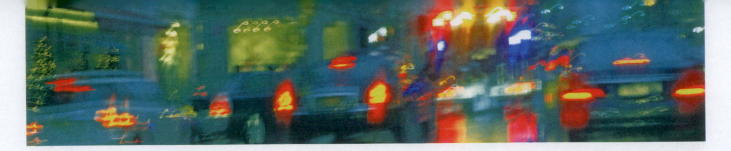

Glossary

abduction   movement of a body part away from the midline.

abrasion   scraping or abrading away of the superficial layers of the skin; an open soft tissue injury.

abruptio placentae   a condition in which the placenta separates from the uterine wall.

absolute zero   the temperature at which all molecular motion stops (–273°C or –459°F).

acceleration   the rate at which speed or velocity increases.

acclimatization   the reversible changes in body structure and function by which the body becomes adjusted to a change in environment.

adduction   movement of a body part toward the midline.

afterload   the resistance a contraction of the heart must overcome to eject blood; in cardiac physiology, defined as the tension of cardiac muscle during systole (contraction). Also called *peripheral vascular resistance*.

aggregate   to cluster or come together.

alpha radiation   low-level form of nuclear radiation; a weak source of energy that is stopped by clothing or the first layers of skin.

ampere   basic unit for measuring the strength of an electric current.

amphiarthroses   joints that permit a limited amount of independent motion.

amputation   severance, removal, or detachment, either partial or complete, of a body part.

anaerobic   ability to live without oxygen.

anaphylactic shock   form of shock in which histamine causes general vasodilation, precapillary sphincter dilation, capillary engorgement, and fluid movement into the interstitial compartment.

aneurysm   a weakening or ballooning in the wall of a blood vessel.

anterior cord syndrome   condition that is caused by bony fragments or pressure compressing the arteries of the anterior spinal cord and resulting in loss of motor function and sensation to pain, light touch, and temperature below the injury site.

anterograde amnesia   inability to remember events that occurred after the trauma that caused the condition.

aqueous humor   clear fluid filling the anterior chamber of the eye.

arachnoid membrane   middle layer of the meninges.

arterial gas embolism (AGE)   an air bubble, or air embolism, that enters the circulatory system from a damaged lung.

arteriole   a small artery.

artery   a vessel that carries blood from the heart to the body tissues.

articular surface   surface of a bone that moves against another bone.

ascending reticular activating system   a series of nervous tissues keeping the human system in a state of consciousness.

ascending tracts   bundles of axons along the spinal cord that transmit signals from the body to the brain.

atelectasis   collapse of a lung or part of a lung.

autonomic hyperreflexia syndrome   condition associated with the body's adjustment to the effects of neurogenic shock; presentations include sudden hypertension, bradycardia, headache, blurred vision, and sweating and flushing above the point of injury; a medical emergency in which seizures, stroke, or death may result.

autonomic neuropathy   condition that damages the autonomic nervous system, which usually senses changes in core temperature and controls vasodilation and perspiration to dissipate heat.

autoregulation   process that controls blood flow to brain tissue by causing alterations in the blood pressure.

avulsion   forceful tearing away or separation of body tissue; an avulsion may be partial or complete.

axial loading   application of the forces of trauma along the axis of the spine; this often results in compression fractures of the spine.

axon   extension of a neuron that serves as a pathway for transmission of signals to and from the brain; major component of white matter.

ballistics   the study of projectile motion and its interactions with the gun, the air, and the object it contacts.

barotrauma   injuries caused by changes in pressure. Barotrauma that occurs from increasing pressure during a diving descent is commonly called "the squeeze."

basal metabolic rate (BMR)   rate at which the body consumes energy just to maintain stability; the basic metabolic rate (measured by the rate of oxygen consumption) of an awake, relaxed person 12 to 14 hours after eating and at a comfortable temperature.

Baux score   scoring system for burn severity that takes into account the burn victim's age, percentage of surface area burned, and significant respiratory involvement, with a resulting score reflecting seriousness/ mortality.

beta radiation   medium-strength radiation that is stopped with light clothing or the uppermost layers of skin.

bilateral periorbital ecchymosis   black-and-blue discoloration of the area surrounding the eyes. It is usually associated with basilar skull fracture. (Also called *raccoon eyes*.)

blast wind   the air movement caused as the heated and pressurized products of an explosion move outward.

blepharospasm   uncontrolled muscle contraction of the eyelids, resulting in tightly closed eyelids.

blood–brain barrier   the characteristic thickness of central nervous system capillary walls that makes them less permeable than other capillaries, which has the effect of reducing the interstitial flow of proteins and other materials to the brain and spinal cord.

blunt trauma   injury caused by the collision of an object with the body in which the object does not enter the body.

body surface area (BSA)   percentage of a patient's body affected by a burn.

brainstem   the part of the brain connecting the cerebral hemispheres with the spinal cord. It is composed of the medulla oblongata, the pons, and the midbrain.

Brown-Séquard syndrome   condition caused by partial cutting of one side of the spinal cord, resulting in sensory and motor loss to that side of the body.

bursae   sacs containing synovial fluid that cushion adjacent structures. Singular, *bursa.*

caliber   the diameter of a bullet expressed in hundredths of an inch (0.22 caliber = 0.22 inches); the inside diameter of the barrel of a handgun or rifle.

callus   thickened area that forms at the site of a fracture as part of the repair process.

cancellous   having a latticework structure, as in the spongy tissue of a bone.

capillary   one of the minute blood vessels that connects the ends of arterioles with the beginnings of venules; where oxygen is diffused to body tissue and products of metabolism enter the bloodstream.

cardiac contractility   the ability of the heart to contract; the strength of the heart's contractions.

cardiogenic shock   shock resulting from failure to maintain the blood pressure because of inadequate cardiac output.

cartilage   connective tissue providing the articular surfaces of the skeletal system.

catecholamine   a hormone, such as epinephrine or norepinephrine, that strongly affects the nervous and cardiovascular systems, metabolic rate, temperature, and smooth muscle.

cauda equina syndrome   condition caused when nerve roots at the lower end of the spinal cord are compressed, interrupting sensation, movement, and function in the lower body.

cavitation   the outward motion of tissue due to a projectile's passage, resulting in a temporary cavity and vacuum.

central cord syndrome   condition usually related to hyperextension of the cervical spine that results in motor weakness, usually in the upper extremities, and possible bladder dysfunction.

cerebellum   portion of the brain located dorsally to the pons and medulla oblongata. It plays an important role in the fine control of voluntary muscular movements.

cerebral perfusion pressure (CPP)   the pressure moving blood through the brain.

cerebrospinal fluid (CSF)   fluid surrounding and bathing the brain and spinal cord (the elements of the central nervous system).

cerebrum   largest part of the brain. It consists of two hemispheres separated by a deep longitudinal fissure. It is the seat of consciousness and the center of the higher mental functions, such as memory, learning, reasoning, judgment, intelligence, and emotions.

cervical vertebrae   the seven vertebrae that form the top of the vertebral column, supporting the neck.

chemotactic factors   chemicals released by white blood cells that attract more white blood cells to an area of inflammation.

Cheyne-Stokes respirations   respiratory pattern of alternating periods of apnea and tachypnea.

circumduction   movement at a synovial joint where the distal end of a bone describes a circle but the shaft does not rotate.

closed fracture   a broken bone in which the bone ends or the forces that caused it do not penetrate the skin.

clotting factors   proteins from damaged blood vessel walls and damaged platelets that, when released into the bloodstream, cause chemical reactions that result in the formation of clot-forming fibrin.

coagulation necrosis   the process in which an acid, while destroying tissue, forms an insoluble layer that limits further damage.

coagulation phase third step in the process of hemostasis, which involves the formation of a protein called fibrin that forms a network around a wound to stop bleeding, ward off infection, and lay a foundation for healing and repair of the wound.

coagulopathy condition in which the blood's ability to clot is impaired.

coccyx small bone, formed from four fused vertebrae, that lies below the sacrum at the base of the vertebral column.

collagen tough, strong protein that makes up most of the body's connective tissue.

comminuted fracture fracture in which a bone is broken into several pieces.

commotio cordis lethal cardiac arrhythmia caused by a sharp nonpenetrating blow to the sternum.

comorbidity simultaneous presence of more than one disease or condition.

compartment syndrome muscle ischemia that is caused by rising pressures within an anatomic fascial space.

compensated shock hemodynamic insult to the body in which the body responds effectively. Signs and symptoms are limited, and the human system continues to provide oxygenated circulation to most tissues.

complete cord transection a total severing of the spinal cord.

concussion a transient period of unconsciousness. In most cases, the unconsciousness will be followed by a complete return of function.

conduction moving electrons, ions, heat, or sound waves through a conductor or conducting medium.

conjunctiva mucous membrane that lines the eyelids.

consensual reactivity the response of both eyes to changes in light intensity that affect only one eye.

contralateral opposite side.

contrecoup injury occurring on the opposite side; an injury to the brain opposite the site of impact.

contusion closed wound in which the skin is unbroken, although damage has occurred to the tissue immediately beneath.

convection transfer of heat via currents in liquids or gases.

core temperature the body temperature of the deep tissues, which usually does not vary more than a degree or so from its normal 37°C (98.6°F).

cornea thin, delicate layer covering the pupil and the iris.

coup injury an injury to the brain occurring on the same side as the site of impact.

cramping muscle pain resulting from overactivity, lack of oxygen, and accumulation of waste products.

cranium portion of the skull encasing the brain. Also called the *cranial vault*.

crumple zone the region of a vehicle designed to absorb the energy of impact.

crush injury mechanism of injury in which tissue is locally compressed by high-pressure forces.

crush syndrome systemic disorder of severe metabolic disturbances resulting from the crush of a limb or other body part.

current the rate of flow of an electric charge.

Cushing's reflex response due to cerebral ischemia that causes an increase in systemic blood pressure, which maintains cerebral perfusion during increased intracranial pressure.

Cushing's triad the combination of increasing blood pressure, slowing pulse, and irregular respirations in response to increased intracranial pressure.

deceleration the rate at which speed or velocity decreases.

decompensated shock continuing hemodynamic insult to the body in which the compensatory mechanisms break down. The signs and symptoms become very pronounced, and the patient moves rapidly toward death.

decompression sickness development of nitrogen bubbles within the tissues from a rapid reduction of air pressure when a diver returns to the surface; also called *the bends* or *dysbarism*.

deep frostbite freezing involving epidermal and subcutaneous tissues, resulting in a white appearance, hard (frozen) feeling on palpation, and loss of sensation.

degloving injury avulsion in which the mechanism of injury tears the skin off the underlying muscle, tissue, blood vessels, and bone.

denature alter the usual substance of something.

dermatome topographical region of the body surface innervated by one nerve root.

dermis true skin, also called the corium; it is the layer of tissue producing the epidermis and housing the structures, blood vessels, and nerves normally associated with the skin.

descending tracts bundles of axons along the spinal cord that transmit signals from the brain to the body.

devascularization loss of blood vessels from a body part.

diaphysis hollow shaft found in long bones.

diarthroses synovial joints.

diffuse axonal injury type of brain injury characterized by shearing, stretching, or tearing of nerve fibers with subsequent axonal damage.

digestive tract internal passageway that begins at the mouth and ends at the anus.

direct pressure method of hemorrhage control that relies on the application of pressure to the actual site of the bleeding.

dislocation complete displacement of a bone end from its position in a joint capsule.

drag the forces acting on a projectile in motion to slow its progress.

drowning the process of experiencing respiratory impairment as the result of submersion or immersion in liquid.

dura mater tough layer of the meninges firmly attached to the interior of the skull and interior of the spinal column.

dyspnea labored or difficult breathing.

ecchymosis blue-black discoloration of the skin due to leakage of blood into the tissues.

electrical alternans alternating amplitude of the P, QRS, and T waves on the ECG rhythm strip as the heart swings in a pendulum-like fashion within the pericardial sac during tamponade.

emboli undissolved solid, liquid, or gaseous matter in the bloodstream that may cause blockage of blood vessels.

emergent phase first stage of the burn process, characterized by a catecholamine release and pain-mediated reaction.

energy the capacity to do work in the strict physical sense.

environmental emergency a medical condition caused or exacerbated by the weather, terrain, atmospheric pressure, or other local factors.

epicardium serous membrane covering the outer surface of the heart; the visceral pericardium.

epidemiology the study of disease to determine its prevalence, course, and seriousness.

epidermis outermost layer of the skin composed of dead or dying cells.

epidural hematoma accumulation of blood between the dura mater and the cranium.

epiphyseal fracture disruption in the epiphyseal plate of a child's bone.

epiphyseal plate area of the metaphysis where cartilage is generated during bone growth in childhood. Also called the *growth plate*.

epiphysis end of a long bone, including the epiphyseal, or growth, plate and supporting structures underlying the joint.

epistaxis bleeding from the nose resulting from injury, disease, or environmental factors; a nosebleed.

epistaxis nosebleed.

epithelialization early stage of wound healing in which epithelial cells migrate over the surface of the wound.

erythema general reddening of the skin due to dilation of the superficial capillaries.

erythrocyte peripheral blood cell that contains hemoglobin; responsible for transport of oxygen to the cells.

eschar hard, leathery product of a deep full thickness burn; it consists of dead and denatured skin.

evaporation change from liquid to a gaseous state.

event amnesia inability to remember circumstances of a traumatic event.

evisceration a protrusion of organs from a wound.

exertional metabolic rate rate at which the body consumes energy during activity. It is faster than the basal metabolic rate.

exsanguination blood loss sufficient to cause death.

extravascular space the volume contained within the cells (intracellular space) and the spaces between the cells (interstitial space).

extrinsic pathway the activation of clotting factors from damaged blood vessel walls and surrounding tissue.

fascia a fibrous membrane that covers, supports, and separates muscles and may also unite the skin with underlying tissue.

fascicle small bundle of muscle fibers.

fatigue fracture break in a bone associated with prolonged or repeated stress.

fatigue condition in which a muscle's ability to respond to stimulation is lost or reduced through overactivity.

fibrin protein fibers that trap red blood cells as part of the clotting process.

fibroblasts specialized cells that form collagen.

flail chest defect in the chest wall that allows for free movement of a segment. Breathing will cause paradoxical chest wall motion.

flechettes arrow-shaped projectiles found in some military ordnance.

fluid shift phase stage of the burn process in which there is a massive shift of fluid from the intravascular to the extravascular space.

force strength or energy.

frostbite environmentally induced freezing of body tissues, causing destruction of cells.

full thickness burn burn that damages all layers of the skin; characterized by areas that are painless and often dry; also called a third-degree burn.

galea aponeurotica connective tissue sheet covering the superior aspect of the cranium.

gamma radiation powerful electromagnetic radiation emitted by radioactive substances with powerful penetrating properties; it is stronger than alpha and beta radiation. Similar to X-rays, which are generally less energetic.

gangrene deep-space infection usually caused by the anaerobic bacterium *Clostridium perfringens*.

Glasgow Coma Scale scoring system for monitoring the neurologic status of patients with head injuries that considers 15 elements of eye-opening, motor, and verbal response.

Golden Period the 60-minute period after a severe injury; it is the maximum acceptable time between the injury and initiation of surgery for the seriously injured trauma patient.

granulocytes white blood cells charged with the primary purpose of neutralizing foreign bacteria.

Gray   a unit of absorbed radiation dose equal to 100 rads.

great vessels   large arteries and veins located in the mediastinum that enter and exit the heart: the pulmonary artery, the aorta, the inferior vena cava, and the superior vena cava.

greenstick fracture   partial fracture of a child's bone.

guarding   protective tensing of the abdominal muscles by a patient suffering abdominal pain.

Haddon Matrix   a framework for classifying factors associated with injury, death, or events that may cause injury or death. The matrix is used to identify factors that can be modified and interventions that can be taken to prevent or reduce the severity of such events.

hairline fracture   small crack in a bone that does not disrupt its total structure.

haversian canals   small perforations of the long bones through which the blood vessels and nerves travel through the bone itself.

heat cramps   acute painful spasms of the voluntary muscles following strenuous activity in a hot environment without adequate fluid or salt intake.

heat exhaustion   a mild heat illness; an acute reaction to heat exposure.

heat-related illness   increased core body temperature due to inadequate thermolysis.

heatstroke   acute, dangerous reaction to heat exposure, characterized by a body temperature usually above 105°F (40.6°C) and central nervous system disturbances. The body usually ceases to perspire.

hematemesis   vomiting of blood.

hematochezia   passage of stools containing red blood.

hematocrit   the percentage of the total blood volume consisting of the red blood cells, or erythrocytes.

hematoma   collection of blood beneath the skin or trapped within a body compartment.

hematuria   blood in the urine.

hemoglobin   an iron-based compound found in red blood cells that binds with oxygen and transports it to body cells.

hemopneumothorax   condition in which air and blood are in the pleural space.

hemoptysis   coughing up blood that originates in the respiratory tract.

hemorrhage   an abnormal internal or external discharge of blood.

hemostasis   the body's three-step response to local hemorrhage, comprising a vascular phase that reduces blood flow, a platelet phase in which aggregating platelets form a weak clot, and a coagulation phase that results in the formation of fibrin, creating a strong clot.

hemothorax   blood within the pleural space.

homeostasis   the natural tendency of the body to maintain a stable, steady, and normal internal environment.

hydrostatic pressure   the pressure of liquids in equilibrium; the pressure exerted by or within liquids.

hyperbaric oxygen chamber   recompression chamber used to treat patients suffering from barotrauma.

hyperemia   increased blood flow into and through injured or infected tissue, responsible for the reddish skin color, or erythema, associated with inflammation.

hypermetabolic phase   stage of the burn process in which there is increased body metabolism in an attempt by the body to heal the burn.

hyperthermia   unusually high core body temperature.

hyphema   blood in the anterior chamber of the eye, in front of the iris.

hypoperfusion   inadequate perfusion of body tissues, resulting in inadequate supplies of oxygen and nutrients to body tissue; also called *shock*.

hypotension   lower-than-normal blood pressure.

hypothalamus   portion of the diencephalon producing neurosecretions important in the control of certain metabolic activities, including body temperature regulation.

hypothermia   state of low body temperature, particularly low core body temperature.

hypovolemia   reduced volume in the cardiovascular system.

hypovolemic shock   shock caused by loss of blood or body fluids.

impacted fracture   break in a bone in which the bone is compressed on itself.

impaled object   foreign body embedded in a wound.

incendiary   combusting easily or creating combustion.

incision   very smooth or surgical laceration, frequently caused by a knife, scalpel, razor blade, or piece of glass.

index of suspicion   anticipation of the severity of an injury based on the events and circumstances that appear to have caused the injury.

inertia   tendency of an object to remain at rest or in motion unless acted on by an external force.

infection   invasion and multiplication of pathogenic microorganisms in a body part or tissue.

inflammation   complex process of local cellular and biochemical changes as a consequence of injury or infection; an early stage of healing.

insertion   attachment of a muscle to a bone that moves when the muscle contracts.

integumentary system   skin, consisting of the epidermis, dermis, and subcutaneous layers.

interstitial space   the space between cells.

intervetebral disk   a pad of fibrocartilage that lies between adjacent vertebrae, allows slight movement of the spine, and acts as a cushion or shock absorber.

intracerebral hemorrhage   bleeding directly into the tissue of the brain.

intracranial pressure (ICP) pressure exerted on the brain by the blood and cerebrospinal fluid.

intravascular space the volume contained by all the arteries, veins, capillaries, and other components of the circulatory system.

intrinsic pathway the activation of clotting factors from damaged platelets within blood vessels.

ionization the process of changing a substance into separate charged particles (ions).

ipsilateral same side.

iris pigmented portion of the eye. It is the muscular area that constricts or dilates to change the size of the pupil.

irreversible shock final stage of shock in which organs and cells are so damaged that recovery is impossible.

J waves ECG deflections found at the junction of QRS complexes and the ST segments. They are associated with hypothermia and seen at core temperatures below 32°C, most commonly in leads II and V_6; also called *Osborn waves*.

Jackson's theory of thermal wounds explanation of the physical effects of thermal burns.

joint capsule chamber formed by ligaments surrounding a joint that holds a small amount of synovial fluid to lubricate articular surfaces.

joint area where adjacent bones articulate.

Joule's law the physical law stating that the rate of heat production is directly proportional to the resistance of the circuit and to the square of the current.

keloid a formation resulting from overproduction of scar tissue.

kinematics the branch of physics that deals with motion of a body or system of bodies without consideration to its mass or forces acting upon it. *See also* kinetics.

kinetic energy the energy an object has while it is in motion. It is related to the object's mass and velocity.

kinetics the branch of physics that deals with motion, taking into consideration mass, velocity, and force. *See also* kinematics.

laceration an open wound, normally a tear with jagged borders.

lacrimal fluid liquid that lubricates the eye.

lactic acid compound produced from pyruvic acid during anaerobic glycolysis.

Le Fort criteria classification system for fractures involving the maxilla.

ligaments bands of connective tissue that connect bone to bone and hold joints together.

ligamentum arteriosum cordlike remnant of a fetal vessel connecting the pulmonary artery to the aorta at the aortic isthmus.

liquefaction necrosis the process in which an alkali dissolves and liquefies tissue.

lumbar vertebrae the five vertebrae that lie between the thoracic vertebrae and the sacrum, helping to support the lower back.

lumen opening, or space, within a needle, artery, vein, or other hollow vessel.

lymphangitis inflammation of the lymph channels, usually as a result of a distal infection.

lymphatic system a system of vessels that pick up excess tissue fluid and purify it before returning it to the circulatory system.

lymphocyte white blood cell that specializes in humoral immunity and antibody formation.

macrophage immune system cell that has the ability to recognize and ingest foreign pathogens.

malleolus the protuberance of the ankle.

mammalian diving reflex a complex cardiovascular reflex, resulting from submersion of the face and nose in water, that constricts blood flow everywhere except to the brain.

mandible the jawbone.

mass a measure of the matter that an object contains; the property of a physical body that gives the body inertia.

maxilla bone of the upper jaw.

mean arterial pressure (MAP) the diastolic blood pressure plus one-third the pulse pressure (systolic pressure minus diastolic pressure).

mechanism of injury (MOI) the processes and forces that cause trauma; the manner in which an injury occurs.

medulla oblongata lower portion of the brainstem containing the respiratory, cardiac, and vasomotor centers.

medullary canal cavity within a bone that contains the marrow.

melena black, tarlike feces due to gastrointestinal bleeding.

meninges three membranes that surround and protect the brain and spinal cord: the dura mater, pia mater, and arachnoid membrane.

mesentery double fold of peritoneum that supports the major portion of the small bowel, suspending it from the posterior abdominal wall.

metaphysis growth zone of a bone, active during the development stages of youth. It is located between the epiphysis and the diaphysis.

microcirculation blood flow in the arterioles, capillaries, and venules.

midbrain portion of the brain connecting the pons and cerebellum with the cerebral hemispheres.

motion the process of changing place; movement.

myocardium muscular tissue of the heart.

myotome muscle and tissue of the body innervated by spinal nerve roots.

nares the openings of the nostrils.

necrosis tissue death, usually from ischemia.

negative feedback   homeostatic mechanism in which a change in a variable ultimately inhibits the process that led to the shift.

neovascularization   new growth of capillaries in response to healing.

neurogenic shock   type of shock resulting from an interruption in the communication pathway between the central nervous system and the rest of the body, leading to decreased peripheral vascular resistance.

neutron radiation   powerful radiation with penetrating properties between that of beta and gamma radiation.

nitrogen narcosis   a state of stupor that develops during deep dives due to nitrogen's effect on cerebral function; also called "raptures of the deep."

oblique fracture   break in a bone running across it at an angle other than 90 degrees.

oblique   having a slanted position or direction.

ohm   basic unit for measuring the strength of electrical resistance.

Ohm's law   the physical law identifying that the current in an electrical circuit is directly proportional to the voltage and inversely proportional to the resistance.

oncotic pressure   the force exerted by large protein molecules in the plasma that tends to draw fluid into the capillaries, compensating for the loss of fluid that leaks out of capillaries because of hydrostatic pressure.

open fracture   a broken bone in which the bone ends or the forces that caused it penetrate the surrounding skin.

opposition   pairing of muscles that permits extension and flexion of limbs.

orbit   the eye socket.

ordnance   military weapons and munitions.

origin   attachment of a muscle to a bone that does not move (or experiences the least movement) when the muscle contracts.

orthostatic hypotension   a decrease in blood pressure that occurs when a person moves from a supine or sitting position to an upright position.

osteoblast   cell that helps in the creation of new bone during growth and bone repair.

osteoclast   bone cell that absorbs and removes excess bone.

osteocyte   bone-forming cell found in the bone matrix that helps maintain the bone.

osteoporosis   weakening of bone tissue due to loss of essential minerals, especially calcium.

overpressure   a rapid increase, then decrease, in atmospheric pressure created by an explosion.

oxidizer   an agent that enhances combustion of a fuel.

paraplegia   paralysis of the lower limbs and lower trunk.

paresthesia   abnormal sensation such as tingling or prickling ("pins and needles").

partial thickness burn   burn in which the epidermis is burned through and the dermis is damaged; characterized by redness and blistering; also called a second-degree burn.

pelvic space   division of the abdominal cavity containing the organs located within the pelvis.

penetrating trauma   injury occuring when an object pierces the skin and enters the body.

percutaneous cricothyrotomy   a procedure for gaining access to the airway via needle or other puncture device.

perforating canals   structures through which blood vessels enter and exit the bone shaft.

perforating trauma   a form of penetrating trauma that occurs when an object enters and exits the body.

pericardial tamponade   a restriction to cardiac filling caused by blood (or other fluid) within the pericardial sac.

pericardium   fibrous sac that surrounds the heart.

periosteum   the tough exterior covering of a bone.

peripheral vascular resistance   the resistance of the vessels to the flow of blood; it increases when the vessels constrict and decreases when the vessels relax. Also called *afterload*.

peritoneal space   division of the abdominal cavity containing the organs or portions of organs covered by the peritoneum.

peritoneum   fine fibrous tissue surrounding the interior of most of the abdominal cavity and covering most of the small bowel and some of the abdominal organs.

peritonitis   inflammation of the peritoneum caused by chemical or bacterial irritation.

phagocytosis   process in which a cell surrounds and absorbs a bacterium or other particle.

pia mater   inner and most delicate layer of the meninges. It covers the convolutions of the brain and spinal cord.

pinal canal   opening in the vertebrae that accommodates the spinal cord; also called the *vertebral foramen*.

pinna   outer, visible portion of the ear.

platelet phase   second step in the process of hemostasis in which platelets adhere to blood vessel walls and to each other.

platelet   one of the fragments of cytoplasm that circulates in the blood and works with components of the coagulation system to promote blood clotting. Platelets also release serotonin, a vasoconstrictive substance.

pneumomediastinum   the presence of air in the mediastinum.

pneumothorax   a collection of air in the pleural space. Air may enter the pleural space through an injury to the chest wall or through an injury to the lungs. In a tension pneumothorax, pressure builds because there is no way for the air to escape, causing lung collapse.

pneumothorax a collection of air in the pleural space. Air may enter the pleural space through an injury to the chest wall or through an injury to the lungs. In a tension pneumothorax, pressure builds because there is no way for the air to escape, causing lung collapse.

pons process of tissue responsible for the communication interchange between the cerebellum, the cerebrum, the midbrain, and the spinal cord.

precordium area of the chest wall overlying the heart.

preload the pressure within the ventricles at the end of diastole; the volume of blood delivered to the atria prior to ventricular diastole.

pressure wave area of overpressure that radiates outward from an explosion.

profile the cross section of a bullet along its direction of travel; the energy-exchange surface of the bullet when it contacts a target.

projectile an object hurled or projected by the exertion of force.

pulmonary hilum central medial region of the lung where the bronchi and pulmonary vasculature enter the lung.

pulmonary overpressure expansion of air held in the lungs during ascent. If not exhaled, the expanded air may cause injury to the lungs and surrounding structures.

pulse pressure difference between the systolic and diastolic blood pressures.

pulsus alternans drop of greater than 10 mmHg in the systolic blood pressure during the inspiratory phase of respiration that occurs in patients with pericardial tamponade.

pulsus paradoxus alternating strong and weak pulse.

puncture specific soft-tissue injury involving a deep, narrow wound to the skin and underlying organs that carries an increased danger of infection.

pupil dark opening in the center of the iris through which light enters the eye.

pyrexia fever, or above-normal body temperature.

pyrogens any substances causing a fever, such as viruses and bacteria or substances produced within the body in response to infection or inflammation.

quadriplegia paralysis of all four limbs.

rad basic unit of absorbed radiation dose.

radiation transfer of energy through space or matter.

rebound tenderness pain caused by any abdominal jarring, as occurs with percussion or when the pressure of deep palpation is released quickly.

recompression resubmission of a person to a greater pressure so gradual decompression can be achieved; often used in the treatment of diving emergencies.

red bone marrow tissue within the internal cavity of a bone responsible for the manufacture of erythrocytes and other blood cells.

reduction returning of displaced bone ends to their proper anatomic orientation.

remodeling stage in the wound healing process in which collagen is broken down and relaid in an orderly fashion.

resiliency elasticity; the ability to spring back from a force or impact to resume the original condition.

resistance property of a conductor that opposes the passage of an electric current.

resolution phase final stage of the burn process in which scar tissue is laid down and the healing process is completed.

respiration the exchange of gases between a living organism and its environment.

retina light- and color-sensing tissue lining the posterior chamber of the eye.

retinal detachment condition that may be of traumatic origin and presents with patient complaint of a dark curtain obstructing a portion of the field of view.

retroauricular ecchymosis black-and-blue discoloration over the mastoid process (just behind the ear) that is characteristic of a basilar skull fracture. (Also called *Battle's sign*.)

retrograde amnesia inability to remember events that occurred before the trauma that caused the condition.

retroperitoneal space division of the abdominal cavity containing the organs posterior to the peritoneal lining.

rhabdomyolysis acute pathological process that involves the destruction of skeletal muscle.

rhabdomyolysis acute pathological process that involves the destruction of skeletal muscle.

rotation turning along the axis of a bone.

rule of nines method of estimating amount of body surface area burned by a division of the body into regions, each of which represents approximately 9 percent of total BSA (plus 1 percent for the genital region).

rule of palms method of estimating the amount of body surface area burned that sizes the area burned in comparison to the patient's palmar surface.

sacrum triangular bone, formed from five fused vertebrae, that lies between the fifth lumbar vertebra and the coccyx.

sclera the "white" of the eye.

scuba acronym for **s**elf-**c**ontained **u**nderwater **b**reathing **a**pparatus. Portable apparatus that contains compressed air that allows the diver to breathe underwater.

sebaceous glands glands within the dermis secreting sebum.

sebum fatty secretion of the sebaceous gland that helps keep the skin pliable and waterproof.

semicircular canals the three rings of the inner ear. They sense the motion of the head and provide positional sense for the body.

septic shock form of shock caused by massive infection in which toxins compromise the vascular system's ability to control blood vessels and distribute blood.

serous fluid a cellular component of blood, similar to plasma.

shock a state of inadequate tissue perfusion.

Simplified Motor Score (SMS) a simplified scoring system for monitoring the neurologic status of patients with head injuries based on three elements of motor responsiveness, compared to 15 elements of eye-opening, motor, and verbal response in the Glasgow Coma Scale.

skeletal muscle contractile tissue organized in large bundles that provides locomotion and movement for the body.

spasm intermittent or continuous contraction of a muscle.

spinal clearance protocol set of criteria for discontinuing spinal precautions.

spinal canal cavity that runs through all the vertebrae and contains the spinal cord.

spinal cord central nervous system pathway responsible for transmitting sensory input from the body to the brain and for conducting motor impulses from the brain to the body muscles and organs.

spinal meninges protective structures that cover the spine, consisting of the dura mater, the arachnoid membrane, and the pia mater.

spinal nerves 31 pairs of nerves that originate along the spinal cord from anterior and posterior nerve roots.

spinal shock the loss of spinal reflexes after injury of the spinal cord that affects muscles innervated by the cord segments below the site of the injury.

spiral fracture a curving break in a bone as may be caused by rotational forces.

sprain tearing of a joint capsule's connective tissues.

strain injury resulting from overstretching of muscle fibers.

stroke volume the amount of blood ejected by the heart in one cardiac contraction.

subcutaneous tissue body layer beneath the dermis.

subdural hematoma collection of blood directly beneath the dura mater.

subglottic referring to the lower airway.

subluxation partial displacement of a bone end from its position in a joint capsule.

sudoriferous glands glands within the dermis that secrete sweat.

superficial burn a burn that involves only the epidermis; characterized by reddening of the skin; also called a first-degree burn.

superficial frostbite freezing involving only epidermal tissues, resulting in redness followed by blanching and diminished sensation; also called *frostnip*.

supine hypotensive syndrome inadequate return of venous blood to the heart, reduced cardiac output, and lowered blood pressure resulting from pressure on the inferior vena cava by the fetus and uterus late in pregnancy.

supraglottic referring to the upper airway.

surfactant a compound secreted by cells in the lungs that regulates the surface tension of the fluid that lines the alveoli, which is important in keeping the alveoli open for gas exchange.

sutures pseudojoints that join the various bones of the skull to form the cranium.

synarthroses joints that do not permit movement.

synovial fluid substance that lubricates synovial joints.

synovial joint type of joint that permits the greatest degree of independent motion.

tendons long, thin, very strong collagen tissues that connect muscles to bones.

tension lines natural patterns in the surface of the skin revealing tensions within.

tension pneumothorax buildup of air under pressure within the thorax. The resulting compression of the lung severely reduces venous return, cardiac output, and the effectiveness of respirations.

tetanus a rare wound infection caused by the bacterium *Clostridium tetani*. Also called *lockjaw*.

thalamus switching station between the pons and the cerebrum in the brain.

thermal gradient the difference in temperature between the environment and the body.

thermogenesis the production of heat, especially within the body.

thermolysis the loss of heat, especially from the body.

thermoregulation the maintenance or regulation of a particular temperature of the body.

thoracic vertebrae the 12 vertebrae that lie between the cervical and lumbar vertebrae, helping to support the thorax.

tilt test measuring the blood pressure before and after moving the patient from a supine to a sitting position; a drop in the systolic blood pressure of 20 mmHg or an increase in the pulse rate of 20 beats per minute after the patient is moved to a sitting position is a finding suggestive of a relative hypovolemia.

tone state of slight contraction of muscles that gives them firmness and keeps them ready to contract.

tourniquet a constrictor used on an extremity to apply circumferential pressure on all arteries to control bleeding.

tracheobronchial tree the structures of the trachea and the bronchi.

trajectory the path a projectile follows.

tranexamic acid (TXA) a drug that inhibits fibrinolysis (the breakdown of blood clots); an antifibrinolytic.

transection a cutting across a long axis; a cross-sectional cut.

transverse fracture a break that runs across a bone perpendicular to the bone's orientation.

trauma center a hospital that has the capability of caring for acutely injured patients; trauma centers must meet strict criteria to use this designation.

trauma registry a data retrieval system for trauma patient information, which is used to evaluate and improve the trauma system.

trauma triage criteria guidelines to aid prehospital personnel in determining which trauma patients require urgent transportation to a trauma center.

trauma a physical injury or wound caused by external force or violence.

trench foot a painful foot disorder resembling frostbite and resulting from exposure to cold and wetness, which can eventually result in tissue sloughing or gangrene; also called

vascular phase first step in the process of hemostasis, in which smooth blood vessel muscle contracts, reducing the vessel lumen and the flow of blood through it.

vein a blood vessel that carries blood toward the heart.

velocity the rate of motion in a particular direction in relation to time.

vertebra one of 33 bones making up the vertebral column.

vertebral column the main support for the axis of the body, consisting of 33 bones (vertebrae); also called the *spinal column*.

vertebral foramen *see* spinal canal.

vitreous humor clear watery fluid filling the posterior chamber of the eye. It is responsible for giving the eye its spherical shape.

voltage the difference of electric potential between two points with different concentrations of electrons.

xiphisternal joint union between xiphoid process and body of the sternum.

yaw swing or wobble around the axis of a projectile's travel.

yellow bone marrow tissue that stores fat in semiliquid form within the internal cavities of a bone.

zone of coagulation area in a burn nearest the heat source that suffers the most damage and is characterized by clotted blood and thrombosed blood vessels.

zone of hyperemia area peripheral to a burn that is characterized by increased blood flow.

zone of injury in association with projectile wounds, the maximum area of injured tissue, usually extending beyond the permanent cavity formed by the projectile.

zone of stasis area in a burn surrounding the zone of coagulation that is characterized by decreased blood flow.

zygoma the cheekbone.

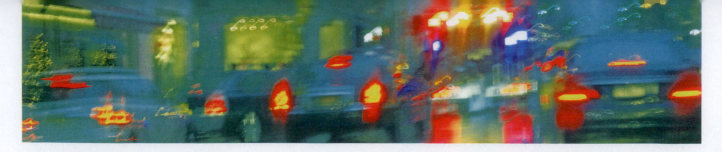

Index